Detection of New Adverse Drug Reactions

FOURTH EDITION

Edited by
M.D.B. Stephens, J.C.C. Talbot
and P.A. Routledge

Detection of New Adverse Drug Reactions

FOURTH EDITION

Edited by
**M.D.B. Stephens, J.C.C. Talbot
and P.A. Routledge**

Published in the United Kingdom by
MACMILLAN REFERENCE LTD, 1998
25 Eccleston Place, London, SW1W 9NF
and Basingstoke

Companies and representatives throughout the world.

http://www.macmillan-reference.co.uk

Distributed in the UK and Europe by
Macmillan Direct,
Brunel Road, Houndmills,
Basingstoke,
Hampshire, RG21 2XS, England

ISBN 0-333-693914

A catalogue record for this book is available from the British Library.

Published in the United States and Canada by
GROVE'S DICTIONARIES INC, 1998
345 Park Avenue South, 10th Floor
New York, NY 10010-1707, USA

ISBN 1-56159-190-4

Typeset by Pure Tech Ltd, India

Printed and bound in the UK by
BPC Information Ltd, Exeter, Devon

Contents

Foreword

When a new drug (new active substance) is launched into widespread clinical use prescribers and their patients can be assured of its pharmaceutical quality and efficacy. Any assessment of its safety, however, must inevitably be provisional. Nevertheless, all those concerned with the development of new drugs—whether in industry, academia or the health services—need to make strenuous efforts to ensure that the adverse reaction profile of a new drug is as fully defined as possible at the time it is authorized for marketing. Furthermore, prescribers generally have a professional responsibility to inform the appropriate authorities if they suspect that a patient under their care has suffered an adverse reaction. It is only by such concerted action that the safety of new drugs can be evaluated.

Dr Myles Stephens has devoted much of his professional life to the assessment of the safety of new pharmaceutical products. Previous editions of this book have enabled him to share his interests, knowledge, skills and enthusiasm with a wide audience in the pharmaceutical industry, regulatory authorities, academia and beyond. Dr Stephens has thus had a profound influence on the conduct of drug development and this new edition will unquestionably continue this fine tradition.

Michael D. Rawlins
Chairman, Committee on Safety of Medicines, London
Professor of Clinical Pharmacology, Newcastle upon Tyne

Purpose of this Book

Identification of the ADR profile of a new drug *before* marketing lies entirely within the sphere of the pharmaceutical company whose staff have the responsibility for providing adequate information on a new drug to the licensing authorities and later prescribing physicians and patients. After a drug is marketed, the responsibility for extending knowledge of the adverse reactions spreads to all prescribers of that drug, as well as to specific organizations set up for that purpose. The originating company, however, retains the prime responsibility for collecting adverse reaction data for the prescribers, assessing its validity and informing the medical world and regulators of its evaluation.

This book reviews the available methods used for detecting adverse drug reactions both within and outside the pharmaceutical industry. The theme is of a progressive integrated programme for the detection and evaluation of possible ADRs from the time a new drug is first used in man and throughout its subsequent worldwide usage.

Preface to the Fourth Edition

Since the third edition there has been a rapid expansion in the work undertaken by the pharamacovigilance staff in the industry with a subsequent increase in staff numbers. At the same time two diploma courses in pharmacovigilance have been set up. The fourth edition hopes to cover the syllabus for these diplomas in addition to acting as a reference book for those involved in pharmacovigilance in the pharmaceutical industry and drug regulatory authorities.

Each chapter is written to stand on its own and hence there is some repetition where different authors have looked at the same subject from different perspectives. It is hoped that the extensive references, the further reading suggestions and the bibliography will enable the reader to cover the whole subject in depth.

Acknowledgements

It is a pleasure to thank:

1. Professor J. A. Lewis of the *Medicines Control Agency* and Elsevier Biomedical Press for permission to reproduce his statistical tables on the numbers of patients required for post-marketing surveillance.
2. Dr E. Miller of the PHLS and Dr W. Shepherd and Ms L. Maskell of Glaxo Wellcome for their help with vaccines.
3. Ms E. Meldrum, Amgen Ltd, for permission to use her Diploma Clinical Science dissertation on 'The potential impute of the proposed USA regulation on the safety monitoring of pre-approval drugs. An original survey and overview of drug safety' for the list of drugs removed from the market (Appendix 1).
4. Dr S. N. Linder-Ciccolunghi, for the use of the 'Ciccolunghi-Fowler-Chaudri Method'.
5. Dr B. D. Dinman, University of Pittsburgh, and JAMA for permission to reproduce his tables of risk 'The reality and acceptance of risk', *JAMA*, 1980, **244** (11), 1226–1228. Copyright 1980, American Medical Association.
6. Dr J. Haller, Dr J. Ward and Dr R. Amrein and the editors for permission to reproduce the table on page 148 from *Drugs and Driving*, J. F. O'Hanlon and J. J. de Gier (eds), and also the publishers, Taylor and Francis.
7. Dr J. Cott, National Institute of Mental Health, Clinical Treatment Research Branch, for information on the *Early Clinical Drug Evaluation Program (ECDEU)* manual.
8. Dr G. Venning and Dr J. P. Griffin for permission to reproduce the graph on page 137, which originally appeared in *Adverse Drug Reactions and Acute Poisoning Review*, 1984, **3**, 113–121.
9. Dr J. A. Tangrea for the details of the basal cell carcinoma prevention trial.
10. Ms M. Small, Amgen Ltd, for the figures of the 'box and whisper' and 'X-Y' plots.
11. Miss M. Rees, Syntex Research, for details of their laboratory data methods.
12. Dr R. D. Mann for information on Prescription Event Monitoring (Appendix 4).
13. The staff of International Drug Surveillance, Glaxo Group Research Ltd for their contributions over the years 1980–1992.
14. Mr J. Freeman, Amgen Ltd Cambridge for comments on biologicals.
15. Dr M. Hadoke, Glaxo Wellcome, Germany, for details of the German books on pharmacovigilance.
16. Dr P. Harrison for information on Mediplus (Appendix 4).
17. Dr T. M. MacDonald and Ms J. M. M. Evans for information on Medication Events Monitoring Organization (MEMO) (Appendix 4).
18. Dr F. Mackay and Ms J. Hollowell for the section on the General Practice Research Database (GPRD) (Appendix 4).

19. Dr R. M. Martin for the section on the Doctors' Independent Network database (Appendix 4).
20. Dr D. Lewis, Glaxo Wellcome for 'Taiwan' (Appendix 3).

Chapter 1

Introduction

M. D. B. Stephens

Pharmacovigilance has been defined as 'All methods of assessment and prevention of adverse drug reactions. The framework of pharmacovigilance is broader than that of post-marketing surveillance and includes clinical and even pre-clinical development of drugs' (Bégaud, 1993). It has been more fully defined by an EEC directive as 'System set up to collect information useful in the surveillance of medicinal products, in particular with regard to adverse reactions in human beings. The system contributes to ensuring the adoption of appropriate regulatory decisions concerning the medicinal products authorised within the Community, having regard to information obtained about adverse reactions to medicinal products under normal conditions of use' (Directive 75/319/EEC. Article 29A). The latter phrase implies that it applies to the post-marketing period.

The aims of pharmacovigilance are:

- Identification and quantification of previously unrecognized adverse drug reactions (ADRs).
- Identification of subgroups of patients at particular risk of ADRs (the risk relating to dose, age, gender and underlying disease).
- Continued monitoring of the safety of a product throughout the duration of its use, to ensure that its risks and benefits remain acceptable. This includes safety monitoring following significant newly approved indications.
- Comparing the ADR profile with those of products within the same therapeutic class.
- Detection of inappropriate prescription and administration.
- Further elucidation of a product's pharmacological/toxicological properties and the mechanism by which it produces ADRs.
- Detection of significant drug–drug interactions between new products and co-therapy with agents already established on the market, which may only be detected during widespread use.
- Communication of appropriate information to health care professionals (Rawlins *et al.*, 1992).
- To permit refutation of 'false positive' ADR signals arising in the professional or lay media or from spontaneous reports (Rawlins and Payne, 1997).

History of Pharmacovigilance

The first ADRs must have occurred when man first used plants as medication and learnt to brew alcohol and to smoke tobacco. The history of ADRs is, however, sparse until this century when it slowly gathered pace until the end of the Second World War; there has since been an explosion of new drugs and a consequent increase in drug ADRs. Important events in the history of ADRs are listed in Table 1.

Table 1 Important events in the history of ADRs

Year	Event
c. 2000 BC	The Babylonian Code—a physician who caused the death of a patient should lose his hands.
c. 1300 BC	The use of inhaled smoke (opium) to reduce pain was mentioned in Ebrus Paprus (Atkins, 1995).
c. 950 BC	Homer said 'Many drugs were excellent when mingled and many were fatal'.
c. 500 BC	Hippocrates said 'Primum non nocere'. Like many pithy epithets there is a nucleus of truth; but further thought reminds us that any drug can cause harm.
230	Hoa-Tho (Wei dynasty) administered fumes of aconite, datura and hyoscyamus (Atkins, 1995).
c. 994	'New remedies should first be tried in animals' (Haly Abbas).
1538	Paracelsus (Teofrasto Bombasto di Hoenheim) said 'All things are a poison and none is without poison, only the dose makes that a thing is a poison'. Obviously he did not know about type B reactions.
1662	The original randomized clinical trial (Rose, 1982).
Late 1700s	Friedrich Hoffman (1660–1742) described adverse effects of ergot (Borghi and Canti, 1986).
1700s	Voltaire 'They poured drugs of which they knew little into bodies of which they knew less'.
1785	William Withering wrote 'Account of the foxglove and some of its medical uses', including 'Foxglove when given in large and quickly repeated doses occasions sickness, vomiting, giddiness, confused vision, objects appearing green or yellow'.
1796	Jenner first 'vaccinated' against smallpox.
1799	Introduction of nitrous oxide (Atkins, 1995).
1839	First observation of anaphylaxis in rabbits by Magenta (Borghi and Canti, 1986).
1846	First use of chloroform and ether (Turk, 1994).
1877	British Medical Association met to investigate the sudden deaths associated with chloroform (Royal, 1973). Introduction of phenacetin.
1880	Toxicology of anaesthetics reported (*Br. Med. J. leader*, 1880).
1883	First use of paracetamol.
1899	Introduction of acetyl salicylic acid (aspirin).
1902	Biologics Control Act passed following deaths of 10 children in St Louis, USA, caused by diphtheria antitoxin contaminated with live tetanus bacilli (Roberts, 1996).
1903	Introduction of barbital.
1906	Pure Food and Drugs Act (USA) concerning labelling and adulteration.
1922	Insulin discovered.
1925	Therapeutic Substances Act (USA) regulating the manufacture and sale of substances requiring biological testing.
1933	Dinitrophenol found to cause weight reduction but also caused sclerosing cataracts leading to blindness and fatal hyperthermia. Forced off the market by the Food and Drug Administration (FDA) in the USA in 1935 (Hecht, 1987).
1935	First use of prontosil red (sulfamidochrysoidine) (Turk, 1994)
1937	Elixir sulfonamide containing 72% diethylene glycol given to 353 patients during a period of a week. There were 105 deaths (including 34 children) due to renal failure caused by the diethylene glycol (DEG). In 1969 in South Africa seven children died of renal failure due to DEG. In 1986 14 deaths in Bombay and in 1990 47 children died in Nigeria due to DEG (Okuonghae *et al.*, 1992; Wax, 1995). In 1995 there were 51 deaths due to DEG (Hanif *et al.*, 1995). *(contd.)*

Year	Event
	In Haiti 88 children died as a result of paracetamol syrup being contaminated with 14.4% DEG (O'Brien *et al.*, 1998). And so it goes on.
1938	Federal Food, Drug and Cosmetics Act (USA) as a result of the DEG epidemic.
1941	First use of penicillin.
1948	Introduction of chloramphenicol.
1948	First modern randomized clinical trial of streptomycin by the Medical Research Council (MRC).
1952	First book on ADRs ('Meyler's').
1953	Suspected renal damage by phenacetin.
1954	'Stalinon' (an organic compound of tin used in the treatment of boils) alleged to have killed 102 patients (*Br. Med. J.*, 1958).
1961	McBride reported phocomelia due to thalidomide (Distillers Company, 1961; McBride, 1961; Mellin and Katzenstein, 1962; Burley, 1988). The FDA delayed marketing approval of thalidomide because its toxicity in acute animal studies was questioned in view of clinical reports of polyneuritis (D'Arcy and Griffin, 1994).
1961–1967	Asthma deaths due to high dose isoprenaline nebulizer (Inman and Adelstein, 1969).
1962	Kefauver–Harris Amendments (USA). All clinical testing of investigational drugs to be reviewed and subject to veto by the FDA. New drugs to be effective as well as safe before marketing. This resulted from the thalidomide disaster.
1964	Committee on Safety of Drugs (CSD) formed in the UK 'to advise whether a new drug should be submitted for clinical trials, to advise whether a drug should be released for marketing and to study adverse reactions to drugs already in use' (Mann, 1988).
1967	World Health Organization (WHO) resolution 20.51 laying basis for international system of monitoring ADRs (Venulet, 1993).
1968	WHO pilot research project for international drug monitoring set up in Alexandria, USA.
1968	Medicines Act (UK). Both the CSD and the Medicines Act were responses to the thalidomide disaster.
	MER/29 (Triparanol) cataract disaster (Rheingold, 1968).
1970	Thromboembolic disease with high dose oestrogen oral contraceptives discovered (Inman *et al.*, 1970).
	Subacute myelo-optic neuropathy (SMON) due to halogenated hydroxyquinolones given for nonspecific gastroenteritis (Tsubaki *et al.*, 1971; Kono, 1980).
1971	Diethylstilboestrol given for threatened abortion produced vaginal carcinoma in the daughters of the recipients 10–20 years later (Herbst *et al.*, 1971).
	Committee on Safety of Medicines (CSM) replaced CSD to advise the licensing authority on the safety, efficacy and quality of the medicinal products on which advice was needed.
	WHO Research Centre for monitoring ADRs set up (Mann, 1988).
1973	French pharmacovigilance system implemented.
1974	Pertussis vaccine and encephalopathy (see page 24).
1975	European Committee for Proprietary Medicinal Products (CPMP) set up.
	Practolol caused oculomucocutaneous syndrome (Wright, 1975; Nicholls, 1977; Tierny, 1977).
1978	WHO ADR monitoring moved to Uppsala, Sweden.
1979	Halcion (triazolam) fiasco. Dr C. Van der Kroef gave details of four patients with severe psychiatric symptoms including anxiety, derealization and paranoid ideas (Van der Kroef, 1979; Lasagna, 1980). Subsequent studies showed that it could cause anxiety (Oswald, 1989) and next-day memory impairment (Bixler *et al.*, 1991). Company and FDA criticized (Barnett, 1996).
1982	Opren/Oraflex disaster (Abraham, 1995).
	Deaths in premature neonates due to benzyl alcohol used as a preservative for injectable drugs not being metabolized by the immature liver (Roberts, 1996). Fatalities in neonates due to untested parenteral vitamin E preparation containing benzyl alcohol (Martone *et al.*, 1986) and also benzyl alcohol in saline and water used for irrigating through IV catheters (Hiller *et al.*, 1986). Its toxicity had been reported earlier (Gershanik *et al.*, 1981; Brown *et al.*, 1982).
1988	European Rapid Alert system started (Wood, 1992). *(contd.)*

Year	Event
1993	Fialuridine caused hepatic deaths in patients with chronic hepatitis B (An FDA task force, 1993; Horton, 1994; Manning and Swartz, 1995; McKenzie *et al.*, 1995). Sorivudine, an antiviral agent for shingles, interacted with 5–fluouracil causing severe neutropenia and the death of 15 patients. (Ross, 1994; Hirokawa, 1996).
1995	Establishment of the European Medicines Evaluation Agency (EMEA).
1996	Third generation oral contraceptives and venous thromboembolism controversy (McPherson, 1996) led to an increase in the number of abortions—over 800 and 6 of every 10 patients on oral contraceptives in the UK stopped taking them (Wilson, *Daily Telegraph*, 1996a; Leader, 1996a). In Norway abortions rose by 8.2% compared with the same period the previous year (Andrew *et al.*, 1996) and in the UK abortions rose by 6.7%, which was 2688 more than for the first quarter of the year (Feger, *Daily Express*, 1996; *Daily Telegraph*, 1996b). This figure was later amended to 14.5% (Hall, *Daily Telegraph*, 1997). The original findings that there was a doubling of the rate of thromboembolism have been disputed (Lewis *et al.*, 1997; Suissa *et al.*, 1997; Szarewski, 1997).

Drug Withdrawals

There have been three surveys of drugs withdrawn from the market:

- The first covered 24 drugs from the US and UK over the period 1964–1983 (Bakke *et al.*, 1984).
- The second covered 126 drugs from the UK, Germany and France over a 30-year period (Spriet-Pourra and Auriche, 1988, 1994).
- The third covered 29 drugs from the US, UK and Spain from 1974–1993 (Bakke *et al.*, 1995). See appendix 1 for futher details.

The median period of market life for 97 products was 8 years with the market life for 25 drugs equal to or less than 2 years, for 23 drugs more than 2 years but less than 8 years, and for 49 drugs more than 8 years. Most of the reactions were type 'B' involving the hepatic, haematological and neuropsychiatric systems. The commonest drugs were non-steroidal anti-inflammatory drugs (NSAIDS), which accounted for double the number of withdrawals when compared with antibiotics/anti-infectives, analgesics/antipyretics, and antidepressants (Spreit-Pourra and Auriche, 1994). The results of these surveys have been combined in a table in Appendix 1.

The decision to take a drug off the market for safety reasons is frequently very difficult, with different countries taking different decisions. Both the manufacturers and the regulatory bodies collect data on suspected ADRs, but with varying success. The main problem is that health professionals tend to underreport suspected ADRs on marketed drugs.

Underreporting

One might expect that reporting of adverse events (AEs) during clinical trials would be complete, but some investigators fail to document and report AEs and there have been cases where the investigator has chosen not to report AEs because it was too much effort or in a deliberate attempt to defraud. In addition some investigators are confused as to what constitutes an AE (Mackintosh and Zepp, 1996).

It has been suggested that once a drug is marketed only about 10% of its ADRs are reported (Inman, 1972). This estimate was based on the pertussis vaccine ADRs and thromboses with the oral contraceptive. There is evidence that the deaths attributable to excessive use of bronchodilating aerosols were underreported (Inman and Adelstein, 1969), as were the thromboembolic deaths due to the oral contraceptive (Beral, 1977; Crooks, 1977) and the practolol eye problems (Tierney, 1977). Poor reporting is not confined to the UK. The USA (Hemminki, 1980), France (Bader,1981), Spain (Alvarez-Requejo *et al.*, 1994), Italy (Conforti *et al.*, 1995), Denmark (Hallas *et al.*, 1992) and Germany (Schonhofer, 1981) have reported similar, if not worse underreporting.

Studies

It is only rarely that the number of cases of a reaction that really occurred as opposed to reported reactions can be known, but with certain diseases this is possible:

1. Aplastic anaemia with phenylbutazone/oxyphenbutazone—only 5 of 44 deaths (11%) were reported (Inman, 1986) and of the 32 fatal blood dyscrasias with phenylbutazone only 4 (12.5%) were reported (Inman, 1977a).
2. Practolol—only one case of conjunctivitis was reported in clinical trials and this was soon followed by nearly 200 cases within 5 weeks of the first publication of a series of cases.
3. In Uppsala, Sweden all known cases of cytopenias were collected from hospital discharge notes. Only 33% of thrombocytopenias, 34% of aplastic anaemias and 25% of agranulocytoses in the years 1966–1970 were reported. Several assumptions had to be made in order to derive these figures (Bottiger and Westerholm, 1973). Of the 84 hospitalized cases of drug associated neutropenias only 29 (35%) had been reported (Arneborn and Palmbled, 1982).
4. Oral contraceptives and fatal thromboembolism—only 15% of cases were reported.
5. A Rhode Island (USA) survey cited in a recent report suggests that the average physician sees one serious ADR and seven moderate ADRs per year. The FDA receive only 12 reports of any type for every 100 physicians in the USA involved in patient care (Baum *et al.*, 1988).
6. In Sweden 80% of all children who developed osteitis after *bacillus Calmette-Guérin* (BCG) vaccination were reported. This was derived from the number of positive *Mycobacterium bovis* BCG cultures in bacteriology laboratories (Bottiger *et al.*, 1982).
7. The use of protamine in patients undergoing cardiopulmonary bypass was monitored in a hospital in the USA during 1990–1991. The incidence of serious ADRs was 6.6% (CI: 5.1–8.4). The chart records showed 1.7% (CI: 1.0–2.8). The incidence of ADRs reported to the hospital ADR program was 0.3% (CI: 0.07–0.9) (Kimmel *et al.*, 1995).
8. Monitoring an Italian 72–bed ward for a year disclosed 89 AEs (7.4% per 100 patients). None had been reported to the official national drug surveillance system in the previous year. Of 120 randomly chosen patients 22 AEs were considered as constituting the expected AEs but only nine were actually reported (Maistrello *et al.*, 1995).

9. In the UK 14 cases of fibrosing colonopathy with high-strength pancreatic enzyme preparation were all reported on 'yellow cards' (Smyth *et al.*, 1995).

10. There may be underreporting by the patient to the doctor. A study in the Netherlands compared the responses from a questionnaire sent to all drug dispensing GPs and also to all their patients who had been prescribed sumatriptan. The doctor response was 86% and the patient response was 70%. Among the doctors there were 30 (1.7%) reports of dizziness, 26 (1.5%) reports of nausea/vomiting, 25 (1.4%) reports of drowsiness/sedation and 23 (1.3%) reports of chest pain. Among the patients there were 96 (8.1%) reports of dizziness, 94 (7.9%) reports of chest pain, 139 (11.7%) reports of paraesthesia and 95 (8%) reports of a feeling of heaviness (Ottervanger *et al.*, 1995).

11. Patients in general practice were asked ' Have any medicines or tablets ever disagreed with you or caused an allergy?' 'Are you able to take aspirin or penicillin?' These questions identified 97 reactions. Of these 76% were likely to be related to the drug. The doctors only recorded 50% of them and did not preferentially record well-established reactions (Cook and Ferner, 1993).

12. In order to discover the degree of underreporting in UK general practice a survey was undertaken in 1986 of 24 training practices south of the Thames. Only 6% of AEs were reported. (Lumley *et al.*, 1986). It is not possible to extrapolate from training practices to all practices and even this figure is doubtful since the general practitioners (GPs) knew that they were being monitored and were asking the patients leading questions. It also depended upon the GP's diagnosis of a suspected ADR.

13. A random sample of 100 French GPs was surveyed to obtain data on observed AEs. Overall, 81 GPs agreed to enter data during three consecutive days and these were compared to the spontaneous reports received from GPs at the Bordeaux pharmacovigilance centre during the reference period. The average number observed per day was 1.99. The underreporting coefficient was 24 433 (95% confidence interval 20 702–28 837). This was equivalent to only one out of every 24 433 ADRs being reported to the centre (Moride *et al.*, 1997) (see page 8).

14. A survey of hospital records in five English districts showed that five times more cases of idiopathic thrombocytopenic purpura occurred following mumps, measles and rubella (MMR) vaccination than were reported to the UK CSM (Farrington *et al.*, 1995).

Factors Affecting Reporting

The following factors have been suggested as affecting direct reporting to the FDA in the USA:

(a) Severity of the reaction.
(b) Length of time that the drug has been on the market.
(c) Attribution by the patient.
(d) Whether the reaction has previously been seen by the doctor.
(e) Legal implications.
(f) Unusual nature of the event (Milstein *et al.*, 1986).

However, 90% of the reports in the USA come from the pharmaceutical companies and there is considerable variation between them (Baum *et al.*, 1987). Other factors affecting direct reporting are:

(g) Religion of the area. Countries with a predominant catholic population report less than those with a predominant protestant population (Dukes and Lunde, 1979).

(h) Regulations of the country (Griffin and Weber, 1986).

(i) Year of reporting (Sachs and Bortnichak, 1986). Weber plotted the mean number of ADR reports for seven NSAIDs over the first five years of marketing and showed that they peaked at two years and then declined rapidly. This has been called the Weber curve (Weber, 1984). When 10 drugs on the French market, which gave rise to approximately 100 spontaneous reports each during the first four years of marketing, were examined the reports peaked at one year and then decreased (Haramburu *et al.*, 1997).

(j) Physician's age, specialty and years qualified (Spiers *et al.*, 1984).

(k) Nationality (Sachs and Bortnichak, 1986; Belton *et al.*, 1997). For one Pfizer product the relative reporting rate (patients per 10^6 patient months) was Germany 1, Sweden 9.8, UK 6, USA 3 (Gordon, 1985).

(l) Media publicity (Rawlins, 1988a).

(m) Seriousness of the adverse event (Griffin and Weber, 1986).

(n) The ADR mechanism (Milstein *et al.*, 1986).

(o) The cumulative total of prescriptions (Rawlins, 1988a).

(p) Doctor's familiarity with the regulations (Scott *et al.*, 1990).

(q) Local health district (Bateman *et al.*, 1991).

In 1986 the relatively large number of reports for piroxicam produced a defensive report from Pfizer in which they gave evidence that there were the following reporting biases:

1. The first few years of marketing.
2. Launch after 1980 in the USA or 1976 in the UK.
3. Vigorous marketing by the sales force.
4. Publicity.
5. Distribution by one manufacturer worldwide.
6. Used on a long-term basis.
7. Used in a population with a high background risk.
8. Used in conjunction with other therapy (Sachs and Bortnichak, 1986).

Calculation of the Degree of Underreporting

The underreporting coefficient (U) is equal to the expected number of AEs divided by the observed number. The expected number can be calculated from a study of a sample of the target population where a known number of doctors (n) collect all AEs (m) over a standard period (T) and then knowing the total number of doctors in the target population (N) the proportionate number of AEs can be calculated (M) as follows:

$$\text{Expected number of AEs for target population} = m \times N/n \times T$$

$$\text{Reported number of AEs for target population} = K$$

$$\text{Underreporting coefficient} = U = \frac{m \times N/n \times T}{K}$$

Instead of N/n, the ratio of doctors in the sample to the number in the target population, one can use the ratio of incidence rates, but this involves calculating the number of patients prescribed the drug in the target population from the number of prescriptions multiplied by the average duration of treatment.

Recommended reading is *Analyse d'incidence en Pharmacovigilance-application á la Notification Spontanée*, 2nd edition, ARME-Pharmacovigilance, 1992. The 'comité de rédaction' is headed by Professor B. Bégaud, Hôpital Pellegrin, 33076 Bordeaux Cédex, France.

In Bordeaux the number of cases of cough with angiotensin converting enzyme (ACE) inhibitors was estimated at 3925 for the region based on a pilot study of 60 practitioners, but only three cases were reported to the pharmacovigilance centre. The underreporting coefficient (U) was 1305 (Bégaud *et al.*, 1994), but for all AEs the underreporting rate was 24/433 and was lower for severe AEs and for recently marketed drugs (Moride *et al.*, 1994) whereas the same figure (U) for Spain was 1144 (95% CI 941–1347) (Alvarez Requejo *et al.*, 1994). When the Bordeaux team looked at a sample of ADRs seen by 81 GPs during three non-consecutive days the underreporting coefficient was 24 433 (i.e. only one case out of every 24 433 ADRs were reported to the local pharmacovigilance centre). The figure for serious and unlabelled effects was 4610 and for recently marketed drugs 12 802 (Moride *et al.*, 1997).

Conclusion

It is clear that no general figure can be given for underreporting and that the best estimate can be obtained by a study in a sample of the relevant population.

- There are too many factors involved in underreporting to be able to quote a general figure

---

Incidence of ADRs

General Practice

A survey of a Yorkshire (UK) general practice showed that 1 in 40 consultations were for an ADR (Mulroy, 1973). Another survey, this time in Derbyshire (UK), showed that 25% of the practice population may have had an ADR or 41% of the patients receiving drugs had a certain or probable ADR, 90% occurring by the fourth day (Martys, 1979). Extrapolating from a Dutch study in general practice approximately 2.6% of the population were seen with an ADR, only 4.8% being serious. Almost all the ADRs were known (Hoek *et al.*, 1995). The figure given by a group of French GPs was two ADRs per day per doctor (Moride *et al.*, 1997).

Hospital Admissions

ADRs have been reported to cause between 2% and 19% of all hospital medical admissions (see below), resulting in 300 000 admissions per year in the USA (Atkin and Shenfield, 1995) and as many as 160 000 deaths each year in hospitals in the USA (Shapiro *et al.*, 1971). A review of studies of hospitalizations for ADRs gave a figure of 2% for children (USA), for general medicine 4.1% (Israel) 6.2% and 8.8% (UK), 5.7% (Germany) and 8.6% (Sweden), for general medicine and geriatrics 15.3% (UK), for psychiatry 7.5% (Israel), for intensive care 12.6% (France) and for cardiology 11.5% (Denmark). Approximately 75% of the ADRs were type 'A' (Wiholm, 1990). In Australia and Canada the figures were 23–24%, and in the UK 12.4%. A study in two hospitals in the USA gave a figure for ADRs of 6.5% of which 28% were judged to be preventable (Bates *et al.*, 1995; Leape *et al.*, 1995). Another review this time in the elderly gave a range of 3–17%. The latest figure based on 25 original studies in six developed countries shows that 5.8% of all admissions to medical wards were due to ADRs, including relative overdosing (Muehlberger *et al.*, 1997). A further review of 13 publications gave a figure of 5.5%.

The problems with all these surveys is the variation in admission policy from one hospital to the next and different criteria for drug relatedness (Atkin and Shenfield, 1995).

Hospitals in the USA

Of 1024 patients in the medical wards of a 350-bed hospital, 23% had ADRs with 29.6 % of elderly patients having ADRs. Independent factors in the elderly were female gender, decline in renal function and polymedicine. This paper includes a table giving results of 24 surveys from 1964–1991 (Bowman *et al.*, 1996).

A survey of 1000 patients in the USA showed that 15% indicated that they had had a side effect on medication (Drug Information CPE study 67, 1983). Almost 4% of patients hospitalized in New York State in 1984 suffered an AE due to medical treatment (Brennan *et al.*, 1991) and 19.4% of these were due to drugs (Leape *et al.*, 1991).

A survey of two large hospitals in the USA showed that there were 6.5 adverse drug events per 100 admissions during the hospital stay (Bates *et al.*, 1995). In a Salt Lake City hospital (1989–1990) 36 653 patients were monitored for AEs. There were 731 AEs occurring in 648 patients (1.76%). Of the AEs 96% were moderate or severe and 91% were type A reactions. The causal agent was not stopped for over 76% of verified ADR cases until the study personnel informed the physician of the ongoing ADR. This study quotes that 30% of hospitalized patients will have an ADR and that 0.31% of all admissions will have a fatal ADR (Classen *et al.*, 1991). In the same hospital during the following period, 1990–1993, the ADR rate had increased to 2.43 per 100 admissions. There was an almost twofold increase in deaths.

Approximately 1.5% of all hospitalizations for the elderly to the Mayo clinic were due to ADRs (Silverstein *et al.*, 1994). The figure for admission of children is 2% from a survey of five hospitals in the USA (Mitchell *et al.*, 1988).

A review of 39 studies of ADRs in hospitals in the USA has shown that 2 216 000 patients suffered ADRs and of these 106 000 died during 1994. This represented 4.6% of all deaths and was ranked the 4–6th most common cause of death (Lazarou *et al.*, 1998).

Canadian Hospitals

A survey of patients aged 50 years or over in a Winnipeg hospital showed that 19% of admissions were for drug-related events (Grymonpre *et al.*, 1988). Among elderly patients (over 50 years of age), ADRs accounted for 19% of admissions (Grymonpre *et al.*, 1988).

In an internal medicine group practice 5% of ambulatory outpatients had a probable or definite ADR (Hutchinson *et al.*, 1986).

Hong Kong Hospitals

Drug related problems were responsible for 9.5% of admissions and 6.2% were ADRs (Chan and Critchley, 1995).

UK Hospitals

A survey of 437 patients in a Birmingham hospital revealed 97 AEs (22%) and most were due to a drug (76%), but the doctors had only recorded 50% of these reactions in the patients' notes (Cook and Ferner, 1993).

In an analysis of inpatient ADRs 23% of patients had an ADR and 37.5% of these patients were elderly (Bowman *et al.*, 1996). This last paper also gave the results from 23 similar studies carried out between 1964 and 1991, showing the average ADR rate to be 15.6% and the range 1.5–35%.

French Hospitals

Excluding attempted suicides 3% of admissions were drug related and 6.6% of inpatients had significant ADRs (i.e. necessitating changes in drug treatment or prolonged hospitalization) (Moore *et al.*, 1995a). At another French hospital the respective figures were 6% of admissions and 8.4% of inpatients (Moore *et al.*, 1995b).

Dutch Hospitals

One in six elderly patients had an ADR on admission and 24% of these were severe, severe being defined as potentially life-threatening or had led to admission. A comparison between patients with a severe ADR and those without showed that the significant factors were:

- A fall before admission.
- Presence of gastrointestinal (GI) bleeding or haematuria.
- Use of three or more drugs (Mannesse *et al.*, 1997).

Outpatient Visits

Drug-related visits to an Italian multidisciplinary hospital emergency department in Milan over a 3-month period were 4.7% for drug-related illnesses (Raschetti *et al.*, 1997).

Conclusions

This enormous variation in hospital admission rates for ADRs is partly due to different survey methods but the following are probably factors:

- Causality assessment methods.

- ADR/ADE/AE definitions (see pages 32–34).
- Hospital admission policies.
- Length of hospital admission.
- Type of hospital (mixture of wards).
- Country (most surveys are from the USA).
- Number of new chemical entities used.
- ADRs on admission or developed during admission?

> **ADR Hospital Admissions**
> - There are too many factors involved to give an accurate overall figure

Risk factors identified in some studies were age, number of drugs being taken, sex, previous medical history, race, country, weight, alcohol intake, renal function, length of stay and infections. These risk factors need to be examined in more detail.

ADR Risk Factors

Age

The relationship between age and ADRs is ambiguous. On the whole older people are likely to have more ADRs because of the increased number of medications taken by the elderly, but elderly patients may be at less risk of depression with beta blockers than young patients. There is a threefold increase in the incidence of ADRs in patients over 60 years of age compared with patients under 30 (Swafford, 1997).

A group of 1 026 ambulatory patients seen in an internal medicine practice over one year were monitored for ADRs by intensive telephone surveillance. When the analysis examining the frequency of ADRs was controlled for the number of courses of drug therapy there was no age effect (Hutchinson *et al.*, 1986; Bégaud *et al.*, 1996); the number of drugs is directly related to the number of coexisting diseases (Grymonpre *et al.*, 1988). In the intensive drug monitoring in Heidelberg from 1980–1987 when the incidence of ADRs in various age groups was analysed in relation to prescription data there was no age effect (Jacubeit *et al.*, 1990).

> **Age as a factor**
> - There is no evidence that age by itself is a factor in ADRs

The metabolism, distribution and excretion of drugs may decrease with age and these factors may be responsible for ADRs. Individual physiological parameters are far more important than any chronological measure in predicting ADRs (Gurnitz and Avorn, 1990). At the other end of the age scale, neonates and children up to 2 years of age may be more susceptible due to different pharmacokinetics and pharmacodynamics (Güdeke, 1972; Ashton, 1981). There is an excellent review of the subject from Australia (Atkin and Shenfield, 1995).

Sex

Females appear to be more susceptible to ADRs than males (Hurwitz, 1969; Hoigné *et al.*, 1984; Jacubeit *et al.*, 1990; Bowman *et al.*, 1996). This remained so after consideration of the duration of hospitalization, number of drugs, age, and the presence of liver and renal disease (Domecq *et al.*, 1980). The increases may be due to pharmacokinetic factors and hormonal influences (Kando *et al.*, 1995). Another study gave figures of 37.5% for women and 29.6% for men (Domecq *et al.*, 1980). In seven phase 1 studies females reported spontaneously 2.3 times more frequently than males and side effects due to laboratory abnormalities were higher in women (26%) than men (15%) (Vomvouras and Piergies, 1995). There may also be differences in pharmacokinetics (e.g. serum propranolol levels are twice as high in women as in men) (Walle *et al.*, 1994).

Medical History

Patients who have already had an adverse reaction to a drug are more likely to have reactions to other drugs (Hurwitz, 1969), but atopy is not a factor either for ADRs in general or allergic ADRs (Hoigné *et al.*, 1984). However, that does not exclude the possibility that an individual ADR may be more common in atopic patients (e.g. anaphylactoid reactions to radiocontrast media are more common in atopic patients) (Lieberman, 1991).

Race

'Ethnic factors in the acceptability of foreign data' is the title of one of the International Committee of Harmonization (ICH) projects. For about 80 products the pharmacokinetic variability seems to be no greater than the intraindividual variability, but there is evidence of differences in both pharmacokinetics and pharmaco dynamics and susceptibility to ADRs. The factors can be divided into intrinsic and extrinsic:

1. Intrinsic. These are inborn (e.g. height, weight and metabolic genetic polymorphism).
2. Extrinsic. These are acquired (e.g. medical practice, smoking, alcohol and diet). These factors tend to become more important later in the drug development programme (Flicker, 1995).

Pharmacokinetic Factors   These are illustrated by the following:

(a) 88–93% of Japanese are fast acetylators compared to 50% of Caucasians and blacks.
(b) 32% of Canadian Chinese are poor metabolizers for debrisoquine-sparteine oxidation compared with 7% of people in the USA, 0.5% in Japan, 9–10% in Switzerland and Hungary and 3.8% of Nigerians.
(c) 18–22% of Japanese are poor metabolizers of mephenytoin compared with 3–5% of people in the USA and Europe.

Pharmacodynamic Factors   The Chinese are more sensitive to beta blockade than Caucasians as well as more sensitive to neuroleptic agents.

Safety   Racial factors are also involved in drug safety as follows:

(a) The Japanese are more susceptible to hepatitis with isoniazid than Caucasians or blacks.
(b) Ashkenazi Jews with schizophrenia are more susceptible to clozapine agranulocytosis (20%) than the general schizophrenic population (1%) (Flicker, 1995).

(c)   There are higher rates of cholestatic jaundice with the oral contraceptive in Scandinavian and Chilean women than in women elsewhere (Sherlock, 1972).

(d)   Methyldopa induced haemolytic anaemia has a low occurrence in Indians, Negroes and the Chinese (Seedat and Varoda, 1968; Burns-Cox, 1971).

(e)   Black people have a poor response to ACE inhibitors and beta blockers (Temple, 1996).

Country

Comparison of the AEs occurring in a series of gastroenterological clinical trials, using the same protocol for the collection of AEs showed a reporting rate of more than 50% for Australia, Canada, Sweden and the UK, 35–45% for Denmark, Finland, France, Hong Kong, the Netherlands and Norway and less than 30% in Belgium, Germany and Italy. Different countries put different emphases on different types of AE (Joelson *et al.*, 1997).

Genes

It is worth reading 'Genetic factors in adverse reactions to drugs and chemicals' in *Pseudo-Allergic Reactions*, Vol. 1, pp. 1–27 by D. A. Price Evans (*see Bibliography*). Examples illustrating the role of genes in ADRs are as follows:

1.   Acetylator status—slow acetylators are more prone to hydralazine-induced systemic lupus erythematosus (SLE) and fast acetylators are more prone to isoniazid hepatotoxicity (Perry *et al.*, 1967; Bechtel, 1995).
2.   Glucose-6-phosphate dehydrogenase (G6PD) deficiency can result in haemolytic anaemia with oxidant drugs (Mitchell *et al.*, 1975).
3. · Blood group—there is a link between venous thromboembolic disease and ABO grouping (Jick *et al.*, 1969).
4.   Porphyria metabolism (see Chapter 2) (Moore, 1980).
5.   Human leucocyte antigen (HLA) status, (e.g. those with DRW4 status are more prone to hydralazine-induced SLE) (Batchelor *et al.*, 1980).
6.   Plasma pseudocholinesterase, (see Chapter 2).

These factors are explored more fully in Chapter 2 on pages 65–67.

Drugs

There is a direct linear relationship between the number of drugs taken and the rate of ADRs (Jacubeit *et al.*, 1990).

Disease

There is a high frequency of drug allergy in Sjögren's syndrome (43%). The syndrome is linked with HLA DR3. Drug allergy is associated with an impaired lymphocyte response after mitogenic stimulation which, like Sjögren's syndrome, is linked with HLA DR3 (Katz *et al.*, 1991). Renal function, as indicated by a high serum creatinine, is an independent factor (Bowman *et al.*, 1996).

Memory

A retrospective survey of adverse events (i.e. symptoms, illnesses, ADRs and hang-overs), among a group of 190 volunteers from a pharmaceutical company showed a

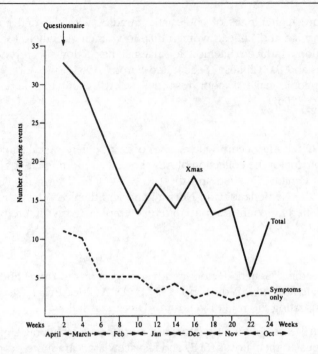

Figure 1   Loss of memory of volunteers for adverse clinical events over time

rapid drop in reported events over time. The results from the 111 replies are seen in Figure 1. The symptoms alone (no diagnosis) fell over a 14-week period and then reached a plateau. The latter, judging by the accuracy of the dates, was due to reporting by diarists. There were relatively few symptoms without diagnoses, which perhaps reflects the medical bent of the volunteers. The relevance of these findings to clinical trial protocols is in the timing of patient visits. Minor events are quickly forgotten and if one wishes to capture them the visits need to be frequent, every 1–2 weeks and at equal intervals. The practical alternative is to collect minor events only over the first week since 90% of ADRs occur within four days and only 4% after one week (Martys, 1979). Major events will not only stick in the memory, but are also more likely to be recorded in the patients' notes.

When patient recall of past drug use was compared with a pharmacy database it was influenced by demographics (age and level of education) and past drug use (recency of use and number of different drugs used in the past) and varied with the type of drug and its chronicity of use (West *et al.*, 1995).

All patients in a radiotherapy for cancer study gave their consent, but 22% had no recollection of consenting, 24% could not recall being told about any side effects from radiotherapy, and 44% believed that by consenting they would be unable to complain subsequently about side effects (Montgomery *et al.*, 1997).

Infectiousness of ADRs

A trial involving 28 chronic psychotics who had been shown to be stable over a period of five months, compared placebo and nicotinic acid, 100 mg. The latter produces flushing of the skin with a sensation of heat and sometimes skin irritation, appearing within 30 minutes and disappearing within a further 30 minutes. The patients had either schizophrenia or depression and had had no recent psychiatric treatment. The nurses were told that it was a trial of a new preparation. They were questioned about each patient before, during and after the nine-week trial with particular reference to changes in habit, amount of activity and occupation. They were also asked to report at once any unusual signs or symptoms and a number of likely ones were listed including giddiness, nausea or vomiting, headaches, paleness or flushing, drowsiness, fits or faints, loss of appetite, abdominal pain, jaundice and restlessness. Of the nicotinic acid group 10 had flushing, 2 during the first week, another 2 during the second week, and a further 2 during the third week, 3 during the fourth week and 1 during the seventh week. Of the 14 patients in the placebo group 5 also had flushing, 2 during the fourth week, 2 more during the eighth week and 1 during the ninth week. There were also many other reports of symptoms, of which 50 reports involved the 15 patients with flushing and 28 of those without flushing (i.e. a ratio of nearly 2:1). These results suggested that the placebo patients 'caught' the flushing from the patients on nicotinic acid and that once a side effect is noticed more attention is focused on those patients or volunteers. The slow recognition of the flushing is also noticeable (Letemendia and Harris, 1959).

Another study among psychiatric patients, mostly schizophrenics and all female, compared placebo and chlorpromazine. After a two-week baseline period on the usual chlorpromazine dose the patients in group A were changed to placebo, but only the pharmacist knew of the change. Two weeks later the patients in group B was changed to placebo. After a further week when group A patients had been on placebo for one month and group B for one week, the nurses were told to administer placebo, previously believing that they had been on chlorpromazine. After a further week the placebo was withdrawn and the patients themselves knew that they were without medication. The AE reports are shown in Table 2.

It can be seen that substitution of placebo produced no deterioration, but on the nurses being told the reports trebled. Six patients were described as unmanageable. One ward sister who had predicted that withdrawal of chlorpromazine would have no effect experienced no increase in the number of reports of disturbances while for another ward sister who had foretold problems if chlorpromazine was withdrawn the number of disturbances per week rose from one to 17 and she threatened to resign (Le Vay, 1960). It would appear that the placebo by itself was as effective as

Table 2   AE reports among psychiatric patients in chlorpromazine / placebo study

Trial week	Group A reports	Group B reports
1	Chlorpromazine 4	Chlorpromazine 8
2	Chlorpromazine 6	Chlorpromazine 6
3	Placebo 5	Chlorpromazine 9
4	Placebo 5	Chlorpromazine 5
5	Placebo 4	Placebo 4
6	Placebo 4	Placebo 9
7	Prescribed placebo 17	Prescribed placebo 23
8	No drugs 18	No drugs 27

chlorpromazine, but that its adverse effect on withdrawal was in the mind of the observer.

A three-way comparison of aspirin, sulfinpyrazone and placebo in patients with unstable angina took place at three different centres A, B and C, and a questionnaire was used to collect AEs. Minor GI were reported by 65% of patients at centre A, 66% at centre B and 39% at centre C ($p < 0.001$). The only difference between the three centres was that the consent form omitted mentioning GI symptoms at centre C (Myers *et al.*, 1987). Levine suggested that the way round the problem was to introduce some false side effects into the consent form (Levine, 1987). This would, however, only introduce more problems and cannot be recommended.

The possibility that a patient package insert (PPI) might encourage patients to report more side effects was excluded in a study in the USA of 249 mild hypertensives given thiazides (56% black and 33% Spanish Americans). Of these, two-thirds were given a PPI and one third were not. There was no difference in the number of AEs reported by the two groups, but those given the PPI attributed more of them to the drug (Morris and Kanouse, 1982).

Causal factors for ADRs:
- ?Age • Gender • Medical history • Race • Genes • Number of drugs
- Disease • Memory • Contact with others with ADRs

Risk–benefit ratio

Risk–benefit ratio is a poor term as it should be either 'risk of harm–risk of benefit ratio' or 'harm–benefit ratio' (Veatch, 1993), but the commonest term used is risk–benefit ratio (Ernst and Resch, 1996). The use of the word 'ratio' implies the use of figures and exact measurement. A better word would be 'analysis' or 'assessment' or 'evaluation'.

Risk–benefit Analysis

Three methods can be used:
1. Formal analysis.
2. Comparative analysis.
3. Comprehensive analysis (Rawlins, 1989).

Formal Analysis

A randomized well-controlled clinical trial   Ideally if this is of sufficient power it will give an exact answer. This can be expressed as the number of AEs caused for each case of disease successfully treated or prevented—for example, a Medical Research Council (MRC) trial of treatment of mild hypertension showed that for each cardio-vascular event prevented, 33 men experienced ADRs (mostly impotence and fatigue) and 20 stopped treatment (Robson, 1997; MRC Working Party, 1985).

Utility Analysis   This is not too dissimilar to the use of Bayes' theorem for causality assessment in that the risks and benefits can be broken down into their constituents and the alternative possibilities expressed numerically. The numerous probabilities can be calculated (Lane and Hutchinson, 1987). This method, like the Bayesian Adverse Reaction Diagnostic Instrument (BARDI) (see page 308), requires a large amount of data and is therefore too complicated to use except for very important decisions.

Merit Analysis   This uses a general 'principle of threes structure'. Seriousness, duration and incidence of the disease, level of improvement produced by the drug and AEs of the drug are each graded as high, medium or low (Edwards *et al.*, 1996). This method, however, is too crude to use for important decisions.

Remaining Methods   These have been outlined by Rawlins as:

1.   Trade-offs: human capital—is an economic assessment where the financial costs of goods and services diverted from other areas are set against the output costs by premature death or retirement through ill health, but this is inadequate for dealing with human parameters; willingness-to-pay—again in financial terms (proportion of the patient's income in exchange for degrees of cure); standard gamble—what risk of death will patients take for a complete cure (see page 19).
2.   Comparative analysis (so-called 'bootstrapping'). Drugs used for similar purposes are compared. Rawlins describes its limitations as the assumption of similar efficacy in the compared drugs and insensitivity to changing standards over time.
3.   Judgement analysis. This is the intuitive integration of all known factors. Its equivalent in causality assessment is clinical judgement or 'global introspection'. The main problem with clinical judgement is that it is not usually possible to say which factors have been included and which have not, nor what weight has been given to each factor. It will depend upon factors such as training, clinical experience, subjective bias, degree of investigation of the literature, time available. This is an inadequate précis of Rawlins's chapter in '*Risk and Consent to Risk in Medicine*' (*see Bibliography*). This is the commonest method used, but an attempt should be made to explain the factors responsible for the decision.

Further reading: *Formal Methods for Risk Assessment.* Fischoff, B., Lichtenstein, S., Slovic, P., Derby, S. Z., Keeney, R. L. (1981). In *Acceptable Risk*, Cambridge Univ. Press.

Perception of Risk

If time and money are available then all the necessary figures can be obtained from the literature or studies can be set up to obtain them. The various facts needed are dealt with later in this chapter. However, humans are not necessarily logical creatures when it comes to balancing risks and benefits. 'A bird in the hand is worth two in the bush'—a benefit or gratification of a desire now is worth more than the distant probability of retribution or payment. How else can we explain the number of youngsters taking up smoking or other addictive drugs? Many human decisions are made emotionally and justified intellectually. Lee has listed the factors that distinguish between objective risk and perceived risk:

1. Voluntary risks vs involuntary risks—the 3000 embryopathies per year due to alcohol abuse in pregnancy compared with the thalidomide disaster (Slovic, 1987).
2. Familiar vs unknown—AIDS deaths have a lot of publicity, but tobacco-related cardiovascular deaths are rarely publicized.
3. Immediate vs delayed effect—the explosion of the TWA Boeing 747 flight 800 on the 17th July 1996 killed 230 people and produced a worldwide reaction, while nearly five times that number die in the USA each day (1096 in 1990) due to tobacco (Longo *et al.*, 1996) (i.e. about 20% of the total deaths in the USA), and in China the ministry of health estimates that smoking may kill 50 million children and young people in the country today (Goldsmith, 1996).
4. Threat to self vs threat to society—the unexpected death of a contemporary reminds one of one's own mortality whereas the 12.2 million children under five years of age dying due to famine in the world produce little reaction (Kevany, 1996).
5. Catastrophic vs chronic—the Chernobyl nuclear explosion caused far more alarm than the world total of 500 deaths due to mining each year (Heilman, 1988).
6. Fates worse than death vs clean sharp death (Lee, 1987).

When asked to choose between two treatments, A and B, a group consisting of patients, students and physicians were told that with treatment A the one-year survival rate was 90% while for treatment B there was a 10% mortality rate, but otherwise the drugs were the same; most respondents showed a preference for treatment A (McNeil *et al.*, 1982).

There is also the 'my baby is the most beautiful' attitude. In the same way that mothers think that their baby is the most beautiful so people in clinical research tend to consider that the drug that they are working on is more unique than it is. 'Scientists who work for the pharmaceutical industry get steeped in corporate culture and slip into biases of their own drugs' (Ramsay, 1990). This is a good reason for separating drug safety from efficacy clinical research, but it tends to pervade all staff at all levels.

Groups interested in the cost–benefit ratio include:

1. Patients.
2. Prescribing physicians.
3. Pharmacists.
4. Clinical pharmacologists.
5. Pharmaceutical companies.
6. Regulatory authorities.

Patients
Sources of information will include the patients' information leaflet, the prescribing physician, the pharmacist, the media and the patient's friends. None of these is satisfactory from the point of view of making a valid cost–benefit judgement.

The leaflet will mention possible ADRs, but will give no guide to severity or frequency nor is it the intention that the patient should be able to make a cost–benefit judgement from it. Its prime aim is to improve patient understanding of the use of the medicines—Association of the British Pharmaceutical Industry (ABPI) guidelines. Patients will rarely have the knowledge and background to be able to make an adequate assessment of the cost–benefit ratio. However, that does not mean that they will not attempt to make such a judgement on whatever information is available. Their assessment may be expressed in non-compliance (e.g. 14.5% of patients failed to have their prescription dispensed in a UK general practice) (Beardon *et al.*, 1993). Provision of verbal and written information about the side effects of antidepressant medication did not reduce compliance or increase reporting of side effects by patients treated with the drug (Myers *et al.*, 1987, 1993).

When patients with rheumatoid arthritis (RA) were asked what risk they were prepared to take for a cure of their disease they said that they would accept a 27% risk of death for a guaranteed cure (Thompson, 1986). Another paper mentions that patients would accept a median risk of death of no more than 1/10 000 000 for a 90% probability of a complete cure, while their physicians would accept a risk of 1/10 000. The risk of death with NSAIDs is between 1/260 and 1/360 over a course of a patient's treatment for RA (Pullar *et al.*, 1990). It seems that the answer depends upon how the question is worded. Suggested further reading is: 'Benefit/risk assessment; what patients can know that scientists cannot' (Veatch, 1993).

Prescribing Physicians

Prescribing physicians will not discuss with patients all the elements necessary to make a judgement; they simply do not have the time and very rarely have enough information. There is a presumption that physicians know all the relevant factors and have weighed up the probability of ADRs and the probability of benefit before prescribing drugs for particular patients. However, there is evidence that doctors are not necessarily better at judging probabilities than the patients (Kee, 1996). The UK NHS physician will usually have the following sources of drug information—MIMS, *ABPI Data Sheet Compendium, National Formulary, Current Problems* and the *Prescribers Journal.* Physicians in other countries will have their equivalent texts. There are other specific journals, which are not supplied free of charge unlike the above, for example *Prescrire International*, which deals specifically with cost–benefit ratios of new drugs.

The benefit half of the equation consists of the chance that the patient in question will be cured or relieved by the drug. This involves extrapolation from all the clinical trial patients to the individual patient or, more likely, extrapolation from the drug company representative's spiel to the individual patient.

The cost half of the equation can be assessed from the drug's adverse reaction profile (see page 44), but comparative data on drugs of the same class are rarely available. Unfortunately the necessary information is not available to the average prescriber and the data sheet is totally inadequate for this purpose.

In a study of the factors influencing general practitioners' decisions about whether or not to prescribe 51% mentioned side effects as a source of concern (Bradley, 1992). Of prescribing changes, 48.6% initiated by a random sample of 340 physicians in 15 American and Canadian metropolitan areas were initiated as a result of information supplied by pharmaceutical manufacturers (Putnam, 1990).

Pharmacists

Hospital pharmacists depend upon the available literature, and this may be quite extensive. They are likely to be in the best position to advise the prescriber, but of course will not know details of the patient's case unless they attend ward rounds or review case notes. District or community pharmacists may have little more information than the prescribing physicians.

Clinical Pharmacologists
These people have all the necessary information and experience, but not necessarily the time to answer queries on the cost–benefit ratio.

Regulatory Authorities
These have a continuous responsibility to the public to monitor the risk–benefit ratio throughout the life of a product. They have the ability and authority to obtain any relevant data. However, many are understaffed and therefore unable to fulfil their mandate.

Before allowing marketing of a new drug 'consumers can expect regulatory authorities to use six types of assessment of the supporting data submitted by the manufacturers' in balancing risk and benefit:

1. Regulatory authorities should establish that the product is of satisfactory quality and that this will be maintained during post-marketing manufacture.
2. Regulatory authorities should ensure that the product is efficacious for all the clinical indications that the manufacturer wishes to promote. With a combination product each ingredient should contribute to its overall therapeutic activity and the ingredients should be pharmaceutically and pharmacokinetically compatible.
3. Regulatory authorities will expect the animal and clinical studies to have rigorously explored the likely toxicological hazards to man during therapeutic use. Regulatory authorities, prescribers and consumers should be aware, however, that at the time a new drug is marketed only rough estimates of risk can be made because of the relatively short duration of treatment and limited numbers of patients involved in clinical trials.
4. Consumers expect regulatory authorities to carry out an objective and impartial risk–benefit assessment from the evidence of safety and efficacy. With non-narcotic analgesics used in the symptomatic relief of pain, formal analysis is impossible and regulators must use their professional judgement in making their assessment. The subjective nature of this form of risk–benefit evaluation, however, makes it inevitable that no decision will go unchallenged.
5. Regulatory authorities should ensure that prescribers are provided with sufficient objective unbiased information to enable them to exercise proper professional judgement on when and how to use the product. Prescribers will also wish to know how the product compares with others in the same therapeutic class; such information is not usually provided either by regulatory authorities or by manufacturers and may be more appropriately the responsibility of professional organizations (e.g. national drug or formulary committees) or consumer groups (e.g. *Drug and Therapeutics Bulletin*).
6. Regulators should have sufficient legal and executive powers to ensure that they can enforce actions against manufacturers that make exaggerated claims of efficacy or safety for their products (Rawlins, 1986).

Before treating a patient, a doctor must balance the expected benefits of a drug against its potential risks (i.e. evaluate the risk–benefit ratio). The situation is similar for the licensing authority in that its decision about whether to allow a drug to be marketed must depend upon the risk–benefit ratio for the whole population at risk.

In its assessment the CSM considers:

1. Quality.
2. Efficacy—new evidence for lack of efficacy, uniqueness of therapeutic properties, uniqueness of efficacy in small subgroups.
3. Safety—spontaneous reports, cohort studies, case–control studies, animal carcinogenicity.

The CSM does **not** consider:

1. Impact on company or competitors.
2. Unknown/unsuspected benefits.
3. Decisions by other regulatory authorities.
4. Misuse—potential or actual.
5. Pressure—from parliament, media, pressure groups (Rawlins, 1985).

The question arises 'Should the regulator consider the alternative therapies?' 'Before regulatory action is taken, the risk associated with available alternative therapies should ideally be evaluated and compared with the risk at issue. Moreover, the benefits of the actual and alternative therapies should be evaluated and weighed in the final evaluation of the situation' (Wiholm, 1991). 'Furthermore the substances being evaluated must be compared with the alternatives (benefit–benefit and risk–risk evaluation)' (Bass, 1987). Is this synonymous with 'uniqueness of therapeutic properties'? Presuming that alternative therapy is considered in the final analysis, 'Does a new drug have to be as good as or better than current alternatives'? Direct comparative studies, of sufficient size with the main competitors are unlikely to have been performed before a drug is approved. Like the prescribing physician, a regulatory authority must make its decision on inadequate evidence.

Pharmaceutical Companies

Although all the relevant information will be or should be available to the research company it will rarely have been analysed or assembled into a readable package for the marketing company to pass onto enquiring prescribers. It should be the pharmaceutical industry's aim to provide the information necessary such that these decisions can be made (i.e. undertake the first five assessments mentioned above).

The International Medical Benefit Risk Foundation (IMBRF) was established in 1991 to evaluate medical benefits, risks and costs. It was funded by the pharmaceutical industry in Europe, USA and Japan. It produced the international drug benefit–risk assessment data resource handbook in four volumes. It was originally named *Risk/benefit Assessment of Drugs—Analysis and Response (RAD-AR)*. Its work has been published in:

The Perception and Management of Drug Safety Risks. Editors: B. Horisberger and R. Dinkel. Proceedings of the 1988 Wolfsberg conference, Springer, 1989.

Improving Drug Safety—A Joint Responsibility. Editors: R. Dinkel, B. Horisberger and K. W. Tolo. Proceedings of the 1990 Wolfsberg conference, Springer-Verlag, 1991.

Databases for Pharmacovigilance. Editor: S. Walker. Centre for Medicines Research, 1996. (Copies available from CMR, Woodmansterne Rd, Carshalton, Surrey, SM5 4DS, UK.)

Unfortunately due to reduced funds the IMBRF had to close its secretariat in 1996 and reduce its activities.

The Two Opposing Factors in the Risk–benefit Ratio

These are:

1. Benefits (i.e. efficacy).
2. Risk (i.e. the side effect liability).

Benefits—measurement of Efficacy

The efficacy of a drug in the treatment of a disease needs to be considered compared with the following three alternatives:

1. No treatment and, therefore, the natural progress of the disease.
2. Placebo, which is the same as the above plus a psychological effect and a nonspecific trial effect, which may produce objective benefits or costs.
3. The standard treatment for the disease. If there is more than one standard treatment, then a comparison with each may be necessary.

If it is presumed that the healing rate for the standard therapy is greater than the natural healing rate or that induced by placebo and take as an example a healing rate of 60% for the standard therapy, the number of patients required in the trial can be calculated. In order to be approximately 95% certain of detecting a 5% difference between the standard therapy (60%) and the new therapy (55% or 65%), 500 patients would be required (Bulpitt, 1983). If the results are accepted as an adequate indication of the drug's efficacy, would this number of patients give an adequate indication of the safety of the drug? It should be able to establish the incidence of very common side effects, but what chance would one have of detecting a more rare serious side effect? There would be a 95% chance of finding a side effect with a true incidence of 1% if the background rate of the AE is 1 in 1000.

Risk of Harm—the Statistical Background to ADRs

With a sample size of 5000 patients there would be more than 99% certainty of finding one case of an ADR with a true incidence rate of 1 in 1000. If more than one case is required on which to base a decision as to whether this drug is safe to market, then the chance of finding them diminishes rapidly, there being only a 73% chance of finding four such cases in the sample of 5000 patients. The proviso mentioned earlier that the ADR is identified as being due to the drug is, however, important. If the ADR cannot be clearly differentiated from naturally occurring disease, then the problem is formidable. For instance, if the drug produces a 10% increase in a disease with a natural incidence of 1 in 1000, then to be 95% certain of detecting this some 1 100 000 patients would be required and for doubling of the incidence of the disease approximately 16 000 would be needed. For a given number of patients there will be more certainty about a drug's efficacy than its safety.

The reason for this situation is 'that a standard treatment nearly always means that it is efficacious in more than 10% of the population ($p_1 = 0.1$) and may even be effective in 50% of the population ($p_1 = 0.5$), the increase to 11% ($p_2 = 0.11$) or doubling to 20% ($p_2 = 0.2$) in the first instance and from 50% to 55% ($p_2 = 0.55$) and doubling to 100% healing ($p_2 = 1.00$) in the second instance. All these are relatively large figures compared with the figure for adverse reactions that would be of interest (e.g. a background death rate of approximately 1 in 10 000 ($p_1 = 0.0001$) doubling due to treatment to 2 in 10 000 ($p_2 = 0.002$); (Table 3). The increase from 50% efficacy to 55% efficacy would need a total of 3 280 patients in the study, while to detect a doubling of the rate of 1 in 10 000 of an ADR the figure required would be 474 000. To pick up a rarity like the aplastic anaemia caused by chloramphenicol,

Table 3 Number of observations needed in each group (populations p_1 and p_2) to detect given change in proportion (power 80%, significance level 5%)

p_1	p_2	n
0.5	0.55	1 640
	1.00	20
0.4	0.44	2 490
	0.80	30
0.3	0.33	3 890
	0.60	50
0.1	0.11	15 130
	0.20	240
0.01	0.011	168 000
	0.020	2 700
0.001	0.0011	1 684 000
	0.0020	23 000
0.0001	0.00011	11 860 000
	0.0002	237 000

Table 4 Number of observations needed in each group to detect a given difference in the group means in a parallel group trial (power 80%, significance level 5%, SD approx. 14)

Difference in means	Number of observations
2	700
5	120
10	30
15	15
20	8

1 500 000 observations would be needed (Melmon and Nierenberg, 1981). At the other end of the spectrum only 16 patients would be needed to compare a new hypertensive drug with placebo with an 80% certainty of finding a difference of 20 mm Hg in blood pressure (significance level 5%) (Table 4). It is obvious that absolute safety is unobtainable, even in the relatively short term. The problem of the changing risk–benefit ratio in the long term is even more difficult. Practolol introduced the medium-term ADR problem with a mean time to onset of eye signs of 23 months (Wright, 1975), while the delay between the use of diethylstilboestrol and the appearance of vaginal adenocarcinoma in the children of its recipients of at least 21 years (Herbst *et al.*, 1971) represents the long-term problem. The problem of long-term evaluation of the risk–benefit ratio has been illustrated by clofibrate where ultimately the risk exceeded the benefits, but the reasons why are not known (Committee of Principal Investigators, 1978, 1980). It is clearly essential that maximum advantage is taken of clinical trials to establish the side effect burden of a drug and that great effort must be made to collect side effects presenting after marketing and that these must then be correctly assessed.

The Risks of Harm

There is no way of establishing the complete safety of a new drug before it comes into widespread use. As the number of patients increases so the risks can be defined with greater accuracy and this will continue until the drug is marketed, when there is no longer a 100% reporting on the fate of each patient treated. The decision as to how many patients should be treated before allowing a drug onto the market will depend upon several factors. A relatively small number may be required for a new drug for a rare fatal disease for which there is no treatment, but several thousands may be required for a drug which needs to be taken on a long-term basis for a common chronic disease or an antibiotic for an infection that is rarely fatal and for which there are already acceptable treatments (McMahon, 1983). In the UK for the years 1987–1989 the median number was 1528 patients with 95% confidence interval of 1194–1748, with a range from 43–15 962 (Rawlins and Jefferys, 1993).

The regulatory authority will be influenced by the government, which in turn will be influenced by the general opinion within parliament, which should reflect public opinion. There have been several occasions when the reaction to the publication of an ADR has resulted in the unjustified condemnation of a medication.

False Alarms

Oxygen and Retrolental Fibroplasia   The discovery in 1953 that 100% oxygen given to neonates could cause retrolental fibroplasia, produced a change in practice which caused a large number of neonatal deaths from hypoxia. Cross and Bolton (Cross, 1973; Bolton and Cross, 1974) suggested that there were about 200 000 deaths in England and Wales and over 180 000 deaths in the USA over the subsequent two decades. These numbers were 16 times higher than the estimated number of babies who would have been blinded by a more liberal oxygen policy.

Pertussis Vaccine and Encephalopathy   The reports of neurological illness following the use of pertussis vaccine resulted in decreased immunizations in the UK—

immunizations of neonates dropped from 80% to 31% (Miller *et al.*, 1981), resulting in the largest epidemic of pertussis for 20 years (Meade, 1981). Of children in the encephalopathy study 3.5% had had triple vaccine within seven days, compared with 1.7% of controls. The relative risk was 2.4; if the child had previously been neurologically normal, the relative risk was 3.3, but there was no significant risk if the child had diphtheria and tetanus vaccine alone. The risk of serious impairment within seven days was 1 in 110 000 and the risk of permanent impairment was 1 in 310 000 (Anon, 1981a).

Teratogenicity of Debendox (Bendectin)   There remain some controversies concerning ADRs where publicity has not helped to resolve the problem. Although on three occasions the CSM has carefully examined all the available data on the issue of whether debendox for the treatment of morning sickness in pregnancy has produced an increased incidence of congenital abnormalities in the offspring of mothers treated with the drug, it found no evidence that there was an increased risk of fetal damage with the use of this agent (Fleming *et al.*, 1981). The adverse publicity produced such a large fall in sales that it was no longer viable commercially and it was withdrawn from the market. It was the first drug victim of trial by the media (Austrian, 1996). It has subsequently reappeared in Canada and Spain (Einarson *et al.*, 1996)

Cancer in Children following Vitamin K Administration   A case–control study in 1992 reported an increase in cancer and leukaemia in children given intramuscular vitamin K for prevention of haemorrhagic disease of the newborn (Golding *et al.*, 1990, 1992). The British Paediatric Association then recommended oral vitamin K, but in 1993 there were five reports of late haemorrhagic disease in infants receiving the oral form. Two later studies could find no association between intramuscular vitamin K and cancer (Klebanoff *et al.*, 1993; Von Kries *et al.*, 1996) or leukaemia (Ansell *et al.*, 1996). It was suggested that there were design flaws in the Golding study (Zipursky, 1996).

A further four studies have confirmed that there is no link between vitamin K and solid tumours but a small risk of leukaemias cannot be ruled out (von Kries, 1998).

Cancer and Depression Caused by Reserpine   This originated from a study by the Boston Collaborative Drug Surveillance Program—(Cohen, 1974; Jick, 1984; Porter *et al.*, 1986; Lawson, 1986b) and later there was contrary evidence (Fraser, 1996).

MMR Vaccination and Autism 1998   A paper produced the hypothesis that of 12 children with bowel abnormalities and serious developmental regression (nine had autism), eight of these children developed the disease after receiving MMR and that there was a causal relationship (Wakefield *et al.*, 1998). This was subsequently denied (Nicholl *et al.*, 1998; Chen and Destephano, 1998).

Risks We are Prepared to Take
It is very difficult to find out what risks the general public would be prepared to run for an effective drug, but one can study the risks they are prepared to take in everyday life and with certain common social drugs (Table 5).

The actions that various risks provoke give an idea as to whether the public considers them acceptable or not:

1. Fatal accidents present a risk of 1 in 1000/person/year and are infrequent. As immediate action is taken to reduce such hazards it is suggested that this level of risk is socially unacceptable.
2. At lethal accident levels of 1 in 10000/person/year public money is spent to control the cause.
3. Mortality risks of 1 in 100000/person/year are still considered candidates for some action, but Knox argues that if the probability from a procedure is less than 1 in 100000 public concern ceases and it can be regarded as 'safe' and therefore acceptable (Knox, 1975).
4. Fatal accidents with a probability of 1 in 1000000/person/year are not of concern to most people. Just to put this figure into context the incidence of fatal ADRs to prescription only drugs is just less than 1 per 1000000 prescriptions dispensed (O'Brien, 1986).

These figures show that the boundaries of acceptable risk lie between 1 in 1000000 (those associated with natural hazards) and 1 in 1000 (i.e. the annual per capita illness and disease risks). Society appears to accept voluntary risks with orders of magnitude greater than involuntary risks (Dinman, 1980a) (see Tables 5 and 6). Dinman (1980b) points out that a country (the USA) that accepts 200000 excess deaths a year associated with smoking (the figure given in 1996 is 400000) and 20000

Table 5   The risks of common voluntary activities

Voluntary risks (Dinman, 1980a,b; *Daily Telegraph*, 1981; Pochin, 1975)		Death/person/year (odds)
Smoking (20 cigarettes per day)	1 in	200
Drinking (1 bottle of wine per day)	1 in	13300
Soccer*	1 in	25000
Car racing	1 in	10000
Car driving* (UK)	1 in	5900
Motorcycling (see footnote)	1 in	50
Rock climbing**	1 in	7150
Taking contraceptive pills	1 in	50000
Power boating	1 in	5900
Canoeing	1 in	100000
Horse-racing*	1 in	740
Amateur boxing*	1 in	2000000
Professional boxing**	1 in	14300
Skiing	1 in	1430000
Pregnancy (UK)	1 in	4380
Abortion (legal less than 12 weeks)***	1 in	50000
Abortion (legal more than 14 weeks)***	1 in	5900

  * Based upon deaths/per million participants/year
 ** Based upon deaths/per million hours/year spent in sport
*** Based upon deaths/per million pregnancies per year
A figure of 1 death per 1056 registered motorcycles is quoted by Urquhart and Heilmann in *Risk Watch*.

Table 6 Rare risks in life (involuntary)

Involuntary risks (Dinman, 1980b)		Risk of death/person/year (odds)
Struck by auto (USA)	1 in	20 000
Struck by car (UK)	1 in	16 600
Floods (USA)	1 in	455 000
Earthquakes (California)	1 in	588 000
Tornados (Mid West)	1 in	455 000
Lightning (UK)	1 in	10 000 000
Falling aircraft (USA)	1 in	10 000 000
Falling aircraft (UK)	1 in	50 000 000
Explosion pressure vessel (USA)	1 in	20 000 000
Release from atomic power station at site boundary (USA)	1 in	10 000 000
at 1 km (UK)	1 in	10 000 000
Flooding by dikes (Holland)	1 in	10 000 000
Bites of venomous creatures (UK)	1 in	5 000 000
Leukaemia	1 in	12 500
Influenza	1 in	9 000
Meteorite	1 in	100 billion

These figures are only approximate and may have been calculated using different assumptions. Any individual figure should be treated with reserve.

excess deaths from not buckling seat belts will not, and to be consistent, should not pursue extreme risks posed by environmental contaminants. There was considerable opposition to the parliamentary bill that made the fastening of front seat belts mandatory, a move that the British Medical Association (BMA) had suggested would save more than 700 lives per annum and prevent serious injuries to 11 000 per annum (*Daily Telegraph*, 1981).

Recommended reading on this subject includes:

1. The BMA guide *Living with Risk*, Wiley medical publications, 1987, which is a paperback that is also suitable for patients.
2. *Risk and Consent to Risk in Medicine*. Editor: R. Mann, The Parthenon Publishing Group, 1989.
3. *Risk Watch. The Odds of Life* by J. Urquhart and K. Heilmann, Facts on File Publications, New York and Bicester, England (or in the original German *Keine Angst vor der* Angst, Kindler Verlag, Munich, 1983).

The authors of the latter suggest the use of safety degree units, which is the number of noughts in the unicohort size (i.e. 5 = 1 in 100 000). They also give the number of premature deaths caused or accelerated by cigarette smoking in the USA as the equivalent of three fully loaded Boeing 747 Jumbo jets (over 1 500 people) crashing every day. This is a useful comparison to use when discussing the incidence of fatal ADRs.

Terms Used to Describe Risks
These are as follows:

Negligible—less than 1 AE per 1 000 000 (e.g. death due to being struck by lightning or death due to release of radiation by nuclear power).

Minimal—1 in 1 000 000 to 1 in 100 000 (e.g. death due to a railway accident or vaccination-associated polio).

Very low—1 in 100 000 to 1 in 10 000 (e.g. death at football, at home or at work or death due to homicide or leukaemia).

Low—1 in 10 000 to 1 in 1000 (e.g. death from 'flu or road traffic accident or all kinds of violence and poisoning).

Moderate 1 in 1000 to 1 in 100 (e.g. death from smoking 10 cigarettes daily or from all natural causes at the age of 40 years).

High—over 1 in 100 (e.g. transmission of measles/varicella or risk of GI effects of antibiotics) (Calman, 1996).

Risks:
- Negligible < 1 in 1 000 000   • Minimal 1 in 1 000 000 to 1 in 100 000   • Very low 1 in 100 000 to 1 in 10 000   • Low 1 in 100 000 to 1 in 1 000   • Moderate 1 in 1 000 to 1 in 100   • High > 1 in 100

Risks We Take With Drugs

To compare these death rates with those of deaths caused by drugs is extremely difficult since there is gross underreporting of the latter and therefore the following figures must be considered in this light and also bearing in mind the source of the figures (i.e. seriously ill patients). In the BCDSP 0.9 patients per 1000 were considered to have died as a result of drugs. The rates varied from 0 in Israel and Italy to 1.4

Table 7   Numbers of deaths reported as possibly due to drugs over a $7\frac{1}{2}$ year period or less (Girdwood 1974)

Oral contraceptives	332	Acetylsalicylic acid	72
Phenylbutazone	217	Oxphenbutazone	69
Chlorpromazine	102	Indomethacin	68
Corticosteroids	94	Halothane	57
Isoprenaline	84	Amitriptyline	50
Phenacetin	77		

Table 8   The ratio of reports per annum of deaths/millions of prescriptions (Girdwood, 1974)

Sodium aurothiomalate	164.3	Indomethacin	4.4
Phenindione	30.0	Imipramine	3.6
Warfarin	28.3	Chloramphenicol	3.6
Phenelzine	17.2	Phenytoin	3.0
Oxyphenbutazone	14.3	Chlorpropamide	3.0
Tranylcypromine	13.7	Amitriptyline	2.3
Adrenaline	9.6	Trifluoperazine	2.0
Chlorpromazine	8.6	Methaqualone/diphen.	1.9
Isoprenaline	7.9	Frusemide	1.3
Propranolol	7.4	Methyldopa	1.3
Phenylbutazone	7.1	Corticosteroids	0.84
Orciprenaline	6.2		

per 1000 in New Zealand (Porter and Jick, 1977). The figures for the UK are given in Table 7, from Girdwood (Girdwood, 1974). These figures, however, do not give any idea of the population at risk. The same author also gives a table based on the ratio of reports of deaths per annum compared with the number of millions of prescriptions (Table 8). These figures have shown the involuntary risks that patients have to run and those voluntary risks they are prepared to exchange for various pleasurable pursuits. At lethal accident rates of 1 in 10 000/person/year public money is spent to control their causes and at 1 in 100 000/person/year mothers warn children of the dangers of playing with fire, of drowning and of poison, and some people accept inconvenience, such as avoiding air travel (Dinman, 1980a). Where should we draw the line as acceptable risk with, say, a treatment with a new antihypertensive drug? It has been suggested (Anon, 1981b) that at the time of marketing, risks of 1 in 100 should be known, but this figure is not the risk of deaths, but only of ADRs. It would seem that a similar figure for post-marketing surveillance (PMS) of 1 in 1000 (Inman, 1981a) – 1 in 10 000 is acceptable (Shapiro, 1977b) and this would require a cohort of 10 000–20 000 individuals. If a side effect is exceedingly rare, say 1 in 50 000, no formal system will be sufficiently cost-effective to discover it.

Table 9 Number of patients required with no background incidence of adverse reactions (Lewis, 1981)

Expected incidence of adverse reaction		Required number of adverse reactions		
		1	2	3
1 in	100	300	480	650
1 in	200	600	900	1 300
1 in	1 000	3 000	4 800	6 500
1 in	2 000	6 000	9 600	13 000
1 in	10 000	30 000	48 000	65 000

Table 10 Number of patients required in drug treated group when background incidence exists (Lewis, 1981)

Size of control	Background incidence of adverse reaction	Additional incidence of adverse drug reaction		
		1 in 100	1 in 1 000	1 in 10 000
Infinite (background incidence known)	1 in 10	10 000	980 000	98 000 000
	1 in 100	1 600	110 000	11 000 000
	1 in 1 000	500	16 000	1 000 000
5 times as big as treated group	1 in 10	12 000	1 200 000	120 000 000
	1 in 100	9 000	130 000	13 000 000
	1 in 1 000	700	19 000	1 400 000
Equal to treated group	1 in 10	20 000	2 000 000	200 000 000
	1 in 100	3 200	220 000	22 000 000
	1 in 1 000	1 300	32 000	2 300 000

Number of Patients Needed to Assess Risks   The phrase 'risks of 1 in 100' needs clarification. It probably refers to those distinct drug reactions for which there is no background incidence. There are two classifications of ADRs from the statistical point of view:

1. The adverse reaction that is clearly an ADR and for which there is no naturally occurring background (e.g. the oculomucocutaneous syndrome with practolol) (see Table 9).
2. The adverse reaction that either simulates disease or produces an increase in a naturally occurring disease (e.g. dry eyes caused by beta blockers) (see Table 10).

All these tables are based on a 95% probability of success, so our 10 000 population will give a greater than 95% chance of having at least three recognizable ADRs with an incidence of 1 in 1 000 and a 95% chance of discovering two recognizable ADRs with an incidence of 1 in 2000. So 10 000 patients will give a 95% chance of discovering an additional incidence of 1 in 100 where the background incidence is 1 in 10, but a less than 95% chance of discovering an additional incidence of 1 in 1000 when the background incidence is 1 in 1000 (see Table 10).

The Rule of Three   If no AEs occur in N patients the upper limit of the 95% confidence interval for the frequency of events is approximately 3/N. The numerators for the 95% confidence interval upper limits for observed numerators of 0, 1, 2, 3 and 4 are about 3, 5, 7, 9 and 10 (Newman, 1995).

Monitoring for Multiple ADRs   The figures so far presume that one is only monitoring for one type of ADR, whereas in most cases we will be monitoring for an unknown number of ADRs. Since the 5% level of significance is used, of every 100 possible ADRs examined five could be expected by chance (Table 11). It must be

Table 11   Number of patients required in drug treated group to allow for examination of 100 adverse reactions (Lewis, 1981) (significance $p < 0.05$)

Size of control	Background incidence of adverse reaction	Additional incidence of adverse drug reaction		
		1 in 100	1 in 1 000	1 in 10 000
Infinite (background	1 in 10	23 000	2 200 000	*220 000 000
incidence known)	1 in 100	3 100	250 000	24 000 000
	1 in 1 000	800	32 000	2 500 000
5 times as big as treated	1 in 10	27 000	2 600 000	260 000 000
group	1 in 100	4 000	300 000	29 000 000
	1 in 1 000	1 300	40 000	3 000 000
Equal to treated group	1 in 10	46 000	4 400 000	440 000 000
	1 in 100	7 200	510 000	48 000 000
	1 in 1 000	2 900	73 000	5 100 000

* This is approximately the combined total population of France, Italy, Germany and the United Kingdom.

realized that this type of PMS (i.e. without concurrent randomized controls) is searching for hypotheses and not testing them. If it is accepted that nothing will be published until a hypothesis testing study is finished, then this risk is not important, except from the point of view of cost; however, if as it seems, possible hypotheses are published, the level of significance must be increased if we are to prevent more widespread apprehension (see Table 11). These figures presume that the drug is given to the same population as has the known background incidence of the disease. It is very unlikely that the background incidence will be known in the particular subset of the population who will be prescribed the drug. Another presumption is that there will be no drop out of patients over the monitoring period.

Conclusions   Very many fewer patients are required to detect an ADR that has no background incidence than one that mimics or increases a known disease. Many ADRs mimic known diseases and the means of differentiating between them often does not develop until several years have passed. If a new drug causes a modest increase (10%) in the incidence of a common disease (1 in 100 per annum), the number of patients needed for monitoring to discover this is prohibitively large (250 000) (Spriet-Pourra *et al.*, 1982).

Financial Cost of ADRs

The new science of pharmacoeconomics has grown rapidly in the last few years. The financial cost of a disease (e.g. hospitalization) is balanced against the cost of intervention (e.g. cost of drugs or operations). One factor in the cost of drugs is the cost of dealing with ADRs. In general terms the following problems occur:

1. Definition of the AE for search purposes.
2. Causality assessment of the AE. Few AEs are definitely ADRs or definitely not ADRs.
3. If ADRs occur in hospitalized patients there is difficulty in judging the prolongation of hospitalization due to the ADR or additional hospital costs.
4. The hospitalized patient is not representative of the general population.
5. Frequently there is no satisfactory control group (Abadie and Souetre, 1993).

Cost is paid by:

1. The patient. This will vary from nil for a mild transitory ADR, lost earnings for a temporarily incapacitating ADR, to many thousands of pounds for a permanently incapacitating ADR.
2. The physician. Depending upon circumstances, the additional cost of diagnosis and management in general practice may be claimed from a private patient or considered part of a health service commitment and therefore has to be absorbed by the practice/partnership. There may be additional cost in trying to either avoid ADRs or insure against those caused by negligence.
3. The manufacturer. This will include the cost of a pharmacovigilance department and the additional costs of detecting ADRs in clinical trials as well as insurance and/or possible litigation and compensation costs. If there is evidence that may affect the stock market price then the evidence must be reported to the stock

exchange and thence to the press and there may then be a large fall in share price (Richman, 1996; Senard *et al.*, 1996).

4. The nation. This will include part of the social insurance costs and a proportion of the cost of a nationalized health service as well as the cost of pharmacovigilance. Drug related morbidity and mortality have been estimated to cost more than $136 billion a year in the USA and a major component of these costs derives from ADRs (Classen *et al.*, 1997). An estimate of the direct costs of hospital admissions due to ADRs in Germany is 1050 million DM per year or £374 million or $619 million (Goettler *et al.*, 1997).

Moving from vague generalizations to more specific costs:

Stenoses and gut perforations due to potassium chloride in Nancy over a period of 42 months amounted to 14 perforations and 3 stenoses at a direct cost of 2 160 530 fr (Royer *et al.*, 1990).

Again in France, in a 36-bedded ward over two months 52 patients were admitted with an ADR, 27 patients developed an ADR while in hospital, and five patients fell into both categories. Total costs were 695 134 fr (£89,810, $136,512, 206 114 DM) (Moore *et al.*, 1996).

The yearly cost of the excess duration related to ADRs in a French 29-bedded was 758 016 fr (£94,752, Euro 113 136) (Moore *et al.*, 1998).

In a hospital in the USA over a 2-year period 109 patients suffered clinical consequences due to ADRs or medication related errors at a cost of US$1.5 million in 1994 (Reactions No. 578, 1995; Schneider *et al.*, 1995).

A two-hospital study in the USA gave a figure of $2595 per ADR and patient stay was prolonged by 2.2 days. The estimated annual cost for a 700-bedded hospital was $5.6 million or £3.45 million (Bates *et al.*, 1997).

In a further study in the USA (1990–1993) the excess cost of hospitalization attributable to an ADR occurring in the hospital was $2013, (£1266, DM 3279, 11 027 fr) and the stay in hospital was prolonged by 1.74 days (Classen *et al.*, 1997).

The total direct charges for severe ADRs leading to hospital admission in Germany totalled $656 million (£409 million/3785 million fr/DM 1124 million) in 1965 (Schneeweiss *et al.*, 1997).

Computerized ADR detection reduced the numbers of ADRs by 30% and reduced one hospital's costs in the USA by US$ 300 000 per year (James, 1997).

It is important that figures for drug-related costs are broken down into their various constituents since they may include drug underdosage, suicides, untreated indications, failure to receive drugs and drug use without indication. Bearing in mind all the variables mentioned above studies cannot be compared unless they use the same definitions and methods.

Definitions and Classifications of Adverse Reaction Terms

Some of the terms used by the FDA were altered in October 1997 and these are dealt with in Chapter 13.

Adverse Event

Finney, who originally suggested that AEs should be collected rather than adverse reactions, defined an AE as a "Particular untoward happening experienced by a patient, undesirable either generally or in the context of the disease" (Finney, 1965; Skegg and Doll, 1977).

The definition used by Inman in *Prescription Event Monitoring* (Inman, 1981b) is "An event is any new diagnosis, any reason for referral to a consultant or admission to hospital (e.g. operation, accident or pregnancy), any unexpected deterioration (or improvement) in a concurrent illness, any suspected drug reaction, or any other complaint which was considered of sufficient importance to enter in the patient's notes".

Kramer *et al.* (1979) define an AE as 'An abnormal sign, symptom or laboratory test or a cluster of abnormal signs, symptoms and tests'.

The CPMP working party on efficacy of medicinal products in *Notes for Guidance 111/3976/88–EN (Final)* quote "Any undesirable experience occurring to a subject during a clinical trial, whether or not considered related to the investigational product(s)". This is for Good Clinical Practice (GCP) for trials on medicinal products in the European Community, which came into operation on the 1st July 1991.

The WHO definition (September 1991) is "Any untoward medical occurrence that may present during treatment with a pharmaceutical product but which does not necessarily have a causal relationship with this treatment".

The Commission of the European Communities definition (MCA EuroDirect Publication No.337/93) also ICH guideline on Clinical Safety Data Management, Topic reference E2, 1994, also US Federal Register Part XIII Vol. 60, No.40 (March 1st 1995). ICH Guideline for GCP (step 5) (1996) is as follows: an AE (or adverse experience) is "Any untoward medical occurrence in a patient or clinical investigation subject administered a pharmaceutical product and which does not necessarily have a causal relationship with this treatment".

The CPMP notes for guidance (CPMP/PhWP/176/95) defines AE (or adverse experience) as "Any undesirable experience occurring to a patient treated with a pharmaceutical product whether or not related to the medicinal product".

Adverse Drug Experience (USA)

"Any adverse event associated with the use of a drug in humans whether or not considered drug related including the following: an adverse event occurring in the course of the use of a drug product in professional practice, an adverse event occurring from overdose whether accidental or intentional, an adverse event occurring from drug abuse, an adverse event occurring from drug withdrawal and any significant failure of expected pharmacological action" (Nelson, 1988). Under the ICH process adverse drug experience (ADE) becomes synonymous with adverse event (Kessler, 1993). The wording for biologicals is similar (Ellenberg, 1995).

Adverse Drug Reaction

"A response to a drug that is noxious and unintended and occurs at doses normally used in man for the prophylaxis, diagnosis or therapy of disease, or for modification of physiological function"—WHO Technical Report No. 498, 1972 and *Note for Guidance on Clinical safety Data Management: Definitions and Standards for Expedited Reporting* (CPMP/ICH/377/95). A modified version of this has been suggested adding "excluding failure to accomplish the intended purpose" (Karch and Lasagna, 1975). The latter also give "An adverse reaction is any undesirable effect produced by a drug".

Kramer *et al.* (1979) give "An undesirable clinical manifestation consequent to and caused by the administration of a given drug".

An ADR is any undesirable effect of a drug. The effect may be an extension of the drug's pharmacological action or of an idiosyncratic nature (Porta and Hartzema, 1987).

An ADR can be defined as a noxious and unintended response to a drug that occurs at usually recommended doses (Stolley, 1981).

The FDA in the USA (1979) used a completely different definition: 'Any experience associated with the use of a drug whether or not considered drug-related and includes any side effect, injury, toxicity or sensitivity reaction or significant failure of expected pharmacological action'. This definition could be more suitable for 'adverse event' than for 'adverse drug reactions' (see page 33).

The EEC's version in *Notes for Guidance* (CPMP/PhWP/176/95) is "A reaction which is harmful and unintended and which occurs at doses normally used in man for the prophylaxis, diagnosis or treatment of disease or for the modification of physiological function. In the case of clinical trials injuries by overdosing, abuse/dependence and interactions with other medicinal products should be considered as ADR" (Council Directive 93/39/EEC, Article 29b of Official Journal of the European Communities, Vol. 36, pp. 22–30, 24 August 1993). Within Europe there are several more different versions and these can be found in *Report on Pharmacovigilance in the European Community* (111/3577/89).

The Council for International Organization of Medical Science (CIOMS) definition was "An undesirable effect suspected of being caused by a drug" (Faich *et al.*, 1990).

The CPMP (MCA EuroDirect Publication No.337/93) also US Federal Register Part XIII, Vol. 60, No. 40, March 1st 1995 and now synonymous with the *ICH Harmonised Tripartite Guideline* (step 5) 1996 has a different definition for premarketing and post-marketing. Pre-approval it is "All noxious and unintended responses to a medicinal product related to any dose should be considered adverse drug reactions". The phrase 'responses to a medicinal product' means that a causal relationship between a medicinal product and an AE is at a least reasonable possibility (i.e. the relationship cannot be ruled out). This is a contradiction in terms. An ADR is an AE caused by a drug. The new definition is equivalent to a possible, probable or definite ADR. Post-approval the definition is 'A response to a drug which is noxious and unintended and which occurs at doses normally used in man for prophylaxis, diagnosis, or therapy of diseases or for modification of physiological function'.

Unexpected
Unexpected adverse drug reaction—Medicines Control Agency (MCA) EuroDirect Publication No.337/93, also US Federal Register Part XIII, Vol. 60, No.40, March 1st 1995, also *ICH Guideline for Good Clinical Practice* (step 5), 1996—"An adverse reaction, the nature or severity of which is not consistent with the applicable product

information (e.g. investigator's brochure for an unapproved investigational medicinal product or package insert/summary of product characteristics for an approved product)".

In *Notes for Guidance on Procedures for Competent Authorities or the Undertaking of Pharmacovigilance Activities* (CPMP/PhWP/176/95) "An unexpected ADR is an adverse reaction which is not mentioned in the summary of product characteristics".

For biological products in the USA the wording is different: "An adverse experience associated with a biological product that is not listed in its current labelling and includes an event that may be symptomatically and pathophysiologically related to an event listed in the labelling; but differs from the event because of greater severity or specificity" (Ellenberg, 1995).

CPMP (MCA EuroDirect Publication No. 3375/93)

The following documents or circumstances will be used to determine whether an AE (reaction) is expected:

1. For a medicinal product not yet approved for marketing in a country, a company's investigator's brochure will serve as the source document in that country.
2. Reports which add significant information on specificity or severity of a known, already documented serious ADR constitute unexpected events, for example, an event more specific or more severe than described in the investigator's brochure would be considered 'unexpected'. "In general, information that might materially influence the benefit–risk assessment of a medicinal product or that should be sufficient to consider changes in medicinal product administration or in the overall conduct of a clinical investigation represent situations that necessitate rapid communication to regulatory authorities" (MCA EuroDirect Publications No. 3375, 93).

Unexpected AE "means any adverse experience that is not identified in nature, severity, or frequency in the current investigator's brochure or, if an investigator's brochure is not required, that is not identified in nature, severity, or frequency in the risk information described in the general investigational plan or elsewhere in the current application, as amended" (21CFR312.32) (CFR, US Code of Federal Regulations).

Life-threatening—investigational new drug (IND) definition—means that the patient was, in the view of the investigator, at immediate risk of death from the reaction as it occurred (i.e. it does not include a reaction that had it occurred in a more serious form, might have caused death) (21CFR312.32).

Serious

A serious AE (experience) or reaction is any untoward medical occurrence that at any dose:

*   Results in death.
*   Is life-threatening. (This implies that the patient was at risk of death at the time of the event; it does not refer to an event which hypothetically might have caused death if it were more severe).
*   Requires inpatient hospitalization or prolongation of existing hospitalization.
*   Results in persistent or significant disability/incapacity.
*   Is a congenital anomaly/birth defect.

(*ICH Guideline for Good Clinical Practice*, Step 5, 1996).
(CPMP/ICH/377/95)

Proposed new definition (Federal Register, October 27th, 1994) is "An AE occurring at any dose that is fatal or life-threatening, results in persistent or significant disability/incapacity, requires or prolongs hospitalization, necessitates medical or surgical intervention to preclude permanent impairment of a body function or permanent damage to a body structure, or is a congenital anomaly".

For biological products it is "An AE associated with the use of a biological product that is:

- Fatal or life-threatening, is permanently disabling, requires inpatient hospitalization, or
- A congenital anomaly, cancer or overdose" (Ellenberg, 1995).

Medical and scientific judgement should be exercised in deciding whether expedited reporting is appropriate in other situations, such as important medical events that may not be immediately life-threatening or result in death or hospitalization but may jeopardize the patient or may require intervention to prevent one of the other outcomes listed in the definition above. These should also usually be considered serious (MCA EuroDirect Publication No. 3375/93 also US Federal Register Part XIII, Vol. 50, No.4). *Guideline on Clinical Safety Data Management; Definitions and Standards for Expedited Reporting* (March 1st 1995) is the same as the ICH guidelines—a "Serious adverse drug reaction that is fatal, life-threatening, disabling, incapacitating or which results in or prolongs hospitalization" (from draft notice to applicants Chapter V (*Pharmacovigilance of Medicinal Products for Human Use*, December 1994, 111/5944/94) and is also in *Notes for Guidance on Procedures for Competent Authorities or the Undertaking of Pharmacovigilance Activities* (CPMP/PhWP/176/95). Note that at the moment 'congenital anomaly' is not there.

There are still problems with the definition of 'serious'. The FDA regulations as opposed to the guidelines mentioned above still (June 1997) have 'cancer and overdose'. Japan excludes 'hospitalization'. The EEC have not yet added 'congenital anomaly'.

It is important that all adverse medical events rather than ADRs or side effects are collected, since the latter two terms imply that they were caused by drugs and if the recorder is not certain if the event was caused by a drug, it would not be recorded. The term 'adverse event' is preferable and should be used in clinical trials (Skegg and Doll, 1977; Weintraub, 1978; Simpson *et al.*, 1980) and postmarketing (WHO Euro Report, 1978; Anon, 1982a). There are seven different types of classification of adverse reaction and all are necessary for different purposes. Several different classifications are available for each type of classification. These have been chosen as the most appropriate for this purpose.

Other Significant Adverse Events

The ICH wording (see page 334) includes another category that requires expedited reporting under the heading of serious adverse events.

These include any clinical or laboratory event that has led to:

- An intervention, including withdrawal of drug treatment.
- Dose reduction.
- Significant additional concomitant therapy (*CPMP/ICH/137/95 Structure and Contents of Clinical End of Study Reports*).

The ICH wording is, however 'important medical events that... may require intervention to prevent one of the other outcomes listed' i.e. already mentioned as serious. The interventions being as listed above.

Side Effect

This is any unintended effect of a pharmaceutical product occurring at doses normally used in man which is related to the pharmacological properties of the drug effect (WHO letter ref: M10/372/2(A), 1991).

Signal

This is reported information on a possible causal relationship between an adverse event and a drug, the relationship being unknown or incompletely documented previously. Usually more than a single report is required to generate a signal, depending upon the seriousness of the event and the quality of the information (WHO, 1991; Delamothe, 1992).

Associated

'Associated' with the use of the drug means that there is a reasonable possibility that the experience may have been caused by the drug (21CFR312.32). This differs from the *Concise Oxford Dictionary* meaning 'A thing connected to another'. Types of association are:

1. None (independent).
2. Artefactual (spurious or false)—due to chance (unsystematic variation) or bias (systematic variation).
3. Indirect (confounded).
4. Causal (direct or true) (Strom, 1994).

The definition quoted by Linberg refers to 'a possible causal association' and ignores the other types. Most of the associations occurring in pharmacovigilance are temporal in nature and our task is to decide to which of the four groups a particular association belongs. (See Chapter 13 for the latest FDA version).

Idiosyncrasy

This implies an inherent qualitatively abnormal reaction to a drug (Hoigné, 1997).

Unexpected

An 'unexpected' ADR is one for which the nature or severity is not consistent with information in the relevant source document(s) (CPMP/ICH/377/95) Step 5. Reports that add significant information on specificity or severity of a known, already documented serious ADR constitute unexpected events.

Causality Classification

Karch and Lasagna Classification (Karch and Lasagna, 1975)

Definite A reaction that follows a reasonable temporal sequence from administration of the drug or in which the drug level has been established in body fluids or tissues, follows a known response pattern to the suspected drug and is confirmed on stopping the drug (dechallenge), and reappearance of the reaction on repeated exposure (rechallenge).

Probable A reaction that follows a reasonable temporal sequence from administration of the drug, follows a known response pattern to the suspected drug, is confirmed by dechallenge and cannot be reasonably explained by the known characteristics of the patient's clinical state.

Possible A reaction that follows a reasonable temporal sequence from administration of the drug; that follows a known response to the suspected drug but that could have been produced by the patient's clinical state or other modes of therapy administered to the patient.

Conditional A reaction that follows a reasonable temporal sequence from administration of the drug, but does not follow a known response pattern to the suspected drug and could be reasonably explained by the known characteristics of the patient's clinical state.

Doubtful Any reaction that does not meet the criteria above.

Modified Karch and Lasagna Classification

The above definitions need some modification for use in pharmaceutical research. The word 'definite' is too absolute as it is possible to conceive of a non-drug-related adverse event which could fit this definition, and the fact that experienced physicians find, on occasion, that they need to re-rechallenge supports this opinion. 'Almost certain' is more applicable. One attribute of this definition 'that follows a known response pattern to the suspected drug' would preclude its application to new drugs, so this attribute should be left out when used with new drugs. The category of 'conditional' is suggested as a way of preventing the loss of previously unsuspected drug reactions, which implies that all that is 'doubtful' is lost. All classifications should be reviewed in accordance with any new evidence so the classifications 'conditional' and 'doubtful' can be combined under the heading of 'unlikely'.

The whole subject of causality assessment is dealt with in Chapter 11 and also in a paper (Stephens, 1987) and includes other definitions of words used in causality assessment. There has however, been a further paper since then from Germany (Grohmann *et al.*, 1989) giving:

Possible—an ADR not characteristic for the drug in question and/or time sequence, and not in accordance with previous experience or probability of alternative cause for unwanted effect over 5%.

Probably—an ADR to drug in question generally accepted, time sequence in accordance with previous experience and probabilities of alternative cause less than 50%.

Definite—probable plus reappearance of ADR following rechallenge with drug in question.

The latest definitions from the WHO letter ref: MIO/372/2 (A) (1991) are as follows:

Certain—a clinical event, including laboratory test abnormality, occurring in a plausible time relationship to drug administration, and which cannot be explained by concurrent disease or other drugs or chemicals. The response to withdrawal of the drug (dechallenge) should be clinically plausible. The event must be definitive pharmacologically or phenomenologically, using a satisfactory rechallenge procedure if necessary.

Probable/likely—a clinical event, including laboratory test abnormality, with a reasonable time sequence to administration of the drug, unlikely to be attributed to concurrent disease or other drugs or chemicals, and which follows a clinically reasonable response on withdrawal (dechallenge). Rechallenge information is not required to fulfil this definition.

Possible—a clinical event, including laboratory test abnormality, with a reasonable time sequence to administration of the drug but which could also be explained by concurrent disease or other drugs or chemicals. Information on drug withdrawal may be lacking or unclear.

Unlikely—a clinical event, including laboratory test abnormality, with a temporal relationship to drug administration which makes a causal relationship improbable, and in which other drugs, chemicals or underlying disease provide plausible explanations.

Conditional/unclassified—A clinical event, including laboratory test abnormality, reported as an adverse reaction, about which more data are essential for a proper assessment or the additional data are under examination.

Unassessable/unclassifiable—a report suggesting an adverse reaction which cannot be judged because information is insufficient or contradictory, and which cannot be supplemented or verified.

These definitions are commented upon in a WHO letter ref: M10/372/2 (A) (1991).

In April 1991 the Pharmacovigilance Working Party put forward a causality classification for the EEC as follows:

1. Category 'probable' or 'A'—reports including good reasons and sufficient documentation to assume a causal relationship, in the sense of plausible, conceivable, likely, but not necessarily highly probable.
2. Category 'possible' or 'B'—reports containing sufficient information to accept the possibility of a causal relationship, in the sense of not impossible and not unlikely, although the connection is uncertain or doubtful, for example because of missing data or insufficient evidence.
3. Category 'unclassified' or 'O'—reports where causality is, for one or another reason, not assessable (e.g. because of insufficient evidence, conflicting data or poor documentation).

> EEC causality classification
> - Category A—Probable
> - Category B—Possible
> - Category O—Unclassified

This also outlined how the causality classifications for each of the EC countries could be converted to this system (Meyboom and Royer, 1992).

Statistical Classification

This may be:

1. Specific—the ADR has no known natural occurrence.
2. Nonspecific—an ADR that either simulates or increases the incidence of naturally occurring diseases.

Severity Classification

Venulet Classification (Venulet, 1977)
This is as follows:

Mild/minor—no treatment is required, does not significantly complicate the primary disease and suspected drug may or may not be stopped.

Moderate—Symptoms are marked, but involvement of vital organ systems is moderate; there is no loss of consciousness and no cardiovascular failure. Treatment or hospitalization is required, or hospitalization is prolonged by at least one day. Development of definite biochemical or structural changes justifies this classification.

Severe—fatal or life-threatening, lowers the patient's life expectancy and there is a severe impairment of a vital organ system, even if transient; it persists for more than one month.

The Venulet classification mixes two separate qualities of an ADR: severity and seriousness.

Severity   This is the quantification of the reaction symptoms, mild, moderate or severe; these are best used as grades of discomfort and as subjective symptoms will vary from person to person. They have been defined by Tangrea *et al.*, 1991, as:

Mild—slightly bothersome; relieved with symptomatic treatment.

Moderate—bothersome, interfere with activities, only partially relieved with symptomatic treatment.

Severe—prevent regular activities, not relieved with symptomatic treatment.

The Early Clinical Drug Evaluation Program (ECDEU) classification is:

Mild—symptoms do not alter patient's normal functioning.

Moderate—symptom produces some degree of impairment to function but is not hazardous, uncomfortable or embarrassing to patient.

Severe—symptom definitely hazardous to well-being, significant impairment of functioning or incapacitation (Assenzo and Sho, 1982).

A classification used in German psychiatric hospitals is:

Grade 1—ADR did not lead to any change in medication.

Grade 2—ADR led to a change in medication in the form of dose reduction and/or additional treatment to counteract the ADR.

Grade 3—ADR led to discontinuation of the medication suspected of causing the ADR (including cases where the drug would have been discontinued had it not been vital) (Grohmann *et al.*, 1989).

Seriousness   This is an objective assessment of the importance of the ADR in terms of living and dying. The elements of severity and seriousness should, therefore, be separated.

Seriousness Classification

Seriousness may be classified as:

1. Symptomatic only—worries the patient, but not the doctor. The patient stops treatment or complains.
2. Serious—worries the doctor but not necessarily the patient. The doctor stops treatment. (See official definitions above.)

Different countries define 'serious' in different ways (see Chapter 9).

Frequency Classification

The pharmacovigilance team from Bordeaux questioned 300 French general practitioners and found that 'frequent' corresponded to a frequency of 1 in 10, 'rare' to 1 in 200 and 'very rare' to 1 in 3300; however, only 19% of the doctors replied so these figures may not represent the true opinion of the average French general practitioner (Péré *et al.*, 1984).

A Canadian paper (Toogood, 1980) has reported on the use of everyday adjectives to describe medical events as follows:

'Rarely'—ranges 0–17%, (95% confidence limits) mean 5%.
'Occasionally'—0–43%, (95% confidence limits) mean 21%.
'Often'—27–91%, (95% confidence limits) mean 59%.

Two American authors (Roberts and Gupta, 1987) carried out their own survey comparing the house staff's (HS) (juniors) and the full-time attending physicians' (senior) (P) understanding of terminology:

'Frequently'—the HS have a mean of 72.4% and a range of 35–90%; the P gave 65.7% and 40–90%, respectively.

'Often'—the HS gave a mean of 71%, range 61–85% and the P mean 59%, range 30–80%.

'Occasionally'—the HS gave a mean of 21% and a range of 5–40% while the P gave a mean of 17%, range 5–30%.

'Rarely'—the HS gave a mean of 5.2%, range 3–15% and the P mean 8.7%, range 1–30%.

Two French clinical pharmacologists have attempted the same exercise (Marion and Simon, 1984).

'Rarement'—range 2.3–6.1% (95% confidence limits).
'Souvent'—37.5–56.9% (95% confidence limits).

The German regulatory authority (Bundesgesundheitsamt) in their 1986 guidelines (Enstellung, 1986) on how to express established or estimated incidences of adverse events gave:

Incidence over 10%—may occur frequently.
Incidence between 1–10%—has been observed occasionally.
Incidence below 1%—may occur rarely.

The Swiss classification is:

Frequent—> 5%.
Occasional—5–10%.
Rare—< 0.1%.

In Sweden the classification for entry into the Swedish pharmaceutical drug handbook (FASS) is:

Frequent—> 1%.
Less frequent—0.1%–1%.
Rare < 0.1%.

In Japan the *Japanese Pharmaceutical Reference*, 2nd edition, 1991–1992 is used:

Rarely—< 0.1%.
Infrequently—0.1% < 5%.
Greater than 5%—no specific designation'.

In 1996 the chief medical officer at the UK Ministry of Health, suggested the following terminology when discussing risk:

Negligible—< 1 in a million.
Minimal—> 1 in a million but < 1 in 100 000.
Very low—> 1 in 100 000 but < 1 in 10 000.
Low—> 1 in 10 000 but < 1 in 1000.
Moderate—> 1 in 1000 but < 1 in 100.
High—> 1 in 100 (Calman, 1996; 1997).

Since there is considerable variation in the interpretation of the adverbs used to describe frequency it is sensible to choose one of the above and give its reference.

CIOMS Definitions 1995 • Very common (optional category) > 10% • Common (frequent) > 1% and ≤ 10% • Uncommon (infrequent) > 0.1% and ≤ 1% • Rare > 0.01% and ≤ 0.1% • Very rare (optional category) < 0.01%

Adverse Event Classification

This classification accounts for the source of the reported data, the potential clinical importance and the role of the report in the safety profile of the drug:

Class I—machine findings or findings made by humans using machines.
Class II—findings of study observers related to the patient's physical condition.
Class III—reports by the subject or patient.

Each of these may be subclassified by somebody with clinical knowledge as:

Subclass A—may lead to morbidity or mortality either acutely or in the near term.
Subclass B—may have historically been associated with the class of drug and have expected benign outcomes.
Subclass C—have undetermined significance at the time of reporting (Alexandra, 1991).

Pharmacological Classification

This is as follows:

Type A (augmented)—those that result from an exaggeration of a drug's normal pharmacological actions when given in the usual therapeutic dose and are normally dose dependent; sometimes referred to as Type l.
Type B (bizarre)—those that represent a novel response not expected from the known pharmacological action (Rawlins and Thompson, 1977); sometimes referred to as Type 2, and their characteristics are listed in Table 12.
Type C (chronic)—adaptive changes, rebound phenomena and other long-term effects.
Type D (delayed)—carcinogenesis, effects concerned with reproduction (impaired fertility), teratogenesis (adverse effects on the fetus during the early stages of pregnancy), adverse effects on the fetus during the later stages of pregnancy, drugs in breast milk (Aronson and White, 1996.).

Table 12 Characteristics of Type A and B drug reactions

Type A (augmented)	Type B (bizarre)
Pharmacological	Hypersensitivity or idiosyncratic
Dose related	Not dose related
Predictable	Unpredictable
Common	Rare
Usually not serious	Usually serious
Majority discovered before marketing	Majority discovered after marketing
Relatively low mortality	Relatively high mortality

The latter two definitions are rarely used.

An excellent review of the ADR mechanisms and their relationship to these classifications has been published (Royer *et al.*, 1997).

Reaction Time Classification

This is:

Acute—0–60 minutes; 4.3% of reactions.
Subacute—1–24 hours; 86.5% of reactions.
Latent—1 day–several weeks; 3.5% of reactions.

Reaction time is defined as the time between the last drug exposure and the appearance of the first symptom (Hoigné *et al.*, 1990).

Adverse Reaction Profile

Ideally an adverse reaction of a drug should have a profile consisting of the following elements:

1. Manifestation (clinical or laboratory) both subjective and/or objective.
2. Grading for both severity and seriousness.
3. Frequency or incidence, both absolute and relative to similar drugs with confidence intervals.
4. Mechanism of action.
5. Causality.
6. Predisposing factors, (e.g. renal function, pharmacokinetic factors).
7. Treatment and its effect.
8. Reversibility or sequelae.

It will be apparent that the present data sheets and the proposed modifications in the CIOMS III report do not provide these data and if they did the amount of information even on a single drug would grossly overload the prescriber. However, there is a hope that in the near future they will be available on a CD-ROM at an affordable price and this would make it user friendly.

Adverse Events in a Patient's Life

The adverse event must be discussed in the context of the many adverse events in the patient's life as follows:

1. The adverse event is one of many minor abnormalities that affect normal people (Reidenberg and Lowenthal, 1968) (see below).
2. The adverse event is part of a disease or is a complication of a disease, which is either that for which the drug was prescribed or another disease.
3. The adverse event may caused by a manmade chemical. This may be an environmental chemical. Systemic toxicity can be caused by 220 environmental chem-

icals of which 149 are neurotoxins. The signs and symptoms are usually non-specific (Grandjean *et al.*, 1991).

4. Effect of drugs of abuse.
5. Over the counter (OTC) drugs. Many countries are encouraging the transfer of drugs from Prescription Only Medicines (POM) to OTC to relieve the costs of their health services, so we must expect a large increase in their usage.
6. Herbal medicines. There has been a move towards making these require a special licence (De Smet, 1995a), but meanwhile their usage is increasing and some are dangerous as follows: ephedra also known as Ma Huang but better known as ephedrine has caused deaths (Josefson, 1996); respiratory distress with royal jelly (Peacock *et al.*, 1995); hepatitis (Carlsson, 1990) with horse chestnut leaf and lactone, which is sometimes adultered with other drugs (De Smet *et al.*, 1996); chronic nutmeg psychosis (Brenner *et al.*, 1993); an outbreak of fibrosing interstitial nephritis in 70 Belgians caused by a herbal slimming preparation. Others are dangerous because they have been adulteratated with metals (Pb, As, Hg, Cd, Ti) or pharmaceuticals (e.g. NSAIDs, corticosteroids or benzo-diazepines) (De Smet, 1995b). Further details can be found in *Adverse Effects of Herbal Drugs (see Bibliography)*; Huxtable, R. J. (1990) The harmful potential of herbal and other plant products. *Drug Safety*, **5** (Suppl. 1), 126–136; De Smet, P. A. G. M. (1997) Adverse effects of herbal remedies. *Adverse Drug React. Bull.*, **183**.
7. Food allergies. Peanut and nut allergy are probably the leading cause of fatal food allergy (Sampson, 1996); shellfish and eggs can also cause acute allergic reactions (Finn, 1992).
8. Food additives (see below).

Symptoms in Healthy Persons

Reidenberg (Reidenberg and Lowenthal, 1968) investigated 414 healthy students and hospital staff of Temple University, USA, who were taking no medication, and surveyed their symptoms retrospectively using a questionnaire. Only 19% stated that during the previous 72 hours they had experienced none of the 25 symptoms listed. The median number of symptoms experienced per person was two and 30 people experienced six or more symptoms. The symptoms listed varied from pains in muscles and joints, headaches, skin rashes and urticaria to mental symptoms and changes in bowel function, all of which have been described as ADRs. Their order of frequency was fatigue, inability to concentrate, excessive sleepiness, bleeding from the gums after brushing teeth, irritability, headache, nasal congestion, pain in the muscles, insomnia, lack of appetite, pain in joints, faintness on first standing up, skin rash, bad dreams, dry mouth, constipation, palpitations, bleeding or bruising, giddiness or weakness, diarrhoea, nausea, fever and urticaria. These findings were repeated in a futher study in Germany 30 years later. Here there were two personality groups: the first were not nervous, were emotionally stable and were success motivated and these had fewer AEs, whilst the second group were nervous, emotionally unstable and had lack of motivation and these had more AEs (Meyer *et al.*, 1996).

Symptoms Due to Food Additives

Food additives causing symptoms include:

1. Sulphiting agents. These can cause flushing, itching of the mouth and skin, and asthma. About 5% of asthmatics are susceptible. They may be present in wines, other drinks, shrimps and processed potatoes.
2. Nitrates (E249–E252). These can cause flushing and giddiness. They give preserved meats their pink colour.
3. Colouring agents. Details of these are given on page 55 when dealing with drug excipients.
4. Flavouring agents. These may exacerbate eczema.

Adverse reactions to common foods occur in 1.4–1.9% of the population (Lessof, 1992).

Results of a Questionnaire Survey of Normal Patients, Untreated Hypertensives and Treated Hypertensives

The variety of symptoms that can be caused by a disease or any of its complications is vast, but taking the specific area of hypertension, an AE questionnaire (Bulpitt *et al.*, 1976) has been used in a survey of normal subjects, untreated hypertensives and treated hypertensives (Bulpitt *et al.*, 1976). The normal patients were randomly selected from a local general practice register and the untreated patients were newly referred hypertensives at the Hammersmith Hospital. Although the survey showed that headaches, unsteadiness, lightheadedness or faintness, and nocturia could actually be caused by raised blood pressure, this was so in only a proportion of those patients complaining of these symptoms (Table 13). Many of the symptoms are common in all three groups and in any one person complaining of a symptom who was on treatment, it is clearly difficult to allocate the symptom to a particular group (Joubert *et al.*, 1977).

Adverse Reactions to Placebo

Definition

A placebo can be defined as 'any component of a therapy (or control in experimental studies) that is without specific activity for the condition being treated or being evaluated' (Joyce, 1982).

Symptoms that are in some part caused by treatment must be divided into those effects caused by the chemical constituents and those caused by the giving of a 'medication', even though the 'medication' is known not to cause side effects by its chemical nature. The latter are referred to as 'placebo responses or effects' and have specific characteristics, which resemble those of active chemicals. In clinical trials with a placebo group the 'placebo response' is made up of several factors:

1. The natural course of the underlying disease (indication for treatment).
2. Any other incidental medical event unconnected either with the underlying indication or the placebo medication (e.g. a cold).

Table 13   Symptoms in normal persons, untreated hypertensives and treated hypertensives (Bulpitt *et al.*, 1976)

Symptom	Normal (%)	Untreated hypertensives (%)	Treated hypertensives (%)
Sleepiness	**31.4**	**43.2**	51.4**
Dry mouth	20.5	**23.7**	**40.2***
Unsteadiness on standing or in the morning	7.9***	**35.4**	**33.5**
Nocturia	**45.3***	**68.4**	73.2
Diarrhoea	**15.5**	25.8	**30.4**
Depression	**34.3**	44.7**	29.4
Blurred vision	14.7	29.8*	20.6
Weak limbs	**18.4**	34.0	**26.4** n.s.
Nasal stuffiness	**26.8**	**29.7** n.s.	– n.s.
Poor concentration	**4.0**	**12.8** n.s.	– n.s.
Vivid dreams	**25.3**	**27.8** n.s.	– n.s.
Nausea	**12.0**	**19.8** n.s.	– n.s.
Impotence	**6.9**	**17.1**	24.6***
Slow walking pace	**9.5***	24.2***	**37.0***
Waking headache	**15.1**	**31.3***	15.5
Failure of ejaculation	0	7.3	25.6***

Asterisks within table refer to χ^2 comparisons between one result and the result in bold in other columns
* $p < 0.05$
** $p < 0.01$
*** $p < 0.001$
n.s. Not significant

3. Regression towards the mean. This phenomenon is due to the probability that patients on presentation to the doctor are likely to be at the peak of their problems and since there is fluctuation of all biological variables the odds will be on the problem not being so intense at the next visit. This has been put forward as a cause of the placebo effect on efficacy, but with an AE it may be a factor in a positive dechallenge (see pages 304–5).

4. The effects of being in a clinical trial. These may be mental (e.g. increased anxiety), or physical (e.g the wearing off of 'white coat hypertension' as the patients become used to the trial circumstances) (i.e. the patient's blood pressure is lower on the second occasion). In hospitalized volunteers there was a 10% increase in heart rate and blood pressure remained unchanged, but there were increases in the time to sleep initiation and asthenia self-rating, suggesting poor neuropsychiatric tolerability (Rosenzweig *et al.*, 1995). The general beneficial effect of being the object of special attention as in a clinical trial is known as the 'Hawthorne effect'. It was named after the town in Illinois where the effect was noted during work studies at the Western Electric plant (Mayo, 1949).

5. The true additional affect of adding the placebo medication (Ernst and Resch, 1995).

The first four of these type of events are those of the untreated disease and the fifth factor is the true placebo factor. It is extremely unusual to have a placebo control group and an untreated control group in clinical trials. This is because the difference between the active drug group and the placebo group represents the effect of the active drug. The other factors should be equally distributed in both the active drug group and the placebo group (Ernst and Resch, 1995).

Commonest Complaints

A review of 67 publications for unwanted or toxic side effects that occurred during the administration of a placebo showed that drowsiness was the most common side effect, followed by headache. Stimulation of the central nervous system manifested as daytime nervousness or insomnia was the third most common effect, followed by nausea and constipation (Pogge, 1963). In 80 healthy volunteers taking a single dose of a drug when first used in man there were 50 AEs. In order of frequency they were:

Headache—17.6%.
Rhinitis—7.1%.
Bruising at injection site—4.7%.
Pharyngitis—3.5%.
Coughing—2.4% (Kitchener *et al.*, 1995).

The numbers and types of AEs will depend upon all the factors previously mentioned plus those due to the physical circumstances of the study.

Physical Changes

Although the symptoms are activated via the mind they can produce physical changes to the nose, skin, bladder, oesophagus, stomach, colon, heart and blood vessels, and kidneys (Wolf, 1950, 1959a; Wolf and Pinsky, 1954) such as vomiting, sweating, diarrhoea, constipation, eosinophilia, hyperacidity and skin rashes (Joyce, 1982). One case has been reported of a patient meeting the definition of being 'dependent' upon a placebo (Vinar, 1969). Others caused by placebo include: dermatitis medicamentosa, anaphylactoid reaction, urticaria and angioneurotic oedema and hallucinations (Thompson, 1982).

Frequency of Placebo Reactions

Placebo tends to increase the severity of pre-existing symptoms and females tend to have more frequent and severe placebo reactions than males (Domecq *et al.*, 1980). When placebos were administered to professional people, 58% complained of one or more side effects and, contrary to expectations, some symptoms decreased in the institutionalized aged when they were given placebo (Wolf, 1950).

Variation With Age and Sex

On the whole the incidence of placebo reaction rises linearly with age (Green, 1964). However, it is not known whether adjustment had been made for the number of drugs taken in addition to placebo since with active drugs the same rise with age was found to disappear when adjusted for the number of drugs taken (Weber and Griffin,

1986). The occurrence is higher in females than in males (Green, 1964); again, could this be due to the females taking more drugs?

Variability in Type of Effects

Placebo side effects, when the placebo is used as a control for an active drug, are often similar in type to the side effects of the active drug itself (Letemendia and Harris, 1959): throbbing headaches after placebo in a hydralazine study; 'closed' nose after reserpine placebo (Wolf, 1959b); diminished perception of high tones after streptomycin placebo (Tucker, 1954). Once a patient on placebo or active drug has complained of an adverse event, an observer will note that these patients have more symptoms than those who did not complain of the adverse event, suggesting that there is an increased interest in those patients who show change (Thompson, 1982).

Psychological Differences in Placebo Reactors

Lasagna and his colleagues (Lasagna *et al.*, 1954) were able to show differences of attitude, habits, educational background and personality structure between the people who consistently responded to placebo and those who did not, but reactors were not 'whiners' or 'nuisances', not typically male or female, not younger or old and had the same average intelligence as the non-responders. In volunteers, placebos can cause effects in 66% of subjects (Knowles and Lucas, 1960) and 35% of patients (Beecher, 1955).

When healthy French volunteers were tested with the Bortner rating scale the majority were found to have type A personalities, that is they were 'hurried, hard-driving, competitive and aggressive' and 50% of type A personalities had AEs on placebo compared with 17% of type B volunteers (Drici *et al.*, 1995).

Placebo Pharmacology

It has also been shown that the placebo has its own pharmacology with peak effects, cumulative effects, carry-over effects and a varying efficacy, depending upon the severity of the complaint being treated (Lasagna *et al.*, 1958). Symptoms generally become more frequent and severe with an increase in the number of placebo tablets (Green, 1964). Placebos can relieve postoperative dental pain and naloxone blocks this effect, suggesting that the placebo acts through endorphin release (Levine *et al.*, 1978; Fields and Levine, 1981). However, a leader in *The Lancet* (Leader, 1983), quotes that there is no evidence for an opioid component in placebo analgesia and goes on to say that there is no reason to believe that the placebo effect has a single specific mechanism.

The former statement is supported by a recent study using naloxone with dipipanone and placebo analgesia for tourniquet pain (Posner and Burke, 1985). It has been argued that most improvements attributed to the placebo effect are actually instances of statistical regression (i.e. a tendency of extreme measures to move closer to the mean when repeated) (McDonald and Mazzuca *et al.*, 1983). This may account for the adverse effect of placebo where what was normal becomes abnormal (see page 276).

Severity of Placebo Reactions

The fact that placebo reactions can be severe has been noted by several authors (Wolf and Pinsky, 1954; Green, 1964). In a Norwegian multicentre study (Norwegian

Table 14 Important side effects of placebo (from Schindel, 1972)

Symptom	Number with symptom	Total number of treated patients	Percentage of treated patients
Numbness	36	72	50
Headache	23	92	25
Fatigue	10	57	18
Sensation of heaviness	14	77	18
Inability to concentrate	14	92	15
Drowsiness	7	72	10
Nausea	9	92	10
Dryness of the mouth	7	77	9
General weakness	5	57	9
Flushes	6	77	8

Multicenter Study Group, 1981) comparing timolol and placebo in inducing reduction of morbidity and reinfarction in patients surviving acute myocardial infarction, many patients were withdrawn due to an adverse reaction and were subsequently found to be on placebo.

Range of Placebo Reactions
In a study of more than 1000 cases of side effects of placebo there were 35 different symptoms. The most important are given in Table 14 (Schindel, 1972).

It will be apparent that it may well be impossible to tell whether a side effect that has occurred while on active treatment is due to that treatment or might have occurred if a placebo had been given instead.

Influence of the Placebo Administrator
After extraction of teeth under a local anaesthetic patients assessed their pain using a McGill pain questionnaire at 1 hour and 10 minutes before and after an intravenous injection or no treatment. Clinicians knew that one group had placebo or analgesic antagonist (Group PN) and the other group (Group PNF) would receive placebo plus analgesic or analgesic antagonist. The trial was double blind. The two placebo groups differed only in the clinicians' knowledge of the possible double blind treatments. The change in pain score for the PN group was +6 and for the PNF group −2 ($p < 0.01$). This suggests that the analgesia was dependent upon the clinicians' expectations (Gracely *et al.*, 1985).

The strongest predictor of placebo ADRs found in 490 patients in a multicentre clinical trial was the centre, presumably via the investigator, despite strict control of the management of the AEs. None of the baseline characteristics were helpful (Tangrea *et al.*, 1994).

Withdrawal or Rebound Phenomena

Some adverse effects of drugs can be produced after the drug has been stopped and for this reason may not be considered as possibly drug related (e.g. pseudomembranous—antibiotic associated—colitis or aplastic anaemia). Some hypersensitivity reactions to drugs are delayed and may appear within 2–3 weeks of dechallenge. Drugs causing dependency may cause withdrawal effects even when their dosage has been kept within the recommended limits (e.g. opiates, alcohol, barbiturates and benzodiazopines). Others may cause withdrawal effects due to atrophy of the adrenal glands following suppression of the hypophyseal–pituitary axis (e.g. corticosteroids) and yet others cause a rebound effect due to changes in the receptor density (e.g. beta blockers). These post-dechallenge ADRs pose several problems:

1. Previous drug therapy is frequently stopped on admission to hospital with a new illness that requires drug treatment that will coincide with withdrawal symptoms.
2. Some drug withdrawal effects are difficult to distinguish from their indication (e.g. anxiety).
3. Patients are not always aware of the names of their drugs or may try to hide their dependency on drugs or alcohol.

A pre-marketing clinical trial programme must be planned with these possibilities in mind (i.e. post-study visits included in all trial protocols).

These different forms of withdrawal or rebound phenomena are considered in turn below and are:

1. Delayed hypersensitivity ADR.
2. Sedative/hypnotic dependence.
3. Antidepressant withdrawal symptoms.
4. Alcohol withdrawal syndrome.
5. Corticosteroid withdrawal.
6. Rebound phenomena.
7. Neonatal drug withdrawal syndrome.
8. Miscellaneous.

Delayed Hypersensitivity

Examples are jaundice after chlorpromazine and aplastic anaemia (see Appendix 3).

Sedative/hypnotic Dependence

Barbiturate Withdrawal Syndrome

The major symptoms are tonic–clonic seizures, acute organic brain syndrome, delirium similar to alcoholic delirium tremens and hyperpyrexia. Minor symptoms in approximate order of appearance are anxiety, involuntary muscle twitches, coarse intention tremor of hands and fingers, progressive weakness, dizziness, persistent tinnitus, visual illusions, depersonalization, nausea, vomiting, insomnia, weight loss, orthostatic hypotension, and an increase in pulse rate of 20 beats per a minute on standing.

The probability of developing a withdrawal reaction depends upon the daily dose, duration of therapy and drug half-life. The onset usually occurs when the drug has been nearly eliminated from the body. Benzodiazepine withdrawals are usually recognized by the onset of fits. Lorazepam fits occur between 1–4 days (median 64 hours) mean half-life 14 hours. Diazepam fits occur at 2–17 days (median 5 days) mean half-life 31 hours. Diazepam's active metabolite, desmethyldiazepam has a mean half-life of 51 hours. Fits occur more frequently after withdrawal of short-acting benzodiazepines rather than after the long-acting kind and with a shorter period of chronic use and at lower dosages. Lorazepam fits occurred after 2–12 mg/d (median 7.5 mg) used for 3–4 weeks (median 3 months); 75% occurred with drugs in the therapeutic range of 1–10 mg/d. Diazepam fits occurred after 20–170 mg/d (median 77.5 mg) used for 3 weeks to 12 years, median 7.5 months. One third of the patients were receiving dosages within the therapeutic range.

Low-dose Withdrawal Syndrome

It has been suggested that benzodiazepines given within the recommended dosage may induce idiosyncratic dependence in predisposed persons (i.e. alcoholics, those with a positive family history of alcoholism, those taking other sedatives). The syndrome takes a long time for all symptoms to resolve (up to six months) and is most intense during the withdrawal of the last few milligrams. Episodic symptoms occur in 2–10-day cycles and include anxiety, panic, tachycardia, mydriasis, hypertension, memory and concentration difficulties, paraesthesia, derealization, altered sensations, insomnia, muscle spasms and occasionally psychosis (Perry and Alexander, 1986).

The onset of symptoms (not fits) in a group on short-acting benzodiazopines were 0.75 + or −0.7 days with peak symptoms at 1 + or −0.5 days, while for long-acting benzodiazopines it was 5.1 + or −4.1 days to onset with peaking of symptoms at 9.6 + or −5.1 days. In this latter group, in order of frequency, the symptoms were anxiety and headaches in about 80%, insomnia and tension in about 70%, and sweating, difficulty in concentrating, tremors, sensory disturbances, fear and fatigue in about 60%. Although these were quite different studies and protocols the minor symptoms were not too dissimilar, but in the latter second study there were no major symptoms. The minor symptoms in the second group that distinguished them from patients with anxiety were persistent tinnitus, involuntary movements, paraesthesia, perceptual changes and confusion (Busto *et al.*, 1986).

Antidepressant Withdrawal Symptoms

Withdrawal reactions are distinct from recurrence of the primary psychiatric disorder and usually start abruptly within a few days of stopping the antidepressant and resolve within one day to three weeks whereas depressive relapse is uncommon in the first week after stopping the drug (Haddad *et al.*, 1998).

Withdrawal symptoms such as nausea, dizziness and sweating have been reported after missing a single dose of imipramine after only two weeks on the drug. These are a few similar reports for desipramine and chlomipramine (Stern and Mendels, 1980). Other tricyclics are discussed in R490 (reports in *Reactions* are given as R followed by the volume number). Similarly, new antidepressants: fluoxetine R596, paroxetine R492, R583, sertraline R497, R603, fluvoxamine R454, R391, mianserin R283, venlafaxine R599.

Withdrawal symptoms have been collected using a self-rating scale and a withdrawal symptom questionnaire (Schmaurs *et al.*, 1987). Other scales that have been used are:

(i) Ashton Scale (Ashton, 1984).
(ii) Tyrer Withdrawal Scale. (Tyrer *et al.*, 1981).
(iii) Lader Tranquillizer Withdrawal Scale (Lader and Olajide, 1987).

Alcoholic Withdrawal Syndrome

This occurs 6–8 hours after a substantial fall in blood alcohol. The symptoms are nausea, vomiting, sweating, tremor, agitation and easy startling. The signs are tachycardia, hypertension, hyperreflexia, hypokalaemia, hyponatraemia and hypophosphataemia. It may progress over 24 hours leading to grand mal seizures, hallucinations, fever, a raised erythrocyte sedimentation rate (ESR) dilated pupils and leucocytosis (delirium tremens).

Corticosteroid Withdrawal

Sudden high-dose withdrawal can cause:

(a) Steroid pseudorheumatism—a syndrome of anorexia, nausea, lethargy, pain in joints and muscles and skin desquamation,
(b) Panniculitis, characterized by painful itchy skin nodules.
(c) Aseptic conjunctivitis and rhinitis.
(d) Confusional state without localizing signs (Bhowmick, 1991).

Minor symptoms are fatigue, weakness, arthralgia, anorexia, nausea, desquamation of the skin, orthostatic hypotension, fainting, dyspnoea and hypoglycaemia, as well as flare-ups of the underlying disease (Byyny, 1976).

Beta Blocker Withdrawal

Sudden withdrawal may cause increased angina or myocardial infarction in the ensuing fortnight (Lancet leader, 1975b). It can also cause ventricular arrhythmias and left ventricular failure. Signs and symptoms usually begin within 24–72 hours (Bhowmick, 1991).

Neonatal Drug Withdrawal Syndrome

Benzodiazepines, barbiturates, alcohol, tricyclic antidepressants, and phenothiazines can all cause withdrawal symptoms (Koren, 1990).

Miscellaneous

These include:

(a) Clonidine—rebound hypertension (Bhowmick, 1991).
(b) Fenfluramine—depression.
(c) Diuretics—rebound oedema.
(d) Analgesia—rebound headaches after prolonged use for headaches, mainly in the first four days, with nervousness, restlessness, nausea, vomiting, insomnia, diarrhoea and tremor, as well as increased headaches (Matthew *et al.*, 1990).

(e) Calcium antagonists—severe angina.

(f) Anti-anginal therapy—severe angina and myocardial infarction.

(g) Levodopa withdrawal causing neuroleptic malignant syndrome (Rainer *et al.*, 1991).

(h) Caffeine withdrawal—can cause headaches, drowsiness and fatigue (Hughes *et al.*, 1991).

(i) Anticholinergic drugs—myalgia, depression, anxiety, insomnia, headaches, GI symptoms, vomiting, nightmares and malaise (Marken *et al.*, 1994).

(j) Parkinson's disease therapy—severe exacerbation of symptoms and signs with akinetic crisis (Bhowmick, 1991).

(k) Anticonvulsants—may precipitate a series of convulsions.

(l) Nicotine withdrawal—can cause anxiety, irritability, restlessness and depression with a fall in heart rate and blood pressure, electroencephalogram changes and weight increase (Ashton, 1991).

(m) Octreotide—can cause biliary colic due to calculi 12–16 hours after dechallenge.

(n) Amantidine and fluphenazine can cause neuroleptic malignant syndrome (R498).

At least two weeks of monitoring are required after drug withdrawal with the use of a withdrawal symptom scale to study all aspects of potential withdrawal (Merz and Ballmer, 1983).

Suggested further readings: George, C.F. and Robertson, D. (1987) Clinical consequences of abrupt drug withdrawal. *Med. Toxicol.*, **2**, 267–382.

Adverse reactions to drug withdrawal. *Adverse Drug React. Bull.* 1997, **187**, 711–714. P. A. Routledge and M. C. Bialas.

Excipients and Formulation

Before passing on to the main part of the book a mention must be made of the possibility that the excipients of a product may be the cause of an ADR and that placebos may, therefore, produce ADR due to the excipients. Throughout the remainder of the book the word drug refers to the total product: active principal plus excipients. Once a product has been shown to cause an ADR consideration must be given to the possibility of the excipient playing a role (see pp. 727–737, Appendix 2 in *Davies' Textbook of Adverse Drug Reactions*, 3rd edition. (Oxford University Press). It is also discussed by Napke in the 'Side effects of drugs essay' in the *Side Effects of Drugs Annual* No. 7, 1983. Allergic reactions to drug excipients are reviewed by Smith in the *Practitioner*, **231**, 579–583, 1987. Three other reference books are cited in the *Bibliography*.

The first major ADR to cause public concern was produced by elixir of sulphanilamide, which caused at least 76 deaths in 1937 due to the toxic solvent diethylene glycol (Geiling and Cannon, 1938). In 1968–1969 the change in capsule filler from calcium lactate to lactose in phenytoin caused an outbreak of phenytoin intoxication in Australia (Tyrer *et al.*, 1970). Two years later an interaction between para-aminosalicylic acid (PAS) and rifampicin resulted in impaired absorption of the latter due to bentonite in the PAS granules (Boman *et al.*, 1975). In 1972–1973 overdigitalization in previously stable cardiac patients was traced to increased bioavailability due to changes in size of the particles of digoxin (Johnson *et al.*, 1973). More recently, in 1983, controlled-release indomethacin (Osmosin) resulted in dumping in the intestines, leading to ulcers and perforation of the gut (*Current Problems*, 1983). In 1989 six women reported severe local reactions following intramuscular injections of vitamin A. On investigation it appeared that the formulation had been changed from an oil base to a water base plus Cremophor RH and the bioavailability had increased 50-fold (McCormick *et al.*, 1990). These examples emphasize the importance of considering the possibility that an ADR might be due to the formulation or to an excipient. The following are the main categories of excipients (Smith, 1985):

1. Colouring agents.
2. Sweetening or flavouring agents.
3. Surfactants and solubilizing agents.
4. Anti-oxidants.
5. Aerosol propellants.
6. Preservatives and antibacterials.
7. Thickening, suspending and binding agents.
8. Solvents.
9. Disintegrants and lubricants.
10. Perfumes.
11. Fats and oils.

Suggested recommended reading is a slim paperback in the *Topics in Pharmacy* series entitled *Formulation Factors in Adverse Reactions*. Editors A. T. Florence and E. G. Salole, Wright 1996. Professor D'Arcy has written a chapter on ADRs to excipients, which is the source of the above details.

The following drug additives have been reported as causing ADRs:

Colourings (Pollock *et al.*, 1989).
Amaranth.
Black PN.
Blue (Colour index 12196 and 16383).
Brilliant blue FCF.
Brown FK.
Brown HT.
Brown (colour index 18285).
Buff (colour index 17175).
Carmoisine.
Disperse blues.
Disperse pinks.
Erythrosine BS.
Green S.
Indigo carmine.
Patent blue V.
Ponceau 4R.
Quinoline yellow.
Red 2G.

Sunset yellow FCF.
Tartrazine.
Yellow 2G.
Various commercial mixtures containing the above.

Aerosol Propellants and Preservatives

Most propellants in metered-dose inhalers have until recently been chlorofluorocarbons and high-dose nebulizer solutions usually have one of three preservatives—ethylenediamine tetraacetic acid (EDTA), benzalkonium chloride or chlorbutol. All have been shown to produce bronchoconstriction in asthmatics. Both hypotonic and hypertonic aerosols cause bronchoconstriction in asthmatics and in animals sensitize the myocardium to circulating catecholamines and can precipitate arrhythmias (Snell, 1990).

Preservatives and Antioxidants (Pollock *et al.*, 1989)

These include:

Benzoates.
Butylated hydroxyanisole.
Butylated hydroxytoluene.
Sulphites.

   Full details of the AEs associated with inactive ingredients in drug products can be found in a paper of the same title in *Med. Toxicol.*, 1988, **3**, 128–165 and 209–240 (Golightly *et al.*, 1988). Generic drug products may not have the same excipients as the branded product and different brands of the same drug may also have different excipients. This may give rise to an AE not seen previously when the same drug but a different brand has been prescribed or where there has been product substitution. This may also give rise to false positive and negative rechallenge tests (Napke and Stevens, 1984).

   Suggested further reading is 'Excipients and additives: hidden hazards in drug products and in product substitution'. *Can. Med. Assoc. J.*, 1992, **131**, 94–111.

Summary

It should be clear from this chapter that separating the AEs due to a drug from the many other similar AEs due to normal physiological variation, disease, environmental chemicals, placebo, food allergies, food additives, drug excipients, drug withdrawal and rebound reactions is a difficult and complicated task. The drug disasters of the past and the number of drugs removed from the market because of their ADRs indicate that too often their discovery is delayed until too many patients have suffered. The subsequent chapters attempt to describe the methods currently available for detecting new ADRs as soon as possible.

   It has been estimated that the average research and development cost for each new drug including capital costs and the cost of failures is $359 million (Allport, 1994;

Wierenga and Beary, 1995). The time from start of research until marketing is a minimum of 12 years, usually 15 years and may be up to 30 years and of those that reach the market 80% fail to cover their development costs (Gittins, 1996). Only five of 5000 compounds ever make it to human testing (Sylvestri, 1996). Only 23% of drugs that begin clinical testing receive marketing approval (DiMasi, 1991). Since 1972 3–4% of new active substances licensed in the UK have been withdrawn for safety reasons (Rawlins, 1995).

Chapter 2

Adverse Drug Reactions and Interactions: Mechanisms, Risk Factors, Detection, Management and Avoidance

P. A. Routledge

Department of Pharmacology, Therapeutics and Toxicology, University of Wales College of Medicine, Health Park, Cardiff, Wales, UK

Adverse drug reactions, of which adverse interactions are a special case, are a major cause of morbidity in the community. They are also reported to account for up to 5% of all medical admissions to hospital (Grahame-Smith and Aronson,1992; Aronson and White, 1996) and, of course, they are occasionally fatal. ADRs are sometimes difficult to differentiate from non-drug related disease. Many factors such as concomitant treatment and disease can cloud their identification and there are few specific laboratory or clinical methods to confirm them. In clinical practice it is thus often difficult to separate adverse events from adverse reactions, particularly in the case of previously unrecognized reactions. Most doctors often rely on their own experience or the experience of others of similar problems before accepting that a drug might have caused the event.

Classification of Adverse Drug Reactions

Type A Versus Type B

Adverse drug reactions can occur in two forms: commonly they are 'Type A' or 'dose related' adverse reactions, which are an 'accentuation' of normal drug effect (Dollery

Table 1   A classification of adverse reactions (revised from Rawlins and Thompson, 1977)

	Type A—'Accentuated'	Type B—'Bizarre'
Dose relationship	Yes	No
Frequency	Common	Rarer
Mortality	Low	Higher
Morbidity	High	Lower
Treatment	Stop drug or reduce dose	Stop drug

and Rawlins, 1977; Rawlins and Thompson, 1977). Thus digoxin slows the heart rate in a dose-dependent fashion, but this may become an adverse effect if the heart rate becomes too slow. Type A reactions make up perhaps 75% of all adverse reactions, but are proportionately less likely to have fatal consequences than Type B reactions (Table 1). Nevertheless, because their onset is often gradual, they may remain unrecognized for some time and produce considerable morbidity to the patient.

Type B reactions are unpredictable and often 'bizarre' reactions to a drug, which may be present at an extremely low concentration. These reactions tend to be sudden and often dramatic in onset and are usually quickly recognized, altough some, particularly those involving anaphylaxis, may be fatal.

Grahame-Smith and Aronson (1992), in an excellent chapter on ADRs, have extended the original Rawlins and Thompson classification described above to include Type C adverse drug reactions and Type D reactions. In Type C (chronic) reactions are long-term drug effects including adaptive changes (e.g. drug tolerance) and withdrawal (rebound) effects. Type D (delayed) reactions involve carcinogenesis and effects associated with reproduction. Although this classification highlights ADRs that may have been given inadequate consideration in the past, it relies on both temporal and mechanistic features. In this chapter, these issues will be addressed within the context of the original classification.

Risk Factors for Type A Adverse Reactions

Type A reactions, being an extension of the normal pharmacological effect of the drug, occur when the concentration of the drug at the site(s) of action is increased above the normal therapeutic level (Table 2). This may occur when the dose administered is excessive for that individual either because:

- Elimination mechanisms are compromised (pharmacokinetic causes).
- The target organ is excessively sensitive to a given drug concentration (pharmacodynamic causes).

Both of these mechanisms tend to go hand in hand and are seen at the extremes of life, as well as in patients with renal or liver disease. Other individuals may be at increased risk because of genetically inherited factors and these will also be described.

Table 2   Risk factors for Type A adverse drug reactions
Pharmacological/pharmaceutical
Pharmacokinetic
Renal disease
Liver disease
Cardiac failure
Extremes of age
Pharmacogenetic
Pharmacodynamic
Renal disease
Liver disease
Cardiac failure
Extremes of age

Pharmacological and Pharmaceutical Factors

Certain drugs are associated with an increased risk of adverse reaction or interaction. These tend to be agents with a low therapeutic ratio (i.e. the difference between a therapeutic and toxic dose is low) and include oral anticoagulants, oral hypoglycaemic agents, some antihypertensives, many cytotoxic agents, corticosteroids, non-steroidal anti-inflammatory drugs (NSAIDs) and digoxin.

In addition to these pharmacological factors, the pharmaceutical formulation may predispose to ADRs. Changes in formulation have in the past been associated with increased bioavailability of certain drugs with a low therapeutic ratio (e.g. phenytoin and digoxin) and subsequent type A toxicity. The likelihood of this problem is now low because of the strict bioequivalence criteria insisted upon by national licensing bodies. Nevertheless, the formulation may cause local toxicity, for example the intestinal perforation seen in association with a certain form of indomethacin in the early 1980s (Day, 1983) or the colonic strictures recently reported in association with high-dose pancreatic enzyme supplements (Fitzsimmons *et al.*, 1997). It is also rare now for the fillers, binders, surfactants, dyes or other excipients, which constitute around 90% of the mass of many formulations to cause type A toxicity, although serious problems have recently occurred, such as fatal renal failure in Bangladeshi children caused by diethylene glycol in paracetamol elixir (Hanif *et al.*, 1995).

Pharmacokinetic Risk Factors

These include several situations when elimination mechanisms are impaired. These include reduction in renal excretion of drugs as well as impaired drug metabolism (largely due to liver disease) (Routledge, 1997).

Renal Disease
Most drugs are lipid-soluble and are therefore first metabolized to more polar (water-soluble) compounds before the metabolites can be excreted in the urine.

Several clinically important compounds (e.g. digoxin, aminoglycoside antibiotics, lithium, captopril and potassium-sparing diuretics) are already relatively water-soluble and are not markedly bound to plasma proteins so undergo glomerular filtration. In other cases, the active metabolite of an inactive drug (prodrug) may be excreted lagely unchanged by the kidney—examples include oxypurinol, the active metabolite of allopurinol, and enalaprilat, which is the active metabolite of enalapril. In renal failure, glomerular filtration rate (GFR) declines progressively and is a useful marker of renal dysfunction. Normally the GFR in an adult is around 120 ml/min and the clearance of drugs exclusively by this process cannot exceed this value. Mild renal failure is defined by a GFR of 20–50 ml/min, moderate renal failure by a GFR of 10–20 ml/min and severe renal impairment by a GFR of less than 10 ml/min. Drugs for which glomerular filtration is an important pathway may accumulate in renal failure unless the dose is reduced accordingly.

Active tubular secretion is the other important excretory process in the kidney. Weak electrolytes (acids and bases) are secreted into the proximal tubular fluid and digoxin may be secreted by the distal tubule. This is an energy-dependent process and drugs can be effectively cleared, with a tubular secretion of ampicillin of around 400 ml/min in subjects with normal renal function. Tubular secretion is relatively spared in renal impairment so dose reduction of those drugs for which this process contributes significantly to total clearance may not be necessary unless renal impairment is severe.

Liver Disease

The liver is the largest metabolic organ and quantitatively the most important, although the skin, gut, lungs, kidney and white cells have some limited metabolic capacity. Many drugs are lipid soluble, and even if a substantial proportion was not protein-bound in the blood and could therefore undergo glomerular filtration, they would be passively reabsorbed through the renal tubular cell down a concentration gradient. Several metabolic pathways are present to convert these agents to more water-soluble metabolites, which are generally less active than the parent compound, although there are several important exceptions.

Phase 1 metabolism involves the monooxygenase system in the smooth endoplasmic reticulum of the hepatocyte. Here, a variety of subtypes of cytochrome P450 enzymes catalyse oxidation, reduction, hydrolysis and dealkylation reactions. These enzymes are not specific and drugs may compete with each other for metabolism via one particular pathway and a given drug may be metabolized via several routes mediated by several subtypes of P450. Some of the most clinically relevant sub-types and substances for which they are quantitatively important metabolic pathways are shown in Table 3.

Phase 2 metabolism involves the conjugation of parent drug or metabolite with a water-soluble molecule such as glucuronic acid (glucuronidation), sulphate, amino acid such as glutathione or glycine or acetyl coenzyme A (acetylation). As with phase 1 reactions, the metabolites are generally less active and therefore of low toxicity, but these are important exceptions.

Finally, drugs with a high molecular weight (e.g. rifampicin) may be excreted in the bile, particularly as conjugates. The drug or its conjugate may be reabsorbed, either directly or after deconjugation by intestinal microflora, resulting in an enterohepatic recycling, which offsets the effects of biliary excretion. In obstructive jaundice enterohepatic circulation is impaired leading to an accumulation of drugs excreted in the bile (e.g. rifampicin and fusidic acid).

Table 3 Some clinically important subtypes of cytochrome P-450, and some important substrates and inhibitors of metabolism

Cytochrome P450 subtype	Some important substrates	Some important inhibitors
CYP1A2	Clozapine R-warfarin Tacrine Theophylline	Cimetidine Ciprofloxacin Erythromycin
CYP2C9	Amitriptyline Phenytoin S-warfarin	Amiodarone Cimetidine Fluconazole Metronidazole Sulphapyridine
CYP2C19	Diazepam Mephenytoin Omeprazole	Fluoxetine Fluvoxamine
CYP2D6	Codeine Haloperidol Imipramine Paroxetine Risperidone Thioridazine Venlafaxine	Amiodarone Fluoxetine Fluvoxamine Quinidine
CYP2E1	Ethanol Isoniazid Paracetamol	Disulfiram
CYP3A4	Astemizole Carbamazepine Corticosteroids Cyclosporin Erythromycin Lignocaine Nifedipine Quinidine Terfenadine Verapamil	Cimetidine Clarithromycin Erythromycin Grapefruit juice Ketoconazole

In liver disease, phase 1 metabolism is often relatively more affected than phase 2 metabolic reactions. The effect of liver disease is most marked for those drugs that are normally efficiently removed by hepatic metabolism (high-clearance compounds). These agents normally have high presystemic (first pass) metabolism resulting in low bioavailability after oral administration despite complete absorption. Important examples include morphine and chlormethiazole (a drug advocated by some for alcohol withdrawal). Not only is the metabolic activity of the liver affected in liver disease but intra-and extrahepatic shunting results in a smaller proportion of the drug being metabolized on its first passage through the liver.

There is no ideal marker of the likely reduction in drug metabolic processes in chronic liver disease. The simplest clinical marker is the serum albumin, although strictly speaking this is a marker of biosynthetic rather than metabolic function. Although the serum albumin gives a measure of the likely degree of liver damage and also the patient's prognosis, it is relatively crude. However, serum bilirubin, transaminases and alkaline phosphatase may be normal, even in the presence of severe chronic liver dysfunction and may therefore be unhelpful. In acute liver damage, the albumin concentration may be normal at first because of the long half-life of the protein (20 days) and the reduction in vitamin K-dependent clotting factors, particularly factor VII, which has a half-life of 4 h, is a more useful guide. The International Normalized Ratio (INR), a derivative of the one-stage prothrombin time that is particularly sensitive to changes in factor VII, is normally used for this purpose.

In cardiac failure, cardiac output (normally around 6 l/min) is reduced. This results in a disproportionate reduction in hepatic blood flow (normally around 1.5 l/min) and a reduction in the systemic clearance of compounds that are normally efficiently cleared (e.g. lignocaine) for which hepatic blood flow is a major determinant of clearance. In addition, the liver can be affected by the increased venous back pressure caused by failure of the right side of the heart consequent to left ventricular failure (biventricular or congestive heart failure). This results in increased size and congestion of the liver and derangement of liver function, which can progress in severe cases to jaundice. Drug metabolism can decrease so that clearance even of drugs that are normally poorly cleared (e.g. theophylline) may be further decreased. In addition, the increased venous pressure may result in intestinal mucosal oedema and reduced absorption of relatively inefficiently absorbed drugs (e.g. frusemide).

Extremes of Age

Neonates   The neonatal period covers the first 30 days of life. Prematurity amplifies many of the problems encountered in the drug treatment of this group, but even the healthy full-term neonate is prone to ADRs because of the immaturity of pharmacokinetic processes (Routledge, 1994a). Absorption of drugs may be more complete in the neonate as transit delays are compensated for by increased mucosal contact times. If a rapid drug response is needed, routes other than the oral route should be used. Reduced gastric acidity may result in increased absorption of drugs such as amoxycillin. Reduced body fat and increased body water result in changes in the volume of distribution (Vd) for lipid- and water-soluble drugs. Other influences include reduced plasma albumin and α-1-acid glycoprotein concentrations resulting in reduced plasma protein binding affinity and increased competition for binding from free fatty acids and bilirubin. These effects tend to prolong the half-life of the drug. Despite increased hepatic size relative to body size, phase I and most phase II metabolic enzyme systems are immature so hepatic metabolism of drugs may be reduced. Chloramphenicol produces the 'grey baby' syndrome via inefficient glucuronidation for example. Renal function is globally reduced in neonates with the GFR being about 40% of the normal adult value. This results in delayed excretion of drugs such as digoxin and gentamicin. In general smaller weight-related doses of all drugs are required in the neonatal period (Rylance and Armstrong, 1997).

The Elderly The increased risk of ADRs in the elderly is well described, and around 10% of all admissions to geriatric units are directly due to an ADR, generally a type A reaction (Williamson and Chopin, 1980).

Pharmacokinetic factors are important contributors to the increased risk of Type A ADRs in the elderly. The GFR tends to decline with increasing age from 30 years onwards (Lindeman, 1992) so that the average GFR of an 80-year-old is 30% less, even in the absence of overt renal disease. This decline does not occur in all elderly subjects and may be partly related to subtle underlying pathophysiological changes rather than the inevitable consequence of age. Nevertheless, the decline in renal function is important in relation to renally excreted drugs with a low therapeutic index, as mentioned on pages 61, 67 and 75.

The relationship between age and drug metabolism is less clearcut. There does tend to be a slow decline in the metabolism of some drugs with increasing age, but wide variability at any age indicates that factors other than chronological age are more important determinants of the rate of metabolism. Perhaps the most important of these is the presence of physical frailty (Owens *et al.*, 1994). Biological (rather than chronological) age more accurately reflects nutritional state and protein–energy malnutrition, which is particularly seen in the housebound or nursing home resident is associated with a reduction in the activity of several important pathways of drug metabolism (O'Mahony and Woodhouse, 1994).

Pharmacogenetic Factors

Genetic factors play a major role in determining drug response and handling as well as susceptibility to ADRs. Although receptors, transport processes and metabolic pathways may all be affected, most is known of the metabolic processes, many of which are responsible for handling foreign substances (xenobiotics), of which drugs are an important group. Allelic variations affecting drug handling (pharmacokinetics) with a frequency of at least 1% are often termed polymorphisms (e.g acetylation) while less common variants are often classified as rare inborn errors of metabolism (e.g. porphyria), but the distinction is relatively arbitrary.

The extent to which an individual metabolizes a drug is often, if only partly, genetically determined. Twins derived from the same ovum (monozygotic) twins metabolize many drugs at a similar rate, while dizygotic twins differ more in clearance values. For most drugs the variability in metabolism is unimodally distributed. A bimodal or trimodal distribution may suggest the existence of separate populations capable of metabolizing those drugs at markedly different rates. Some pathways of drug metabolism showing such polymorphism are acetylation, oxidation (hydroxylation), succinylcholine hydrolysis (de-esterification) and thiopurine s-methylation.

Acetylation This metabolic pathway and its polymorphic distribution was discovered over 40 years ago. Acetylation of some drugs is mediated by the enzyme *N*-acetyltransferase. At least two populations exist with different rates of acetylation. The gene controlling the *N*-acetyltransferase in the liver (NAT2) is on chromosome 8 and the slow phenotype is inherited as an autosomal recessive trait. For reasons that are not clear, the proportion of slow acetylators varies markedly between different races, being 55% in European Caucasians, 10% in Japanese and 5% in the Inuit of Northern Canada and in Egyptians.

Drugs that undergo genetically determined acetylation are dapsone, isoniazid, hydralazine, phenelzine, procainamide and some sulphonamides such as the sulpha-pyridine, which forms part of the sulphasalazine molecule used for the treatment of ulcerative colitis. Slow acetylators require lower doses of hydralazine than fast acetylators in the treatment of hypertension and are more likely to have dose-related toxicity with high doses of sulphasalazine. They are also more likely to develop the lupus erythematosus-like syndrome caused by isoniazid or hydralazine, and the pyridoxine-deficient peripheral neuropathy caused by isoniazid. Phenytoin toxicity due to inhibition of its metabolism by isoniazid occurs more frequently in slow acetylators receiving isoniazid for treatment or prophylaxis of tuberculosis. Drug-related lupus (DRL) is very rarely seen in fast acetylators of hydralazine, but not all slow acetylators develop the complication. It is therefore clear that the mechanism is multifactorial and several studies have examined other causes of susceptibility. Studies of HLA associations with DRL have given conflicting results, but immuno-genetic differences are associated with systemic lupus esythematosus (SLE) and it is likely that they will also pertain to the drug induced form of this condition.

The acetylator status of an individual may be easily assessed by giving isoniazid (200 mg orally) and measuring the ratio of the concentration of acetylisoniazid and isoniazid in a plasma or saliva sample 3 h later (Hutchings and Routledge, 1986). Genotyping only requires a sample of blood without administering a drug and may be available for clinical use in the future.

Oxidation Certain metabolic pathways involving oxidation are polymorphically inherited, with poor and extensive metabolizer phenotypes.

One of the most important examples is the autosomal recessive defect of cyto-chrome P450, CYP2D6. The gene is located on chromosome 22 and the poor metabolizer phenotype is inherited in an autosomal recessive fashion. This pheno-type occurs in about 7 % of Caucasians, but has a lower prevalence in other racial types (e.g. 1% in Oriental populations). The metabolism of codeine, debrisoquine, haloperidol, imipramine, paroxetine, phenformin, propafenone, sparteine and many other drugs (including several neuroleptic agents) occurs via this route. The dose-related adverse effects of some of these drugs (e.g. peripheral neuropathy with perhexiline and central nervous system (CNS) toxicity with some tricyclic antidepres-sants) are more likely in poor hydroxylators. Since codeine is a prodrug and is activated by metabolism to morphine, poor metabolizers may fail to obtain analgesic relief from the drug. Quinidine inhibits this pathway and its concurrent administration may result in a genotypically extensive metabolizer behaving as a poor metabolizer.

The lactic acidosis that has been described in approximately 10% of subjects receiving phenformin was first reported in 1959, 10 years before the drug was marketed in the UK (Walker and Linton, 1959). The drug was not withdrawn until around 1980 after approximately 50 fatal case of lactic acidosis associated with its use had been reported. Despite this, phenformin is still used in some countries outside the USA and Europe and lactic acidosis is still reported. Ultrarapid metabolism may also rarely occur via this pathway due to gene amplification in some subjects, but the clinical relevance is unknown.

The metabolism of mephenytoin (an anticonvulsant drug similar to phenytoin) and the proton pump inhibitor, omeprazole is mediated by cytochrome CYP2C19, whose activity is bimodally distributed. The normal (wild-type) gene is absent in 2–6% of Caucasians and up to 20% of Southeast Asians (Japanese, Koreans and Chinese) in an autosomal recessive inheritance and these people are therefore poor metabolizers. These individuals are more likely to develop drowsiness during mephenytoin treatment. In addition they do not convert the antimalarial prodrug proguanil to the active form (cycloguanil) and may therefore fail to respond to treatment.

Succinylcholine De-esterification Succinylcholine is a depolarizing neuromuscular blocking agent used in induction of general anaesthesia. Normally, it is rapidly metabolized in the plasma by a nonspecific esterase called pseudocholinesterase and has a short half-life and duration of action. Some individuals possess pseudocholinesterase of abnormal affinity or amount, and metabolize the succinylcholine much more slowly, resulting in prolonged neuromuscular blockade. Prolonged apnoea was first recognized in 1953 (Forbat *et al.*, 1953). It is now known that there are three types of abnormalities of pseudocholinesterase, each inherited in autosomal recessive fashion: the dibucaine-resistant, fluoride-resistant and gene types (Kalow and Genest, 1957). The prevalence of the homozygous poor metabolism phenotype is only 1 in 3000 so it is not a common polymorphism like acetylation or CYP2D6 oxidation. The gene for the trait is located on chromosome 3.

In some individuals there is an increase of up to threefold in the concentration of plasma pseudocholinesterase with consequent resistance to the effects of succinylcholine (Cynthiana variant). The prevalence may be as high as 1 in 1000 (i.e. three times more frequent than the deficiency state).

Thiopurine S-methylation Thiopurine methyltransferase (TPMT) is one of three major enzymes responsible for the metabolism of azathioprine and its active metabolite 6-mercaptopurine. TPMT activity is determined by an allelic polymorphism for either high (TPMT H) or low (TPMT L) enzyme activity. Homozygotes for the low activity allele (0.3% of the population) are known to be at risk of profound myelosupression on recommended doses of azathioprine and heterozygotes (11%) may also be at risk. Homozygotes for the high activity allele may be inadequately immunosuppressed with conventionally recommended doses of this drug. The chromosomal location of this gene has yet to be determined.

Pharmacodynamic Risk Factors

In general, many of the groups with pharmacodynamic reasons for susceptibity to ADRs are also those with pharmacokinetic differences. In addition, pharmacogenetically determined differences in pharmacodymamics may increase the risk of adverse reactions.

Renal Disease

In renal failure, there is an accumulation of toxic waste products, resulting eventually in severe uraemia and encephalopathy with confusion, loss of memory and other neurological signs. It is thought that purine metabolites, amines, indoles, phenols and other substances may contribute to uraemia and retained middle molecules (molecular weight 500–5000 Da) may also contribute to the problem. It is likely that subclinical accumulation may contribute to the increased sensitivity to psychoactive drugs, particularly opiates, although pharmacokinetic factors may also be important for several drugs.

Liver Disease

Encephalopathy may occur in severe liver disease. Even before this, however, a subclinical phase may be detected by psychometric or electrophysiological testing. It is thought to be due to decreased hepatic extraction of substances that tend to inhibit neuronal function. The precise mechanism by which psychoactive drugs cause a further deterioration of cerebral function in these circumstances is not yet known; however, in the case of benzodiazepines it is thought to be related to an interaction at the GABA receptor complex. Liver disease (both acute and chronic) is associated with a reduced production of vitamin K-dependent clotting factors, even after parenteral vitamin K administration. This (together with other defects of haemostasis) contributes to an increased risk of bleeding per se; in addition bleeding risk due to drug therapy (e.g. aspirin and other NSAIDs) is increased. The increased sensitivity to warfarin is caused by a combination of this effect and the reduced clearance of warfarin in liver disease, although the pharmacodynamic sensitivity is probably the more important factor.

Extremes of Age

Neonate   The blood–brain barrier regulates the entry of drugs to the brain and is less efficient at birth, especially in preterm neonates, who are particularly sensitive to psychoactive agents such as opiates or lithium.

The Elderly   Increasing age is associated with several pharmacodynamic changes that may increase the risk of drug toxicity. Lamy (1991) has classified these as:

- Primary (physiological) ageing factors.
- secondary (pathophysiological) ageing factors.
- Tertiary (psychological) ageing factors.

All these factors may affect response. Primary factors include the slower metabolic processes, the reduction in brain mass, neurone density, cerebral blood flow and capacity for autoregulation, and possible increased permeability of the blood–brain barrier, all of which occur with increasing age. Secondary factors include the many diseases to which the elderly are more prone. Tertiary factors include the effects that psychological stresses may have upon motivation, nutrition and other aspects of self-care.

Physiological ageing of the CNS contributes to the increased risk of toxicity of drugs acting on the CNS. Reduced ability to respond to stress (reserve capacity) results in reduced ability to maintain homeostasis so that drugs that affect balance (e.g. CNS sedatives), temperature regulation (e.g. phenothiazines), bowel and bladder function (e.g. anticholinergic agents), blood pressure (e.g. vasodilators) may all cause adverse effects at normal adult doses.

Risk Factors for Type B Reactions

Type B reactions are 'bizarre' in that they cannot be predicted from the drug's known pharmacology. They include allergic reactions to drugs and because of their often dramatic onset may be associated with a proportionately higher mortality than Type A reactions, although they are less common. Type B reactions may occur to the excipients, preservative or vehicle in the formulation. This problem is discussed at length by Uchegbu and Florence (1996). The mechanisms of Type B reactions are often poorly understood, but many involve allergic or pseudoallergic mechanisms (Rieder, 1994).

Allergic Reactions

Allergic reactions to drugs are often known as hypersensitivity reactions.

Type I Hypersensitivity
The commonest form of hypersensitivity is the immediate hypersensitivity associated with hay fever and asthma. This was classified by Gell and Coombs as Type I (or immediate) hypersensitivity and certain drugs (e.g. penicillins and cephalosporins) can also cause this problem. Mast cells, which are common in the gut and lung, and basophils have a high affinity receptor for the Fc domain of the immunoglobulin, IgE. When two such IgE molecules bound together as a dimer on the cell wall are crosslinked by an previously circulating antigen molecule, mediators such as histamine, leukotrienes and prostaglandins are released. If these are released in large amounts, systemic anaphylaxis may ensue, with bronchospasm and circulatory collapse, sometimes with fatal consequences.

Type II Hypersensitivity
In Type II or antibody-mediated cytotoxic hypersensitivity, the antigen (rather than the antibody as in Type I reactions) is bound to the surface of a cell membrane, often a red cell or platelet. Circulating immunoglobulin (IgG, IgM or IgA) reacts with the antigen to stimulate complement as well as cytotoxic cells, resulting in lysis of the target cell. This is the mechanism of certain drug-induced haemolytic anaemias (e.g. due to methyldopa) and thrombocytopenias (e.g. due to quinine).

Type III Hypersensitivity
In Type III hypersensitivity reactions, antigen–antibody complexes are deposited in areas of turbulent flow or filtration (e.g. the glomerulus of the kidney). This type of reaction, known as immune complex hypersensitivity, results in complement activation and the lysosomes released by polymorphonuclear cells cause vascular damage. In addition to glomerulonephritis, this reaction may result in fever, lymphadenopathy, arthritis and rashes and may be induced by several drugs including gold and penicillamine.

Type IV Hypersensitivity
Type IV or delayed-type (cell-mediated) immunity occurs in the absence of detectable circulating antigen or antibody. Specific helper T lymphocytes may be

stimulated by a drug that acts as a hapten and has complexed with a tissue macro-molecule to form an antigen. This results in the release of cytokines and accumulation of other cells, particularly monocytes, in the area, and resulting granulomata, oedema or widespread rash, normally several days after exposure to the drug. It appears that people with human immunodeficiency virus (HIV) infection may be more prone to such drug-induced allergic reactions, particularly in response to sulphonamides.

Pseudo Allergic Reactions

Pseudoallergic reactions are so-called because they mimic allergic hypersensitivity, particularly of Type I hypersensitivity. Such reactions, if severe, are often termed anaphylactoid and can occur on first exposure to a drug, particularly a neromuscular blocker or radiographic contrast dye. It is not known why certain individuals are predisposed to such reactions, but asthmatics, especially those with nasal polyps are more likely than others to experience such reactions with aspirin, for example. There is cross-reactivity with other non-steroidal agent and with tartrazine, which was a dye once commonly used in drugs, but is now restricted in use.

Pharmacogenetic Factors

Glucose-6-phosphate Dehydrogenase Deficiency

Some individuals have erythrocytes that are genetically deficient in glucose-6-phosphate dehydrogenase (G6PD), which is at least partly responsible for preventing the oxidation of various red cell proteins. Haemolysis occurs if the abnormal erythrocyte is exposed to oxidizing agents, probably because of unopposed oxidation of sulphydryl groups in the cell membrane. Common causative agents include aspirin, sulphonamides, some antimalarials, antileprotics and pharmacological doses of vitamins K or C. The gene is on the X chromosome and inheritance of the deficiency state therefore occurs in a sex-linked (X) recessive mode. It is relatively common (up to 14%) in African Americans and in Mediterranean races, but the severity of reactions appears to be greater in G6PD deficient Caucasians.

Porphyria

People with hepatic porphyrias (acute intermittent porphyria or porphyria cutanea tarda) have abnormalities of haem biosynthesis and symptoms may be precipitated by many drugs, particularly alcohol, the oral contraceptive, barbiturates and sulphonamides. (For a fuller and up-to-date list, contact the Welsh Drug Information Centre, University of Wales, Cardiff CF4 4XW, UK.)

Malignant Hyperthermia

This is a serious and occasionally fatal condition that may occur in association with general anaesthesia with halothane or methoxyflurane used in conjunction with succinylcholine. It occurs in about 1 in 20 000 anaesthetized patients and is inherited in an autosomal dominant fashion. Body temperature may rise to 41 °C, with increased muscle tone, tachycardia, sweating, cyanosis and tachypnoea. Creatine kinase activity may rise due to muscle damage and muscle death (rhabdomyolysis) may occur. The muscle relaxant, dantrolene, and diazepam, which acts as a general relaxant, are sometimes effective in preventing muscle damage. The gene is thought to lie on the long arm of chromosome 19.

Coumarin Resistance

Coumarin resistance is a very rare defect that has been reported in only two human kindreds. In this condition up to 20 times the usual dose of warfarin or other coumarin anticoagulant may be required to produce satisfactory anticoagulation. It has an autosomal dominant inheritance and the mechanism appears to be resistance of the enzyme vitamin K epoxide reductase in the vitamin K–K epoxide shuttle to the normal inhibitory effect of coumarins. The site of the gene is not known.

Aminoglycoside Antibiotic-induced Deafness

Susceptibility to the ototoxic effects of aminoglycoside antibiotics such as gentamicin may be genetically determined in some individuals. Inheritance is solely through the maternal line and both sexes are equally affected, supporting the evidence that transmission is dependent upon the mitochondrial genome, a rare mechanism for inheritance of disease. The prevalence is thought to be at least 1 in 10 000, and in Shanghai it is thought that 25% of all deaf mutes may have become deaf after exposure to these widely used agents (Hu *et al.*, 1991).

Long QT Syndrome

This condition is characterized by an increased delay between the QRS complex and T wave in the electrocardiogram associated with a susceptibility to life-threatening ventricular arrhythmias occurring spontaneously or during therapy with some drugs (e.g. some antihistamines, antiarrhythmic drugs, neuroleptics and tricyclic antidepressants). There seem to be several forms of the condition with linkages between chromosomes 3, 7 and 11 in three of these. The QT duration and morphology are not always very sensitive and specific diagnostic markers, making the identification of affected individuals and carriers difficult.

Other Pharmacogenetic Disorders

The above conditions are some of the more important pharmacogenetic disorders, but several more exist and are described in the excellent text by Weber (1997).

Genetic Predisposition to Adverse Drug Reactions

Factors associated with an increased risk of ADRs include a history of allergic disorders such as atopic disease or hereditary angioedema (Grahame-Smith and Aronson, 1992).

Human leucocyte antigen (HLA) status may also be important:

- The risk of nephrotoxicity from penicillamine is increased in patients with the HLA types B8 and DR3 while patients with HLA-DR7 may be protected.
- The risk of skin reactions with penicillamine is associated with HLA-DRw6, and the risk of thrombocytopenia is associated with HLA-DR4; patients with HLA-DR4 also have a greater risk of the lupus-like syndrome (see below) associated with hydralazine.

Detection of Adverse Drug Reactions

Vere described the tendency of ADRs to masquerade as natural illness over 20 years ago (Vere, 1976). He gave five main reasons why so many adverse reactions escape unnoticed:

- The reaction may be so odd or bizarre that an often used and apparently innocent drug escapes suspicion.
- The drug-induced disorder can closely mimic a common natural disease.
- There is a long delay in the appearance of the adverse effect.
- The drug evokes a relapse of natural disease or may evoke a disorder in a naturally susceptible subject.
- The clinical situation may be so complex that its drug-related components pass unnoticed.

Even today, iatrogenic disease may still go unrecognized. If the delay in onset of iatrogenic disease is very prolonged, effects are even more difficult to detect. Auto-immune haemolytic anaemia has been described nine years after uneventful antihypertensive treatment with methyldopa for example (Terol *et al.*, 1991), so continued vigilance is required in all patients throughout the course of their treatment.

Another difficulty in identifying drug-induced disease is that there may be a significant prevalence of the non-drug-induced condition in the community. Vere pointed out that the risk of adenocarcinoma of the vagina in female children born to mothers who took high doses of the oestrogen, stilboestrol in pregnancy was probably recognized largely because it is so unusual there was no 'background noise' (Vere, 1976). The same argument applies to the unusual maldevelopment of limbs seen in phocomelia caused by thalidomide, which was therefore recognized reasonably quickly.

Drugs that aggravate already existing disease may escape suspicion for some time, particularly if the natural disease is common. Fialuridine is a nucleoside that was undergoing trials for the treatment of hepatitis B. Unfortunately the major adverse effect of this drug was on the liver and the worsening liver function in treated patients appeared to be explained by the monitoring physicians as worsening of the hepatitis rather than as direct drug toxicity. The incorporation of the nucleoside in patients into the cell nuclear protein ensured that the toxicity was quite persistent, even after withdrawal of the drug and several patients died of the complications of lactic acidosis associated with the hepatitis (McKenzie *et al.*, 1995).

Finally, ADRs may be difficult to detect because of the confounding effects of other treatments being administered at the same time. Some agents (e.g. blood products or contrast media) may be administered for therapeutic or diagnostic purposes while the patient is undergoing treatment and other drugs (e.g. corticosteroids or antihistamines) may affect the natural history of iatrogenic disease and prevent it from being recognized.

Biochemical and Histological Confirmation

There are relatively few specific investigations to confirm the presence of an ADR. Biochemical pictures associated with iatrogenic disease may mimic those from other idiopathic causes. Histological evidence, although often difficult to obtain, may sometimes be more helpful:

● The ductopenia associated with flucloxacillin-induced liver damage is relatively specific for this drug-induced hepatic damage.
● Although not specific for drug-induced glomerulonephritis, the granular deposition of immune complexes shown on immunocytochemical stains of renal biopsy material contrasts with the more linear deposition seen in other forms of immune complex glomerulonephritis such as Goodpasture's syndrome.

Some in-vitro investigations, such as the radioallergosorbent test, (RAST) which detects antigen-specific antibodies in serum, or the histamine release test, may be valuable in determining anaphylactic or anaphylactoid reactions, particularly to anaesthetic induction agents. The histamine release test and basophil degranulation test may have an advantage over RASTs in that they will demonstrate anaphylactoid reactions (i.e. those that are non-IgE mediated) as well as those that are anaphylactic and mediated by IgE. Tryptase is the most important protein in mast cell granules and is released in anaphylactoid as well as anaphylactic reactions. Plasma tryptase concentrations are maximal 1–6 hours after the reaction, but may be detected in concentrations above normal for up to 12–14 hours, making this test a useful but nonspecific confirmatory test in severe reactions, particularly those occuring in anaesthesia. Urine methylhistamine concentrations have also been used for this purpose, but are more difficult to interpret (Association of Anaesthetists of Great Britain and Ireland and The British Society of Allergy and Clinical Immunology, 1995).

Tests using other cellular components of blood such as the basophil degranulation test, passive haemagglutination, lymphocyte transformation and leukocyte/macrophage migration inhibition tests may have some value in certain allergic Type B reactions; however, the sensitivity of these tests is relatively poor and negative tests do not always exclude the possibility of drug-induced disease (Pohl *et al.*, 1988). The major difficulty with many of the in-vitro tests is that the challenge agent is normally the parent drug. Since the responsible compound may be a metabolite or breakdown product and unless this specific agent is present or generated in the in-vitro situation, the test may be falsely negative (Pohl *et al.*, 1988).

Skin Testing and Direct Drug Rechallenge

Skin tests are essentially a form of in-vivo rechallenge at reduced drug dose. Such tests may be insensitive and nonspecific. In addition, they can be potentially dangerous and deaths have been reported with intradermal testing to penicillin, for example, although this is rare with a careful technique and newer reagents. Scratch tests and intradermal tests may be particularly helpful in the investigation of immediate-type anaphylactic/anaphylactoid reactions to drugs used during anaesthesia. Skin patch testing may be helpful in the investigation of fixed drug eruptions, but should not be used in Stevens–Johnson syndrome or toxic epidermal necrolysis (Breathnach, 1995).

Systemic drug rechallenge is fraught with even more potential risk than skin testing. It is generally only considered when a suspected drug is the only agent known to be effective in a particular condition (e.g. aspirin in the secondary prevention of ischaemic heart disease or allopurinol in long-term prophylaxis of gout). For a comprehensive review of this subject, the reader is referred to the excellent review by Stephens (1983).

Other Evidence

Since direct evidence is often difficult to obtain, circumstantial evidence may be important in detecting ADRs. A useful criterion for determining whether a reaction is drug induced is the timing of the onset of the symptoms relative to the start of drug therapy:

- Type A reactions normally occur when the drug has accumulated, thus it may take five half-lives of the drug for the ADR to reach maximum intensity.
- Type B reactions are often immunological in nature and so sometimes require a latent period of up to five days before being seen. Most occur within 12 weeks of initiation of drug therapy.

The time course for Type B reactions may, however, be clouded by several factors. Drug-induced agranulocytosis, for example, may take two or more weeks to occur after initial drug exposure and may therefore present after the drug has been discontinued. The same is true of drug-induced jaundice, particularly when it occurs after the agent is used for short-course therapy (e.g. co-amoxiclav or flucloxacillin). Some Type B reactions (e.g. halothane-induced jaundice) appear more rapidly on re-exposure after a previous reaction has occurred.

The time course to resolution after stopping the drug (dechallenge) may also be of help in assessing causality. Some ADRs take a considerable time to disappear after drug discontinuation, particularly if the drug has a long half-life of elimination (e.g. amiodarone), while others may be associated with irreversible effects (e.g. pulmonary fibrosis after busulphan or nitrofurantoin).

The absence of an alternative explanation is an important criterion in considering a drug-related cause, but the latter should still be considered and relevant information sought without waiting to rule out non-drug-related causes.

Finally, it has been shown that doctors rely to a large extent on whether previous reports of adverse reactions have been published in association with the drug therapy. It is important that clinicians are trained to have a much higher level of suspicion of the possibility of iatrogenic disease since it is a situation in which prompt treatment (e.g. drug withdrawal) may result in a permanent cure.

Management of Adverse Drug Reactions

Type A reactions will generally respond to a reduction in dose of the drug although temporary drug discontinuation may be necessary if the reaction is significant. Unfortunately, some adverse effects are permanent (e.g. lung fibrosis with busulphan or liver fibrosis with methotrexate) although withdrawal of treatment as soon as the condition is recognized may reduce the eventual magnitude of toxicity.

For type B reactions the clinician should withdraw the suspected drug immediately and refer the patient for specialist investigations (e.g. skin testing if appropriate) on recovery. It is sometimes necessary to give supportive therapy, particularly for anaphylactic and anaphylactoid reactions, and corticosteroids may sometimes be used to suppress inflammatory or potentially fibrotic processes.

Part of the management of adverse reactions is to report them to the regulatory authorities. This allows the appropriate bodies to assess risk–benefit of particular medications, which can contribute to safe drug use in susceptible subjects in the future. In the UK, the Committee on Safety of Medicines (CSM) (Medicines Control Agency, MCA) asks health professionals to report all suspected serious reactions to established medicines and all suspected adverse reactions to newly introduced (so-called black triangle ▼) drugs, whatever their severity.

In rare circumstances, when no alternative agents are available for treatment of a particular condition, desensitization by administration of gradually increasing doses of the drug may eventually allow the patient to tolerate the agent at full dose. This approach has been used successfully in some patients with aspirin or allopurinol hypersensitivity, for example.

Avoidance of Adverse Drug Reactions

The goal of therapeutics is to obtain optimum efficacy and minimum toxicity of drug therapy. This ideal is difficult to achieve because of the wide variability in drug response within patients. Bespoke prescribing aims to achieve this by tailoring initial doses to the individual patient and titrating drug dose subsequently to avoid toxicity. Bespoke prescribing has been used for the initiation of warfarin and heparin therapy (Routledge, 1986). The approach is primarily of value in avoiding Type A adverse reactions, although the avoidance of excessive doses of certain drugs in high-risk individuals may also reduce the risk of Type B reactions (e.g. there is a higher risk of severe allergic-type skin reactions with excessive doses of allopurinol in patients with renal disease).

In renal dysfunction, the creatinine clearance is closely related and similar in magnitude to the GFR. Thus GFR can be calculated by measuring the patient's serum creatinine (which has little diurnal variation) and age, gender and body weight. The Cockroft–Gault equation uses the relationship:

$$\text{Equation1 : Creatinine clearance} = \frac{(140 - \text{age(y)}) \times \text{Body weight (kg)}}{0.82 \times \text{plasma creatinine } (\mu\text{mol/l})}$$

For females, who have less muscle mass at any given weight, the result must be multiplied by 0.85. This equation is relevant only when the renal function is relatively constant and in the absence of concomitant liver disease. It is a useful guide to dose adjustment in renal disease and in the elderly when glomerular filtration is the major renal excretory mechanism. The proportional dose adjustment will also depend upon the proportion of the drug excreted unchanged by the kidney (F) (since some drug may be cleared by metabolic pathways) in the following formula:

$$\text{Equation2 : Dose (as proportion of normal)} = \frac{(1 - F) + F \times \text{GFR (patient)}}{\text{GFR (normal)}}$$

This relationship can be used to aid in the calculation of the dose of digoxin or gentamicin, for example. The situation is more difficult if renal tubular secretion is a major excretory mechanism since no clinically applicable direct measurements of this pathway are available.

Dose adjustment is more difficult in liver disease, although the serum albumin concentration is of some help in deciding upon the starting dose. The initial induction dose of warfarin should be reduced by at least 50% if the INR is greater than 1.3 (Fennerty *et al.*, 1988).

Therapeutic Drug Monitoring

Monitoring drug concentration in the plasma is also of value in avoiding some ADRs. The ideal way to monitor drug therapy is to have a simple measure of drug effect (e.g. oral anticoagulant therapy), but this is rarely available. In the absence of a pharmacodynamic measure, and particularly when the only endpoint is the absence of features of the illness (e.g. absence of seizures during anticonvulsant treatment or arrhythmias during antiarrhythmic treatment) the plasma drug concentration is a useful surrogate marker of efficacy and safety. To be applicable, the drug should have a concentration-related and reversible effect without the development of tolerance, and the metabolites should be relatively inactive unless active metabolite concentrations are also measured. Relatively few drugs fulfil these strict criteria, but therapeutic drug monitoring (TDM) is used to adjust the doses of cyclosporin, digoxin, gentamicin and other aminoglycoside antibiotics, lithium, phenytoin and theophylline (Routledge, 1994b).

Since drugs are normally given at fixed intervals, the plasma concentration varies between doses during the processes of absorption, distribution, metabolism and excretion. Samples taken some time after the dose are therefore more reflective of the average concentration between doses and should be taken at least 8 hours after digoxin administration and 12 hours after lithium. Peak levels are sometimes required (e.g. with gentamicin) and occur around 30–60 minutes after an intramuscular injection or immediately at the end of an intravenous infusion. Peak levels of orally administered drugs are achieved at 30–180 minutes after conventional formulations and later after modified-release preparations. For many drugs, a sample taken just before the next dose is due (trough concentration) will correlate best with the average (steady state) concentration.

It takes approximately five half-lives before the plasma concentrations of a drug reach their maximum steady state level. Sampling before this time has elapsed is therefore most valuable if drug toxicity due to excessive accumulation is expected. Ideally, five half-lives should elapse before steady state plasma concentrations are measured, but this make take some time in certain cases (e.g. nine months in the case of amiodarone, which has a half-life of 45 days). Details of sampling time relative to dose, time of last dose change and present daily dose schedule should always be stated on the assay request form to aid interpretation of the plasma concentration.

In clinical practice, total rather than free (active) drug concentrations are measured by conventional assay methodologies. Although in most circumstances, these will correlate with free drug concentrations, this is not always the case:

- In neonates, the frail elderly and in liver disease, plasma albumin may be reduced due to impaired production.
- In renal dysfunction, particularly nephrotic syndrome, plasma albumin may be reduced due to loss into the urine.
- In renal failure, accumulation of inhibitors of protein binding may further reduce binding so measurement of total concentration may underestimate free concentrations in all these conditions.

For some drugs (e.g. phenytoin and theophylline), saliva concentrations may reflect the free drug concentration more accurately and some laboratories can also measure free drug concentrations directly by ultrafiltration or equilibrium dialysis techniques.

α-1-acid glycoprotein (AAG) is an acute phase protein that avidly binds many basic drugs (e.g. lignocaine, disopyramide, quinidine and verapamil).

- In situations where AAG may be raised, for instance after acute myocardial infarction, surgery, trauma or burns, or in rheumatoid arthritis and other inflammatory conditions, total drug concentrations may overestimate free drug concentrations.

Conversely, AAG may be reduced in neonates, nephrotic syndrome and severe liver disease and the opposite holds true. Measurement of free drug concentration may thus be more helpful in such circumstances, although direct measurement of AAG concentration in plasma may allow the free concentration to be calculated with reasonable accuracy (Routledge, 1986).

Surveillance and the Avoidance of Adverse Drug Reactions

Many Type B reactions occur in patients who are prescribed the same drug or a very similar agent to which they have had a previous adverse reaction. For this reason, the general practitioner and hospital medical records and inpatient prescription sheets should all be clearly marked with a bright label so that the prescriber is aware of previous serious ADRs. Computerized systems have been developed to alert physicians to previous Type B reactions to drugs and of appropriate drug administration rates and their use has resulted in a reduced frequency of Type B reactions (Classen *et al.,* 1991; Evans *et al.,* 1994). Unfortunately these systems are not yet widely available and the vigilance of health care professionals is still the most important factor in avoiding such episodes.

Drug Interactions

Interactions between drugs have been observed for nearly 100 years and have been described under the classical headings of antagonism, synergism and potentiation. Many interactions have been and still are deliberately used with therapeutic benefit, but adverse interactions are becoming an increasingly important problem for several reasons:

- Newly introduced drugs are often much more potent than their predecessors and act on fundamental biochemical and enzymatic pathways or receptors.

- Progress in therapeutics, together with an increasingly ageing population, has resulted in increased polypharmacy. Drug interactions have been estimated to account for 6–30% of all ADRs (Orme *et al.*, 1991). Since adverse reactions are relatively common and interactions involve many different types of drugs it may appear at first sight an almost impossible task for any physician to retain a perspective on the subject. Fortunately, although more than 1000 drug interactions have been described, the number that are clinically important is much smaller and involves a relatively small number of pharmacological groups of drugs. It is also important to recognize that perhaps more than 50% of drug interactions result in some loss of action of one or other of the drugs. These are more likely to be overlooked, since alternative explanations such as poor compliance may be considered as reasons for inefficacy of the treatment.

Mechanisms

Interactions may occur outside or inside the body:

- The former are referred to as pharmaceutical incompatibilities and generally occur when two or more agents are mixed in infusions or in the same syringe or when a drug reacts with the infusion fluid itself.
- Interactions occurring within the body result from either an alteration in the delivery of the drug to its site of action (pharmacokinetic interactions) or from a drug-induced alteration in receptor or organ response to another agent (pharmacodynamic interactions). Often these characteristics are altered when other drugs are given.

Both pharmacokinetic and pharmacodynamic interactions are equally important. Pharmacokinetic interactions will be discussed first, because these must generally first be excluded before the possibility of a pharmacodynamic interaction is investigated.

Pharmacokinetic Interactions

These may occur during any one or more of the pharmacokinetic processes whereby drug reaches its site of action and is then eliminated (i.e. absorption, distribution, metabolism and excretion). Such interactions may result in either an increased or decreased drug concentration at the site of action and although the former may result in drug toxicity, decreased efficacy may put the patient at increased risk from the effects of the disease.

Absorption   For most drugs, absorption is a passive process that is dependent upon the properties of the drug and its particular formulation, the pH of the absorption media and the length of time the drug remains at the site of absorption. Drugs may interact with each other during all these processes, as well as directly with each other by formation of poorly absorbed complexes. It is important to distinguish in this context between changes in the rate and extent of drug absorption:

- Alteration of the rate of absorption alone will change the shape of the concentration–time curve after oral administration, but will not alter the average or steady state drug concentration. Such changes may be important, however, in the case of drugs given in single doses and in which a threshold concentration for drug effect exists (e.g. analgesics). A delay in absorption under these circumstances, especially if the rate of elimination of the drug is high, may result in an inability to reach a drug concentration associated with drug efficacy.

- In contrast, a change in extent of absorption will result in a change in variation in delivery of drug to its site of action both after a single and repeated doses.

Drug-induced changes in the pH of the gastrointestinal media may increase or decrease the rate and extent of drug absorption. Alkalis may aid dissolution of poorly soluble acidic drugs (e.g. aspirin) and stimulate gastric emptying. Alterations in gut motility induced by one drug may alter the rate and/or extent of absorption of another. Sparingly soluble drugs (e.g. digoxin) may be unable to undergo complete disintegration and dissolution when gastric emptying and intestinal transit rates are increased by such drugs as metoclopramide and their extent of absorption may therefore be reduced. In contrast, since the greatest proportion of drug absorption occurs in the small intestine, the rate limiting step for absorption of well-absorbed drugs is the rate of gastric emptying. Metoclopramide therefore increases the absorption rate of paracetamol by increasing the gastric emptying rate. Opposite effects are seen with anticholinergic and opiate drugs.

Certain agents may complex with drugs and reduce their absorption. Aluminium, calcium, or magnesium antacids may thus reduce the absorption of several drugs including 4-quinolone antibiotics, tetracyclines and iron. Ion exchange resins such as cholestyramine and colestipol have been shown to bind to and thereby decrease the extent of absorption of warfarin, thyroxine and triiodothyronine, and digitalis glycosides.

Drugs may also interfere with absorption of other drugs more indirectly by causing malabsorption syndromes. Colchicine, neomycin and paraamino salicylic acid (PAS) may impair the absorption of folate, iron and vitamin B_{12} by this means.

The causes of drug absorption interactions are therefore numerous. Their importance may have been underestimated since physicians are more likely to attribute inadequate response to other factors such as poor compliance with prescribed therapy.

Changes in Drug Distribution Most drugs do not merely distribute throughout body fluids, but are bound or in some cases actively transported into blood and tissue elements. Drugs that are relatively inefficiently cleared by the organ of elimination (e.g. liver or kidney) have been termed restrictively-eliminated compounds since their clearance, either by glomerular filtration or by liver metabolism, is limited by their degree of binding in the blood. Restrictive elimination occurs when the extraction ratio of the drug is less than the free fraction of that drug in blood. Displacement of such compounds from plasma protein binding sites will cause an immediate rise in free drug concentration. This increase will only be temporary, however, since the increase in free fraction will allow more of the drug to be eliminated until a new steady state is reached when the unbound (free) concentration returns to its original level. Permanent changes will be seen in the total plasma concentration since total clearance of the drug has been increased. This will only be detected if total plasma concentration is measured (this is the moiety most often measured by laboratories) since the effect at steady state will be unchanged.

The magnitude of the temporary increase of unbound drug will depend upon:

- The original volume of distribution of the displaced drug.
- The original degree of binding in the blood.
- The degree of binding to tissues.

Thus it is likely plasma protein displacement interactions will cause (and then only temporarily,) a significant increase in free drug concentration only when poorly cleared drugs have a high degree of binding in plasma and poor binding to tissues. Although warfarin fulfils these criteria, several drugs that have been shown to displace warfarin from plasma binding sites, such as phenylbutazone, also interact in more important ways with warfarin (e.g. competition for metabolism). It is therefore difficult to estimate what (if any) effect is produced by the transient increase in free drug concentration.

Many drugs are effectively cleared by the body so that the extraction ratio of the eliminating organ(s) is greater than and therefore not limited by the fraction of drug free in the blood. Displacement of these compounds from plasma binding sites will theoretically result in a permanent increase in free drug concentration, but only a temporary increase in total drug concentration in blood. The magnitude of the permanent increase in free drug concentration will also depend upon the relative degrees of initial binding in blood and tissues, being greatest for drugs with high binding in blood and poor tissue binding. To date, no clinically important interactions involving this mechanism alone have been described for highly cleared drugs.

Elimination   Drugs are either excreted directly in the urine or are first metabolized by other organs (e.g. the liver or gut) to more water-soluble products, which can be more easily excreted by the kidney. Interactions may occur during any of these processes and result in enhancement or diminution of drug effect.

Hepatic Metabolism   The chemical reactions involved in drug metabolism are generally classified as either:

- Phase 1 (oxidation, reduction or hydrolysis).
- Phase 2 reactions (conjugation with glucuronic acid, sulphates or acetate).

Any drug may undergo one or more of these types of metabolism before being excreted by the kidney, but the most important of these are oxidation and glucuronic acid conjugation. Because of its size, enzyme content and plentiful blood supply, the liver is the major site of drug metabolism, although the intestine, lung and kidney have been shown to be other minor sites of metabolism.

The major group of drug metabolizing enzymes, the cytochrome P-450 system, is extremely versatile and is responsible for the biotransformation of many drugs and endogenous compounds. Because of the relative nonspecificity of these pathways, several interactions can take place between drugs using this route of metabolism. Cytochrome P-450 is now known to be made up of several subtypes or isozymes and enzyme inhibition interactions have been reported with at least six of these:

- Cytochome P-450, subtype1A2 (CYP1A2) is involved in the metabolism of xanthines, the R-enantiomer of warfarin, clozapine and tacrine.

- CYP2C9 is involved in the metabolism of S-warfarin and phenytoin and the demethylation of amitryptyline, for example.
- CYP2C19 mediates diazepam and omeprazole metabolism.
- CYP2E1 is involved in the oxidative metabolism of alcohol, isoniazid and para-cetamol (acetaminophen).
- CYP2D6 is important in the metabolism of several drugs, including codeine, haloperidol, imipramine and nortryptyline hydroxylation, and metabolism of par-oxetine, venlafaxine, risperidone and thioridazine. Around 8% of Caucasians are genetically deficient in this enzyme and may be particularly at risk of interaction.
- CYP3A4 is involved in catalysing the metabolism of astemizole, erythromycin, terfenadine, carbamazepine, several calcium antagonists, lignocaine (lidocaine), quinidine, erythromycin, several corticosteroids and cyclosporin as well as sev-eral other agents.

Some drugs are metabolized by several of these isozymes, either concurrently or sequentially. In addition, some drugs metabolized by these pathways can act com-petitively to inhibit metabolism of each other via that route. Other drugs (e.g. cimetidine or erythromycin) can inhibit more than one isozyme non-competitively and so act on more than one pathway.

Drug clearance is a measure of the efficiency of removal of the compound and unlike half-life of elimination ($T_{1/2}$) is unaffected by drug distribution. For those drugs in which intrinsic clearance, and therefore efficiency of removal (extraction ratio), is high, systemic (intravenous) clearance is rate-limited by blood flow to the organ. In contrast, the systemic clearance of poorly extracted compounds is limited predominantly by the intrinsic clearance ability of the organ. The lower the initial efficiency of removal, the more a given change in enzyme activity will alter systemic clearance. After oral administration, however, changes in intrinsic clearance will equally affect the clearance of drugs that are both poorly and well extracted by the liver. This occurs despite the fact that the systemic clearance of the oral dose of a highly extracted drug will be much less affected by any change in intrinsic clearance analagous to after intravenous administration. The reason for this phenomenon is that increasing intrinsic clearance will increase the hepatic extraction ratio so that a much smaller proportion (F) of the highly extracted drug will reach the systemic circulation, even for the first time. Thus for all drugs that are completely absorbed from the gut and metabolized by the liver the area under the plasma concentration–time curve (AUC) is independent of changes in blood flow.

Two important consequences emerge from these theoretical considerations:

- In contrast to poorly extracted drugs, changes in enzyme activity caused by other compounds will affect plasma levels of highly extracted drugs much more after oral administration than after the intravenous route. Poorly extracted drugs will be affected approximately equally, whatever the route of administration.
- Secondly, $T_{1/2}$ of orally administered highly extracted drugs will be much less affected by changes in intrinsic clearance than the half-life of poorly extracted compounds.

One example is the difference in lignocaine kinetics between patients with epilepsy receiving enzyme-inducing drugs and drug-free controls given oral and intravenous doses of lignocaine on separate occasions (Perrucca and Richens, 1979). The patients did not differ significantly from controls in $T_{1/2}$ after oral or intravenous administration or clearance after intravenous administration. Despite this, intrinsic (apparent oral) clearance (as measured by the AUC) was increased more than two-fold in the subjects after oral administration. Thus, $T_{1/2}$ may be a poorer indicator of changes in hepatic drug metabolism than clearance or AUC, particularly for already highly efficiently cleared drugs (Routledge and Shand, 1981).

Enzyme Induction Induction of the metabolism of one drug by another is an important mechanism for interactions. Several agents (e.g. phenobarbitone, phenytoin, primidone, carbamazepine and rifampicin) can increase the activity of many isozymes of cytochrome P-450. The delay between commencement of the inducing agent and the full effect (7–10 days) can make recognition of the interaction difficult. The offset of the interaction occurs over a similar period after the inducing agent is stopped, producing similar difficulties in identification (Kristensen, 1976).

Several agents had been implicated as inducers of hepatic drug metabolism. The more important ones are listed in Table 4. It is important to remember that not all patients receiving these agents will necessarily be affected since there is wide inter-individual variation. There is also a lag period of approximately 1–2 weeks before maximum induction occurs. When the drug is stopped, there is a lag period of similar duration for enzyme activity to return to pre-induction levels. These phenomena may disguise the causative relationship between the drug interaction and administration of the inducing agent.

Although interactions involving induction usually result in decreased drug action, toxicity may occur if toxic metabolites production is increased. Phenobarbitone

---

Table 4   Some clinically important drugs that induce oxidative metabolism

Barbiturates
Carbamazepine
Oxcarbazepine
Phenytoin
Primidone
Rifampicin
Cigarette smoke

Table 5   Some clinically important inhibitors of clinically important pathways of drug metabolism

Allopurinol
Amiodarone
Cimetidine
Clarithromycin
Erythromycin
Monoamine oxidase inhibitors
Some 4-quinolones
Some antifungals
Metronidazole
Some selective serotonin re-uptake inhibitors (SSRIs)

increases the demethylation of pethidine to norpethidine, which may cause CNS depression and prolonged sedation in enzyme-induced subjects.

Enzyme Inhibition   Inhibition of drug metabolism is also a well-established and potentially more serious phenomenon since it may lead directly to toxic concentrations of some drugs. As inhibition is in many cases, competitive, two simultaneously administered drugs may inhibit the metabolism of each other. Several of the compounds observed to cause clinically significant inhibition of metabolism are listed in Table 5.

One important interaction illustrating both inhibition and induction of drug metabolism is that between phenylbutazone and warfarin. Warfarin (like many other drugs) consists of a racemic mixture of equal parts of the dextro (R) and laevo (S) enantiomer (stereoisomer). Phenylbutazone increases the clearance of R-warfarin and simultaneously decreases the clearance of S-warfarin. It does not therefore affect the clearance or $T_{1/2}$ of warfarin when it is measured as the racemate. Since S-warfarin is approximately five times more potent as an anticoagulant than R-warfarin, however, the overall effect of the interaction is to increase the anticoagulation produced by the racemic drug.

Renal Excretion   Drugs are excreted by the kidney both by glomerular filtration and tubular secretion. They may then be reabsorbed by active tubular reabsorption. Changes in any of these processes induced by one agent may result in altered excretion of another compound.

Frusemide in low doses may reduce the renal clearance of cephaloridine and gentamicin and this has been attributed to a frusemide-induced reduction in GFR. Other work has indicated, however, that frusemide may increase GFR, so although frusemide may increase the nephrotoxicity of cephalosporins and the ototoxicity of gentamicin the role of altered GFR in these interactions is unclear.

Tubular secretion is an active process by which some acids and bases are transported into tubular fluid against a concentration gradient. Competition for this relatively nonspecific process between two acidic or two basic drugs may lead to diminished excretion of one or both agents. Clinically significant interactions will only occur, however, if this process is responsible for a major proportion of the total excretion of the drug(s).

Probenecid and salicylates can reduce the elimination of methotrexate by this mechanism and may lead to severe toxicity if methotrexate dosage is not adjusted accordingly. Weak bases are less ionized when the urine is alkalinized by other agents. Acetazolamide and antacids, which render urine alkaline, have thus caused toxicity due to impaired excretion of the basic compound, amphetamine, and also reduce quinidine excretion by the kidney. Conversely alkalinization of urine may increase the excretion of acidic drugs such as salicylate and phenobarbitone and this interaction has been put to clinical use in the treatment of poisoning by these agents with forced alkaline diuresis.

Pharmacodynamic Factors
Pharmacodynamic interactions occur when one drug alters the response of another by interaction at the receptor site or acts at a different site to enhance or diminish the first drug's effects.

The interactions that were first recognized were those in which drugs act at the same receptor site:

- Drugs that combine with the receptor to initiate a response are termed agonists.
- Drugs that interact with the receptor to inhibit the action of an agonist, but do not initiate a response themselves are termed antagonists.

Antagonism may be competitive when increasing the agonist concentration restores its effects completely or it may be non-competitive (irreversible). Partial agonists act on the same receptor as the agonist to initiate a minor response, but by occupying a significant fraction of the receptors they antagonize the action of more potent agonists. Thus naloxone is a potent antagonist of the agonist action of morphine. Nalorphine, however, although possessing antagonist activity, is also a partial agonist and may add to respiratory depression produced by morphine.

Many of the interactions at the receptor site are used to advantage clinically, either to antagonize or augment the effect of endogenous mediators or to counteract toxicity due to overdose of administered agents. Unwanted interactions most commonly occur when one fails to realise that a drug acting at one receptor may also act at another receptor. Antihistamines, which block H_1 receptors, also have muscarinic anticholinergic activity, for example, as do some phenothiazines and tricyclic antidepressants; co-administration of two or more of these agents can lead to excessive anticholinergic activity.

Pharmacodynamic interactions may also occur when two drugs act at separate sites to cause potentiation, summation or antagonism of their normal actions. Such interactions are often used clinically in the treatment of:

- Angina (e.g. beta blockers and vasodilators).
- Hypertension (beta blockers and diuretics).
- Malignant disease (combined cytotoxic chemotherapy).

However, these interactions may also occur inadvertently. Several drugs, including anabolic steroids, clofibrate, quinidine and salicylates act on the synthesis of vitamin K-dependent clotting factors or the normal coagulation mechanism to potentiate the anticoagulant action of warfarin. Another long-recognized example is the ability of diuretic-induced hypokalaemia to potentiate digoxin toxicity. Even if the effects are only additive rather than synergistic, they may be sufficient to cause adverse effects in some cases.

Sometimes the effect may be more than additive. The estimated relative risk of peptic ulcer in elderly subjects receiving NSAIDs is around four (Griffin *et al.*, 1991). The relative risk in comparable subjects receiving corticosteroids is only 1.1 (Piper *et al.*, 1991). Patients taking both types of compound concomitantly have a risk for peptic ulcer disease 15 times greater than that of non-users of either drug (Piper *et al.*, 1991).

Pharmacodynamic interactions that occur when drugs act at different sites may also result in a loss of drug efficacy. For example, the use of NSAIDs in patients receiving antihypertensive therapy with beta blockers, thiazides and angiotensin-converting enzyme (ACE) inhibitors can result in a loss of antihypertensive action, probably because NSAIDS promote sodium retention.

Risk Factors for Drug–drug Interactions

It is well known that the potential for drug–drug interaction increases both with age and with the number of medications prescribed. As increasing numbers of effective strategies for primary and secondary prevention of disease are discovered, the number of agents that patients receive is also increasing (e.g. in ischaemic heart disease) so this issue will increase in importance in the future.

It is clear that the more dependent patients in institutionalized settings (e.g. nursing homes or long-stay medical wards) have an increased risk of ADRs, including interactions. This may be explained partly by the fact that patients cared for in these establishment are more frail and ill and therefore receive many drugs. Thus residents of nursing homes are often prescribed an average of 5–8 regular medications.

Increased frailty is an important risk factor for ADRs, even in outpatients, and excessive psychotropic medication, which may be used in such individuals, is a particular concern because of the risk of adverse reactions and interactions.

A recent study showed that the number of prescribing physicians was a determinant of the risk of potentially inappropriate drug combinations. The use of a single primary care physician, but particularly the use of a single dispensing pharmacy lowered this risk significantly (Tamblyn *et al.*, 1996).

Detection and Management

These issues are essentially the same as for adverse reactions in general. The physician should maintain a high level of surveillance, particularly when drugs with a low therapeutic ratio are prescribed to patients with a high risk for an adverse interaction.

Avoidance

Guides to intravenous admixture incompatibility exist, but the possibility of their occurrence can be minimized by taking the following precautions:

- Never add a drug to an infusion fluid unless absolutely necessary.
- Never add more than one drug to the syringe or infusion fluid.
- Do not add drugs to whole blood or blood products, amino acid or lipid solutions, mannitol or sodium bicarbonate.

An inordinate proportion of serious adverse interactions occur with relatively few therapeutic agents. These are generally drugs in which the therapeutic ratio (i.e. difference between effective and toxic concentrations), is small, such as oral anticoagulants, cytotoxic drugs, anticonvulsants, and hypotensive and hypoglycaemic agents. The decision to use these agents should be considered carefully and the patient monitored closely.

Drugs may be prescribed for many years without any assessment of their continuing therapeutic role. The list of drugs a patient receives should therefore be regularly reviewed. On some occasions it may be appropriate to withdraw one or more drugs and subsequently monitor the patient. For example, in the elderly it may be possible to consider stopping:

- Digoxin in some patients in sinus rhythm.

- NSAIDs in osteoarthritis.
- Diuretics for idiopathic oedema.
- Neuroleptics such as prochlorperazine prescribed for nausea or 'dizzy turns'.

Great care is recommended in those situations where patients have been on drugs that can produce dependence (e.g. long-term benzodiazepines or barbiturates) since sudden withdrawal can result in a severe withdrawal syndrome. Similarly, gradual withdrawal may be necessary for many agents (e.g. nitrates or beta blockers used in angina or anticonvulsants used in epilepsy) to avoid rebound, with worsening of the condition. Nevertheless, a shorter drug list is an important factor in reducing the risk of interactions.

Drug–drug interactions may not be immediately obvious when combinations are first prescribed, so patients should be encouraged to form a 'prescribing partnership', alerting doctors and other prescribers to symptoms that occur when new drugs are introduced. Nonspecific complaints such as confusion, lethargy, weakness, dizzy turns, incontinence, depression and falling should all prompt a closer look at the patient's drug list. The patient should be warned of the dangers of taking new medications (particularly over-the-counter remedies) without obtaining advice concerning potential interactions. The fewer people prescribing for the patient, the lower the risk that an interaction will occur iatrogenically (Tamblyn *et al.*, 1996).

On a broader front, more sensitive and reliable parameters of drug effect are needed. It is reassuring to note that when physicians have a reliable and simple measure of drug effect, (e.g. for anticoagulants with the one-stage prothrombin time) drug interactions are often quickly recognized and therapy can be adjusted appropriately.

Conclusions

Adverse drug reactions, of which drug–drug interactions are a special category, are a significant cause of morbidity and occasionally cause fatality. The risk of serious ADRs is highest for only a few drug groups (e.g. cytotoxics, hypotensives, NSAIDs, hypoglycaemics and oral anticoagulants) and in certain groups (e.g. the frail elderly and those with renal or liver disease or heart failure). Adverse drug reactions may be difficult to detect because they can mimic other diseases and may have very few specific features. In addition, there are often few specific or sensitive in-vitro tests and rechallenge to the agent may be precluded because of a possible severe response.

The diagnosis of ADRs reactions may therefore have to rely on circumstantial evidence, based on the time course of onset relative to the introduction of the drug or change in dose and the response to dose withdrawal or drug discontinuation.

Fortunately, many ADRs and adverse drug interactions can be avoided with a knowledge of basic pharmacological principles and judicious choice of drugs and doses. When an ADR is suspected, a report to the regulatory authority will help identify risks and inform decisions about risk–benefit, and thus help to protect others from similar problems in the future.

Chapter 3

Toxicology and Adverse Drug Reactions

A. D. Dayan

DH Dept of Toxicology, St Bartholomew's and the Royal London School of Medicine and Dentistry, Charterhouse Square, London EC1M 6BQ, UK

Toxicology, the study of harmful effects, has two distinct roles in relation to adverse reactions to medicines. One is to use various laboratory procedures to predict toxicity before clinical use of the substance and so to suggest therapeutic circumstances in which adverse actions are unlikely to occur. The other is to find the causes of adverse reactions detected in man in order to understand how to avoid them, or failing that, how to minimize and treat them if the toxic risk is outweighed by the therapeutic benefit of continued prescription of the medicine.

Prediction of Toxicity

Toxicity Testing

This is the familiar role of regulatory toxicity testing of candidate drugs, in which extensive studies are carried out to comply with official requirements, as well as additional investigations adapted to the particular properties of the drug.

The range and purpose of conventional studies are shown in Table 1, together with additional studies, which are not always regarded as part of toxicology, but are essential if the toxic risk of the substance is to be understood. In addition, and of equal importance, are other experiments focused on any special susceptibility of the group being treated (e.g. secondary to the effects of the disease), and on individual physiological factors also specific to particular groups of patients (e.g. extremes of age, pregnancy, malnutrition or race) (Table 2).

Nature of Toxicity

The guiding principles of this very extensive set of required experiments, all of which should conform to the GLP regulations, are to demonstrate toxic actions. It is important to realise that toxicity (considered as chemically induced harmful effects) may be:

Table 1   Nature and purposes of non-clinical regulatory toxicity testing (all conform to good laboratory practice—GLP)

Test type	Special features	Nature of data obtained
Acute toxicity	Single high dose by therapeutic and parenteral route; carried out in rodents and often in non-rodents; follow for up to 14 days	Clinical effects on major physiological systems; indication of possible effects of 'poisoning'
Subacute to chronic toxicity	Control group and three dose levels given by therapeutic route for 2–52 weeks depending on anticipated use; rat and non-rodent species	Many clinical observations, effects on blood cells and clinical chemistry, autopsy and extensive histological survey; measure blood drug levels; shows target organ toxicity and dose (blood level) – toxic response relationship; may include special study of endocrine or physiological effects if appropriate
Carcinogenicity	Control group and three dose levels by therapeutic route (at present) for 2 years; rats and mice	Incidence and nature of neoplasms of solid tissues and blood cells and dose (blood level) – response
Genetic toxicity	Standard set of Ames, cytogenetics *in vitro* and *in vivo*, and point mutation test in mammalian cells; include hepatic S9 metabolizing system *in vitro*.	Indicates harm to DNA and chromosomes
Reproduction toxicity	Segment I—fertility (rat); Segment II—fetal and maternal toxicity and teratogenicity (rat and rabbit); segment III—peri- and postnatal toxicity to dams and pups (rat); all controls and three dose levels	Clinical anatomical and some behavioural observations; dose (blood/milk) level – response data; indicates toxic effects on germ cell production, mating, pregnancy, fetal development, nursing behaviour and postnatal development to maturity
Topical testing for drugs applied locally	Tests of acute–chronic irritancy at site of application; immunological sensitizing potential on skin; local irritancy to skin, eye, airways, etc.; haemolytic and thrombogenic potential	Local effects shown and the dose–response relationship
Further studies for evaluation of toxicity toxicokinetics	In-vivo and increasingly in-vitro studies of metabolism, and of absorption, distribution and excretion of drug and metabolites	Extensive information about handling of substance in animals for comparison with man; species differences; local accumulation; major paths of metabolism and elimination
Safety pharmacology	Classical pharmacological procedures to seek actions on cardiovascular, respiratory, urinary, gastrointestinal and central nervous systems, and on smooth muscle	Functional effects of a range of doses and counter-regulatory responses

Table 2 Special toxicity tests carried out if appropriate

Test type	Special features	Nature of data obtained
Toxicokinetics	Possible effect of genetic polymorphism; effects of physiological variation such as immaturity or age; effect of disease of organ of elimination; *in vitro* or *in vivo*	Demonstrate effects of these factors on metabolic activation and detoxification and on elimination of drug
Drug interactions	Explore effects of other medicines co-administered to the patient	Toxicokinetic and pharmacological interactions to be considered
Treatment of poisoning	Evaluation of available data and possible experimentation	Prove specific antidote; demonstrate supportive measures; show value of generic treatments

- Functional or dynamic—for example a change in blood pressure or cardiac conduction, or in behaviour or other clinically visible effects.
- Biochemical—for example a change in blood glucose or a change in an indicator of damage to a tissue, such as an increase in plasma aspartate aminotiansferase (AST) due to damage to liver cells, in creatinine due to renal damage and in blood clotting factors.
- Structural (i.e. demonstrated pathologically as a change in, for example, liver weight, histological appearance of a tissue, blood cells).

Most toxicity tests, therefore, are general studies that survey a very large number of endpoints in order to detect abnormalities and to relate them to the administered dose, and often to the blood level of the drug or of active metabolites as indices of systemic (internal) exposure.

In reproduction and genetic toxicity experiments, the potential harmful effects may be manifest in the present generation (e.g. loss of fertility or genetic damage as a precursor of tumorigenicity) or in succeeding generations (e.g. teratogenesis and mutation). Time is therefore an important aspect of toxicity, whether as acute, delayed, latent or chronic effects, or related to effects in the present or a succeeding generation.

Acceptance and Interpretation of Toxicity Test Findings

The Valid Experiment

There are a number of essential critical steps between the decision to carry out a toxicity test and acceptance of the final evaluation about the conclusions. Some are concerned with background regulatory or technical factors, and others are critical to the scientific value of the results.

Principal Regulatory and Technical Factors
These are:

- Does the test fully comply with the GLP regulations?

- Is it consistent with current International Conference of Harmonization (ICH) and national guidelines about test type, duration, dose levels, replicates and numbers of animals or appropriate in-vitro system.

Principal Scientific Factors Affecting Validity

The factors to consider are:

- Were appropriate observations made to allow a general survey for toxic actions or investigation of a specific effect?
- Was the duration of the dosing and any recovery phase adequate for effects to occur and to recover (and in relation to the planned period of therapeutic use)?
- Were the dose levels appropriate in relation to the proposed human dose, or better, were blood levels in the test animals (or concentrations in in-vitro systems) sufficient to demonstrate the relationship between dose (systemic or local exposure) and response, and yet not so high as to result in non-linear kinetics or other irrelevant actions?
- At a more subtle level, might toxicity be due to a metabolite rather than the parent drug? If so, and if the metabolism and kinetics in man are known, was the species (or in-vitro system) appropriate because of reasonable similarity of metabolism and kinetics in it?

Once there are suitable answers to all these questions, the finding of toxicity and its converse (the lack of other effects) can be accepted as scientifically valid and potentially useful for regulatory purposes.

Interpretation of Toxicity

There are several sequential and some interactive steps to be considered before concluding that a compound has caused a certain toxic effect under the stated experimental conditions, and that it is relevant to evaluating a risk to man, the ultimate goal of this type of toxicity testing:

- Is there a pattern to the toxic actions?
- What is the relationship between toxicity and the dose (or better the systemic exposure represented by the plasma level of the drug or active metabolite)?
- Is the toxicologist certain that the abnormal findings are not due to chance effects or random variation and are not specific to the test species or in-vitro system.

Toxicity tests, especially those carried out for regulatory purposes, deliberately include many overlapping observations. It is important to decide whether the numerous changes found represent different effects or whether they are different expressions of the same toxic action; for example, suppose that a New Chemical Entity (NCE) was a vasodilator and that it had lowered the blood pressure. This might result in visible reddening of the extremities due to cutaneous vasodilation. If there was marked hypotension, the animal's behaviour would be abnormal, and there would probably be a compensatory tachycardia. Severe hypotension can impair the blood supply to critical organs such as the heart, kidney and brain so severely that their function fails; local necrosis and vascular damage may even ensue, resulting in rises in the levels of the plasma enzyme that denote cell necrosis, for example alanine aminotransferase (ALT) and AST, an increase in plasma urea, changes in the electrocardiogram, histologically detectable necrosis and a reactive polymorphonuclear leucocytosis. Although independent findings, all these effects represent different facets of the same basic effect (i.e. hypotension).

Understanding the pattern of toxicity, if there is one, is essential because it prevents overdiagnosis of innumerable separate effects when all are consequences of the same process. Appreciating the pattern is even more important because its overall nature may suggest the causal mechanism of the toxic effect, and understanding the mechanism will provide a strong basis for extrapolating actions observed experimentally to man—the real purpose of toxicity testing.

Considered expert judgement is required in drawing the final conclusion that compound X causes a particular toxic effect under certain conditions of dosage and route and duration of treatment. If possible, such a conclusion should also indicate the proven or likely toxic mechanism.

The overall strengths and weaknesses of toxicity testing relative to the clinical experience of patients are set out in Table 3.

Table 3   Role of the toxicologist in investigating adverse effects (AEs) caused by drugs

Initial analysis	Pathogenetic evaluation	Possible toxicological investigations
Does the nature or pattern of the effect suggest it is a pathogenetic mechanism? Is it probably a Type A or a Type B AE?	Type A ADRs: Is it due to non-clinical, pharmacodynamic, pharmacological or toxic properties of the drug? Is the ADR due to an overdose or some other cause of excess systemic exposure (e.g. slow elimination, drug interaction etc.)? If not, could the ADR be due to a toxic metabolite or a biological mechanism specific to humans?	Assess plasma/blood drug level; reconsider dose–response data; re-evaluate pharmacokinetics Focused studies of kinetics and metabolism *in vivo* or *in vitro*; interaction experiments, etc.; toxicokinetic–toxicodynamic modelling Experiments on human or animal tissues; search for genetic polymorphisms etc.
Mechanism uncertain because of functional or complex nature of ADR	Examine data and, as available, material from man to try to discover pathogenesis or at least mechanism of abnormality	Broad attempt to reproduce ADR-like process in tissue culture or animals for more detailed study
	Type B ADR: Immunologically-based	Assay specific humoral and cell-mediated immunity and nonspecific immunity; Is there any relation to the patient's genotype or to other physiological factors Try to reproduce the ADR in a laboratory system Consider possible genetic polymorphism and explore a model system
	'Idiosyncratic' or cause not apparent	Evaluate pathological process for clues to mechanism; consider investigating local dysfunctional effects at site of application, if appropriate

It should also be possible to indicate the reversibility (recovery) of toxic actions and to state the 'no observed adverse effect level' (NOAEL), the dose at which no toxic action can be detected.

Extrapolation to Man

Using these conclusions, the following further expert judgement is required to predict effects in patients:

- What is the target dose or plasma level in patients to produce the desired therapeutic effect? How far below the NOAEL in animals is that dose (or plasma level)? This must include consideration of the probable variation in dosing in man, the possibility that there are susceptible individuals due, for example, to genetic polymorphism in metabolism, normal variation in toxicodynamic sensitivity, toxicokinetic and toxicodynamic interactions with age, the effects of the disease, dietary habits (e.g. influencing absorption), or other co-administered medicines.
- Is there previous experience of the chemical or pharmacological class of drug to suggest that the toxicity is specific to certain animal species (e.g. the unique responses of dogs and cats to opiates, the great sensitivity of rodents to coumarin anticoagulants, and the much greater susceptibility of rodents than of man to hepatic enzyme induction and liver tumours)?

Given such precautions, the results of toxicity testing can be used to predict the likelihood and nature of toxic actions in patients at various dose levels, or better in relation to systemic exposure as represented by the plasma concentration.

Care should always be taken not to dose people in such ways that a toxic exposure is achieved, but the experiments, and especially the link between dose and effect, will suggest when harmful effects might occur, and their nature (which will show particular processes to monitor in people), severity and probable reversibility.

The experimentally determined toxic profile of a new chemical entity (NCE), like its pharmacodynamic profile, is a qualitative and partly quantitative prediction of harmful effects in man. Well-designed toxicity tests will suggest what may happen in people under certain circumstances, and careful evaluation of the nature of these actions, possibly supplemented by specific analytical investigations, will suggest the causal mechanisms. Such a set of information will permit a sound and reasonably comprehensive prediction of harmful actions that may occur in the clinic.

Toxicological Investigation of Adverse Effects in Man

General Nature of Adverse Effects

The general nature of ADRs in man is discussed in detail elsewhere in this book. For the toxicologist, they can initially be divided into:

- Type A—dose-related and predictable and due to conventional toxic mechanisms.
- Type B—not related to dose, unpredictable, often rare and usually due to particular individual susceptibility acting via an immunological or other process.

It is also helpful to consider the following general pathophysiological processes involved in causing ADRs:

- Excess of the therapeutic pharmacodynamic action. This may be due to an overdose or sometimes to unusual sensitivity, (e.g. if elimination or protein binding of the drug is impaired in certain subjects). These ADRs are commonly functional in nature.
- Excess of other pharmacological actions of the drug. The causes are similar to those mentioned above. Again, the adverse effects are commonly functional.
- Target organ toxicity. This is the 'standard' type of effect that is commonly regarded as toxicity (e.g. damage to the liver, skin, blood cells, etc.).
- Hypersensitivity. The more frequent form, albeit a rare type of ADR, is due to true immunological hypersensitivity and so requires previous exposure to cause sensitization and subsequent challenge to elicit the response. The ADR may be mediated via antibodies (IgE > IgG > IgM) or sensitized T cells. Common examples include skin rashes, asthma-like reactions and peripheral neuropathy. Often included in this group are a few 'idiosyncratic' responses which may be associated with the first dose (so previous sensitization cannot have occurred), but which may produce a similar spectrum of clinical disorders; for example a skin rash, but possibly even the acute and more serious anaphylactoid reaction. There is no evidence of an immunological basis to the reaction.

The Toxicologist's Role in Adverse Drug Reactions

When an ADR has been detected, it is essential to find out what has caused it, as well as deciding upon its severity and recoverability, and how to treat and prevent it. The toxicologist can help in several ways, working in conjunction with clinicians, other clinical scientists and pharmacologists (see Table 3). The objective is to discover the causal process and the mechanism of the ADR so that it is then possible to decide on rational grounds what the true risk is to man. If firm proof of the toxic action cannot be obtained, the pragmatic approach of showing that there is a threshold exposure below which it does not occur may help to define circumstances in which there will not be harm to humans, but it is better to reveal the pathogenetic mechanisms involved. Accordingly, the role of the toxicologist in relation to dealing with AEs detected in man can be summarized as investigation of the cause; mechanism, prevention and treatment of an ADR.

Investigation of the cause of an ADR involves:

- Examination of the relationship to dosing and exposure.
- Comparison with known actions of the NCE and dose–response relationship.
- Consideration of species-specific kinetics and metabolism.
- Establishing a model system.

Investigation of the mechanism of an ADR involves:

- Examination of the process by which the AE is produced (e.g. necrosis of cells in an organ, dysfunction of a secretory process).

Table 4   **Strengths and weaknesses of animal toxicity tests and adverse effects in man**

Strengths	Weaknesses	Comments
Carefully structured experiments	Variable ways in which patients take medicines	Many important variables controlled
Defined animals (restricted gene pool)	Random, outbred human population	Considerable experience and background knowledge; interindividual variation
Sufficient numbers for precision and power	Limited numbers	As there are millions of patients tests may not reveal rare effects
Commonly use young animals		Age range of patient population
Commonly use healthy animals		? effects of diseases
Understanding of toxicodynamics and toxicokinetics		Species differences
Wide range of controlled doses	Limited control over timing and in relation to meals	Do patients follow instructions?
Effect of reversibility and recovery explored		
Biochemical and pathological effects studies > dysfunction	Limited range of functional endpoints	Disorders of function more important as causes of ADRs in man
Reveal Type A dose-related toxicity	Do not show Type B 'idiosyncratic' toxicity	Type A more common than Type B
Adaptable to new understanding	Slow incorporation of novel procedures under GLP	Slow uptake of new knowledge
Wide range of activities assessable	GLP approach may restrain adoption of new toxic effect detection	Must adapt endpoints to actions of NCE
Explore mechanism	Possible species specificity	Understanding mechanism not always essential for extrapolation of toxicity
Examine any route and duration of dosing	Difficulty of certain routes (e.g. intrathecal and intrauterine)	Problems posed by novel routes and slow-release preparations
	Limited understanding of toxicity affecting immune system, behaviour and development	Basic knowledge also limited in humans
Show carcinogenicity and genotoxicity	Species differences	May risk overprediction of risk; limited knowledge in man
Qualitative and quantitative risk assessment possible	Limited power	Quantitative modelling of toxicity rarely feasible
Ethics—protect humans	Ethics and understanding limit experiments	Ethics, professional needs and legal codes enforce controlled experimentation

- Exploration of the dose–response relationship.
- Establishing a model system.

The toxicologist may also be able to advise on the most sensitive or appropriate indicators of the toxic action suitable for monitoring in man.

In investigation of the prevention and treatment of an ADR, broad toxicological data and understanding the processes involved may make it possible to advise on the most suitable means to treat the ADR, as well as on suitable indicators of progression and increasing severity that might justify more vigorous treatment. Such advice may involve:

- Preventing or limiting exposure.
- Altering route or timing of treatment.
- Specific antidote.
- If an ADR is severe, consideration of oral adsorbent therapy or haemodialysis as appropriate.
- Advice on the appropriate general supportive therapy.
- In the exceedingly unlikely event of findings suggestive of a late and severe or transmissible ADR, such as tumorigenesis, teratogenesis or mutagenesis, clinical advice, counselling and follow-up of exposed subjects may be suggested.

Overview

The toxicologist concerned with drug development and usage has to steer a careful path between carrying out the minimum studies to meet limited regulatory requirements and following more analytical investigation of the toxic effects observed in the laboratory. The first goal, however, is to detect toxic actions and to understand the circumstances under which they may occur in humans in order to predict the toxic risks of a given treatment.

If AEs are detected in man the toxicologist's primary concerns are to understand enough of their causes to know whether their occurrence can be predicted from available non-clinical and early clinical data. If not, investigation is needed into why the AE occurred and its mechanism to be able to predict the risk in future patients. Thus, toxicology has both a predictive and an analytical role in dealing with adverse drug effects in man, as well as providing guidance on treatment, and especially on prevention.

Chapter 4

Methodology for the Collection of Adverse Event Data in Clinical Trials

M. D. B. Stephens

Chapter 1 has reviewed all of the types of symptoms and signs that may occur in healthy volunteers and patients. A specific illness does not preclude ill patients from experiencing many of the same AEs as a healthy person in addition to those due to their illness. Should details of all AEs be collected? This will depend upon several factors:

- The indication for the drug. If the drug is given for a mild illness then even very mild AEs may be relevant. If the drug is given for a disease that leads to death such as secondary cancer or acquired immunodeficiency syndrome (AIDS) then minor discomforts may be less relevant.
- The stage or phase of the clinical trial programme. Exact details of minor symptoms are usually relevant for phase I studies but once an adverse drug reaction (ADR) has been characterized (see ADR profile on page 44) counting the numbers of events may suffice.
- The type of potential ADRs. Standardized enquiry is often needed for psychiatric studies and specialized laboratory examinations are necessary for some drug-induced diseases.
- A signal (the first hint of an ADR) of a possible ADR halfway through a clinical trial programme may require changes to the methods of collecting data.
- The ADR profiles of other drugs of the same class or for the same indication may indicate the type of AE to be expected. The animal toxicology or pharmacology will also be a guide to possible ADRs and indicate the methods suitable for collecting AEs.
- It is important that the clinical trialist makes a diagnosis wherever possible, rather than just listing of signs and symptoms. When the diagnosis is in the form of a

syndrome, such as an organ failure, the cause should be given whenever possible (e.g. left sided cardiac failure due to hypertension; Nickas, 1995).

• AE collection during a clinical trial programme does not need to be standardized throughout the programme, but must be consistent. The addition of a questionnaire to one study should not disrupt the analysis as long as the other standard methods of collection are not missed out. Different questionnaires for a single drug programme should only be used if the drug programme is for two separate indications.

Factors Affecting Collection of Adverse Events

In order to collect AEs efficiently it is necessary to know which factors might hinder their collection so that they can be circumvented. Between the advent of an AE and its final assessment as an ADR the AE must be communicated. Factors preventing this communication include failure of the patient to recognize the AE or to communicate it to the doctor and failure of the doctor to recognize it as a possible ADR or to report it as an ADR.

The patient may fail to recognize the AE for the following reasons:

(a)   There are no symptoms, (i.e. biochemical change, hypertension, etc.).
(b)   There is a change in mood, *which is* only recognized by relatives or friends.
(c)   There is a lack of intelligence or mental illness (Petrie and Levine, 1978).

The patient may fail to communicate the AE to the doctor because:

(a)   The patient does not connect the AE with the drug and therefore does not consider it to be relevant.
(b)   The patient recognizes the event as a possible ADR (e.g. from the patient leaflet), but presumes that one has to put up with it.
(c)   The patient recognizes the event as a possible ADR and stops the drug, but does not mention it to the doctor.
(d)   The patient does not inform the doctor for fear of being thought neurotic or because the doctor inhibits the patient by tone of voice, interruptions or poor bedside manner.
(e)   The patient has a poor memory. Volunteers' memories have been shown to be poor for minor events after two weeks (see pages 13–14).

The doctor may fail to recognize the AE as a possible ADR because:

• The doctor does not give the patient the opportunity to communicate the AE due to a poor relationship with the patient.
• The doctor listens to the patient, but fails to consider the possibility of an AE.
• The doctor fails to take positive steps to look for well-known side effects (i.e. does not ask questions and/or examine patient).

The doctor recognize the AE as a possible ADR, but does not report it because of:

• Complacency, thinking that it is too minor to report.
• Fear of litigation.

- Guilt at causing the patient to suffer.
- Ambition to collect and publish a series. (This is more relevant to post-marketing spontaneous reporting.)
- Ignorance of the mechanism of reporting. Does this happen in clinical trials?
- Diffidence in reporting doubtful ADRs.
- Lethargy—too busy, etc. (Inman, 1986).

Filtration of Adverse Events Using Protocols and Forms

Bearing in mind the factors that can prevent the reporting of an AE to the pharmaceutical company, steps can be taken to overcome them during any company organized studies by using a study protocol and forms for collecting data as well as an explanation by a clinical research associate (CRA). The wording of the protocol and the form design need to be appropriate to the stage in the drugs development. The overall framework necessary is outlined in Table 1.

This framework is not intended to be comprehensive, but to give a general outline of the changes required during the development of a drug. Stage 1 represents the early part of the drug's development with relatively small, closely controlled, clinical trials. The numbers involved in each study increase with progression through the stages, finishing at stage 5, which is suitable for post-marketing surveys involving very large numbers of users and may be exemplified by the asthma deaths surveys (Inman and Adelstein, 1969). The studies progress from stage 1, where there is no filtration of AEs, to stage 2 where only the replies to a standard question and spontaneously reported events are recorded, and then to stage 3, when symptoms alone are filtered out and only clinical diagnoses are reported. In stage 4 general practitioner diagnoses are filtered out and only events severe enough to require hospital attention or having possible sequelae are reported. Stage 5 is the ultimate: only deaths are reported, all else having been filtered out. When a study is planned, the aim of the study must be worded so that the appropriate AEs and diagnoses are collected and recorded.

Collection of Adverse Events

During Treatment

The basic principle is to collect AEs that have appeared while the patient is on the drug and in the immediate period after stopping the drug as well as any AE that was present at baseline but has become worse on treatment (Skegg and Doll, 1977). These are sometimes called 'treatment emergent signs and symptoms' (TESS). A recent history of an AE immediately before the study may influence the assessment if a related event occurs on treatment. For example the sudden onset of blindness in a patient in the early days of a clinical trial led three professors to conclude that it was due to the drug since there had been some ocular changes in animals. However, the patient had recently come from a different part of the country and follow-up at the previous hospital revealed three episodes of amaurosis fugax (transient episodic blindness, before the study and unknown to the trialists.

Table 1 Collecting adverse events at different stages of clinical studies

Stage	Adverse events to be collected	Doctor's action (clinical trialist)	Protocol design	Form design
1 Suitable for phase 2–3–4 studies. Double blind controlled studies.	Mild symptoms but forgotten if not prompted. Will include a lot of non-drug non-disease events.	Not mentioned spontaneously to doctor.	Adverse event reporting to be stressed and will include the working of a standard question	(a) Patients' diary card (b) Patient questionnaire (c) Doctor's checklist + (d) Standard question
2 Suitable for uncontrolled studies.	Mild symptoms. Remembered but will only be mentioned spontaneously if given the opportunity.	Doctor must give patient the opportunity to report adverse events by the use of a standard questionnaire.	Should include a standard patient question at each visit.	Adequate space for patient's reply at each visit.
3 Suitable for GP surveys or uncontrolled studies.	Moderate symptoms. Remembered and mentioned to doctor.	Doctor must be encouraged to take full history and examine patient and make clinical diagnosis.	Requests all doctors to report clinical diagnosis.	Space for clinical diagnosis.
4 Suitable for certain monitored release studies.	Moderate to severe illness.	1. Referred to hospital or second opinion. 2. Serious illness with possible sequelae. 3. Death.	1. Requests all details of hospital or out-patient visits. 2. Defined illnesses. 3. Requests details.	1. Space for final diagnosis. Hospital name and address, and consultant's name. 2. Details.
5 Suitable for certain case–control studies and epidemiological surveys.	Death.	Death certificate (unreliable as a source of diagnostic data even when certified by hospital clinicians) (Cameron and McGregor, 1981).	Epidemiological surveys.	Details can be obtained from Office for Census and Surveys but death certificates are rarely reliable when filled in by general practitioners. (Gau and Diehl, 1982)

It is now common for companies to collect AEs with a specially designed company form and Astra Hassle in Sweden was one of the pioneers in this area (Wallander and Palmer, 1986). However, the company discovered that a substantial number of AEs were recorded not on the special form, but elsewhere in the case record book (73.7% were on the correct form, 26.3% were found elsewhere). In older studies the percentage found elsewhere was 33–36% while for studies starting in 1986 the figure was only 13%. Moreover in the older studies, those found elsewhere were often serious events, 42% compared with 26% on the correct form. This ratio subsequently reversed so that by 1989 no serious AEs and only 14% of non-serious AEs were not on the correct form. It therefore behoves drug safety staff to make certain that the whole of the clinical trial record book is searched for AEs and that there is a satisfactory clinical record form (CRF) design, instructions and investigator training (Wallander *et al.*, 1992).

If a checklist or questionnaire is going to be used it needs to cover the same time interval on each occasion and since minor events are soon forgotten the interval should not be longer than two weeks. Wallander found that a questionnaire revealed events primarily from the preceding week despite asking about the previous month (Wallander *et al.*, 1991). This means that there should be a baseline question, questionnaire or checklist that covers the previous one or two weeks followed by the same question, questionnaire or checklist one or two weeks later. This allows easy recognition increased frequency of headaches for example. The subsequent intervals between visits should preferably be the same; but this is not essential since it is possible to compare the events occurring with the trial drug and comparator over the same period. If the intention is to pick up minor AEs the intervals should not exceed two weeks and preferably one week. If the study is for longer than four weeks it is preferable to have at least two visits while on the drug (one in the middle of treatment and another on the last day of treatment) and a post-treatment visit. In a long study weekly questionnaires may overburden the patient and their enthusiasm to fill them might diminish. The only way to circumvent this problem might be to use the questionnaire to highlight crucial points (i.e. the week before adding the study medication and the week after so as to pick up the most common type A ADRs). Other crucial points are the start of the run-in period and dechallenge.

The Post-treatment Visit

Little has been published in the literature on post-treatment visits following therapeutic clinical trials. Spilker considers their main purpose is to check for any withdrawal effects and to ensure the patient's safety, but says they may also be used to study residual effects of treatment (Spilker, 1984). He lists five factors that should govern whether or not a post-treatment period is needed:

1. Previous experience with the drug in similar patient populations.
2. Whether the drug dosage is being tapered slowly or stopped abruptly.
3. The clinical status of the patient.
4. Whether patients are in a secure and/or controlled environment.
5. The pharmacokinetic characteristics of the drug.

Friedman *et al.* (1985) describe two types of post-study follow-up. The first is a short-term follow-up, which should be considered when 'intervention' is stopped at the last treatment visit in order to find out how soon laboratory values or symptomatology return to baseline. The second type is a long-term follow-up, monitoring possible toxicity or benefit.

The authoritative guidelines of the Fogarty Conference (1979) for the detection of hepatotoxicity recommend that in early clinical trials of new drugs (phase 2) laboratory tests should be performed at 24 hours, 5–7 days and 4–6 weeks after the last dose. In short-term studies (less than six months) the follow-up should be for two months and that following long-term studies (six months or more) should be for two years, and 20 years in a small subset of patients. This rather draconian regimen has not been challenged in the literature. These recommendations are obviously intended to detect adverse reactions with a very delayed onset such as fibrosis, cirrhosis, vascular lesions or neoplasms.

Leaving aside the use of a post-treatment period for further observation of the efficacy or lack of efficacy, in drug studies and also the need for a long post-treatment period of observation under special circumstances for specific purposes (e.g. carcinogenesis), routine post-treatment visit that includes examination and a routine laboratory screen is essential for all pre-marketing studies for the four reasons outlined below.

To Review the Laboratory Data from the Samples Taken at the Last Visit while on Treatment

The results of a laboratory test may take a week or more to reach the clinician: if it is abnormal it may or may not be of clinical significance. If it is of clinical significance it needs to be followed up until it is normal or a definite cause is found since it may represent an ADR or a new disease or complication of an underlying disease. If it is abnormal but of no clinical significance it may be an early sign of an ADR or new disease or complication of an old disease or a chance variation from normal. A repeated individual test value is unlikely to be abnormal by chance (1 in 40). Clinical enquiry, and if necessary an examination and further tests, may resolve whether or not the abnormality is due to the drug or disease. These arguments are usually countered by saying that the clinician only needs to send an appointment for a further visit if the final result on treatment is abnormal and thereby avoids wasting the patient's time and money. Unfortunately, experience shows that clinical trialists do not always recall the patient unless the result is of 'clinical significance'; this 'elastic' term is not defined and varies with many factors.

To Detect any Delayed ADR

A rare type B ADR may not appear until after a drug has been stopped, for example jaundice (Isaacs *et al.*, 1955) or aplastic anaemia (Pisciotta, 1978). The fialuridine disaster in which five of 15 patients with chronic hepatitis B died from drug-induced hepatotoxicity that developed 9–13 weeks after treatment will have repercussions for many years (McKenzie *et al.*, 1995). The Food and Drug Administration (FDA) said that the pharmaceutical company had violated federal rules (*Reactions*, 1994; *Scrip*, 1994) including those involving informed consent forms (Horton, 1994). There was considerable media coverage (Cimons, 1993; Hilts, 1993; McGinley, 1994) and a review of all studies with the drug (Manning and Swartz, 1995). The FDA set up a task force, which produced a report issued in November 1995 (Witt *et al*, 1993). Meanwhile the FDA issued certain rules in October 1994 (Federal Register, 1994), that the Pharmaceutical Research and Manufacturers of America (PhRMA) objected to (*Scrip*, 1995). These were subsequently withdrawn, but will be replaced by guidelines (still awaited, August 1998). In the meantime there has been an open letter to the FDA regarding changes in reporting procedures (Meinert, 1996).

It can be countered that a post-treatment questionnaire would detect any ADR of which the patient was aware and could be followed up by a further appointment. This is true and may well be necessary if the patient lives a long way from the clinical trial centre, but this will not allow early detection of laboratory abnormalities, which may presage a serious AE (e.g. as with fialuridine). If only one of the laboratory parameters investigated at the post-treatment visit is abnormal and all previous values related to the relevant organ have been normal, further follow-up is probably not justified if the abnormality is less than 25% of the reference range beyond the limit of normal (*Reactions*, 1994). This extended range is the equivalent of the mean plus or minus three standard deviations, so a chance abnormality beyond this range should not occur more often than three cases in every thousand.

To Detect any Signs or Symptoms Due to Drug Withdrawal or a Rebound Phenomenon

It is important that it is shown that drugs used in psychiatric disease are not followed by drug withdrawal symptoms similar to those with benzodiazepines (Busto *et al.*, 1986). Any rebound phenomena should occur during the first week after stopping treatment, for example beta blocker rebound (Lancet leader, 1975).

To Ascertain the Response of any Adverse Medical Events to Dechallenge

The response to dechallenge is an important factor in the assessment of an AE occurring while on treatment (Stephens, 1985; Stephens, 1995). If there has been a positive dechallenge then the possibility of a rechallenge should be considered if it is both feasible and ethical. The terms 'reversible' or 'transient' should not be used in the data sheet without a positive dechallenge after drug-induced abnormal laboratory parameters or adverse medical events unless tolerance has been shown to occur to the extent of reversing the AE completely.

Disadvantages of a Post-treatment Visit

The visit is an additional inconvenience for both the patient and the clinical trialist and an additional cost for the patient and the pharmaceutical company. These are counterbalanced by the assurance that no lasting harm has been caused to the patient. However, if a chronic disease requires replacement of the trial drug by another treatment then this latter treatment may cause an ADR by itself and it may be difficult to distinguish between a delayed ADR due to the trial drug and that caused by the replacement treatment. This problem could be overcome by replacement with placebo or a well-known drug with known side effects. A more frequent problem occurs when the AE itself is treated, thereby confounding the response to dechallenge, but this should only occur rarely since most ADRs reverse rapidly when treatment is stopped. It could also be argued that in placebo-controlled studies only those who have been on active treatment require a further visit, but the placebo control may also be necessary in this part of the study if abnormalities are present after the active treatment and to avoid unblinding the study. Also any complications or sequelae of the underlying disease may be difficult to differentiate from a delayed ADR. These can be countered as there should be an equal incidence in the control group.

The reasons for the post-treatment visit dictate the duration of the follow-up period.

The results of the laboratory tests must be available at the time of the visit and sufficient time must be given for AEs to reverse tangibly and for any withdrawal symptoms and any rebound phenomena to manifest themselves. These events should have occurred within one week; a delayed ADR may take longer, and two-week interval is probably a reasonable compromise. However cholestatic hepatitis may appear up to four weeks after stopping treatment and in the case of co-amoxiclav up to five weeks later. This suggests that a visit at one month would be more reasonable. Since pseudomembranous colitis may develop up to three weeks after stopping an antibiotic one month would be suitable despite the short period of treatment. When the study has a crossover design the intermediary washout period should act as a post-treatment period following the first drug and be equal in duration to the post-treatment observation periods following the second drug. In phase 2 studies where treatment is continued for less than one week, a 24-hour visit followed by a 5–7-day visit may suffice if the patient is told to notify the clinical trialist of any delayed AEs. Few would challenge the expertise of the Fogarty Conference, but long-term follow-up introduces new problems. Rather than reassuring the patient the long-term follow-up may cause the patient to worry unnecessarily about the possibility of long-delayed AEs. Following up a cohort of patients for two years pose great practical problems, even with a nationalized health service, and must be more difficult in other circumstances.

It is also reasonable to recommend a routine post-treatment visit following post-marketing clinical trials for subgroups of patients who may be prone to ADRs such as the young, the elderly and those with organ failure. There may also be hypotheses arising from animal testing or from clinical events with similar drugs that will require long-term follow-up for specific purposes. Long-term follow-up to ensure that no serious ADRs such as aplastic anaemia or a fialuridine-type problem have occurred (i.e. at about nine months) might be accomplished by regular telephone interviews with the patient and/or general practitioner.

Conclusion

The increased protection for the patient, the additional information required for assessment of any AEs and better knowledge of the safety of a drug that should result from routine post-treatment visits make them essential and they may need to be repeated under certain circumstances.

Separation of Adverse Reactions from Placebo Reactions

Since adverse non-drug symptoms are common (Reidenberg and Lowenthal, 1968) and are not easily separated from drug-induced symptoms, both must be collected for analysis if a complete profile of adverse reactions is to be made. However, this technique can only be used in controlled studies, ideally with placebo, as well as with other standard drugs. The temptation to subtract the number of the particular AE in the placebo group from the number in the active drug group as follows:

Drug group−Placebo group=Number of adverse reactions to drugs. (Lasagna, 1984)

should be resisted because:

- The difference may not be statistically significant and may have arisen by chance.
- Although the total number of events may be statistically different in the two treatment groups, it is also necessary to establish whether the numbers of patients afflicted with the AE are different and vice versa.
- Having established that there is a significant difference between the two treatment groups for the number of events and the number of patients afflicted, the severity of the ADRs in the two groups should be compared.

A further problem is that due to classification. Some terms may include more than one type of abnormality (e.g. the incidence of 'blurred vision' may be equal in both groups, but there may be several cases of tunnel vision with the trial drug but because there is no code for tunnel vision it is coded under a more general term). Another problem is that the symptoms forming a syndrome are often coded separately and individually there may be no difference between two drugs, but when the cases are examined there may be a combination of symptoms with one drug that warrant being called a syndrome. It is therefore essential to read the individual original description of the AEs before making a judgement. This area has been explored more fully by Bernstein and he has added to the equation with the addition of bias:

$$\text{Attributable AEs} = \text{Drug group AEs} - \text{Placebo group AEs} + / - \text{Bias}$$

Bias is equal to the base line (B) frequency and severity of the AE multiplied by pharmacological clinical activity of the drug (AD) minus the pharmacological clinical activity of the placebo (AP):

$$\text{Bias} = \text{B} (\text{AD} - \text{AP})$$

The argument is that the disease or a symptom or sign of the disease and the drug ADR may interact as follows.

- Compliance. Early improvement may cause the patient to stop the drug and the improvement of the ADR may be inappropriately assigned to tachyphylaxis of the ADR; failure of the disease to improve may persuade the patient to add a rescue drug or increase the dose of the study drug or even stop the drug; impaired mental or cognitive function due to the disease may affect compliance.
- The disease may alter the absorption, distribution, metabolism or elimination of the drug (e.g. alteration of the blood−brain barrier by the disease may allow the drug to affect the brain).
- Observational bias of convalescence (e.g. severe pain causing insomnia may require morphine causing compensatory hypersomnia in excess of that caused by morphine alone).
- Observational bias by halo effects. Perception of an ADR may be swamped by the symptoms of the disease, thus as the disease symptoms resolve the ADR becomes apparent.
- Unblinding. If the patient or physician are unblinded due to rapid improvement of the disease or an ADR they may be led to expect ADRs with the active treatment.

- Pharmacological clinical activity bias. An AE that is already present due to the disease may be increased if is also an ADR of the drug or vice versa. For example the diarrhoea of gastroenteritis may be alleviated by codeine-containing preparations given to relieve pain while the inertia of a severely depressed patient may be sufficiently resolved by an antidepressant to enable the patient to commit suicide. Is this an ADR due to the drug or due to the disease (Bernheim, 1994)?

Adverse drug reactions that are similar to common non-drug AEs are rarely described or investigated sufficiently for a causal relationship for each individual event to be established. If they cannot be distinguished qualitatively, the correct quantitative procedure is to compare them using non-parametric statistics, giving the confidence limits for the incidences of ADRs. Small studies ($n < 30$) have little chance of separating ADRs from placebo or non-drug events unless they are very common and specific to the drug (Simpson *et al.*, 1980). The situation is worsened by the fact that members of a placebo group have a tendency to 'catch' AEs from the active drug group, therefore changing a relatively specific ADR to a non-specific event (Wolf, 1959b; Green, 1964) (see page 14).

Methods for Collecting Symptomatic Adverse Events

Collection of all AEs or symptoms should only be done if:

- It is possible, to compare the AEs of one group with those of another, since the 'background noise' of the non-drug symptoms can overwhelm the drug-induced symptoms in un-controlled studies.
- The use of a questionnaire or checklist makes statistical comparison valid.
- They can be collected at the beginning and end of a study as a minimum.

Methods for Collecting Adverse Events
- Diary card
- Questionnaire
- Checklist
- Standard question

The patient can be prompted to report all adverse symptoms if the doctor uses either a diary card, a patient questionnaire or a checklist with a standard question. Since the majority of ADRs occur within the first week of drug treatment, the first visit should be within a week or so of starting treatment if all the minor events are to be collected. There is a steep fall-off in recollection of minor events, even in young intelligent volunteers and this is likely to be greater in the elderly sick (see page 13).

Patient Diary Cards

In trials where a patient diary card is used for recording patient information (e.g. daily peak flow rates in an asthma trial), it can also be used for recording of AEs (Harlow, 1972). It is, in fact, the equivalent of answering a daily standard question or checklist. If sufficient space is allotted to the daily recording of any AEs in sufficient detail the diary card is likely to be unmanageably large. The large amount of unstructured data that is likely to be collected over any period longer than a few days would be difficult to manage. Daily recording of objective data with weekly recording of AEs makes the data easier to handle without the loss of important events. In cancer studies the known side-effects due to chemotherapy vary from day-to-day and diary cards have been used very successfully. The Medical Research Council (MRC) Tuberculosis and Chest Diseases Unit, the Clinic of Oncology and the Radiotherapeutic Unit diary card has three pages, one for each week (Fayers and Jones, 1983; Jones *et al.*, 1987). The five standard questions asked each day relate to:

1. Sickness (vomiting).
2. Activity.
3. Mood.
4. Anxiety.
5. Overall condition.

Each of these questions is given a range of five answers:

1. Sickness—(i), none; (ii) poor appetite; (iii) felt sick but wasn't; (iv) sick once; (v) sick more than once.
2. Activity—(i) normal work/housework; (ii) normal work, but with effort; (iii) reduced activity, but not confined to home; (iv) confined to home or hospital; (v) confined to bed.
3. Mood—(i) very happy; (ii) happy; (iii) average; (iv) miserable; (v) very miserable.
4. Anxiety—(i) very calm; (ii) calm; (iii) average; (iv) anxious; (v) very anxious.
5. Overall condition—(i) very well; (ii) well; (iii) fair; (iv) poor; (v) very ill.

On the bottom half of every page there is space for any other problems or changes in health.

Many of the problems of a patient diary have been eliminated with the electronic patient diary (Donovan *et al.*, 1996) and it has been successfully used for rheumatology, urology, Parkinson's disease, psychiatry and pulmonary disease. It works like a daily questionnaire rather than a diary since it does not need to allow free text entries. It can have a built-in alarm to remind the patient to fill it in. It has multiple choice questions and a visual analogue scale (VAS) can be added. Electronic patient diaries have been found to be cost-effective and do not present problems for elderly patients (Lundström, 1993).

An intermediate method incorporating features of a diary card and those of a questionnaire has been used in a large-scale general practitioner study comparing dimethylchlortetracycline and placebo (Howse and Clark, 1970). Patients were supplied with six reply-paid postcards for recording for each day of the six months of the trial the presence of cough, spit, purulent spit, purulent nasal discharge, attendance with the doctor, work loss (both with and without insurance certificate) and whether trial tablets were taken. The cards included a request to indicate other medication taken and any side-effects of treatment. A 'record card', also reply-paid, was enclosed for immediate return, indicating occupation, smoking habits, family size, house type, work loss due to respiratory illness the previous year and age. This card was identified, as were the monthly morbidity cards, by a code number. Patients whose monthly reply card had not been received by the middle of the next month were sent a reminder, which was repeated, if necessary, one month later. After three reminders, no further action was taken. The reply rate was 92%. There is no reason why a diary card should not include a few questions regarding AEs. The questions should concern only common type A reactions. The advantage of a diary card is that it circumvents the loss of AEs due to a poor memory and prompts the patient to answer questions at a critical time.

Differences in Reporting Rates with Different Instruments

Studies with temafloxacin showed the following reporting rates:

- Spontaneous reporting 1.5–5.1%.
- Standard question 29–49%.
- Diary cards 41.5%.
- Not using diary cards 23.5% (Norrby and Pernet, 1991).

Questionnaire or Checklist?

Whereas some forms of diary card collect the AEs experienced by the patient in an unstructured fashion on a daily basis, the questionnaire or checklist collects the AEs in a structured fashion so that statistical comparisons can be made between an active drug group and a control group. When the patient diary is limited to answering set questions it loses one of its snags and acts as a daily questionnaire. In many earlier

Table 2   Self-administered questionnaire

Advantages	Disadvantages
1. They can be given directly to the patient and returned to the organizer bypassing the prescribing doctor.	1. Needs more organization and the costs to print, distribute, collect and analyse are greater.
2. Questions involving sexual behaviour can be answered more frankly than by any other method.	2. If the questionnaire bypasses the prescribing doctor the patient may forget to report important adverse events to the doctor, forgetting that the latter does not see the answers to the questionnaire. (The method for avoiding this is shown on page 125).
3. The involvement of the prescribing doctor can be minimal.	3. Greater care is needed in the wording of questions since there is no interpretation by the doctor (Bulpitt *et al.*, 1976).
4. Answers to very precise questions can be given and there is almost no limit to the number of questions posed.	4. Tends to overestimate the real incidence of adverse events (Fisher *et al.*, 1987).
5. Confidentiality can be guaranteed by the use of the patient trial number.	5. May suggest symptoms to patients.
6. It is more likely to lead to the conclusion that the incidence of side effects resulting from a given drug is higher than that resulting from placebo (Bulpitt, 1983).	

Table 3 Checklist (questionnaire administered by a third party)	
Advantages	Disadvantages
1. The actual words used to the patient can be tailored according to the patient's intelligence and background.	1. Unless the administrator reads out the question to the patient there will be individual variations in terminology, etc., and therefore the resulting answers may not be comparable. 2. The number of questions is more limited since it involves the administrator's time. 3. Questions involving sex may cause more embarrassment than with the self-administered questionnaire.

papers the terms 'questionnaire' and 'checklist' have been used loosely to mean any question, whether delivered directly to the patient (self-answering questionnaire) or via a third person (i.e. doctor, nurse, social worker). The advantages and disadvantages of these two approaches are outlined in Tables 2 and 3.

There are advantages and disadvantages to using any form of multiple questionnaire compared with the use of a single standard open question such as 'Have you had any medical problems since your last visit?' (see page 124).

The multiple questionnaire will collect symptoms present in normal healthy subjects in addition to those due to disease or drugs. A comparison between an open question and a 38–item checklist showed that 15% of healthy persons had symptoms in the previous three days when the open question was used compared to 82% when the checklist was used, the latter figure confirming Reidenberg's figures (Reidenberg and Lowenthal, 1968) (see page 45). The parallel figure for patients who had been ill or taken medication in the previous three days was 69% for the open question and 87% for the checklist. An open question tends to collect only the more severe symptoms, whereas the incidence of irrelevant complaints is higher with the multiple questionnaire (Ciccolunghi and Chaudri, 1975).

The multiple questionnaire is likely to lead to the conclusion that the incidence of AEs with a given drug is higher than that resulting from placebo (Downing *et al.*, 1970) and this is especially true for neurotic patients (Rickels and Downing, 1970; Lapierre, 1975) and with depressed patients, 5–10 times more side effects will be listed with the multiple questionnaire than with the open question. Relevant side effects are more likely to be detected if a checklist is not used (Huskisson and Wojtulewski, 1974; Fisher *et al.*, 1987). In Sweden known side effects were recorded more frequently using active questioning whereas unknown side effects were more likely to be described by spontaneous reports (Hagman *et al.*, 1977).

These comments are not as contradictory as they may first appear if one relates the use of the open question and the multiple questionnaire to the phase of drug development. During phase 1 and phase 2, before the nature of any side effect is known the open question is probably more appropriate (with the exception of 'me-too' drugs), whereas in large scale phase 3 and 4 studies where the relative incidence of common side effects of the new drug can be compared with those of its main competitor the multiple questionnaire is more likely to differentiate between the two drugs.

Questionnaire

There are two types of questionnaire:

- The first is a generic questionnaire that has been developed for use over a wide field (e.g. quality of life questionnaires). Its disadvantage is that it needs to be very extensive if it is to cover the range of possible AEs. If it has a restricted number of questions then it must have an open question 'Were there any other AEs?' or just 'Other...'?
- The second is designed specifically for a trial with particular drugs. Use of such a questionnaire is only advised for early randomized clinical trials when the new drug is a variant of a standard drug since a questionnaire designed to pick up the known side effects of the standard drug may be inadequate for identifying the as yet unknown side effects of a new type of drug. This may well bias the study in favour of the new drug since the well known side effects of the standard treatment will be well represented in the questionnaire.

Construction of Questionnaires

Three suggested books on the construction of questionnaires are:

1. *Le Questionnaire Médical* by N. Laferrière, A. Tenaillon, J. C. Saltiel, A. Smagghe, F. J. Chicou, J. Cretien and J.L. Portos, published by Inserm, Paris, 1977.
2. *Guide to Questionnaire Construction and Question Writing* by C. A. Woodward and L. W. Chambers, published by Canadian Public Health Association, Ottawa, 1983.
3. *Asking Questions: a Practical Guide to Questionnaire Design* by S. Sudman and N. M. Bradburn, published by Jassly-Bass, San Francisco, 1982.

Designing a Questionnaire

The ten stages in this process are:

1. Read Stone (1993).
2. Decide what data you need.
3. Select items for inclusion.
4. Design individual questions.
5. Compose wording.
6. Design layout.
7. Think about coding.
8. Prepare first draft and pretest.
9. Pilot and evaluate.
10. Perform survey (Stone, 1993).

Quantification of Symptoms

The two main methods for quantifying a symptom are:

1. Descriptive scales.
2. Visual analogue scales (VAS).

Quantification of Symptoms
• Descriptive scale
• Visual analogue scale

Descriptive Scales (or fixed interval scales) (Likert scales)   These are graded descriptive terms:

- Absent or present (score 0 or 1). This is the method used by most questionnaires, but it may lack sensitivity when comparing two similar drugs in a relatively small trial.
- If present is it mild, moderate or severe? (score 2, 3, 4). Patients' understanding of the words mild, moderate and severe is likely to differ so it might be worth including the definitions on page 40. The Japanese have a three-grade scheme similar to the World Health Organization (WHO) scheme for both clinical and laboratory adverse events (see Chapter 6, page 174).
- A five-point scale (i.e. very drowsy, slightly drowsy, normal, more alert, very alert) (Yuen *et al.*, 1985). The WHO handbook for reporting the results of cancer treatment has a five-grade scheme (0–4) for both clinical and laboratory AEs (WHO, 1979).
- A seven-point scale (Jaeschke *et al.*, 1990)—(i) extremely short of breath; (ii) very short of breath; (iii) quite a bit short of breath; (iv) Moderately short of breath; (v) some shortness of breath; (vi) A little shortness of breath; (vii) not at all short of breath. Another seven-point scale can be used for the frequency of the event (Guyatt *et al.*, 1987)—(i) all of the time; (ii) most of the time; (iii) a good bit of the time; (iv) some of the time; (v) a little of the time; (vi) hardly any of the time; (vii) none of the time. A further seven-point scale has been used with the SAFETEE general inquiry questionnaire. Patients were asked to rank each of the 76 possible symptoms on a scale of 1–7. The rankings were based upon the patients' willingness to exchange their current disease state for a situation where they would now be afflicted with that symptom, a rank of 1 would indicate a complete willingness to exchange while a rank of 7 would be an absolute refusal. Using weighted values for the SAFETEE symptoms obtained from the ranking procedure, an index was created to measure the impact of non-life threatening adverse effects associated with drug therapy. This adverse drug effect index has been validated (Levine *et al.*, 1990). There is also an 'Adverse Symptom Index', which ranges from 'Present but not bothersome' to 'Present and intolerable'. The index was still in the validation stage (Levine *et al.*, 1990).
- A 10-point scale (Lewis *et al.*, 1985a). The patient is asked to allocate a score between 1 and 10 for different symptoms.

Visual Analogue Scales   A VAS (Aitken, 1969; Bond and Lader, 1974; Huskisson, 1976; Nicholson, 1978) is shown in Figure 1. It is a 10-cm VAS, which may be vertical or horizontal with perhaps some practical advantage with the horizontal scale (Scott and Huskisson, 1976; Scott and Huskisson, 1979a; Dixon and Bird, 1981; Sriwatanakul *et al.*, 1982). There should not be any intermediate points (Aitken, 1969; Scott and Huskisson, 1976) that might cause clustering. However, there is always a tendency towards clustering at the extremes of the scale, at the midpoint and at 6.18 cm (Benjafield and Adams-Webber, 1976). It has been suggested that patients should see their previous scores when making serial assessments, but others disagree (Joyce *et al.*, 1975; Scott and Huskisson, 1979b; Carlsson, 1983). Some 7% of patients find the VAS difficult to understand despite instruction (Lewis, 1987; Jaeschke *et al.*, 1990) and

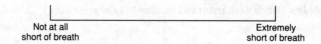

Figure 1   A visual analogue scale (VAS)

it has been suggested that patients who score inaccurately for all symptoms should be screened out (Lewis *et al.*, 1985c). Drug effects were significantly more marked for volunteers who were not depressed compared with those who were depressed (Peat *et al.*, 1981). A VAS has been found to be more sensitive than a 10-point scoring system when used for testing beta adrenoceptor blockers (Lewis *et al.*, 1985c) a five-point scale or a standard question when used to measure sedation (Yuen *et al.*, 1985), a sleep and mood scale (Lundberg, 1980), and a four-point pain scale (Joyce *et al.*, 1975). Errors can occur using a VAS and Maxwell has suggested that it should be combined with either a four-point scale or a simple global assessment (Maxwell, 1978). When a VAS was used in the assessment of angina using 'No pain at all' and 'Pain as bad as I could ever bear' and afterwards the patients were asked which of the following did they use: number of attacks, duration of attacks, severity of an individual attack or a combination of these, it was found that the patients' VAS scores correlated best with the severity of the pain, which was considered the least clinically important variable. It is therefore important to take care in phrasing the question (Vandenburg, 1987). An alternative to using a scale is the use of a VAS meter, which gives an immediate reading without the need for subsequent measurement and this produces a similar assessment to the conventional VAS (Hounslow *et al.*, 1987).

The VAS has been used for:

- Pain (Huskisson, 1974; Joyce *et al.*, 1975; Scott and Huskisson, 1976; Carlsson, 1983; Vandenburg, 1987; McCormack *et al.*, 1988).
- Quality of sleep (Parrott and Hindmarsh, 1978).
- Dyspnoea (Jaeschke *et al.*, 1990).
- Subjective sensation of resistance to breathing (Aitken, 1969).
- Depression (Zealley and Aitken, 1969; McCormack *et al.*, 1988).
- Anxiety (McCormack *et al.*, 1988).
- Beta blocker side effects (Lewis *et al.*, 1984; Lewis *et al.*, 1985a; Lewis *et al.*, 1985b; Lewis, 1987; Dimenäs *et al.*, 1989).
- Quality of life (Jaeschke *et al.*, 1990; Guyatt *et al.*, 1987).

Bulpitt and Fletcher (1990) do not use a VAS because of the difficulty in explaining the concept to many patients, the lack of data on validity and repeatability, and the difficulty in interpreting the results. Several others mention the problems of analysis (Zealley and Aitken, 1969; Maxwell, 1978; Jaeschke *et al.*, 1990) as does the reply to Maxwell (Stubbs, 1979).

Comparison of Fixed and Visual Analogue Scales   Both the fixed scale and the VAS have been mentioned only in regard to the severity of the symptom. The total discomfort of a patient might be better assessed if a time element is involved (i.e. total discomfort = severity × duration; Guyatt *et al.*, 1987). These authors have compared use of a seven-point fixed interval scale and a VAS in chronic respiratory disease using the question 'Please indicate how often you have had a feeling of fear or panic when you had difficulty getting your breath' by choosing one of the following options:

- All of the time.
- Most of the time.
- A good part of time.
- Some of the time.
- A lot of the time.
- Hardly any of the time.
- None of the time.

The alternative VAS had 'None of the time' and 'All of the time' at the extreme ends. On the grounds of ease of administration and interpretation they favoured the seven-point scale. Perhaps the use of two fixed interval scales, one for severity and another for duration would be more discriminatory.

Conclusions The VAS is best used as an efficacy assessment when the symptom is due to the underlying disease and the drug is likely to improve the symptom (i.e. a change in severity). In a large-scale placebo-controlled clinical trial using a questionnaire for AEs there are advantages in having just absent or present (i.e. a tick in a box if present). It is only if the trial compares a new drug and the standard therapy under similar circumstances and it is important to detect a difference that it is worth using a four-point scale. If a large-scale study is not possible and a limited questionnaire is used yet it is vital to discover whether the two treatments differ then it is worth using a VAS, but only in a single centre study with an enthusiastic investigator.

Questionnaire / checklist

A questionnaire can qualify a symptom by asking further questions about the type of sensation, location, duration, quality, etc., but if the questionnaire hopes to cover all body sensations then it will be prohibitively long. Questionnaires devised for one clinical trial may not be suitable in a different context and therefore the trialist needs to check:

1. Is the questionnaire acceptable to the study population?
2. Is it easily completed?
3. Will it produce responses consistent with those obtained in normal doctor–patient interviews?
4. Is it reproducible when administered on two separate occasions?
5. Will it be of value or use when completed (Lewis *et al.*, 1984).

Questionnaires are likely to pick up milder symptoms than those volunteered spontaneously or in answer to a general question and will include body sensations experienced by normal subjects. This increases the background noise and may entail the use of larger groups if ADRs are to be distinguished (Borghi *et al.*, 1984).

Types of Questionnaire

Questionnaires used in clinical trials can be divided into two groups:

1. Specific questionnaire designed for a specific trial(s) or for a specific drug where possible side effects are elicited by individual specific questions.
2. Generic questionnaires, which can be divided into ADR questionnaires and quality of life (QoL) questionnaires.

The ADR questionnaires are designed to cover all reasonable ADRs. Rare ADRs are too specific and cover too many areas to be covered in a questionnaire of limited size. Quality of life questionnaires cover the physical state, emotional wellbeing, sexual and social functioning, and cognitive acuity of patients (Croog *et al.*, 1986). In general an ADR questionnaire is used for picking up the AEs suffered by the patient while the Q of L assessment indicates how the adverse and beneficial events have affected the patient's general wellbeing (see Chapter 5).

Generic Adverse Drug Reaction Questionnaires
Generic Questionnaires (All diseases)
1) The Systematic Assessment for Treatment of Emergent Events
(SAFTEE) (Levine & Schooler, 1986).
SAFTEE was developed over the period 1980–83 and uses a standardized enquiry procedure by a doctor or nurse. There are two versions: general and specific.

General Inquiry—Systematic Assessment for Treatment Emergent Events (SAFTEE-GI) This uses a standard general question (discussed on pages 124 and 206), which is basically 'Have you had any physical or health problems during the past week?' followed by several subsidiary questions resulting from the general enquiry. At the bottom of the page there is space for three possible diagnoses.

Specific Inquiry—Systematic Assessment for Treament Emergent Events (SAFTEE-SI) There are 23 specific questions in addition to the general inquiry series. Each question has further subsidiary questions, such as 'Have you had any trouble with your heart such as beating too fast, pounding or skipping?' with three subsidiary questions:

*   Rapid heart beat?
*   Irregular heart beat?
*   Other?

The questions in both the general inquiry and specific inquiry are answered by ticking boxes or filling in numbers. For each event there are ten columns, each headed by the relevant question(s):

1. Date of event onset.
2. Duration in days.
3. Pattern.
4. Current status.
5. Severity.
6. Functional impairment.
7. Possible contributory factors.
8. Relationship of drug to event.
9. Action taken.
10. Comments, descriptions and additional specifications.

Each of these headings is now taken in turn.

1. Date of event onset. The minimal unit is one day so pharmacologically induced AEs may be difficult to assess from the time to onset.
2. Duration. The same comment applies as for date of event onset.
3. Pattern. This can be 'isolated', 'intermittent' or continuous'. The term 'intermittent' is not broken down further, so events occurring with each dose are described in column 10 under comments.
4. Current status. The alternatives are 'continuing', 'recovered no sequelae', 'recovered with sequelae' and 'indeterminate'. Details of sequelae go in column 10.
5. Severity. This can vary from 'minimal' via 'mild', 'moderate', 'severe' to 'very severe'.
6. Functional impairment. This uses the same alternatives as for severity.
7. Possible contributory factors. The alternatives are: 'current disorder (being treated)', 'intercurrent illness', 'other previous disorders', 'previous history of event', 'protocol drug', 'other drug/drug interaction', 'other' or 'none apparent'. These possibilities are not mutually exclusive.
8. Relationship of drug to event. The possibilities are 'dose response', 'dechallenge/rechallenge', 'timing of onset', 'seen in other patients in this trial', 'known drug effect', 'laboratory data', 'other' or 'not applicable'; again these are not mutually exclusive. In many cases this information will not be sufficient for an individual assessment.
9. Action taken (by clinician). The alternatives are 'none', 'increased surveillance', 'contra-active prescription plus change dose', 'suspend prescription', 'discontinue prescription', 'other (specify)' and 'don't know'.
10. Comments, descriptions, additional specifications. This can be used to provide further characterization of the event especially where requested.

At the back of the manual there are two blank pages for further comments, a laboratory test sheet and a drug dosage record sheet. The basis of the system is the collection of all events, whether considered to be drug related or not over a set period using 76 preferred-event terms. The SAFTEE-SI takes about 20 minutes for psychiatric patients. There is a comprehensive manual for the use of the scale and a copy can be obtained from the National Technical Information Service, Department of Commerce, Washington DC (Dr J. Levine). The reliability and validity of SAFTEE are documented in a further paper (Guy, 1986) and compared with the Association for Methodology and Documentation in Psychiatry (Germany) (AMDP)-Somatic Signs (SS) system (see page 118). Another paper reports on the use of SAFTEE in nine clinical trials and says that the SI version collects three times as many kinds of events as the GI version, but that the GI portion of the SI version collects events which have a higher mean severity and impairment than the events elicited during the SI portion. The overall inter-rater reliability coefficient was not impressive (Jacobson *et al.*, 1986). A pilot study using SAFTEE suggested that more clinically meaningful information is obtained using the SI version than the GI version (Rabkin and Markowitz, 1986). It has been suggested that extreme caution should be used if attempting to detect new ADRs or to estimate true ADR incidences by systematic inquiry. This conclusion was made following a comparison of spontaneous reporting and the use of SAFTEE.

A Systematic Assesstment for Treatment Emergent Events (SAFTEE)-based Study   Part of this large-scale pilot study, developing new methods of Post-Marketing Surveillance (PMS), was the use of computer-assisted interviews for outpatients receiving either a tricyclic antidepressant or an antibiotic. The interview was based on SAFTEE. Of the patients 50% were chosen randomly as 'experimental', the remainder being controls. The 'experimentals' had a printed notice attached to their drugs by the pharmacy requesting them to report any 'new or unusual symptoms' during the following two weeks via a toll-free telephone number. The controls were interviewed by telephone two weeks later without previous warning. The key question in the latter interviews was: 'Have you noticed any new or unusual symptoms during the past ten days or so?' followed by a systematic inquiry. Then, using a list of ten known antibiotic ADRs and 14 known tricyclic ADRs, they coded the patient answers as either 'positive' if a tricyclic patient mentioned a known tricyclic ADR and similarly for antibiotics, and 'negative' if a tricyclic patient mentioned an antibiotic ADR and again similarly for antibiotic patients. They then created an ADR index, which measured the sensitivity comparing the presence of 'positives' relative to 'negatives' with each group of patients. Spontaneous reporting accurately identified ADRs at 17.4% for antibiotics and 11.1% for tricyclics. When the ADRs elicited by systematic inquiry are added, the discrimination of true antibiotic ADRs was destroyed. This did not occur with the tricyclics, although the systematic inquiry did not detect any new ADRs that had not been found with spontaneous reporting. This confirms that use of a checklist or questionnaire can obscure real ADRs by swamping patients with 'background noise' and that they should only be used when an adequate control group is used (Fisher *et al.*, 1986; 1987).

Based on the United States Pharmacopeia Dispensing Information   This comprises 24 areas as follows:

- Skin.
- Scalp, hair or nails.
- Muscles, bones or joints.
- Head or face.
- Vision.
- Eyes.
- Hearing or ears.
- Nose.
- Mouth, lips, gums, teeth or tongue.
- Changes in colour of the mouth, lips, gums, teeth or tongue.
- Sense of taste.
- Throat, voice, neck.
- Breasts.
- Breathing or lungs.
- Heart or circulation.
- Stomach or digestive system.
- Rectum or bowel movements.
- Kidney or urinary system.
- Sexual function.

- Reproductive organs.
- Nervous system.
- Mental health.
- General complaints.
- Injection site.

Each of these areas contains up to 106 separate questions including the essential 'any other?'. Despite the number of questions they only occupy four sheets of A4 paper (Corso *et al.*, 1992).

All Body Organs and Functions Questionnaire (ABOF) for volunteers This (Nony *et al.*, 1994) consists of:

1. A general standard question 'Since the beginning of the treatment have any uncomfortable symptoms appeared (or worsened) or resolved (or decreased)'?
2. Pain question—if positive six further questions.
3. Vision question—if positive seven further questions.
4. Hearing question—if positive three further questions.
5. Smell question—if positive four further questions.
6. Appetite, mouth, swallowing question—if positive eight further questions.
7. Changes of position question—if positive three further questions.
8. Hair, nails, sweat question—if positive six further questions.
9. Hands and feet question—if positive five further questions.
10. Physical activities question—if positive five further questions.
11. Muscular question—if positive five further questions.
12. Cardiac palpitations question—if positive one further questions.
13. Respiratory question—if positive six further questions.
14. Digestive, stomach question—if positive five further questions.
15. Urinary question—if positive four further questions.
16. Sexual question—if positive three further questions.
17. Sleeping question—if positive four further questions.
18. Concentration or memory question—if positive four further questions.
19. Bleeding problems question—if positive five further questions.

Generic Specific Diseases Questionnaires

There are several systems for the collection of AEs in psychiatric drug trials.

Early Clinical Drug Evaluation Unit (ECDEU) Assessment Manual The ECDEU produced the ECDEU assessment manual in 1970 and updated it in 1976 (Guy, 1976). It is still used in this format and further updating has not yet occurred (personal communication, 1997). This 590-page manual consists of separate packets (described below), each of which contains a number of scales.

Demographic Packet This contains four parts:

- A children's personal data inventory.
- A children's symptom history.
- An adult's personal data inventory.
- A prior medication record.

Psychiatric Packet This is divided into three separate scales:

1. Paediatric scale containing five separate scales.
2. Adult scale containing six scales—(a) brief psychiatric rating scale; (b) depression status inventory; (c) Hamilton depression scale (Hamilton, 1960); (d) Hamilton anxiety scale; (e) anxiety status inventory; (f) Wittenborn psychiatric rating scale.
3. Universal scale containing three scales: (a) clinical global impressions; (b) dosage record and treatment emergent symptom scale (DOTES); (c) patient termination record.

Nurses' Packet This contains four scales dealing with childrens' behaviour, inpatient evaluation, a geriatric scale and global impression.

Independent Paediatric Packet This has four scales for parents and teachers.

Independent Adult Scales These are three self-rating scales—a symptom inventory, a depression scale and an anxiety scale.

Independent Adverse Drug Reaction Scales There are seven scales:

1. Treatment emergent symptom scale (TESS): write-in scale.
2. Subject's treatment emergent symptom scale (STESS).
3. Laboratory data.
4. Clinical laboratory standards in paediatric psychopharmacology.
5. Clinical laboratory test standards for schizophrenics.
6. Physical and neurological examination for soft signs.
7. Manual for scored examination for soft signs.

Psychologist's Packet This comprises:

1. Paediatric scales: seven scales including the Porteus mazes, figure drawing and the Bender Gestalt test-Koppitz scoring.
2. Adult scales: (a) Wechsler adult intelligence scale; (b) Porteus mazes; (c) Bender Gestalt test; (d) Wechsler memory scale; (e) Friedhoff task behaviour scale.

Documentation (The Data Package) This contains details of the processing system and methods of documentation such as graphic displays, as well as narrative summary, comments on statistical procedures and research completion report.

Appendices These comprise:

1. Occupation categories.
2. American Psychiatric Association 3rd edition of the *Diagnosis and Statistical Manual* (DSM-111) and WHO diagnostic codes.
3. Formats for non-standard instruments:
   (a) Profile of mood states (POMS).
   (b) Frostig developmental test of visual perception (FROST).
   (c) Abnormal involuntary movement scale (AIMS).
   (d) Crichton geriatric rating scale.

(e) Beck depression inventory (Beck *et al.*, 1961).
(f) Guild memory test.
(g) Physician's questionnaire.
(h) Inpatient multidimensional personality scale.
(i) Physician's outpatient psychopathology scale.
(j) Memory for designs test.
(k) Phillip's scale of premorbid adjustment in schizophrenia.
(l) Sandoz clinical assessment-geriatric.
(m) Clyde mood scale.
(n) Hopkins symptom checklist.
(o) Self-rating symptom scale.
(p) Global assessment scale.
(q) Tartu psychometric battery.

Methods for Estimating the Incidence of Adverse Drug Reactions using ECDEU Methodology Many of the symptoms of psychiatric disorders are also potential ADRs and various other methods have been used to try and separate them. Four methods for estimating the incidence of ADRs have been suggested by the biostatisticians from Upjohn, USA (Assenzo and Shu, 1982) using the methodology with checklist used by ECDEU. Symptoms are graded: 0 = none, 1 = mild, 2 = moderate, 3 = Severe.

Method 1 This is essentially the ECDEU method called 'incidence of treatment emergent symptoms'. For each specified event subtract the pre-score from the post-score.

Method 2 Count the number of occasions that the investigator has:

(a) Increased surveillance.
(b) Reduced dose.
(c) Stopped drug.
(d) Treated the AE.

Method 3 This relates change in disease state (measure of efficacy) to AE severity. The disease state is evaluated as:

- Very much improved = +1.
- Much improved = +2.
- Improved = +3.
- I.S.Q. = +4.
- Worse = +5.
- Much worse = +6.
- Very much worse = +7.

Measure event severity by Method 1 and then for each patient and event calculate the average increase in event severity and average change in disease state over all visits. Then draw up a two-way table and the ADRs are those shown in Table 4. An

Table 4 Average change in event severity

	Average change in disease state		
	$\leqslant$ 2–3.5	> 3.5–4.5	> 4.5
$\leqslant$ 0.33	–	–	–
> 0.33–1.33	ADR	–	–
> 1.33–2.33	ADR	ADR	–
> 2.33	ADR	ADR	ADR

event is assumed to be disease related if an average increase in severity of the ADR is accompanied by an average worsening of the disease state.

Method 4 For each event calculate the proportion of patients having an average change in AE severity of more than one within the average change in disease state category of Method 3 (row incidences). The row incidences are calculated for active drug and placebo. The placebo row incidences are subtracted from those of the active drug. Row differences are then combined, weighting by the number of patients. Then 95% confidence limits are calculated for this weighted estimate of the difference in incidence between the drug and placebo. If the upper and lower limits are positive and they do not contain zero it is a side effect of the drug.

Wellcome's 28-item Checklist The clinical research department from Wellcome, USA described their method using a 28-item checklist in an antidepressant versus placebo study (Cato *et al.*, 1983). The trial lasted one month with weekly visits and assessments. First they calculated the number of AE reports (a maximum of five per patient) as a percentage and subtracted the baseline figure from the treatment figure. Second, the trialists were asked to assesss the event as to the likelihood that it was caused by the drug. There were five possible grades: 'none', 'remote', 'possible', 'probable' and 'definite'. Third, they calculated the percentage of patients with an AE and again subtracted the baseline from the treatment value. If the active drug minus placebo figure was positive for the percentage of patients and this concurred with the opinion of the trialist then the event was declared to be an ADR. The ratio of percentage of patients with an AE to the percentage of reports was used to help distinguish whether the event was due to drug or a spontaneous background event. This ratio gives less information than studying the event patterns individually. The five causality judgements are reduced to two—'drug related' or 'not drug related'—and there is no measure of the severity of the event, which is an advantage of the Upjohn method.

Manual for Assessment and Documentation in a Psychopathology System (AMDP System) According to Guy *et al.*, (Guy & Ban, 1982) this AMDP system (Woggon *et al.*, 1986) was designed to be used routinely in conjunction with a psychopathological symptom scale and was developed by the European AMDP. The AMDP-SS is part of an assessment battery and the scale consists of 44 symptoms each rated on a five-point scale of severity. A semi-structured inquiry procedure is used to collect the data. The paper says that it has been used for a decade and that a number of validity and reliability studies have been published.

The UKU (Udvalg Kliniske Undersogelser) Side Effect Rating Scale A comprehensive rating scale to use with psychotropic drugs has been developed in Scandanavia. It consists of:

- A single symptom rating scale comprising a total of 48 items.
- A global assessment of the influence that the patient's side effects have on daily performance. This assessment is done by the patient and an observer.
- A statement of the consequences that the patient's side effects have for the continuing of the medication (Lingjaerde *et al.*, 1977). Its use in a 44-hospital study in Scandinavia has been published (Denkers *et al.*, 1976). This scale is available in all Nordic languages, English, German and French from Symposium International, Karlebogogård, Karsbovy 9, DK-3400 Hillerød, Denmark.

The scale covers 48 items divided into four categories:

1. Psychic—10.
2. Neurological—8.
3. Autonomic—11.
4. Other—19.

Each item is rated from 0–3 for severity as follows:

- 0 = not or doubtfully present.
- 1 = present to a mild degree.
- 2 = present to a moderate degree.
- 3 = present to a severe degree.

Each item is also rated as either improbable, possible or probable for its relationship to the drug. There is also a global assessment of the interference by existing side effects with the patient's daily performance, again graded as follows:

- 0 = no side effect.
- 1 = mild.
- 2 = moderate.
- 3 = markedly.

There are also four possible actions:

- 0 = no action.
- 1 = more frequent assessment.
- 2 = reduction in dose and/or continuous drug treatment of the ADR.
- 3 = discontinuation of drug or change to another drug.

The scale does not cover all possible side effects of psychiatric drugs and in a drug trial consideration should be given to additional items.

The Liverpool University Neuroleptic Side Effect Rating Scale (LUN-SERS) This is a 51-item scale taking only 5–20 minutes for patients to complete. It has been used in a controlled study with 50 schizophrenics and 50 control subjects (*Reactions*, 1994).

Older Simpler Systems   These include:

1. The Swedish symptom scale for schizophrenics.
2. The side effects scale for schizophrenics.

These systems use five-point scales with operationally defined steps (Andersen *et al.*, 1974).

The DVP scale is another scale and questions are scored between 0 and 4 (Vinar, 1971).

Other Disease-based Questionnaires   It is difficult to separate scales that are disease specific from those for side effects and those for Q of L assessment

Hypertension   These include:

(a) The Bulpitt and Dollery questionnaire. There are 26 questions, mostly of the 'yes', 'no' type. Some questions use three or more alternative answers. It is self-administered (Bulpitt *et al.*, 1974, 1976) and has been used in several trials (Sanders *et al.*, 1979: Nicholls *et al.*, 1980).
(b) The Subjective Symptoms Assessment Profile. (SSAP). There are 42 questions using both a Likert scale and a VAS. The VAS was found to be more sensitive than the Likert scale, but elderly patients found the VAS more difficult to understand. It is self-administered. (Dimenäs *et al.*, 1990) and has been used for measuring QoL with felodipine (Dimenäs *et al.*, 1991; Wallander *et al.*, 1991).
(c) A Swedish questionnaire with 19 questions (Andersson, 1979).

Central Nervous System-related Questionnaires

These include:

1. The Minor Symptoms Evaluation Profile (MSEP). There are 24 items with a VAS (Dimenäs *et al.*, 1989).
2. The extrapyramidal rating scale. This has four parts: (a) Parkinsonism, dystonia and dyskinesia—questionnaire and behavioural scale—12 items; (b) Parkinsonism—physician's examination—eight items; (c) Dystonia—physician's examination—two items; (d) Dyskinetic movements—physician's examination—seven items. Its use has been validated (Chouinard *et al.*, 1980).
3. The Simpson Angus extrapyramidal rating scale (Simpson and Angus, 1970).
4. The short-form health survey (SF-36) (Jenkinson *et al.*, 1995).
5. The Parkinson's disease questionnaire (PDQ-39) (Jenkinson *et al.*, 1995; Peto *et al.*, 1995).

Alcohol Abuse Questionnaire   The CAGE questionnaire consists of four questions:

● Have you ever felt you should Cut down on your drinking?
● Have people Annoyed you by criticizing your drinking?
● Have you ever felt bad or Guilty about your drinking?

• Have you ever had a drink first thing in the morning to steady your nerves or to get rid of a hangover? An 'Eye-opener'.

A positive answer to three or four questions has a 51% sensitivity and a 99.8% specificity (Sackett, 1996).

How to use Questionnaires

An early evaluation of side effects should take place at baseline and within 1–2 weeks of the start of a trial since most side effects are evident within that period. The long-term effects on the Q of L should be assessed 3–6 months later when adaptation has occurred and placebo effects have worn off. The period covered by the questionnaire should be identical throughout the study. Where and how the questionnaire is completed is important; answering a questionnaire in the home setting may not have the same results as within the hospital environment. It is rarely possible to organize a prospective randomized study of an ADR, due to ethical problems, but it has been done with the angiotensin converting enzyme (ACE) cough and the study illustrates a method for doing this (Ramsay and Yeo, 1995).

Drawbacks of Adverse Drug Reaction Questionnaires

In all structured systems for the collection of AEs there is a tendency to lose information. A patient's graphic description of an event may help to separate the drug-induced event from naturally occurring events, but will not be suitable for computerization. In the early studies the quality of the patient's description must be retained. Although in a structured system there should be space for additional description there will inevitably be loss of descriptive information. There is a continuum from the individualized approach with a single event reported spontaneously to the counting of events in epidemiological surveys (see Figure 2). There is a need to characterize the AEs in detail early in the clinical development of a new drug until an accurate description of the events is developed; thereafter they can be counted.

Quality of Life Questionnaires

Although questionnaires can establish whether a patient has suffered an AE it does not ask what effect the AE had on the patient. Most type A AEs are transient since the

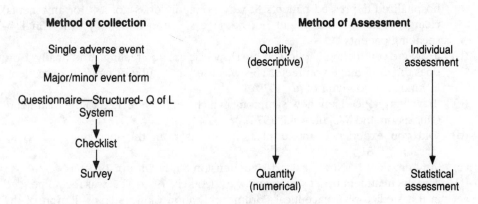

Figure 2   Relationship of assessment to the method of collection of adverse events

patient either stops the drug or reduces the dose, but if the AE applies to a whole class of drugs and one of that class is clinically necessary the patient may have to have a persistent AE—sleepiness with tricyclic antidepressant drugs/tranquillizers or gastrointestinal irritation with non-steroidal anti-inflammatory drugs (NSAIDs), which itself may require treatment. Elderly patients requiring polypharmacy may have one or more ADRs that reduce the pleasure of living on top of the problems due to the underlying diseases. The effect of an ADR on a patient can be assessed by use of a Q of L questionnaire. This whole subject has expanded exponentially in the last few years and now merits a chapter to itself. (see Chapter 5).

Suggested further reading is *Quality of Life and Pharmacoeconomics in Clinical Trials*. 2nd edition, ed. B. Spilker, Lippincott-Raven, 1996, £114.50, 1259 pages. This was reviewed in *Pharmaceutical Medicine* 1996, **10**, 45–46.

Standard or Open Question

This should be the standard method for all clinical trials and some of its character-istics have been mentioned. A common approach in double-blind controlled trials as well as in other studies is to record only 'spontaneously volunteered side effects'. When the list of factors that can prevent reporting of AEs is studied (see page 6) in relationship to this method, it can be seen that it has the following disadvantages compared with a standard question:

- The doctor may not give the patient the opportunity to mention an AE.
- If the doctor assessing the spontaneously volunteered AE judges that it was not definitely due to the drug, it does not need to be recorded.

The standard question should be unambiguous and worded in such a way that it is not mistaken for a social courtesy.

Examples of Standard Questions from Clinical Studies
These include:

(a) 'Have you noticed any change in body function or had any physical complaints in the past week? (Avery *et al.*, 1967). This was used in a study in America in hospitalized depressed patients. It very pointedly does not ask for any mental changes. The wording might not be so easily understood by other English-speaking patients.

(b) 'How are you feeling?', followed by 'How else are you feeling?' and finally 'How does the drug make you feel?'. This was used in a study of neurotic outpatients in America (Downing *et al.*, 1970).

(c) 'Have you noticed any new symptoms which might be related to the treatment?' (Huskisson and Wojtulewski, 1974).

(d) 'Did you experience any unpleasant effects from the medicine you took?' (Lasagna, 1981).

(e) 'Any problems?' (New Zealand Hypertension Study Group, 1979).

(f) 'Has the treatment upset you in any way?' (Aitken, 1969).This was recommended in the Medico-pharmaceutical Forum publication Clinical Trials' Report of the Working Party on Clinical Trials of the Medico-pharmaceutical Forum, 1987.

(g) 'Have you noticed any symptoms since your last examination?' (Jackson, 1990).
(h) 'Have you had any health problems since we last met?' (Wallander, 1991).

Examples (c), (d) and (f) imply that patients make decisions as to causality and will therefore, vary in their interpretation of AEs. These examples should be avoided.

Two alternative standard questions are suggested:

1. 'Have you had any medical problems since your last visit?' (Lapierre, 1975) or 'Have you had any problems since your last visit?', or 'Have you had any problems during the last week?'
2. 'Have you felt different in any way since your last visit?'

The standard question is a suitable method for all clinical trials, being usable in addition to patient questionnaires or checklists, as well as independently. If the question is worded correctly it should collect all drug-related events, but not stimulate the production of too many non drug-related events. If the standard question is worded to collect all events defined by Finney as 'particular untoward happening experienced by a patient undesirable either generally or in the context of the disease' (Finney, 1965), then it includes non-medical events (i.e. social). The problem of dealing with large amounts of social data in uncontrolled and controlled studies has not yet been solved in the drug trial context. Until the methodology of collecting, recording and analyzing social events has advanced and the pattern established, first for the healthy population and second for disease groups, the definition of AEs should be restricted to medical events.

Sequence for Collecting Subjective Adverse Events (See page 145)

If all three methods of collecting subjective AEs—spontaneous, standard question, checklist questionnaire—are to be used, then instinctively they should be used in the order shown in Figure 3.

After a social greeting the patient needs to be given the opportunity to mention any medical problem bothering him or her. Then the standard question should be asked, preferably before redressing, in case further examination is required and then, lastly, a checklist used. A questionnaire can be handed to the patient on leaving so that it can be filled in either in the waiting room or at home. The alternative, that is usually used with Q of L questionnaires, is to have the questionnaire filled in prior to the consultation on the grounds that the doctor/nurse cannot then influence the filling in of the questionnaire. This approach has the theoretical disadvantage that having mentioned their symptoms on the questionnaire they might think it unnecessary to repeat them to the doctor/nurse and therefore they will not be recorded on the

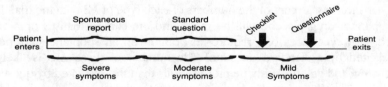

Figure 3 A trial visit

clinical trial record form. However, the influence of a patient-completed symptom checklist on the subsequent reporting of AEs in a clinical trial interview was examined in a study of 128 patients receiving antiepileptic medication. The patients were randomized to receive either a 16-symptom checklist before the clinician assessed the AEs or afterwards. The difference was small and not significant (0.63 AEs vs 0.42 AEs, $p = 0.26$). The authors suggested that giving the checklist first does not affect subsequent reporting (Wagner *et al.*, 1994).

A Comprehensive Method

A very comprehensive method was used in the basal cell carcinoma prevention trial where isotretinoin was being compared with placebo. The trial lasted three years and was followed by a further observation period of two years. After a screening evaluation and a baseline evaluation, clinic visits took place at 2 weeks, 12 weeks, 6 months and 12 months and then every 6 months for the duration of the study (Tangrea and Morge, 1985). The method for dealing with any adverse experiences was as follows:

- Symptom questionnaire at each visit (20 questions including a general question 'Any other symptoms that we haven't mentioned? Specify . . .').
- Study coordinator attempted to attribute any change to study medication or to an alternative cause with the aid of a checklist for determining any alternative cause of the patient's symptoms.
- Investigator assesses the data to evaluate the relationship of the adverse experience to the drug using 'Criteria for determining relationship to test drug' (these are based on those of Karch and Lasagna, see Chapter 1).

Adverse Experience Report

If the experience is thought to be even remotely related to the medication and classified as either moderate or severe, the dose must be modified according to a detailed dose modification scheme and a dose modification report completed. Advice for the clinical management of adverse experiences is also contained in the protocol. The response to any dose modification is reported at the subsequent visit. Details of this method have now been published. (Tangrea *et al.*, 1991) and the results of the first study using this method were published in 1990 (Tangrea *et al.*, 1990).

Clinical Trialists Assessment

Having decided how collection of the AEs occurring in a clinical trial is to be done, a decision must be made as to whether one needs to collect the trialist's opinion about whether the AE was due to the drug. Where a questionnaire or a checklist has been used a statistical assessment of the numbers of each type of AE with the trial drug and the comparator drug/placebo will be made and the clinical trialist's opinion is not required. However, does one require an opinion on all spontaneous reports and those elicited by a standard question? The number of these AEs is likely to be relatively few and will probably be more serious than those elicited by questionnaire or checklist. The clinical trialist knows more about the patients and their diseases, both past and present, and is frequently an expert in the latter. Although the trialist may be an expert in the disease under treatment they may well not be an expert in the area of the AE. Most general physicians have a good knowledge of the common ADRs of the drugs in general use, but physicians who have specialized in a branch of medicine frequently have knowledge of only a narrow range of drugs and diseases; however, their opinion may be invaluable if the AE comes within their specialty. The most sensible decision is to collect the clinical trialist's opinion in all studies except where data have been collected by a questionnaire or checklist.

Evaluation of the Trialist's Opinion

Look at the type B AEs as they come in and check whether this type of AE is within the trialist's expertise. If it is not and it is a serious or important event ask the trialist to obtain a specialist's opinion (at the company's expense). If the AE is not serious or important and is not within the trialist's expertise attach little importance to their opinion.

At the end of the study or trial programme look at each type of event separately: are the clinical trialists consistent in their opinions across centres or studies? An ADR often presents as a pyramid, a broad base of unlikely or possible cases with declining numbers of 'probables' and 'almost certains', for example headache—unlikely, 12; possible, 6; probably, 4; almost certain, 2. In this example if the probables and almost certain cases come from different trialists then examine the clinical pattern of the headaches for further corroborative evidence.

Look at the end of study report: do trialists rate the events similarly to other trialists or do they use 'probably' or 'almost certain' very frequently or is everything assessed as possible?

It comes down to two questions:

1. Should the trialists know what they are talking about?
2. Is their opinion consistent with that of other trialists?

Choice of Alternatives

Two categories include:

(a) Drug related or not drug related.
(b) P (possible or probable) or N (not assessable or unlikely) (used by the Swedish regulatory authorities).
(c) Is there a reasonable possibility that the event may have been caused by the trial therapy? Yes or no.
(d) Do you suspect that the AE was related to drug therapy? Yes or no (Lewis, personal communication).

Three categories include:

(a) Possible, probable or certain.
(b) Probably not, possible, probable.
(c) Improbable, possible, probable (Lingjaerde, 1977) (see page 318).

Four categories include:

(a) Unlikely, possible, probable, definite (Kramer, 1984) (Weber, 1984).

(b) General list—implies unlikely, possible, probable, certain (Mashford, 1984).
(c) Doubtful, possible, probable, definite (Naranjo, 1980).
(d) Unlikely, possible, probable, almost certain. (Stephens, 1984).
(e) Remote, possible, probable, highly probable (Turner, 1984; Ruskin, 1985).

Five categories include:

(a) Unrelated, doubtful possible, probable, almost definite, definite (Emanueli, 1984).
(b) Unrelated, unlikely, possible, probable, definite (Venulet).
(c) Doubtful, coincidental, possible, probable, certain (Blanc).
(d) Appears to be excluded, doubtful, possible, probable, very probable. (French regulatory authority).
(e) Unrelated, conditional, possible, probable, almost definite, definite (Karch and Lasagna).
(f) Negative, coincidental, possible, probable, causative (Irey).
(g) Not related, unlikely, possible, probable, almost certain.
(h) Not related, remote, possible, probable, definite (Tangrea).
(i) None, remote, possible, probable, definite, (Cato).

Six categories include:

(a) Unrelated, very doubtful, possible, probable, almost definite, definite (Cornelli).
(b) Unrelated, unlikely, questionable, possible, probable, definitely related (Sandoz).
(c) Unassessable, conditional/unclassifiable, unlikely, possible, probable/likely, certain (WHO).

Infinite categories include:

• VAS (Venulet) (Lagier).

These categories derive mostly from the different algorithms used in causality assessment (Stephens, 1987).

In a small survey of six major US pharmaceutical companies:

• One company used two alternative terms for causality: related and not related.
• Two used three terms: not related, possible, related.
• Three used five terms: related, probable, possible, probably not, unrelated.

All the companies required the trialists to make a causality assessment (Scott, 1987).

How many Alternatives and which Terms?

There are certain principles as follows:

1. The terms themselves should not require explanation or definition. Their lack of definition is a real advantage.
2. The trialist should not be forced into an either/or situation because of a lack of alternatives. In the clinical world there are all shades of opinion and the choices should cover the whole range.

3. The more alternatives there are the narrower the use of each term becomes.
4. Absolute terms such as: 'unrelated', and 'definitely not', can only be used in exceptional circumstances because they are almost impossible to prove. Therefore, they should be avoided.
5. No term has an absolute meaning and means different things to different people. The very indistinct limits are suitable for an area where differences of opinion are extremely common and the data are very rarely reliable.

Conclusions

Theoretically, the VAS is more accurate; but the measurement of scores gives a very artificial exactness to a vague science. Practically, five categories allows a central mid-range 'possible' with the balancing of two polarized meanings on either side and avoiding absolute terms: (e.g. very unlikely, unlikely, possible, probable, very probable).

Decisions Regarding Collection of Adverse Events

Consider:

(a) Animal toxicology and pharmacology and therefore potential type A effects or class effects.
(b) ADRs of other treatments for the same indication (i.e. AEs of possible control groups).
(c) The drug development plan—phases I–IV. Discuss with the project leader which methods of collection would be suitable, will translation into different languages have to be considered?, and if more than one method is being used can the results be pooled?
(d) All studies should include the opportunity for spontaneous reporting and a standard question. If a diary card or checklist or questionnaire is added to these two standard methods, have the implications been considered?
(e) Check with the data management personnel for design of forms, coding, etc. Will the data be collected by more than one company, for example contract research organizations (CROs)? If so problems of standardization and coordination increase.

Final Questions

These comprise:

*   Does the method of collecting AEs suit the aim of the study?
*   Can the method be simplified?
*   Is the method consistent with the methods used in the rest of the drug programme?
*   Have all the essential staff involved in the study been approached?

Chapter 5

Quality of Life and Drug Therapy

Giuseppe Recchia

Postgraduate School in Medical Pharmacology, University of Milan, Italy

and

Gianfranco De Carli

Glaxo Wellcome, Medical Department, Verona, Italy

The ultimate aim of healthcare is to lengthen the patient's life and/or improve his or her wellbeing and ability to function. Drug evaluation, however, rarely takes into consideration the final outcome of treatment. On the contrary, surrogate endpoints are generally measured (i.e. in the laboratory or using physical symptoms as a substitute for other clinically significant endpoints that directly measure how patients feel, how they function or how long they survive).

Two things are happening at the moment:

- One is the tendency to look for new surrogate endpoints in order to reduce drug development time and hence the time required before an innovative drug is put onto the market.
- The other is the growing awareness that it is only by directly measuring the outcome of a particular treatment that the therapeutic value and use of a drug can be properly ascertained.

The direct measurement of how long a patient survives involves few problems. It is far more difficult to measure health in terms of how he or she feels and functions.

Health, in this context, should be thought of in terms of the definition used by the World Health Organization (WHO) in 1948—'not merely as the absence of illness but as complete physical, psychological and social wellbeing'.

The measurement of a patient's health in addition or alternatively to measuring survival time has become increasingly important clinically over the past few decades. During this time social, scientific and technological progress have allowed physicians to control most acute pathologies and to considerably increase life expectancy in industrialized countries. Healthcare in these countries has shifted towards the treatment of chronic illness and degenerative diseases. This means that the principal aim of treatment nowadays is not to prolong life, but to improve its quality. Consequently, methods for measuring health and, in particular, quality of life (QoL) measurements have been developed for the purpose of assessing and comparing different therapies and rehabilitation treatments.

Definition and Description of the Quality of Life Concept

The expression 'QoL' became widespread both within and outside the scientific community during the 1980s, largely in relation to the ecology and the perception of the degradation of city life. Despite this fact no precise definition of the concept has yet been found.

Researchers attempt to measure QoL by taking an individual as a whole, and considering the sum total of the individual's perceptions about his or her own life. Hence measurements are made of a range of different experimental fields loosely linked with the ability to function (physically, professionally, cognitively, emotionally and socially). The idea of the individual as a whole means that many of these areas overlap and interlink. This phenomenon must be taken into proper consideration when designing a QoL measurement instrument.

One of the most commonly adopted definitions of QoL is the patient's perception of how an illness and its treatment affects his or her ability to function. In 1995 the WHO defined QoL as 'the individual's perception of his/her position in life, within the cultural context and system of values in which he/she lives, in relation to goals, expectancies, models and thoughts' (The WHOQOL Group, 1995).

In practical terms QoL may be measured by investigating an individual's ability to function not merely physically (the effect of symptoms), but socially and psychologically as well (i.e. the individual's ability to enjoy what he or she does in relation to expectancies and self-realization). Each of these areas or 'dominia' can be measured in two ways:

- By objective assessment of the individual's ability to function (y-axis).
- The individual's own subjective perception of health (x-axis).

Clearly, an objective assessment is fundamental when defining a patient's health, but it is the patient's subjective impression of his or her condition and expectations that really give a reading of QoL. Expectancies concerning health and one's ability to adapt to limitations and disabilities have a strong influence on the perception of health and life satisfaction, so people with the same objective condition of health can have quite dissimilar QoL.

QoL can be influenced by many factors related to an individual's experience, such as the environment in which he or she works, personal security, the values of the community in which the individual lives, and so on. This paper will concentrate specifically on health-related QoL as defined by authors in the English-speaking world.

Each dimension of health has a number of components, which need to be measured (Figure 1) (Table 2).

Figure 1   A list of factors that can be measured or assessed with quality of life scales

1. Signs and symptoms of illness
   1. Nature of problems
   2. Severity of problems
   3. Duration and frequency of problems
   4. Amount of treatment required
   5. Adverse drug reactions
2. Function in daily life
   1. Ability to bath, dress and feed oneself
   2. Ability to control physiological functions (e.g. urine, bowel movements)
   3. Ability to ambulate and move in and out of furniture and/or cars
   4. Ability to achieve satisfactory sleep and rest

3. Productivity and economic status
   1. Ability to work productively at the patient's desired (or other) vocation
   2. Ability to support oneself, family, and/or others to a satisfactory standard of living

4. Performance of social roles
   1. With relatives, friends and others
   2. Family relationships
   3. Community relationships
   4. Recreation and pastimes

5. Intellectual capabilities
   1. Memory
   2. Ability to communicate
   3. Ability to make decisions
   4. Overall ability to think, act and react

6. Emotional stability
   1. Mood stability and swings
   2. Concerns about the future
   3. Emotional levels
   4. Religious and/or philosophical beliefs

7. Assessment of satisfaction with life
   1. Level of wellbeing
   2. Perception of general health
   3. Outlook for future

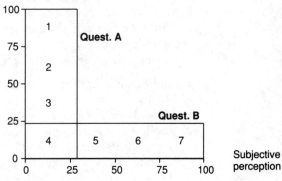

Template for the List of Factors

Modified from Spilker, B. (1986) *Guide to Clinical Interpretation of Data.* 264–267 (Raven Press, New York).

Because of the multifaceted nature of QoL, there is an almost infinite number of states of health, each with various qualities and all independent of the age of the patient.

How Quality of Life is Measured

Converting the different dominia and components of health into a single score representing QoL is a complex process.

Various tools have been developed for the purpose of measuring QoL. In most cases, each dominium is measured separately by questioning the patient about a number of health-related issues—hence these tools are frequently called questionnaires. The number of questions or statements (items or elements of the questionnaire) is a fundamental feature of the tool, since it governs both the patient's sensitivity and his or her acceptance of the questionnaire.

The main difference between questionnaires is the degree to which each dominium is covered and the depth to which it is explored, the relative weighting of the objective and subjective parts, and the different phrasing of the questions, rather than fundamental differences in defining QoL.

Most questionnaires are self-administered by patients since the purpose of the survey is to allow the patient to express his or her point of view without the distorting mirror of the interviewer's attitude to QoL. Tools do exist, however, that use observation, face-to-face interviewing and diary records. Response options can vary in type and can affect the sensitivity of the survey. Options can be binary (yes/no), an analogue bar chart (e.g. 10 cm long with the best possible condition on one side and the worst possible at the opposite side), and multiple choice Likert scales (e.g. excellent, good, moderate, bad, very bad).

The QoL measurement is built up on the basis of the patient's responses to single items in a self-administered questionnaire, grouped together into different areas. Each item has a certain impact on the patient, which he or she considers in the light of experience and then gives an answer. Different answers have different scores and are added up either within the particular area or to all other scores obtained from the questionnaire.

The instruments for measuring QoL can be identified as:

- Individual indicators, covering one health concept or dominium, such as disability, pain, or death.
- Indices. These express a patient's health status numerically. They are particularly useful for assessing the efficacy of different therapies since they allow a quick comparison between the effects of different kinds of treatment; they can also be used to assess cost–benefit ratios.
- Profiles. Unlike the indices, profiles measure different components of QoL separately, providing a series of scores for each dimension; the influence of any modification in individual areas can be assessed.
- Groups. A group of indices or profiles, with overall scores for each individual group.

Measuring tools can be divided into two main groups according to their use and contents as general or generic tools and specific tools.

General or Generic Tools

These measure a patient's basic health status (physical capacity, ability to fulfil family and professional roles, ability to function socially, etc.), without reference to particular illnesses, therapies or the patient's age. They are used to measure overall states of health in large populations and can therefore be used in a wide variety of situations. Theoretically their advantage lies in their broad applicability and the ability to compare the health status of patients with different pathologies; their drawback is that they are not sensitive enough to measure specific clinical situations and do not reveal small, but clinically significant, differences. The most sensitive of these tools are able to show variations in wellbeing and capacity, but are unable to show the reasons for these variations.

Specific Tools

These focus on specific aspects of health in each area of interest. They are therefore specifically related to each dimension of QoL relevant to a particular illness or important in a given population (e.g. the elderly), for a specific function (e.g. emotional or sexual) or a certain problem (e.g. pain). They are able to measure even small variations in states of health related to different kinds of treatment or healthcare and are therefore particularly useful for pharmacological research. Specific tools are available for a range of different pathologies because they are able to distinguish between the different causes of variation in states of health.

Choice of Tool

The choice of a general or specific instrument depends above all upon what is being measured, whether it is the general health status of a population or the degree of morbidity of a specific disease or its evolution after treatment with drugs.

In clinical research the use of specific tools for the pathology under investigation can show statistically and clinically significant differences between different kinds of treatment. This reduces the likelihood of a beta error (i.e. to accept the null error hypothesis when it is false: more simply it means minimizing beta error and thereby increasing the capability to detect differences if the differences really exist) in relation to the health factor affected by the pathology. Specific tools, however, may not show up toxic effects with repercussions on other organs or functions. General questionnaires, on the other hand, can give an indication of all aspects (both positive and negative effects) of an illness and its treatment. They can also be used to compare different treatments with different drugs for different pathologies. This is particularly useful when resources must be allocated to different treatments aiming to improve the health of a certain population. In most studies on specific illnesses where the specific tool is used it is accompanied by a general questionnaire with the least number of items possible in order to reduce the length and complexity of the questionnaire on behalf of the patient.

Choosing the Right Tool for measuring Quality of Life

For an a priori evaluation of whether a particular tool should be used for the measurement of QoL in relation to the aims of an investigation, the investigators should be thoroughly familiar with the principal features of the tool and the way it has been used. They should also consider its design, the study aims and the way it will be used. Nowadays many tools are available for use either independently or in groups, both for the purposes of measuring QoL in clinical studies and for monitoring treatment.

Features of a Tool for Measuring Quality of Life

When evaluating a particular instrument for measuring QoL the following features should be considered:

- Reliability. A tool is defined as reliable if the causal error is the smallest possible. That is, using the tool more than once with variations such as different times and places for responding to the questionnaire and different ways of responding (self-administered or replying to an interviewer's questions) leads to minimum differences. Reliability is therefore related to the accuracy of the tool, in terms of reproducing the same results at different times in the absence of differing treatment factors (minimum variation in patient's circumstances). Similarly, results should be as uniform as possible between different groups, reducing the coefficient for random error to a minimum. The analysis of a particular measuring tool's reliability involves assessing its reproducibility and internal consistency.

- Reproducibility (test/retest reliability). Each item in each dimension of the questionnaire can be checked for reproducibility by using the test/retest technique (i.e. by asking patients to respond twice or more at different times to the same question).

- Internal consistency. This indicates the coherence of the answers within a given dimension. The Cronbach alpha index (Cronbach, 1951) is used to analyse consistency, and the minimum acceptable value in common psychometric practice is 0.7 (comparison between groups) and 0.9 (comparison between one patient's answers at different times).

- Validity. This indicates the instrument's ability to measure what it was designed to measure. Since no 'gold standard' exists the validity of a measuring instrument is established empirically after sufficient use.

- Content validity. This shows whether the conceptual content of the instrument is appropriate. Generally this is established by experts who take a number of aspects into consideration, such as clarity of the questions, how easy they are to understand, and whether there are duplicates, superfluous questions or questions that should be asked and are not included.

- Construct validity. This is a check on the theoretical framework of the replies and the length of the questionnaire. It is carried out after the questionnaire has been filled in generally by using multidimensional statistical analysis (e.g. the analysis of factors, discriminators and principal components, etc).

- Concurrent validity. This indicates how close the results of the questionnaire are to a body of reference, generally consisting in an accepted method of measurement. Content validity must be demonstrated for all uses of the instrument.

- Responsiveness. This is the ability of the instrument to show up changes in the health status of a patient—often called the minimum clinically significant variation—after clinically significant events. Generally it is verified by comparing the results of the questionnaire before and after treatment of a patient that is likely to affect the patient's overall health status. Alternatively it can be verified by comparing the variations in results over time with other parameters that are assumed to differ in the same direction. One method for making such a comparison is to calculate the effect size coefficient (i.e. the relationship between pre- and post-treatment variation and base variation—the relationship between differences and standard base deviation). The responsiveness of a tool has direct implications on the choice of patients to be included in a clinical study that uses the tool as the principal means of measurement.

- Acceptability. This indicates how easy the tool is to apply in a given situation. It includes evaluation of past experience in clinical tests, the length of the questionnaire (number of items), the difficulty of its language, and the time needed to reply to it. Acceptability must be ascertained with regard to both the investigators and the patients in the light of the study population (the elderly, patients with severe disabilities, patients of a generally low educational level).

Another factor is the method for giving patients the questionnaire. Generally a tool is considered valid when given to patients in one or several ways: these may include doctor's observation, face-to-face interview, interview by telephone, the patient filling in the questionnaire on his or her own, and interviewing people close to the patient. The best method depends upon the type of questionnaire and the characteristics of the patient.

The clinical significance of variations in QoL scores and how they should be effectively communicated are two further aspects to be considered. For example, is a difference of 0.5 cm on a scale of 0–10 cm significant or not? In order to answer this question the minimum clinically significant difference should be established for each question. This difference is the smallest difference in score in a given dimension of the questionnaire that a patient experiences as a benefit, which in the absence of disturbing undesired effects or the excessive cost of therapy would lead to a change in the patient's treatment.

The Scientific Advisory Committee of the Medical Outcomes Trust has recently published updated criteria for evaluating QoL measurement instruments. These criteria differ according to whether the tool has been designed to distinguish between the states of health of different groups, to compare differences in states of health and wellbeing over time, or to predict future states of health.

The choice of the right tool for the different applications can only be made if investigators possess the following information:

- Details about all instruments designed for a certain therapeutic area.
- The features of each of these instruments in relation to how they might be used.
- The availability and conditions for using the tool.
- Knowledge about whether the tool has been translated and properly adapted for a different culture, together with the information about the tool that is available in Italy.
- Preceding experience with the tool used for a similar purpose.

Currently, numerous tools for measuring QoL are available. Most of them were designed and developed in Anglo-Saxon countries and in some cases they have been adapted to other cultures.

Table 1 shows a list of tools available to the international scientific community, by therapeutic area, but this is by no means exhaustive. For more detailed information about both general and specific tools for measuring QoL the following sources, among others, may be consulted:

> **Table 1 Quality of life tools**
>
> **GENERAL**
> Medical Outcomes Study short form (SF36)
> Nottingham Health Profile (NHP)
> EuroQoL
> Sickness Impact Profile (SIP)
> Duke UNC Health Profile (DUHP)
>
> **SPECIFIC**
> Respiratory diseases
> Neoplastic diseases
> Cardiovascular diseases
> Gastrointestinal diseases
> Psychiatric diseases
> Aids
> The elderly
> Metabolic diseases
> Epilepsy

- *Compendium of Quality of Life Instruments*, published by the Centre for Medicines Research Unit (CMR), UK.
- The databank *On-Line Guide to Quality of Life Assessment—OLGA*, developed by the Mapi Research Institute. The On-Line Guide to Quality of Life Assessment (OLGA) 11404, Lund Place, Kensington, Maryland 20895, USA (Erikson, 1995).
- The databank *Quality of Life Bibliography*, published at regular intervals in the magazine *Quality of Life Research*, available on floppy disk for research purposes.
- The CD-ROM *Quality of Life Assessment in Medicine*, developed by Dr Marcello Tamburini and published by Glamm Interactive srl, Milan, Italy.
- The Internet site *www.glamm.com/ql/guide.htm* (*Clinician's Computer-Assisted Guide to the Choice of Instruments for Quality of Life Assessment in Medicine*), which was created in 1997 by Glam Interactive srl, Milan, Italy.
- *Quality of Life* newsletter, ed. K. I. Johnson, publisher MAPI Research Institute, 27, Rue de la Villette, 69003 Lyon, France. E-mail-institut@mapi.fr.

Questionnaires designed in other (generally Anglo-Saxon) countries can be used in order to measure QoL in other countries, provided these instruments have been adapted to the local Italian culture; where no instruments have been published in the scientific literature or the available instruments are unsuitable, new instruments may be designed *de novo* in the local setting.

Adapting a Questionnaire to a Different Culture

Although research into costs can to some extent be transferred from one country to another, it is far less easy to extend the results of QoL studies across national boundaries. This is because the results are based on subjective evaluations and these are related to value systems that are culturally specific. Very few QoL tools have been adapted to different cultures, and only these can be used in international multicentre studies.

If the tool is not available outside the country where it was designed (either for international studies or for research in one country alone) it must be translated and adapted to the new culture, validated and supported by data enabling investigators to interpret results correctly, particularly where scores differ due to treatment. Each of these processes must follow a standard methodology, such as the one used in the IQOLA project or others currently used in Italy (Figure 2) (Apolone *et al.*, 1997; Apolone and Mosconi, 1997).

Before using tools for measuring QoL during the development phase of a new drug the tools must be fully supported by documentation concerning their psychometric features, the process of validation and the lessons learned from using each tool. Without this documentation it is not possible to convince regulatory authorities of the correct use of the tool and hence to persuade them of the validity of the data presented for registration purposes or to inform the scientific community about the drug.

Designing a New Questionnaire

Several methods can be adopted in designing a new questionnaire to measure QoL. The most commonly used method in Italy is described below.

On the basis of the fact that QoL represents a series of perceptions about one's own health status, the design of a questionnaire should include:

- Identification of medical items. These are chosen after a meeting of experts in the pathology under examination for the purpose of establishing the most common symptoms and behavioural characteristics of patients with the pathology. After this it is possible to make a first draft of questions (draft 1).
- Identification of patient items. Patient items are chosen after several informal meetings (focus groups) with patients who have the pathology under examination. These patients should be of both sexes, different ages and have had the pathology for different periods of time; some should be receiving treatment and some not. The meetings should be coordinated by an expert. During each meeting patients should fill in draft 1 and be encouraged to talk freely about other relevant aspects of their illness. In this way new items are added to the first draft and items that are consistently viewed as irrelevant are dropped. Each new focus group receives the update of draft 1.
- Preparing the questionnaire. After the focus groups, the medical items and patient items are used to produce a second draft of the questionnaire (draft 2). At this stage the scales for each reply are designed on the basis of the findings of the focus groups. Draft 2 is then given to a representative group of the overall population to ensure that the questions are clear and that the questionnaire can be filled in relatively easily and rapidly.
- Validation of the questionnaire. Draft 2 is given to a representative group of the overall population who have the pathology under examination for validation and standardization. (i.e. to evaluate the characteristics given in the preceding paragraph). The data obtained is analysed and a third draft is produced. Draft 3 may then used in the clinical study.
- Subsequent development. Draft 3 may also be modified on the basis of the experience of other investigators or data collected during its use. Studies integrating

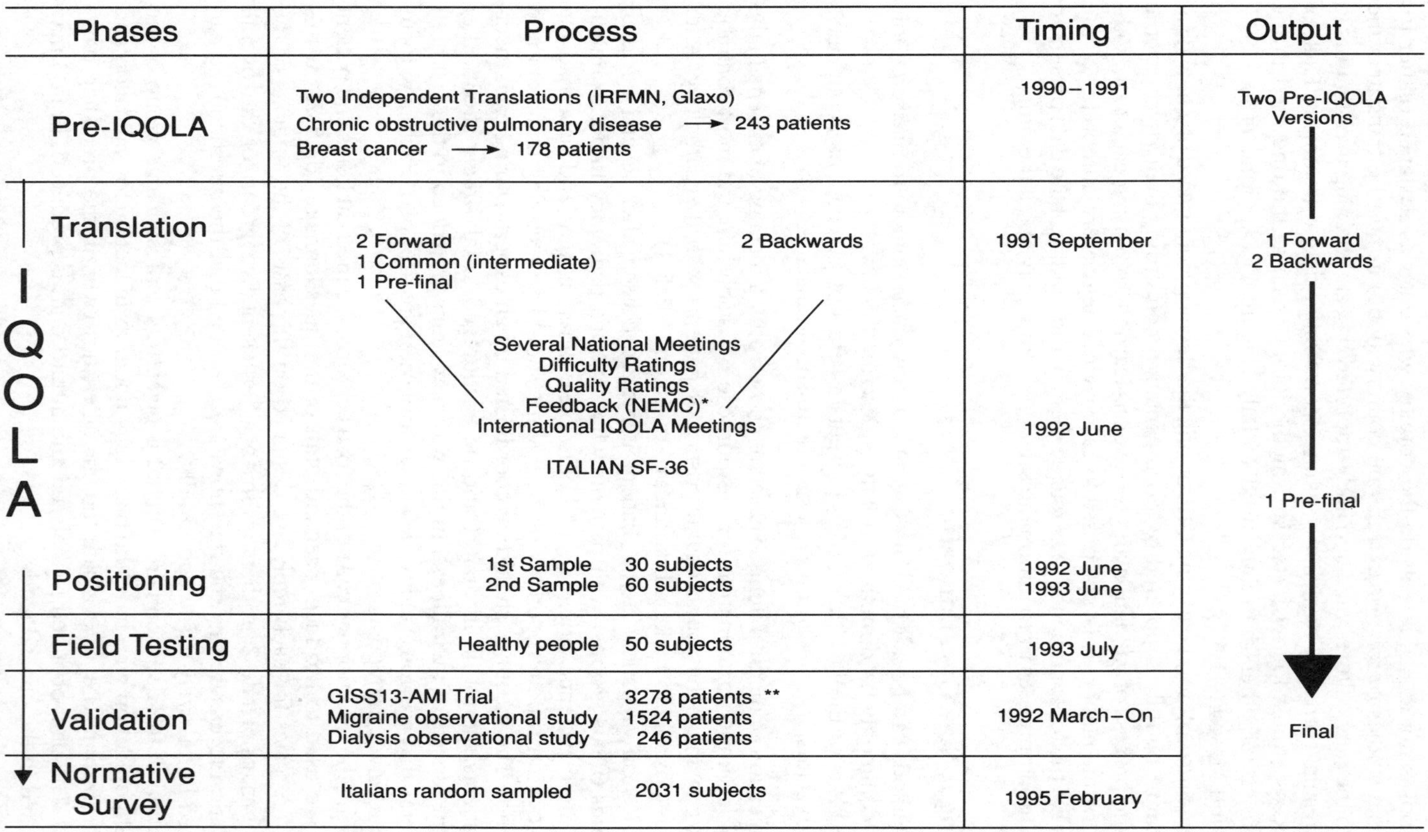

Phases	Process	Timing	Output
Pre-IQOLA	Two Independent Translations (IRFMN, Glaxo) Chronic obstructive pulmonary disease → 178 patients Breast cancer → 243 patients	1990–1991	Two Pre-IQOLA Versions
Translation	2 Forward 1 Common (intermediate) 1 Pre-final 2 Backwards	1991 September	1 Forward 2 Backwards
	Several National Meetings Difficulty Ratings Quality Ratings Feedback (NEMC)* International IQOLA Meetings ITALIAN SF-36	1992 June	1 Pre-final
Positioning	1st Sample 30 subjects 2nd Sample 60 subjects	1992 June 1993 June	Final
Field Testing	Healthy people 50 subjects	1993 July	
Validation	GISS13-AMI Trial 3278 patients ** Migraine observational study 1524 patients Dialysis observational study 246 patients	1992 March–On	
Normative Survey	Italians random sampled 2031 subjects	1995 February	

Figure 2   Cross Cultural Adjustment Process

*New England Medical Center, The Health Institute; **Only in 18 items
Reproduced with permission from Apolone et al., 1997.

Table 2   Scales of short form questionnaire SF 36 (36 items)

Physical functioning (10 items).
Ability to carry out different physical functions in day-to-day life

Role impairment due to physical functions (4 items).
How health status interferes with ordinary daily functions

Physical pain (2 items)
Sensations of physical pain in the past 'four' weeks

General health status (5 items)
Perception of one's own health

Vitality (2 items)
Vital energy or tiredness in last four weeks

Social life (2 items)
How health status interferes with social life

Role impairment due to psychological problems (3 items)
How psychological problems (anxiety and depression) interfere with day-to-day activities

Mental health (5 items)
General tone of mood and affections: depression, anxiety or wellbeing in past four weeks

Change in health status (1 item)
Change in health status in past year

Modified from Apolone *et al.*, 1997, with permission.

the definition of the different characteristics of each tool may also be carried out during this phase.

Application of measurements of Quality of Life

Questionnaires can be used in various ways according to how the results will be used (Table 3).

Application Range

The different ranges of application of the questionnaire require different tools and different methods for collecting the data.

Clinical Research
In recent years one of the primary aims in the development of a new drug has been to compile information about the drug's clinical efficacy (i.e. its ability to improve a patient's health status) and the economic benefits of its use.

One of the objectives of clinical pharmacological research has thus become assessment of the drug's impact on QoL (improved health status or fewer disadvantages compared to other treatments). Clinical research already produces 9% of all articles on QoL. In most cases measuring QoL is a secondary aim of the study (assessing

---

Table 3   Applications of quality of life measurements

Applications
Clinical research
Observational clinical research
Ambulatory or hospital assistance to patients

Use
For clinical decisions
Registration, reimbursement of a drug
Inclusion in handbook
Technical and scientific drug information
Economic assessment

---

efficacy and tolerability are generally the primary aims), but sometimes it is one of the primary aims. In these cases choosing the size of the population means taking into account normal variations in the distribution of QoL scores and the size of clinically significant variations.

Some authors believe measuring QoL is suitable in the following types of clinical study:

- Where QoL is the principal endpoint of the study (above all where treatment is palliative or where patients are incurable).
- Where treatments are presumed to have the same efficacy but different impacts on QoL.
- Where the new treatment may slightly lengthen life expectancy, but have a severely detrimental impact on QoL.
- Where different treatments have very different degrees of efficacy in the short term, but do not produce appreciable long-term clinical differences.

Measuring the impact of a drug on QoL may be done in absolute terms (comparison to base value) or comparative terms (comparison with standard treatment) without needing to change the experimental procedures (randomization, double-blind, etc.) used for traditional parameters, such as efficacy and tolerability, in clinical studies. Generally, because of the time needed to reveal changes in QoL measurements are made in two parallel groups of patients.

In a clinical study the most important feature of a questionnaire measuring QoL is the responsiveness—that is, ability to show up variations induced by the therapy and therefore to identify the cause(s) of the variation(s). In order to achieve this result the full versions of specific tools designed for given pathologies should be used. Some general tools can be used provided their ability to show up variations induced by the therapy has been verified, albeit with the limitations described later in this chapter.

Patients should not be given the questionnaire too many times since they may learn to recognize the questions and remember previous answers; after the initial (base value) measurement the questionnaire can be repeated 2–3 months into therapy to show up variations caused by the treatment, and then 6–12 months later to show the long-term effect on QoL. Scores should be calculated on the basis of the guidelines written by the authors of the questionnaire, which should include instructions about how to handle missing data and how to calculate scores in each dimension, with weighted values and method of standardization.

If a clinical study has the primary aim of measuring QoL, each dimension of the questionnaire should be analysed separately. This means increasing the likelihood of running into false positive readings, since significant correlations are more likely to be found simply by chance the more comparisons are made. In order to correct this statistical bias closed-tests, the Bonferroni-Holm correction method and a global statistical approach can be adopted, each of which considers individual dimensions independently of all others.

The degree and significance of treatment-induced variations in QoL can be assessed by calculating the 'effect size', which represents the standardized measure of variation within a group or the difference in variations between two groups. Although the effect size can be calculated in different ways, all methods involve dividing the average differences in a single variable by the standard base deviation of that variable.

Observational Clinical Research and Surveys of Health Status

The measurement of QoL in general populations, in sample groups or groups of patients with different pathologies can be carried out by surveys of states of health or observational clinical research. In most cases a cross-sectional tool is used and given to patients once only; sometimes a prospective questionnaire is used for repeated measurements with the same patient.

The principal aim of these studies is to ascertain the health status of a certain population, general or specific, such as the elderly (Figure 3) or the impact of a certain disease on the state of patient health. Generally these measurements are made using general tools, even for patients with specific diseases. This is because with this type of tool it is possible to compare the effects of the disease under investigation with the effects of other diseases, as measured with the same tool at the same time or in other studies.

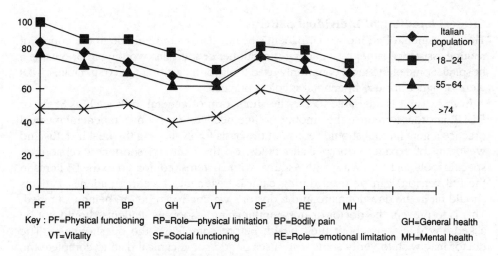

Key : PF=Physical functioning RP=Role—physical limitation BP=Bodily pain GH=General health
VT=Vitality SF=Social functioning RE=Role—emotional limitation MH=Mental health

Figure 3 Health profiles for younger and older adults in Italy

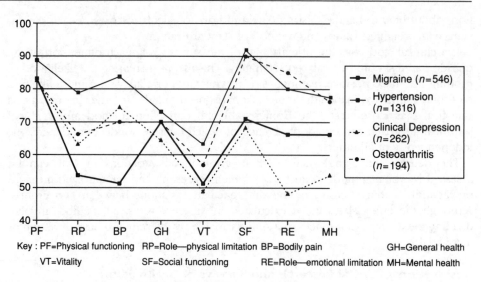

Key : PF=Physical functioning   RP=Role—physical limitation   BP=Bodily pain   GH=General health
        VT=Vitality   SF=Social functioning   RE=Role—emotional limitation   MH=Mental health

Figure 4   Comparison of adjusted SF-36 health status scores for migraine and other conditions (Reproduced with permission from Osterhaus *et al.*, 1994.)

Questionnaires can be given to patients in doctors' waiting rooms (where patients fill in the questionnaire on their own) or at their homes, either by interviewing them face-to-face or on the telephone or by mailing them the questionnaire. It is important for investigators to check that the tool they wish to use is properly designed for the intended use, and that sufficient experience has been gained in the application of the tool for that use. The studies can be used to evaluate the cost (in health terms) of an illness before treatment and the effect of treatments on a given population during healthcare. Figure 4 gives the impact on QoL of some of the most common illnesses in American patients, as measured by the general tool SF 36.

Clinical handling of individual patients
The assessment of an individual patient's health status can be made in the course of routine assistance either by a general practitioner or specialist working in or outside a hospital. Some of the most commonly used tools for measuring QoL (e.g. Duke-UNC) were designed for use in general medical practice.

In this case it is advisable to use the short form of general tools such as SF 36 or DUHP in order to reduce the amount of time needed to respond. In general medical practice a general tool should represent the basis for evaluating the health status and wellbeing of a patient. In specialist fields, on the contrary, shortened versions of specific tools such as 'Living with Asthma' with 20 items (compared to the 63 items in the full version) can be used during clinical treatment of asthma patients. Patients should fill in the questionnaire in the doctor's waiting room before being examined. This is to prevent the doctor or nurse influencing responses. Patients should not be asked any questions about their health before completing the questionnaire. The doctor may wish to verify some responses or add some clinical data to complete the picture of the patient's health status.

Software programmes capable of processing the results of questionnaires are currently being tested. These enable the health status of an individual patient to be monitored by graphic display of scores obtained during the various phases of the study.

How Measurement of the Quality of Life can be used

The QoL scores can be used as the basis of decision-making or to improve understanding. If decisions are taken on the basis of the results, the results should obviously have been obtained with scientifically valid methods and should be as complete as possible. To ensure that this is the case, guidelines and standards should be used for the evaluation of QoL studies according to specific criteria. These guidelines are of help to regulatory bodies, the publishers of medical journals, individual doctors and anyone involved in the purchase or assessment of drugs. They also improve the quality of studies by excluding unreliable data collected with insufficiently documented tools.

Clinical Decisions

One of the most interesting developments recently in the field of general medical practice and in specialist medicine is the application of QoL measurements to evaluate a patient's health status and the variations in his or her health status induced by an illness or treatment.

The QoL tool is a new instrument at the disposal of the doctor in treating his patient. The benefits and risks of a particular treatment are no longer a matter for the doctor to assess alone on the basis of observations and understanding of a pathology; the patient's own assessment and perception of his or her health status can be used to take decisions about what treatment to prescribe. The patient can help the doctor come to the best decision about each individual case. For example, Figure 4 shows how a headache can influence QoL in ways similar to a far more clinically serious condition; pain levels are high as are impairment to social and mental functions; the ability to fulfil one's roles is also severely hampered. This picture would scarcely have emerged from a traditional appraisal of the patient's condition: measuring QoL, in this case, goes well beyond simply registering the patient's level of pain.

Drug treatment may improve or damage a patient's QoL. In the former case it will restore functions impaired by an illness (e.g. allowing an asthmatic patient to function normally in society, where previously the patient avoided social occasions because of the fear of an asthma attack); in the latter case it will limit some of the patient's abilities (e.g. treatment of some allergic conditions by certain antihistamines involves sedation, reducing mental functions and the ability to fulfil social and economic roles). In both cases the most useful treatment for the patient should be identified, not only on the basis of efficacy and tolerability, but also in view of the various dimensions of QoL.

A QoL damaged by a particular treatment (e.g. for hypertension, some anti-epileptic therapy, interferon treatment, etc.) makes patients less likely to accept a given therapy (adverse effect on compliance) and therefore reduces treatment efficacy. In such cases the measurement of QoL may be used to identify the problem and lead to the choice of alternative therapies that are more acceptable to the patient.

Regulatory Aims

Documentation that includes measurement of QoL may be used to apply to regulatory bodies for authorization to sell a drug or may be important to the decision about whether or not the drug's cost can be reimbursed to the patient. QoL is also becoming increasingly important in obtaining authorization to use personal data in medical and scientific literature.

In 1995 a consultative committee of the American Food and Drug Administration (FDA) came to a decision that has been described as epoch-making: for the first time it recommended authorization to sell a new antiblastic drug (gemcitabine) principally on the basis of its effect on QoL.

Regulatory authorities, in particular the FDA, believe that measurements of QoL are made more frequently in clinical studies than in the past because of their high potential for promoting a particular drug; hence rules are currently being drawn up for QoL studies used for regulatory purposes. According to the FDA, declarations about a drug, as with all other variables used in clinical studies, must be based on concrete evidence obtained in controlled and, if possible, randomized clinical studies, carried out double-blind on sufficiently large numbers, and the results should be analysed and where possible repeated.

There are three types of declaration about a drug ('claim' is the expression used worldwide) that catch the regulatory authorities' eye:

- Those that talk about 'improved QoL' (i.e. where the claim is that patients enjoy better health with the drug treatment concerned).
- Those that talk about 'maintaining QoL' (i.e. where the claim is that the patient's condition does not deteriorate when treated with the drug concerned).
- Those that talk about 'relief from negative effects on QoL' (i.e. where the claim is that the drug concerned leads to fewer undesired effects than other drugs).

In 1997 the FDA approved the request to use a declaration about the positive effects on QoL of an anti-asthma drug, salmeterol.

The most recent versions of guidelines published by the European Medicines Evaluation Agency (EMEA) for the clinical development of drugs used for heart disorders, angina pectoris and tumours, include measurement of QoL as one of the parameters for assessing the therapeutic efficacy of a drug.

Economic Evaluation of a Drug

Some authors include techniques for measuring QoL, together with techniques for analysing the cost of a drug, as part of pharmacoeconomic research. Despite efforts by numerous researchers, the attempt to evaluate different states of health and the variations induced by different drug treatments in economic terms has made very little progress.

QoL is nonetheless used in one of the economic analyses used for healthcare — 'the cost-utility analysis' — which compares the relative costs of different treatments in relation to treatment-induced variations in QoL. For this purpose QoL must be expressed as a single number.

On the basis of this model some researchers have developed the concept of 'Quality of Life Adjusted Year' (QALY) (i.e. the number of years of life adjusted for quality as an indication of a healthcare benefit, representing the health status required for survival) (Torrance, 1986).

Health Subsidies and Public Healthcare

The increasing cost of public healthcare and the need to reduce public spending on health has led to a rapid shift towards forms of 'managed care'. This was initiated in the USA and is now rapidly expanding in Europe. At the same time there is an increasing demand for quality healthcare able to solve health problems. Due to this it has become necessary to measure the quality of healthcare (i.e. the 'outcomes' of treatments and illnesses) in order to assess the most effective or least costly treatments and allocate resources accordingly. This has led to 'Outcome Research', which measures clinical, economic and human outcomes of illnesses and their therapies.

Together with patient satisfaction and the patient's preference for one kind of treatment rather than another, QoL is one of the main tools used in health management. Some of the most commonly used QoL tools, such as SF 36, were developed specifically to verify the impact of alternative methods of treatment on the health status of a given population.

Chapter 6

Laboratory Investigations

M. D. B. Stephens

The value of laboratory investigations in the clinical trial programme for detecting new adverse drug reactions (ADRs) has not been explored. A large pharmaceutical company may collect over five million results per year and 50% or more of the database in any new drug application (NDA) is laboratory data (Harkins, 1996). The number and variety of investigations performed must be limited to those that are necessary.

The purpose of the laboratory investigations is twofold:

- Efficacy. To act as an endpoint or surrogate marker for the target disease (e.g. blood sugar in diabetes mellitus or cholesterol in ischaemic heart disease). When this is the case these investigations are the responsibility of the clinical research department
- Safety. The results need to be reported in the Integrated Safety Summary (ISS) of the marketing authorization and as such should be the responsibility of the pharmacovigilance (PV) department. However, the organization of the vene-puncture, transport of the samples and liaison with the investigator comes within the ambit of the clinical research associate (CRA) monitoring the study. There is, therefore, a shared responsibility.

Safety Aims

Screening (phase I and II)

The aims are:

- To protect the safety of the volunteer or patient by excluding those with sub-clinical disease from studies that might expose them to unnecessary risk.
- To protect the drug by excluding patients with subclinical disease that might progress to overt disease during the study and be mistaken for a drug-induced effect.
- To screen out those with a test outside the reference interval (range) and thereby reduce the background noise and increase the power of the study to find any new ADRs (see page 82).

Screening (phase III)

Unless it is intended to have a laboratory exclusion clause in the subsequent data sheet, it is unwise to use laboratory values to screen out patients at the phase III stage.

Monitoring

The aims are:

- To protect the volunteer or patient by detecting the early onset of any drug-related abnormality.
- To detect any unforeseen beneficial effect on a laboratory test.
- In phase III studies to monitor the effect of the drug on any organ function affected by a disease other than the target disease—for example, with thyroid function tests where the hormone is protein bound—the oral contraceptive causes a rise in the thyroxine-binding globulin giving a rise in value of T_3 and T_4 (Ramsay, 1985).

Choice of Investigations

As in monitoring for adverse clinical events there are two types of monitoring of laboratory investigations: specific monitoring and non-specific monitoring.

Specific Monitoring

Animal pharmacology, toxicology or abnormalities seen with drugs of the same class may signal hypotheses concerning changes in laboratory parameters. These will usually be type A adverse events and will be relatively common, although some type A adverse events will be due to genetic abnormalities in a small subgroup of patients and may therefore be quite rare.

Common pharmacological abnormalities can usually be detected in relatively small controlled studies and since most patients will be affected, a comparison of the changes in the mean values is the best way of identifying them. Since these events are predictable it is worth taking special care in monitoring them by ensuring that the patient's condition before sampling is standardized and that the methods of collection, storage and transport of the samples are ideal.

Non-specific Monitoring

Unpredictable adverse laboratory events may precede serious clinical adverse events and are, by definition, type B events. Since they will be relatively rare only one or two events may arise in the whole pre-marketing clinical development programme. Clearly statistical analysis will not be applicable and individual assessment will be required. The choice of investigations to be monitored will depend upon the frequency and seriousness of the possible outcomes. The three most important organs to monitor are the liver, kidney and bone marrow. The choice of tests will be discussed later in this chapter.

Choice of Investigations for Specific and Non-specific Monitoring

Investigations required for specific monitoring will differ from drug to drug, so will not be considered further here. Discussion will be limited to those required for non-specific monitoring. What factors should be considered?

Discomfort and Disturbance of the Patient

Many patients fear needles, so there should be a good reason for every sampling. Some investigations (e.g. blood sugar and cholesterol), require fasting for proper assessment and this usually implies an early morning appointment, and for patients who live far from the clinic the early rise may not be welcome.

Cost–benefit Ratio for a Particular Test

A standard screen will be relatively cheap, but demands for additional individual tests will be much more expensive.

Value in the Detection of Drug-induced Effects

Liver and renal function tests, haematology and urine tests are essential in any monitoring for drug safety, but what is the value of any individual test within these groups? The choice of individual tests depends more upon what is available on the Sequential Multiple Analyzer (SMA) than their value for the detection of ADRs. The Expert Panel on Drug Effects from the Scientific Committee of the International Federation of Clinical Chemistry (IFCC) drew up a list of tests to define the health of volunteers (Table 1). They also gave a list of 72 parameters that may be required in patients (Spiro *et al.*, 1987). The regulatory authorities do not mention any particular tests as being required for adults, but the Food and Drug Administration (FDA) in their guidelines for the clinical evaluation of psychoactive drugs in infants and children have two lists. These lists (the FDA and IFCC) and other alternative lists of tests (a list of tests used by a pharmaceutical company, a list of suggested investigations for general monitoring given by Professor M. Rawlins at a Management Forum meeting in November 1989, the minimal requirements for individual side effects from the rules governing medicinal products in the European Community, Vol. III, Addendum July 1990 and the range of tests available via SMA) are given in Table 1. Unfortunately (in this context) automatic analysers are designed to produce standard outputs which are cheaper than the collection of the individual investigations and this results in tests being performed that are not necessary for safety purposes (e.g. blood urea).

If the range of laboratory investigations undertaken is the minimum possible there will be the possibility that an adverse event occuring during a study may have been developing before the first dose of a new drug, but the limited laboratory tests at screening did not reveal it. If an additional sample of blood is taken at baseline and stored it may be used at a later date to establish a baseline for that particular test, or if no problems occur it can be discarded at the end of the study.

Table 1 Choice of laboratory investions

		1	2	3	4	5	6	7	8	9	10*
Blood	Haemoglobin	x	x	x	x				x	x	x
	Erythrocytes	x	x	x					x	x	x
	Haematocrit—packed cell volume (PCV)	x	x	x	x					x	
	Mean corpuscular volume (MCV)	x	x		x						
	Mean corpuscular haemoglobin (MCH)	x									
	Mean corpuscular haemoglobin concentration (MCHC)	x			x						
	Erythrocyte sedimentation rate (ESR)			x					x	x	
	Leucocytes—White blood count (WBC)	x	x	x	x				x	x	x
	Neutrophils	x	x	x	x				x	x	x
	Basophils	x	x	x	x				x	x	x
	Monocytes	x	x	x	x				x	x	x
	Eosinophils	x	x	x	x				x	x	x
	Lymphocytes	x	x	x	x				x	x	x
	Platelets	x	x	x	x				x	x	x
	Reticulocytes									x	x
Haemostasis	Bleeding time			x						x	
	Prothrombin time			x							
	Activated partial thromboplastin time			x					x	x	
	Blood pH		x								
	Iron					x	x			x	
Liver	Total bilirubin	x	x	x	x	x	x	x	x	x	x
	Alkaline phosphatase (AP)	x	x	x	x	x	x	x	x	x	x
	Gamma glutamyl transpeptidase (GGT)	x		x					x	x	
	Alanine aminotransferase (ALT)	x		x		x	x	x	x	x	x
	Aspartate aminotransferase (AST)	x	x	x	x	x	x		x	x	x
	Lactate dehydrogenase (LDH)			x		x	x	x			
	Glucose-6-phosphate dehydrogenase deficiency (G6PD deficiency)			x							
Kidney	Creatinine	x		x	x	x	x	x	x	x	x
	Urea nitrogen	x	x	x	x	x	x	x			x
	Uric Acid	x		x		x	x	x	x	x	
	Inorganic phosphate/P	x	x			x	x	x			x
	Calcium	x	x			x	x	x			x
	Blood urea nitrogen (BUN)/creatinine ratio					x	x	x			
	Para-amino Hippuric Acid (PAH) clearance	x	x								
	Inulin clearance	x	x								
	Serum electrophoresis	x	x							x	
	Bromosulphalein (BSP) clearance	x	x								
	Creatinine clearance	x	x								
Electrolytes	Sodium	x	x	x	x	x			x	x	x
	Potassium	x	x	x	x	x			x	x	x
	Chloride	x	x		x	x					
	Bicarbonate/CO_2	x	x		x	x					
	Osmolality					x	x				
	Creatine phosphokinase	x									
Nutritional	Glucose	x		x		x	x	x	x	x	x
	Two-hour post-cibum glucose		x								

		1	2	3	4	5	6	7	8	9	10*
	Total proteins	x	x	x		x	x	x	x	x	x
	Albumin	x		x		x	x	x			x
	Globulin					x	x	x			
	Albumin/globulin (A/G) ratio					x	x	x			
	High-density lipoprotein (HDL)	x									
	Low-density lipoprotein (LDL)	x									
	Triglycerides	x		x		x	x			x	
	Cholesterol	x	x	x		x	x	x		x	
	Lipase									x	
	Cholinesterase									x	
	Haemoglobin in plasma									x	
Hormones	Cortisol		x								
	Thyroid stimulating hormone (TSH)		x								
	T3R		x								
	Thyroxine (T)		x								
	Growth hormone		x								
	Luteinizing hormone (LH) or Follicle stimulating hormone (FSH)		x								
	Testosterone		x								
	Cytology for oestrogen effect		x								
	Bone age		x								
	Vanillylmandelic acid (VMA)		x								
Urine	Appearance	x									
	pH	x							x	x	
	Specific gravity	x	x								
	Protein/albumin	x	x	x	x				x	x	x
	Haemoglobin	x		x	x				x	x	x
	White cells	x	x	x					x	x	
	Red cells	x	x	x						x	
	Casts	x	x	x					x		
	Glucose	x	x	x					x	x	x
	Acetoacetate		x	x							
	Ketones	x							x	x	
	Amino acids	x									
	17-Ketosteroids	x									
	Bilirubin									x	
	Osmolality					x					
	Volume					x					

* No. 10 only stipulates urinanalysis

Key

1. Lilly USA (Thompson *et al.*, 1988).
2. FDA Guidelines for the Clinical Evaluation of Psychoactive Drugs in Infants and Children, July 1979.
3. IFCC (Spiro *et al.*, 1987).
4. Professor M. Rawlins, General Monitoring, Management Forum, November 1989.
5. Sequential Multiple Analyser Channel (SMAC) 24.
6. SMAC 20.
7. SMAC 16.
8. Proposals of the clinical pharmacology section of the German Society for Pharmacology and Toxicology (Bethge *et al.*, 1991).
9. Recommendations of Clinical Chemical Association for the performance of clinical chemical studies (*J. Clin. Chem. Clin. Biochem.*, **22**, 1984).
10. Toxicity Tests in phase I and II studies, Evaluation of anticancer medicinal products in man. Minimal requirement of evaluation for individual side effects, guidelines on the quality, safety and efficacy of medicinal products for human use. The rules governing medicinal products in the European Community. Vol. III, Addendum July 1990.

The Value of Individual Laboratory Tests

Liver Function Tests

Aminotransferases

Alanine aminotransferase (ALT)—previously known as serum glutamic pyruvic transaminase (SGPT)—and AST—previously known as serum glutamic oxaloacetic transaminase (SGOT)—both rise with damage to the liver cells; AST also increases with strokes, pulmonary infarction, muscular damage, congestive cardiac failure, myocardial infarction and acute pancreatitis. The ALT is present in relatively low concentrations in other tissues and is therefore more specific for liver damage; it does rise with myocardial infarction, but not as much as AST and similarly ALT may increase in disseminated cancer, muscle disorders, acute renal disease and acute pancreatitis (Helzberg, 1986). Whenever possible both AST and ALT should be used for screening, but if only one is available and there is a choice it is better to choose the more specific enzyme ALT. When the AST/ALT ratio > 1 and the ALT is < 300 a diagnosis of alcoholic liver disease should be considered (Cohen and Kaplan, 1975). The strongest predictor of raised ALT in healthy volunteers on placebo was a baseline ALT > 10 U/l and an AST/ALT ratio < 1 (Merz *et al.*, 1997).

Gamma Glutamyltranspeptidase and Alkaline Phosphatase

These will both increase with obstruction and cholestasis rather than with liver cell damage. The GGT may also rise with pancreatitis, renal cell damage or neo-plasms; but it is used in the context of clinical trials for monitoring excess alcohol intake and obstructive liver damage. There can also be a benign elevation of GGT. The AP is found in liver, bone, intestine and placenta, and is used for monitoring obstructive liver disease and bone disease except in children (in whom it is raised) and pregnancy (when total AP rises, see below). It should be remembered that AP may be elevated after infarction of the myocardium, lung, spleen, kidney or bowel, and in ulcerative colitis, sepsis, hyperthyroidism, congestive cardiac failure, acute bone fracture, carcinoma and benign inherited elevation of AP (Lieberman and Phillips, 1990). If there is a persistent elevation there is usually a clinically obvious cause. The isoenzymes of AP may help in identifying the source of AP. There are four:

- Placental—rises in pregnancy.
- Intestinal.
- Hepatic (also in acute infection)—falls in pregnancy (Parker, 1991).
- Osseous—rises in pregnancy (Moss, 1981).

The isoenzymes are not measured routinely and they cannot be measured by all laboratories, but they may be helpful in cases where the origin of a raised value is unclear.

Both GGT and AP may be elevated due to enzyme induction, and if this can be established it is not necessary to stop the study or enzyme-inducing drug (Davis, 1989). A raised GGT and AP (hepatic isoenzyme) can be seen in rheumatic diseases, possibly due to an acute reaction to inflammation (Akesson *et al.*, 1980).

Lactate Dehydrogenase

This is a very non-specific enzyme and is found in the liver, heart, muscle, lung, brain, kidney, and bone marrow. The isoenzyme LDH1 is significant in myocardial infarction while LDH5 is more specific for the liver (Plaut, 1978). The total LDH is not a useful screening test for liver damage.

Bilirubin

This is raised in diseases involving destruction of red blood cells (RBC) and in liver disease, both obstructive and non-obstructive. If it is raised differentiation between conjugated and non-conjugated bilirubin will help in distinguishing that due to destruction of RBC when the conjugated (direct) bilirubin remains low, usually 5–15% of the total. A rise in unconjugated bilirubin (usually between 20–40 μmol/l or 1.2–2.5 mg/dl and rarely exceeds 80 μmol/l or 5 mg/dl) is frequently seen in an inherited disorder of bilirubin excretion, Gilbert's syndrome, which affects 5% of the population. This is usually an isolated finding (Hegarty and Williams, 1987; Zilva *et al.*, 1988). The total serum bilirubin will be increased in both normal patients and those with Gilbert's syndrome on fasting. After a 12-hour fast the mean total serum bilirubin in volunteers was 14 μmol/l in the non-fasting group and 17.3 μmol/l in the fasting group and after 24 hours 13.7 μmol/l and 35.2 μmol/l, respectively (Meyer *et al.*, 1995). Clinical jaundice is usually detected when bilirubin reaches 34.2–51.3 μmol/l (2–3 mg/dl) (Schimmel, 1968).

Albumin and Total Protein

Serum albumin + serum globulin = Total protein. These are not early indicators of organ damage and may decrease in the nephrotic syndrome or protein losing enteropathy (increased excretion) or severe liver disease or protein calorie malnutrition (decreased production). They are not essential for routine monitoring. Asymptomatic abnormal liver function tests in clinical trials are common and the topic is dealt with in greater depth in a paper in *Pharmacoepidemiology and Drug Safety* (Stephens, 1994).

Renal Function Tests

Blood Urea Nitrogen and Creatinine

These both measure renal function, but if the blood urea rises and the creatinine remains normal a non-renal cause of uraemia, such as increased protein breakdown, haemorrhage or dehydration, needs to be considered. Measurement of the plasma concentration of urea or creatinine is insensitive and can be misleading. Concentrations may remain within the normal range even in the presence of extensive renal damage (Prescott, 1982), but the Siersbaek-Nielsen equation can be used to calculate creatinine clearance and correct for the effects of age, sex and body weight, as can the Cockcroft-Gault equation.

Uric Acid

This rises in renal failure. Urate excretion is diminished by thiazide and loop diuretics and increased by probenecid and corticosteroids. Abnormal purine metabolism or massive nucleic acid turnover can increase uric acid production (e.g. cytolytic cancer therapy can increase it). It is probably worth monitoring in long-term treatments and for drugs used in rheumatic diseases.

Calcium and Inorganic Phosphate
Both of these increase in renal failure, but are not essential for routine non-specific monitoring.

Electrolytes

With potassium and sodium, chloride and bicarbonate help to evaluate fluid and acid–base status. Bicarbonate (P_{CO_2}) is important in respiratory failure. Many drugs can alter the electrolytes resulting in a clinical ADR (e.g. potassium and cardiac arrhythmias) (Brass and Thompson, 1982).

Muscle

Creatine phosphokinase (CPK) is present in cardiac muscle and skeletal muscle as well as the brain. The CPK isoenzymes can be useful for differentiating between brain, heart and skeletal muscle: isoenzyme MM (muscle) and BB (brain).

Brain contains BB, skeletal muscle contains 90% MM 10% MB, while heart muscle contains 60% MM and 40% MB. Rises in MB isoenzyme therefore indicate cardiac damage and rises in MM, skeletal or cardiac muscle damage (Moss, 1981). Since it is not present in liver it can help to distinguish myocardial infarction from liver damage due to congestive heart failure or drugs. Exercise can cause a mild–moderate elevation 2–4 times the upper limit of normal (Widmann, 1987). Yoga alone can cause an elevation 4 times the upper limit of normal (Tamarin *et al.*, 1988). Intramuscular injections can also cause increases. Its principal use is in the detection of myopathies, myositis or rhabdomyolysis (e.g. alcohol or suxamethonium induced). Hypothyroidism can also cause an increase.

Nutritional

Blood Glucose
Random values are not helpful, so when glucose needs to be monitored fasting levels should be arranged. Urine glucose is sufficient for routine non-specific monitoring.

Cholesterol and Blood Lipids
These are important in any long-term treatment and should be checked routinely in any studies continuing for longer than one year; they are probably not worth monitoring for therapies continuing for shorter periods.

Urine

Dipstick testing is adequate for routine screening of urine for glucose, albumin and blood. If there is doubt about the latter two, then microscopy of freshly voided (within two hours) midstream urine is required. The dipsticks for blood testing have a sensitivity of up to 99% but a false positive rate of 16% (Dowell and Britton, 1990). Asymptomatic microscopic haematuria is common with a general prevalence rate in middle-aged men of 2.5%, but detection rates are higher in older people—up to 22% in the over 60s. Dipstick results correlate closely with underlying disease, even in the presence of normal findings on microscopy, with a sensitivity of 91–100% and a specificity > 98% (De Caester and Ballarde, 1990). Dipsticks for proteinuria are mainly sensitive to albumin and are only positive at concentrations > 150 mg/l, which is tenfold higher than the normal urine output (Dawnay, 1990). If there is a prior hypothesis concerning possible renal damage a more sensitive method that identifies the different constituent proteins is necessary—for example sodium dodecyl sulphate-polyacrylamide gel electrophoresis (SDS-PAGE) (Fleming, 1984; Bianchi-Bosisio *et al.*, 1991). Fasting increases the urine ketone level and a delay in urine testing will allow any bacteria to multiply and may reduce the glucose level (Magnani, 1994).

Blood

The MCV is a useful indication of alcohol abuse and also types of anaemia (e.g. macrocytic or microcytic) and is usually measured with the haemoglobin, MCH, MCHC and the haematocrit or PCV. These values are not useful by themselves, but are very useful if there is any blood disorder and are usually included in the routine haematological tests.

Many drugs interfere with the different processes involved in laboratory testing. It is therefore very useful if each clinical trial monitors specifically for one additional parameter as well as the routine monitoring. The effects of drugs on laboratory tests is well covered in:

1. *Drug-Test Interactions Handbook*, 1st edition. Ed. J. G. Salway. Chapman and Hall Medical, 1989. £235.
2. *Drug Interferences and Drug Effects in Clinical Chemistry. 4th edition. Apoteksbolaget AB, Stockholm, 1986.*

Laboratory Test Results—Normal or Abnormal?

The usual presumption is that the 'normal range' covers the central 95% of the measurements in the general population and that the 2.5% at each end of the range are abnormal and that the normal range is the mean +/− two standard deviations due to the Gaussian distribution of values. This is not true. Most physiological variables are skewed (e.g. serum calcium, AP, total proteins, uric acid, and blood urea) so that the mean +/− two standard deviations does not cover the central 95% of values (Wyngaarden, 1988).

Suggested reading is a chapter by the scientists from Lilly Research laboratories USA in *Clinical Drug Trials and Tribulations* entitled 'Routine laboratory tests in clinical trials' (Thompson *et al.*, 1988). The authors point out that most normal ranges are obtained from a small number of healthy subjects, many of whom are young, male and Caucasian. They have defined their own 'reference range' from the results of a single laboratory using patients in clinical trials. Further valuable reading is found in Part xxv 'Laboratory reference range values of clinical importance' in *Cecil's Textbook of Medicine*, 17th edition, W. B. Saunders and Co, 1988.

Ideally all those within the 'normal range' or 'reference interval', as it should be called, would be free of a disease and all those outside these limits would have a disease (Figure 1). Unfortunately the reference interval for 'normal healthy people' usually overlaps that of those with a specific disease, (Figure 2).

The term 'normal range' should be dropped since the values it represents may not be normal nor those outside it abnormal. The term 'reference interval' should be used instead. It covers the same values as the 'normal range' and the population from which it is derived should be stated.

In place of the Gaussian distribution a non-parametric method should be used. Wyngaarden recommends 'percentile estimates'. One takes all the values from the reference population and cuts off the lowest and the highest 2.5% depending upon circumstances. This does not ascribe normality or abnormality and this is important. If the reference intervals are the central 95% they will include the same values as fall within the so-called normal range as already stated, but the central 95% of values with 2.5% outside each end of the reference interval means that 1 in 20 of values from a reference population are outside the reference range. Extrapolating from these values to the clinical trial population and presuming that 20 different parameters are measured, then on average most patients will have at least one 'abnormality'. A clinical trial programme before marketing with, say, 3000 patients with a blood sample taken before, during and at the end of the treatment would involve 180 000 measurements, of which 9000 will fall outside the reference interval purely by chance and this does not include those due to the target disease or any intercurrent illnesses. Clearly this level of false positives is too high to warrant individual examination of each outlier. If the pharmaceutical company changes the reference intervals to, say, the central 98% will the company be accused of decreasing the sensitivity at the expense of specificity? One solution is to use the usual 95% reference interval for a single patient's assessment since as clinicians the

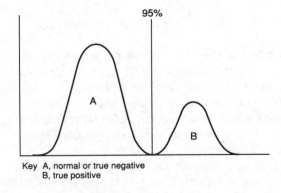

Key A, normal or true negative
      B, true positive

Figure 1   Ideal reference intervals for normal persons and those with a specific disease

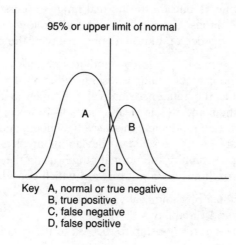

Key   A, normal or true negative
      B, true positive
      C, false negative
      D, false positive

	No disease	Disease
Test normal	A (true negative)	C (false negative)
Test abnormal	D (false positive)	B (true positive)

$$\text{Sensitivity} = \frac{B}{(B + C)}$$

$$\text{Specificity} = \frac{A}{(A + D)}$$

Figure 2   Real-life reference intervals for normals and those with diseases

clinical trialists will be using them in everyday practice, but to use a different central percentage for pooled data.

The Lilly scientists quote using the 95% reference interval and measuring 36 parameters that only 15.8% (95^{36}) of the patients would have no values outside 'normal'. They suggest excluding the 1% of results at each end of a 98% reference interval. A similar figure for 20 parameters is 56% with no values outside 'normal'.

It has been suggested that it would be a waste of time for a clinician to follow up every value outside the 95% reference interval and that approximately 80% of the time unsolicited abnormal chemistry findings do not lead to conclusions with clinical significance for the patient upon follow-up. The Lilly scientists suggest two simple rules.

- First, 'if the finding is outside the normal range as expressed by the mean +/– two standard deviations, but within +/– three standard deviations the physician may follow up the finding if the need for it is suggested by the rest of the medical information about the patient or if the finding alone, in his opinion, may have clinical significance for the patient'.

- Second, 'if the finding is outside the normal range expressed as the mean +/– three standard deviations the physician should follow it up, unless it was expected as a consequence of a known abnormality of the patient'.

A central range of the mean +/– three standard deviations will cover 99.73% of values. The effect mentioned of multiple testing reducing the number of patients without a value outside the reference interval presumes that each parameter is independent of the others and this is clearly not so—for example AST and ALT— but this does not affect the principle discussed (Schoen and Brooks, 1970). In practice using the mean +/– three standard deviations involves adding 25% of the normal range to the upper limit of the normal range (using the old terminology).

A more clinical approach has been put forward which considers:

- The different individual physiological variability.
- The different analytical variability.
- The clinical relevance in relationship to the risk to the patient.

Table 2   Multiplication factors for the 'grey areas'

Test	Lower limit of reference interval	Upper limit of reference interval
AP	–	2
AST, ALT	–	2
CPK	–	1.5
LDH	–	2
GGT	–	1.5
Bilirubin (direct)	–	1.25
Bilirubin (indirect)	–	1.5
Total protein	0.85	1.1
Albumin	0.7	1.3
γ globulin	–	1.4
Glucose	0.8	1.4
BUN	0.5	2
Creatinine	–	1.4
Sodium	0.9	1.1
Potassium	0.9	1.1
Chloride	0.8	1.2
Triglycerides	–	1.5
Total cholesterol	0.75	1.17
HDL cholesterol	–	0.7
WBC	0.70	1.3
Neutrophils	0.9	1.3
Eosinophils	–	1.7
Basophils	–	3
Lymphocytes	0.8	1.2
Monocytes	–	1.5
Platelets	0.7	1.5
RBC	0.8	1.2
Haematocrit	0.6	1.2

After Carmignoto

On either side of the reference interval there are two 'grey areas', which must be considered as requiring attention. The grey areas are bounded by the upper limit of the reference interval and a figure obtained by multiplying this by a factor and similarly for the lower limit. These factors are shown in Table 2 below under the headings of upper and lower limits.

The results are used with the algorithm shown in Figure 3. (Carmignoto, 1991).

Drawing these different approaches together we have:

- Present custom (95% reference interval). However, this is too sensitive when scanning a large number of parameters, but can be used for cases requiring individual assessment when there is support from the rest of the data. The latter can be defined as more than one abnormal value for that parameter over time or when associated with an adverse clinical event or when accompanied by other laboratory abnormalities in the same organ group.
- The Lilly reference interval (98% reference interval), which the Lilley scientists consider as being sufficiently sensitive, but suggest that it can be altered for an analyte if there are special concerns.
- The 99.73% reference interval. General use of this range would be too insensitive. On testing 20 parameters only 5.3% of patients would fall outside this interval by

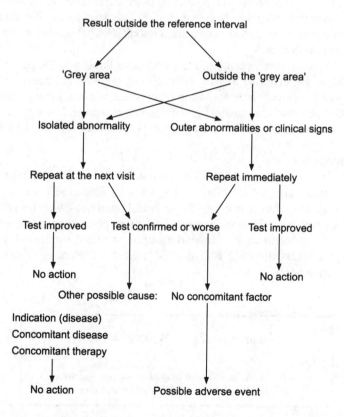

Figure 3   Carmignoto algorithm (Carmignoto, 1991)

chance. This would be sensitive enough for a single unsupported value if combined with the 95% reference interval with the caveats referred to in 1.

Intrapatient Variation

Having discussed the interpatient variation by comparing the values of the patient in a clinical trial with those of a reference population by means of the reference interval, the intrapatient variation should be considered. A value lying at the lower end of the reference interval may increase under the action of a drug by 100% but still lie within the reference interval. Should we also compare the values to an individual's own 'intrapatient reference interval'? If a pharmaceutical company has a panel of volunteers who take part in phase 1 studies it may be possible to draw up individual reference intervals from the previous results in clinical studies (e.g. the Lilly reference interval). This possibility will be discussed further on page 191. However, for patients we are less likely to have more than one or two values taken before the study. There are two methods that may be used for calculating the intrapatient variation.

Delta Limits

The Lilly scientists define 'delta limits' as the distribution of differences between two samples from the same subjects in a reference population taken at an interval of one or two weeks in which 1% of the largest increments are excluded. This, therefore, is a measure of intraperson variation taking the central 98% percentile, again based on their reference population.

Using the 98% reference interval and the 98% delta limits with 36 parameters each sample would be expected to include only 23% of patients/volunteers who do not have at least one abnormal value assuming no correlation among the parameters. The Lilly scientists claim that the method is sufficiently sensitive. There were few influences of patient characteristics on the delta limits (Thompson *et al.*, 1988).

Critical Differences

A leading article in the *British Medical Journal* in 1989 discussing the interpretation of laboratory results drew attention to the use of intrasubject variation and its relevance in clinical decision making (Fraser and Fogarty, 1989). The critical difference allows one to follow the course of one laboratory parameter in one individual in consecutive measurements and is dependent upon the total variation for the single individual. The critical difference is (Figure 4) therefore the change that must occur before significance is claimed.

$$\text{Critical difference} = 2\sqrt{(2(CV_p{}^2 + CV_a{}^2))}$$

where:
CV_p is the coefficient of within subject variation (%)
CV_a is the coefficient of analytical variation (%)

Figure 4   Calculation of critical difference (Costongs *et al.*, 1985)

The critical differences have been measured over one day and six months. Average critical differences (Fraser and Fogarty, 1989) are:

- Sodium 3%.
- Potassium 14%.
- Chloride 4%.
- Urea 30%.
- Creatinine 14%.
- Calcium 5%.
- Albumin 8%.
- Fasting glucose 15%.
- Haemoglobin 8%.
- Erythrocytes 10%.
- Leucocytes 32%.
- Platelets 25%

Intrasubject variation is similar in health and chronic stable disease, in young or elderly subjects and does not vary with nationality.

The use of spontaneous variation for the five most sensitive parameters in phase I studies has been suggested as follows:

- ALT 50%.
- AST 50%.
- AP 30%.
- Creatinine 20%.
- Polymorphonuclear leucocytes 20% increase and 50% decrease.

A laboratory value was considered an AE if it was beyond the normal range and the change from baseline was greater than the critical limit.

These values were tested on 1134 male volunteers (Sibille *et al.*, 1994; Sibille *et al.*, 1997).

The same authors refer to a discriminating threshold for ALT in volunteers, 50 i.u. and an upper limit of spontaneous variation of 50% of the baseline value. Using this in a study of 134 volunteers gave a sensitivity of 1 and a specificity of 1. Further validation is necessary (Sibille *et al.*, 1995).

Reference Change

A paper based on work in Japan uses the term 'reference change' which it defines as the difference between two consecutive test results in an individual that is statistically significant in a given proportion of all similar persons. This paper refers only to healthy volunteers and forecasts problems in adapting it for patients (Harris and Yasaka, 1983). The use of delta limits and critical differences will be mentioned again under the analysis of data.

Pre-analytical Variation

Although delta limits and critical differences are apparently unaltered by patient characteristics, reference intervals are altered to some extent. Changes with age, sex and race for different parameters are given by the Lilly scientists in their paper. Other factors can also make large differences to the results (Statland and Winkel, 1977).

Caffeine

Coffee, tea or soda drinks may affect lipids. Caffeine resulted in a threefold rise in non-esterified fatty acids (NEFA) in plasma. (Both heparin and heparinized saline can also cause a rise in NEFA.) During a three-week period taking normal coffee the average triglycerides rose 16% compared with a fall of 26% during a similar non-caffeine period, with cholesterol doing the opposite.

Alcohol

Prolonged alcohol consumption in non-alcoholics can cause a raised serum CPK and this is also seen in chronic alcoholics. A single episode of taking approximately 6.5 measures of spirit by healthy volunteers caused an increase in CPK, AST and LDH, but a decrease in ALT when the same amount of alcohol was taken on three consecutive evenings. There was a 25% increase in GGT at 60 hours and the ALT peaked at the same time; but there was little change in AP.

Young volunteers frequently prefer beer to spirits. Drinking six pints of beer over three hours produced a small but significant fall in urea and creatinine and a rise in plasma potassium. There were no changes in the AP, GGT, CPK or LDH (Gill *et al.*, 1983).

Alcohol induces hepatic drug metabolism especially involving pathways accomplished by the CYP2E1 isoform affecting metabolism of paracetamol and some anaesthetics, e.g. halothane (Klotz and Ammon, 1998).

It is important to identify chronic alcoholics entering clinical trials for several reasons:

- To find out if they are particularly vulnerable to an ADR.
- So that changes in liver function are correctly ascribed.
- Because alcohol is a risk factor for several diseases.

Liver function tests
GGT is raised in about 50% of alcoholics, while AST is raised in 25–35%. ALT, LDH and AP are also increased in alcoholics, but none has sufficient sensitivity and/or specificity alone for making a diagnosis (Clark *et al.*, 1983).

Mean Corpuscular Volume
The MCV is often raised in alcoholics. Using 98 fl as the upper reference limit, macrocytosis (increased MCV) was observed in ten out of 47 manual workers and ten of 30 company directors admitting to a daily alcohol intake of more than 65 g (Chick *et al.*, 1981).

Serum Uric Acid
This is both insensitive and non-specific, but does correlate with alcohol intake.

Triglycerides
These correlate positively with daily alcohol intake in fasting subjects.

Best Discriminatory Tests

The best discrimination between patients with alcohol-related disease (gastroenterology outpatients) drinking less than 20 g daily and patients with non-alcoholic liver disease was provided by a combination of MCV, $\log_{10}$ GGT and $\log_{10}$ serum AP. These three tests identified over 80% of patients with excessive alcohol intake (Chalmers *et al.*, 1981). In alcoholics the mean GGT was within the reference range when the debauch period was less than two weeks, just above reference range with a debauch of 2–6 weeks and markedly increased when the drinking period exceeded six weeks (Wadstein and Skude, 1979). In order to separate alcoholic liver disease from viral hepatitis the ratio of AST/ALT > 1 with an ALT < 300 is strongly in favour of alcoholic liver disease (Cohen and Kaplan, 1975).

Quadratic multiple discriminant analysis of 25 commonly ordered laboratory tests correctly classified 100% non-alcoholics, 96% of alcoholics with liver disease and 89% of non-alcoholics with liver disease (Ryback *et al.*, 1982). All these tests can be used retrospectively. However, when there is a hypothesis that makes previous identification of alcoholic abuse essential then the use of the CAGE questionnaire (see page 122) and also the quantization of carbohydrate-deficient serum transferrin should be considered (Helander *et al.*, 1995).

Exercise

Transient changes include an immediate fall and then a subsequent increase in free fatty acid (FFA), a 180% increase in the amino acid alanine and a 300% increase in lactate. There are longer lasting effects on CPK, AST, and LDH. There were average increases of CPK of +116%, AST of +41%, LDH of +32% and these remained above baseline for 53 hours or longer (King *et al.*, 1976). These values were obtained after a game of handball. The half-life for CPK varied from 38–118 hours. Short severe exercise (100-yard dash) produced a leucocytosis within 10 seconds, subsiding again in 10–15 minutes, while prolonged exercise causes a threefold increase in neutrophils. Any turbulent increase in cardiac output whether by deliberate effort, convulsions or infusion of adrenaline will cause the neutrophils from the slower moving periphery of the blood vessel (marginal pool) to come into the central (axial) flow and thereby create an apparent increase in neutrophil count (Jandl, 1987).

Smoking

Chronic smoking can cause an erythrocytosis and leucocytosis. The latter varies with the number of cigarettes: An increase of 1000 cells/μl per pack of cigarettes daily (Jandl, 1987). Smokers also have higher haemoglobin values and a higher MCV. Acute changes with smoking are a decrease in eosinophils and monocytes. The cortisol, catecholamines and FFAs acids all rise due to the adrenergic effect of nicotine (Statland and Winkel, 1979).

Diet

A 48-hour fast produced an average increase in bilirubin of 240% in healthy volunteers. Plasma insulin tends to decrease. Ingestion of a meal in healthy subjects caused a significant increase in AST. Another study showed significant increases in glucose, bilirubin, uric acid, calcium, creatinine, total protein, urea, cholesterol, LDH, AP and ALT two hours after a 700-calorie meal; however, these results were not compared with results after fasting. A meal can also cause decreases in FFAs, catecholamines, cortisol and glucagon. Frank obesity increases neutrophils by 1000 cells/μl.

Stress

Examinations produced a rise in cholesterol in medical students and a further study showed that stress could cause leucocytosis (Thomas and Murphy, 1958).

Diurnal Variation

Statistically significant changes have been found for iron, urea, total lipids, total proteins, and albumin while in the fasting state. Haemoglobin and haematocrit are lower in the afternoon and evening compared with morning values. Sodium, chloride and calcium show no change, but phosphate and potassium do. The within-day variation was 6.1% for urea, 4.0% for creatinine and 3.0% for uric acid. Lipids and non-fatty acids fluctuate throughout the 24-hour period. Physiological day to day variation expressed as percentage coefficients of variation were haemoglobin 2.4, haematocrit 2.5, platelets 6.6, total leucocytes 15.6, neutrophils 24.6, lymphocytes 11.0, monocytes 16.2, eosinophils 21.1 and basophils 13.2.

Age

Haemoglobin, PCV, MCH, MCHC, MCV and appearances of the blood film are not affected by age; but serum iron tends to fall and also therefore the iron binding capacity. Serum iron as a percentage of the total iron binding capacity (TIBC) is a more reliable index. The WBC tends to fall with age (Table 3), mainly due to a fall in lymphocyte count (Caird, 1973).

Most liver function tests do not change with age, but AP may increase slightly (Gambert *et al.*, 1982) and albumin falls progressively with increasing age (Woodford Williams *et al.*, 1964)

Table 3 The range of normal values for the leucocyte count in people over 65 years (Elwood and Hughes, 1970)

	Absolute count (cells/mm³ or 10⁹ /l)	Differential count (%)
Total	3100–8900	–
Polymorphs	1800–6500	45–85
Lymphocytes	700–3500	10–50
Eosinophils	–	0–8
Monocytes	–	0–8

Table 4   Normal values for measurements in old age (Andrews *et al.*, 1975) (Values will depend upon the age pattern in the cohort used to determine the reference range)

Measurement	Units	Mean +/– SD	Range
Sodium	mmol/l	141 +/– 3	135–146
Potassium	mmol/l	4.4 +/– 0.4	3.6–5.2
Chloride	mmol/l	102 +/– 3	96–108
Bicarbonate	mmol/l	25 +/– 3	19–31
Total protein	g/l	71 +/– 50	61–81
Albumin	g/l	41 +/– 4	33–49
Globulin	g/l	31 +/– 5	21–41
Magnesium	mg/100 ml	2.0 +/– 0.25	1.5–2.5
	mmol/l		0.75–1.25
Phosphate			
males	mg/100 ml	3.1 +/– 0.5	2.1–4.1
	mmol/l		0.678–1.32
females	mg/100 ml	3.4 +/– 0.6	2.2–4.6
	mmol/l		0.71–1.485
Bilirubin	mg/100 ml	*	0.3–1.5
	μmol/l		5.13–25.65

* Logarithm normal frequency distribution

Table 5   Normal values that differ in old age (Andrews *et al.*, 1975; Gambert *et al.*, 1982; Zilva *et al.*, 1988)

Substance	Units	Mean +/– SD	Range
Urea (> 65)	mg/100 ml	*	22–60
	mmol/l		7.85–21.4
Cholesterol			
males	mg/100 ml	*	160–345
	mmol/l		4.14–8.92
females	mg/100 ml	*	180–435
	mmol/l		4.65–11.25
Calcium			
males	mg/100 ml	9.5 +/– 0.5	8.5–10.5
	mmol/l		2.12–2.62
females	mg/100 ml	9.7 +/– 0.5	8.7–10.7
	mmol/l		2.17–2.67
Uric acid			
males	mg/100 ml	5.5 +/– 1.2	3.1–7.9
	mmol/l		0.184–0.47
females	mg/100 ml	4.9 +/– 1.4	2.1–7.7
	mmol/l		0.125–0.458
AP	K-A units	*	5–20
	units/l		35.5–142

* Logarithm normal frequency distribution

Venepuncture, Storage and Transport

One section of a clinical trial protocol should be devoted to the laboratory investigations and it has been suggested that a meeting between representatives from clinical research, data management and the laboratory is beneficial (Harris, 1994). It is important to speak with investigator concerning the handling of specimens about:

- Identification and method for writing dates.
- Preparation.
- Storage.
- Transportation.
- Analysis (Owen, 1997).

Venepuncture

There are clearly many variables depending upon lifestyle and diet in the day(s) before sampling. It is therefore very important that blood is taken using the same technique at the same time on each occasion and that this should not be changed during a study.

The following factors should be identical:

1. Posture. The concentration of proteins and protein-bound substances increases on standing.
2. Duration of the application of the tourniquet. The longer the duration the more the protein and protein-bound substances increase due to leakage of fluid from the veins. Blood samples for calcium should be taken without stasis. Potassium and phosphate tend to leak out of the cells due to local hypoxia on prolonged stasis (Zilva *et al.*, 1988).
3. Time. To avoid diurnal variation and variation due to meals.

Storage and Dispatch

Plasma values tend to be lower than the serum values for those constituents found in the erythrocytes (i.e. potassium, phosphate, AST, and LDH). The anticoagulant used will also have an effect as follows:

(a) K_2 ethylenediamine tetraacetic acid (EDTA) increases potassium and lowers calcium and affects AP.
(b) Fluoride/oxalate increases potassium and sodium, but lowers calcium.
(c) Lithium heparin. Protein electrophoresis and some immunoassays cannot be performed (Fraser, 1986).

The EDTA (Sequestrene) is used for haematological examination, the fluoride/oxalate is used for glucose determination and lithium/heparin for biochemical examination.

Up to 30% of bloods from general practice have raised potassium concentrations and about 50% of these are due to being left overnight without separation of RBCs from the serum (Johnston and Hawthorne, 1997).

If blood is transported from general practice at ambient temperature falls in potassium may occur during very hot weather (Masters *et al.*, 1996), but cooling the blood to 4°C accelerates the rate at which potassium leaks out of the red cells (Johnston and Hawthorne, 1997).

Should haemolysis occur there are likely to be large rises in LDH, AST, ALT and potassium. A 1% solution of lysed erythrocytes causes a 98% increase in mean creatine kinase activity in sera of healthy subjects (Statland and Winkel, 1979). Prolonged contact of serum with erythrocytes in unseparated blood samples causes a spurious elevation in serum potassium (e.g. mean rise of 0.8 mmol/l in 24 hours) (Moore *et al.*, 1989). The effect of various factors on the mean potassium level is as follows:

- Clotted, centrifuged and serum separated within 30 minutes (3.92 mmol/l).
- Heparinized, centrifuged and plasma separated within 30 minutes (3.77 mmol/l).
- Clotted, left at room temperature sent to hospital and centrifuged there (4.30 mmol/l).
- Clotted, refrigerated at 4°C for one hour (to mimic a cold day) and then as above (4.62 mmol/l).

If a sample is centrifuged before transport the serum potassium will be stable for four days at ambient temperature.

Venepuncture can by itself cause syncope, bradycardia, seizures and cardiac arrest (Roddy *et al.*, 1979), therefore a semirecumbent posture on a examination couch is ideal, and sitting is a good second best. An aliquot of the pre-treatment specimen should be stored to allow additional testing at a later date if this should prove necessary. Attributing cause to changes in laboratory values without a control group can be extremely difficult and will be discussed under analysis (see page 238). An alternative approach is to have a baseline value and only repeat the tests if an adverse clinical event occurs, but this is more suitable for postmarketing studies once the main risks are known.

Transport

Transport of blood specimens is a specialized task and care is required in choosing a carrier. There are three types of carrier:

1. Freight forwarders who specialize in large air cargoes.
2. Express integrators giving a door-to-door service for high volumes at low cost.
3. Specialist couriers for specific industries and low volumes (Wilkinson, 1994).

The International Air Transport Association has two categories for samples that need special handling:

1. Infections.
2. Low risk of infection, diagnostic samples.

Four types of packaging must be considered:

1. Room temperature.
2. Refrigerated (2–8°C), with a choice of wet ice and cooler packs.
3. Frozen (–78°C) carbon dioxide, solid or dry ice.
4. Liquid nitrogen (–196°C) requiring a Dewar flask.

The commonest cause of shipment delays are failure to pick up samples and weather conditions (Dijkman and Querton, 1994). The last two references (Wilkinson, 1994; Dijkman and Querton, 1994) are contained in a single issue of the *Drug Information Journal*.

Laboratories

The UK government controls the standards of laboratories via an External Quality Assessment Scheme. A series of test samples are sent at regular intervals to all the participating laboratories where they are analysed and the results returned to the organizers who notify the laboratories of their performance. Similar schemes operate elsewhere (USA, France, Belgium, Germany) (Ehrmeyer and Laessig, 1994; Libeer, 1994; Peterson *et al.*, 1994).

Central or Local Laboratory

The use of a central laboratory for clinical trials is more common in the USA than in Europe, but their use is increasing steadily. The advantages are:

1. A standardized reference interval.
2. Reduced variation between assay results.
3. Some assays may be performed more rapidly.
4. On-line data transfer is possible.
5. They are Good Laboratory Practices (GLP) accredited.

The disadvantages are:

1. The problem of sample transport.
2. Some local ethical committees may not agree because of delay in results being available for patient care (24–36 hours) or because of the need for two samples, one for local testing (patient care) and the other for the central laboratory.
3. Opposition from local laboratories who might object to arranging transport to a central laboratory when the analyses are possible in their laboratories.
4. Cost (Sturk, 1994).

Core Laboratories

Some advanced assay techniques are best performed by a core laboratory specializing in these assays, which are rarely performed locally. These will often be performed in batches at the end of a study (Sturk, 1994).

With a central laboratory arrangements have to be made for the clinical trialist to be sent the results as soon as possible. The trialist may have problems with the reference range if it differs from his or her usual hospital range.

Dealing with Different Hospital Ranges

In any clinical trial programme there are likely to be different reference intervals in use in the numerous trials. One solution, other than using a central laboratory, is to use a method of standardization and there are several available:

Normalization

Division of each value by the upper limit of normal (ULN) from the reference intervals used by the originating hospitals (Sogliero-Gilbert *et al.*, 1986). This has the following features:

(a) All transformed values are positive.
(b) All parameters have an upper limit of 1.
(c) All values are bounded below by 0.

Values outside the upper limit are easy to interpret. However, this cannot deal with tests where abnormal may be below the lower limit of normal (LLN) (e.g. electrolytes) and the results are not in a format which is familiar to clinicians.

Percentage Transformation

The LLN is made equal to 0% and the ULN equal to 100% (Abt and Krupp, 1986). It is obtained from:

$$\frac{x-LLN \times 100}{ULN-LLN}\% \quad \text{where x is the value} \tag{1}$$

It has the advantage over 'normalization' in that it copes with parameters where the clinical importance lies in values below the LLN or in both directions. The results are given as a percentage and are therefore not in units familiar to a clinician.

Hoffman-La Roche Method

This transformation places the transformed value in the same proportional position relative to the sponsor's range as it was in its untransformed form relative to the investigators range. It is obtained from:

$$LLN(s) + \frac{x-LLN(I)}{ULN(I)-LLN(I)}(ULN(s)-LLN(s)) \quad \text{where x is the value} \tag{2}$$

LLN(s) and ULN(s) refer to the sponsor's range while ULN(I) and LLN(I) refer to the investigator's range.

This is suitable for normally distributed data, but for non-normal data (e.g. LFTs) the original data must be first log transformed. It can also produce negative values where there is a large disparity between the two ranges. The authors describe how to cope with this problem (Smith and Givens, 1993). This method has the advantage of using a range that is familiar to the sponsor.

The above three methods allow all types of analysis of means to be performed, but if only the analysis of the means is undertaken then these can be standardized by using the mean percentage change from baseline throughout all studies.

Chuang-Stein Method

This method is for use with tests that are normally distributed (e.g. haematological tests). The value is obtained from:

$$= \frac{x- \text{the midpoint of the reference interval}}{25\% \text{ of the reference interval}} \tag{3}$$

Finally the values are converted back to the reference interval of the trial with the greatest recruitment (Chuang-Stein, 1992).

Two-stage Adjustment Procedure

Here the standard deviation index (SDI) is obtained from:

$$\frac{x-\text{group mean}}{\text{group SD on same specimen}} \tag{4}$$

Within Group Adjustment The SDI is taken from previous year's proficiency survey and also SD for the group. Take the median SDI and median group standard deviation (SD) and:

$$\text{New value} = \text{old value} - (\text{median SDI} \times \text{median group SD}) \tag{5}$$

Between group adjustment Choose a reference procedure for each analyte (e.g. method used at principle site) (Ga). The mean of the whole group is G. Compute the ratio:

$$\frac{\text{group mean of G}}{\text{group mean of Ga}} \tag{6}$$

Denote the median of these ratios from the last year period by R. The second stage adjusted value is:

$$= (\text{first stage adjusted value} \times \frac{1}{R}) \tag{7}$$

This adjusted value is used for routine summarization (Oliver and Chuang-Stein, 1993).

Monitoring of Laboratory Values Throughout a Clinical Development Programme

A clinical trial programme may take several years before sufficient data have been collected to make an application for an AMM/NDA. During this period it is essential to use a standardized procedure for laboratory data for the following reasons:

- To identify abnormal values of clinical significance that might require intervention during a study (e.g. further investigation).
- To perform interim analyses at critical times.
- To facilitate preparation of the application for a product licence.

If laboratory changes qualify as a serious adverse event (using the regulatory definition) the investigator should notify the company either by telephone or by immediately despatching the adverse event form. Withdrawal of the patient from the trial due to an adverse laboratory result thought to be caused by the drug should also be notified by an immediate letter to the sponsor (see page 219).

A change in a laboratory variable can be considered to be an adverse event if it is considered to be clinically significant by the attending physician or if it causes (or should have caused) the clinician to reduce or discontinue use of the product or institute therapy (Linberg, 1996).

It is important that all results are scanned by 'intelligent' eyes before being computerized so that the drug safety department can be notified of any serious or potentially important events.

There are several advantages in electronic data transfer in reducing errors and speed, but it makes monitoring the data all the more important.

Any one monitor will only see a section of the total laboratory forms and so there has to be a procedure for monitoring the whole laboratory database at regular intervals. There are certain critical periods during the clinical trial programme when an interim analysis of all the safety data is required. The first such period is probably before the beginning of phase 3 studies so that any hypotheses generated in phase 1 and 2 can be specifically targeted in phase 3. The second period is probably half-way through phase 3 so that any significant changes in the rapidly expanding trial data can be recognized and action taken in time to pre-empt any problems with the MAA/NDA. Any interim analysis should be blinded as to the treatment, but the code should be broken by the safety department for serious events notified to the company, keeping the research team blind. However, there will be cases that do not qualify as serious by the FDA definition, but are not of minor importance; hopefully many of these will be identified if there is immediate notification of those patients withdrawn from studies due to adverse events (clinical or laboratory), but important laboratory abnormalities may still go unrecognized. The problem is how to identify clinically significant abnormalities from the many chance abnormalities. Using the expanded reference intervals is a fairly crude method. An alternative is to characterize patterns of clinical significance (e.g. if there are two abnormalities, at any one time in the tests of a single organ group such as the liver function tests). There are various approaches to the problem and these are described below.

The Pfizer Method

Pfizer produced a system in 1979, which they have since updated (Weeks *et al.*, 1986). It is clear that although statistical analysis should detect any type A effects, type B effects require individual assessment. The detection of outliers will indicate a large number of patients whose laboratory abnormalities require clinical review. The Pfizer system aims to reduce this load by:

- Computer identification and categorization of laboratory abnormalities.
- Producing a complete laboratory profile over time for each patient.

The computer is fed with details of the normal range, bearing in mind the age and sex of the patients and all abnormal results are coded according to the degree of severity of the abnormality and its direction—increase or decrease—so that normals = 1, and 3, 5, 7, and 9 indicate results above the ULN; 2, 4, 6, and 8 are results below the LLN. The degree of abnormality is based on expanded limits supplied by the clinician, (i.e. clinically insignificant, clinically significant, clinically important, marked abnormality). Two printouts are provided for the company clinician reviewing the data.

Laboratory Categorization Print
This identifies individual patients with clinically significant laboratory changes. The computer assigns a category to each abnormal value:

- Category 1. Baseline value abnormal; most abnormal value not of clinical significance.

- Category 2. Baseline normal or missing; most abnormal value not of clinical significance.
- Category 3. Baseline normal or missing and there is a single significant abnormal value, which returned to normal during therapy or baseline is abnormal and there is a single divergent value that differed significantly from the baseline, but returned to within these limits during treatment.
- Category 4. The baseline value is normal or missing and there are two or three significant abnormal values, within a six-week period that all lie on the same side of the normal range; no value reaches the level of marked abnormality and the last two values during therapy are within normal limits. Alternatively, the baseline value is abnormal and there are two or more significant abnormal values compared to baseline, within a six-week period, that lie on the same side of the normal range as the baseline. The abnormal values were consecutive, or as they differed significantly from baseline and were interspersed with values differing less than the insignificant percent from baseline.
- Category 5. A documented laboratory error (Pitts, 1993).

The remainder are categorized as 'Provisional 9s' and these are reviewed by the clinician who then allots them as:

- Category 6. Likely to be due to primary or a coexistent disease.
- Category 7. Likely to be due to concomitant therapy.
- Category 8. Clinically insignificant or not due to therapy.
- Category 9. Possibly related to drug therapy.

Patient Profile Print

This shows all clinical laboratory test results for each patient across time and identifies all values falling outside normal limits as well as patient demographic information, concomitant disease and medication. The original paper should be read in its entirety. Pfizer have dealt with data coming from different laboratories by using the 'normalization' mentioned earlier. They also discuss a more debatable manipulation which they call 'Genie score' where the deviations of the parameters from a functional group (i.e. liver function tests) are combined. The Genie score requires a variable weight to incorporate the relative importance of the parameter. It is defined as a summary statistic produced (for a functional group of parameters) from a weighted linear combination of absolute normalized deviations from the normal range in a single patient. The results of four clinical trials using this method have been published (Gilbert *et al.*, 1991).

World Health Organization (Cancer Treatment) Method

The WHO handbook for reporting results of cancer treatment (WHO Offset Publication no. 48) grades for severity all acute and subacute toxic effects of drugs, including laboratory data on a five grade system: grades 0–4. There have been some difficulties with the coding system and there has therefore been a re-evaluation of the system (Franklin *et al.*, 1989). As a result other coding systems have been devised (e.g. M. D. Anderson Comprehensive Criteria, National Cancer Institute Common Toxicity Criteria) (Tombes *et al.*, 1990).

Japanese Pharmaceuticals and Chemicals Safety Division of Pharmaceutical Affairs Bureau—Ministry of Health and Welfare, Japan

This proposes grading for both clinical and laboratory adverse events on a scale of 1–3 similar to the WHO gradings. Further details can be obtained from the Japanese Federation of Pharmaceutical Manufacturers' Association.

The Ciccolunghi/Fowler/Chaudri Method

Ciba-Geigy approached the problem in 1979 when the above authors of the system devised a computer screening of the laboratory data to identify all patients with potentially clinically relevant laboratory abnormalities. The data were first screened and classified by a computer programme. Certain parameters were given arbitrary levels. For haemoglobin these were:

1. Increase or decrease less than 1 g/100 ml.
2. Increase or decrease of 1–2 g/100 ml.
3. Increase or decrease of 2 g/100 ml or more.

Other parameters were:

- Haematocrit—change of +/−< 5%; +/−5–10%; +/−> 10%.
- White count—> 10 000; 5000–10 000; 4000–5000; < 4000 cells/mm^3
- Platelets—> 150 000; 100 000–150 000; 50 000–100 000; < 50 000/mm^3.
- Liver function tests and BUN—normal or above normal.
- Serum glucose—above or below normal range.

Detailed study was restricted to white counts < 4000 cells/mm^3 and platelets counts < 100 000/mm^3.

Each abnormality was then examined in the light of all available information by two Ciba-Geigy physicians using a set classification. The paper by Ciccolunghi, Fowler and Chaudry is worth reading in full (Ciccolunghi *et al.*, 1979) (Table 6).

The Ten-Flag Method

A further possibility, devised by Stephens and Cooper, is to use ten flags to identify different patterns of laboratory abnormalities. One set of ten flags covered the liver and renal systems and a similar set covered haematology and clinical chemistry, with only minor differences between them. The liver flags are given as an example and are as follows:

1. Complete evaluation not possible because some reference intervals are missing.
2. (a) Any test is normal, low or missing pretreatment and becomes abnormally high at any time after starting treatment. (b) Any test is abnormally high pretreatment and at any time after starting treatment. (c) Both (a) and (b).
3. Any test is normal, low or missing pretreatment and shows two or more abnormally high values at any time after starting treatment.
4. More than one test in a group is normal, low or missing pretreatment and has one or more abnormalities (high) at any time after starting treatment.

Table 6 Classification of laboratory abnormalities

Category	Criteria used for assignment
1.1 Spontaneous variation	1. Abnormality present for a maximum of 1–2 visits which was either temporary despite continued treatment or occurred on the last visit only and was minimal. A progressively increasing abnormality over 3–4 visits was never considered to be spontaneous variation.
or	2. No relevant unwanted effects, other laboratory abnormalities or concomitant disease.
	3. No relevant concomitant medication.
	4. No comment or action by investigator.
1.2 Laboratory or recording error	1. Usually a single aberrant value or, if more than one, evidence of centre effect.
	2. No relevant unwanted effects, other laboratory abnormalities or concomitant disease.
	3. No relevant concomitant medication.
	4. No comment or action by investigator.
2. Minimal change of no probable clinical significance	1. Abnormality represents such slight deviation from the norm that it is obviously of no clinical significance.
	2. No relevant unwanted effects, other laboratory abnormalities or concomitant disease.
	3. No relevant concomitant medication.
	4. No comment or action by investigator.
3. Relevant concomitant disease or operation	1. Relevant concomitant disease (recorded by investigator and/or evidenced by pre-treatment abnormality in another laboratory test) or operation present at time of abnormality.
	2. Any unwanted effects or laboratory abnormalities present must confirm this impression.
	3. No relevant concomitant medication.
	4. Confirmatory comment or action by investigator.
4. Possible drug effect 4.1 No relevant concomitant medication taken 4.2 Relevant concomitant medication taken	1. Abnormality progressively increases during trial.
	2. Relevant unwanted effects and other laboratory abnormalities present.
	3. Confirmatory comment or action by investigator. Treatment should not be prematurely discontinued for laboratory abnormality unless relevant concomitant disease or operation present.
	4. Abnormality, other than minimal, present at the last visit only.
5. Probable drug effect	1. Abnormality progressively increases during trial.
	2. Relevant unwanted effects and other laboratory abnormalities present.
	3. No relevant concomitant medication taken or disease present.
	4. Confirmatory comment or action by investigator. Treatment may be prematurely discontinued by investigator for this reason.

5. At any time after starting treatment the patient has a clinical adverse event and one or more laboratory test values become abnormally high were normal, low or missing pretreatment.

6. (a) Any test is abnormal, low or missing pretreatment and shows an abnormally high level of 'minor' clinical significance at any time after starting treatment. (b) Any test is normal, low or missing pretreatment and shows an abnormally high level of 'major' clinical significance at any time after starting treatment.

7. (a) Any test is abnormally high at baseline and increases by 'minor' percentage of its baseline value at any time after starting treatment. (b) Any test is abnormally high at baseline and increases by a 'major' percentage of its baseline value at any time after starting treatment.

8. Investigator's assessment of laboratory changes is (1) Unlikely to be related to test treatment; (2) Possibly related to test treatment; (3) Probably related to test treatment; (4) Almost certainly related to test treatment; (5) Related to test treatment but degree not specified; (A) Abnormal: relationship to test treatment not specified; (U) Missing for one or more variables or the whole organ group; (O) None of the above.

9. For any test the last value recorded, whether on treatment or at follow-up, is outside the reference interval.

10. (a) One test reported at some time on treatment. (b) Two tests reported at some time on treatment. (c) At least one test is reported at some time on treatment. (d) More than one test is reported more than once on treatment.

This combination of flags covers all relevant variations and was designed for computerization

A set of 'minor' and 'major' levels below and above the LLN and the ULN, respectively, were produced, based where possible on the criteria for identifying laboratory values as 'clinically significantly abnormal' set by the FDA (Food and Drug Administration 1986).

In the FDA '*Guidelines for the Format and Content of the Clinical and Statistical Sections of New Drug Applications*', page 41, 'Clinical laboratory evaluation in clinical trials', certain patterns of abnormal laboratory tests are mentioned as possible patterns that may need to be addressed:

- Comparison with patient's own baseline.
- Any clinically significant abnormality.
- Smaller deviations of the abnormality seen above.
- Patients with related abnormalities (e.g. elevated transaminases and bilirubin).
- Those with a specified abnormality on more than one measurement.
- A particular laboratory abnormality with a particular adverse event.

It can be seen that these can be identified using the above flagging system. This method has not yet been put into action.

Laboratory Information Expert System for Safety (Labiess)

It was inevitable that a go-ahead company would develop a system based on artificial intelligence to deal with laboratory data. FIDIA Pharmaceuticals, an Italian company, is first in this field, but the system is still in the early stages of evaluation (Ruggeri *et al.*, 1996).

Laboratory Data Forms

Figure 5 shows a laboratory data form while the instructions for completing it are shown in Figure 6.

The clinical trialist's opinion as to whether an abnormal laboratory value is due to a change in the underlying disease or a new disease is invaluable and the trialist will probably be aware of the common changes which can be brought about in laboratory parameters by standard drugs. It is therefore essential that the trialist's opinion is recorded on the laboratory data form. Various schemes have been used with a varying number of choices for the clinician.

Ten Categories

These are:

0 = Within normal range.
1 = Abnormality probably due to primary diagnosis.
2 = Abnormality probably due to concurrent disease.
3 = Abnormality not evaluable due to concurrent medication.
4 = Probable laboratory error.
5 = Clinically insignificant deviation from normal.
6 = Also has baseline (pretreatment) value abnormal or at limit of normal range.
7 = Transient abnormality resolving on continued treatment.
8 = Inadequate information for interpretation.
9 = Abnormality probably due to test drug.

This system has been used in the USA. Full investigation by the company can be restricted to category 9. Each category excludes the possibility of others, in that only one category can be used. This has the effect of forcing the clinician to say whether the event was probably due to the drug or not. Whatever theoretical merits the scheme may have, in practice the clinical trialists did not fill in the forms.

Five Categories

It can be argued that the clinician' opinion is only required on the question of the relationship of the abnormal investigation(s) to the drug and therefore only this relationship is considered as follows.

0 = Within normal range or outside the normal range but of no clinical significance.
1 = Unlikely.
2 = Possible.
3 = Probable.
4 = Almost certain.

It can also be argued that there should be an additional class of 'almost certainly not' to balance the 'almost certain'. Some have taken this a step further by saying

BATCH FORMAT CODE	PATIENT NO	FOR OFFICE USE ONLY

LABORATORY DATA

Parameters marked with asterisk are optional, but please include if available

	PERIOD	PRE–TREATMENT	Lab. No.		Lab. No.		Lab. No.		Lab. No.		Lab. No.	Clinician's overall assesment
	Sample Date / Parameter	Day Month Year		Day Month Year		Day Month Year		Day Month Year		Day Month Year		
CLINICAL CHEMISTRY	SODIUM											
	POTASSIUM											
	TOTAL PROTEIN*											
	ALBUMIN*											
	CALCIUM*											
	UREA											
	CREATININE*											
	BILIRUBIN											
	SGOT(AST)											
	SGPT(ALT)											
	ALKALINE PHOSPHATASE											
	GGT											
HAEMATOLOGY	HAEMOGLOBIN											
	RBC											
	MCV											
	PLATELET COUNT											
	TOTAL WBC											
	NEUTROPHILS											
	BASOPHILS											
	EOSINOPHILS											
	LYMPHOCYTES											
	MONOCYTES											
URINE	PROTEIN											
	GLUCOSE											
	BLOOD											

COMMENTS: _____

_____

_____

_____

Figure 5 Laboratory data form

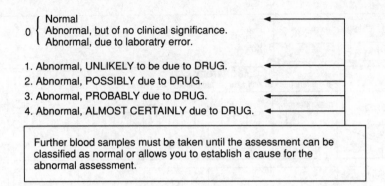

Figure 6 Laboratory data form—instructions

there should instead be a class 'definitely not', but this degree of certainty is rarely found clinically and should not be used.

Three Categories

These are:

0 = Normal value.
1 = Thought to be drug related.
2 = Not thought to be drug related.

Two Categories

These are:

0 = Not due to the drug.
1 = Due to the drug.

Again such certainty of opinion is extremely rare in clinical practice and in my opinion to try and force the clinician into making a decision one way or the other is a subtle way of making it more likely that he or she will say that the drug is innocent rather than say that it definitely did cause the event.

A Further Example with Only Two Categories is

1 = Normal.
2 = Abnormal.

Experience shows that many clinicians do not know the reference intervals for their own hospitals and many errors have been found on checking. It is much better to supply the computer with all the details and it does a far better job than the clinician. There is also the objection made earlier concerning the use of the words 'normal' and 'abnormal' (see page 157).

Boxes to Tick

The final alternative is to have a single box for each parameter and the box is ticked only if the value is of clinical significance. If any individual value(s) is ticked then an overall comment should be given on the complete laboratory data for that patient.

Form Design

It is important that all values from the beginning to the end of the study can be seen at a glance, preferably on a single page. It is possible to fit six different visits on a page. A clinician will not give an opinion on a single value of one parameter, but will judge the parameters in organ groups over time and this should be reflected in the form design. Space also needs to be given so that overall comments can be made and these can be collected by asking for an overall opinion on the likely cause of any outliers. Serious changes in laboratory values which the clinical trialist considers as possibly due to the test drug are likely to precipitate withdrawal of the patient from the study. Arrangements need to be included in the protocol so that withdrawals can be notified to the trial monitor as they occur rather than at the end of the study. First, this is because withdrawals need to be followed up and if they are withdrawn because of an adverse event they will possibly need further investigation. Second, early notification of withdrawals due to adverse events may be the first sign that the dose used is incorrect.

Timing of Laboratory Examinations

There are circumstances in which the number of samplings may need to be curtailed, for example:

1. In studies at very specialized units the patient population may be drawn from a wide area and this would involve some patients in long journeys. In these circumstances the visits and sampling may have to be reduced.
2. In children.
3. Uncontrolled studies. A baseline screen, which is repeated if a serious adverse event should occur or if the patient is withdrawn due to an adverse event, may be all that is required.

    Laboratory investigations are performed:

1. Before the study.
2. During the study.
3. At the end of the study.
4. After the study.

Before the Study

Certain levels of pre-trial investigations may be used to exclude or include patients from the study. The more exclusive these are, the less one is able to extrapolate the results of the study to the general population, but on the other hand, the fewer exclusions there are, the less powerful the study will be in finding toxic effects. This is explained as follows. In a trial of 500 patients with the trial drug and 500 in the control group, the probability of detecting a toxic effect depends upon the amount of background noise in the control group (Table 7).

The background noise can be reduced by having one laboratory examination performed two weeks before the study and a further one week before the study: if either reading is outside the reference interval (the mean+/–two SDs), the patient is excluded from the study. This serves to exclude all patients with abnormal function. Unfortunately, this would make it much more difficult to recruit patients for the study and add greatly to the costs of the study.

A reasonable compromise is a screen 1–2 weeks before the study drug is started so that the results are available before the study and then a baseline screen is carried out immediately before the first dose of the drug is taken, though the results of this will not be known until later. The two samplings show whether patients with chronic disease are stable and therefore less likely to produce abnormalities due to underlying or incipient disease during the trial. This should be the minimum in phase 1 and phase 2 studies.

During phase 2 studies there is an emphasis on exclusions so that the small-scale studies are not embarrassed by problems other than those caused by the target disease and the trial drug. The large phase 3 and 4 studies may have very few exclusions so that the results can be extrapolated to the general population.

It is not desirable to have abnormal laboratory results as an exclusion criterion in a phase 3 study since this implies that once marketed the same exclusions would be valid and requiring normal laboratory values before routine clinical use would be a great deterrent to prescribing the drug.

Pre-trial laboratory screening is only practical in studies where the underlying indication for treatment is a chronic disease. Acute disease requiring immediate treatment will only allow for a single baseline immediately before treatment. The minimum in phase 3 studies is to have just baseline data.

During the Study

Most type A laboratory abnormalities occur within the first week, but not all since the body homeostatic mechanisms tend to rectify abnormalities and these only gradually

Table 7 How power changes with background. Probability (100) of detecting a real toxic effect (POWER) in a controlled study, the agreed risk of reaching a wrong conclusion being 5/100 (Pessayre and Benhamou, 1981)

Prevalence of the anomaly in the control group	Increase in the prevalence of the anomaly in trial drug group	
	1/100	5/100
5/100	17/100	91/100
1/100	37/100	99.5/100
0.1/100	66/100	99.9/100

Example
If the drug increases the toxic effect by 1% and if the 'background noise' in the control group (i.e. toxic effect) is 5%, there is only a 17% chance of finding this difference; but if the 'background noise' is 0.1%, there is a 66% chance of finding it.

fail to maintain the situation. Even if an abnormality appears rapidly one cannot be sure that it will not alter over the long term due to this tachyphylaxis. Some type A reactions are also delayed because the body's protective mechanism only acts under certain specific circumstances (e.g. beta blockers and asthma). Most type B reactions, since they reflect hypersensitivity, are very unlikely to appear before the end of the first week of treatment. A decision on the frequency of patients' visits during a study depends upon many factors including the laboratory side of drug safety. During phase 1 studies on volunteers, laboratory investigations will have been made after a single dose and daily after multiple dose studies. These will usually be sufficient. In phase 2 studies in patients the investigative screening need only be carried out at weekly intervals.

By the time long-term studies are started many of the type A reactions will have been revealed in the short-term studies of phase 1 and 2 where laboratory tests have been performed at frequent intervals. The first test in long-term studies is probably best carried out after two weeks and again at one month, then at 3, 6, 9 and 12 months and then post-treatment. What is probably more important than routine testing after one month is repeating the laboratory screen and taking a sample for drug levels if any serious or severe adverse event occurs or if a patient withdraws from the study due to an adverse event. Even where courses of treatment are short it is best to have two tests while on the drug so that abnormalities early in the study can be contrasted with a result near the end of the study. This will help to reveal laboratory or chance errors (e.g. a single abnormality early in treatment that becomes normal while still on the drug is unlikely to be drug related unless tachyphylaxis has occurred).

The management of severe laboratory abnormalities during clinical trials has been admirably dealt with by Bénichou *et al.*, (1988). It must be remembered that one of the primary objectives is protection of the patients within the study, but it is difficult to decide how often it is necessary to test the laboratory parameters for this purpose. As already mentioned type A reactions are most likely to occur during the first week, depending upon the half-life of the drug, whereas type B reactions involving hypersensitivity develop after five days at the earliest, and usually after one week (unless there has been previous sensitization) and may have a rapid onset. Clozapine produces agranulocytosis in 1–2% of patients and the FDA has therefore required that the distribution of clozapine is linked to WBC monitoring every week (Salzman, 1990). Weekly venepuncture would not be acceptable unless the class of drug was associated with serious type B effects.

At the End of the Study

The laboratory results on blood, etc. taken on the last visit while the patient is taking the new drug or control will not be available to the clinician until some time later.

Post-treatment Visit

It is essential that all drug trials should include a post-treatment visit for the following reasons:

- To examine the patient in the light of any abnormal laboratory tests from the last 'drug' visit. Merely to tell the trialist to recall the patient if there is an abnormality is to 'stretch one's faith in human nature too far'.
- To examine the patient for any delayed AEs, withdrawal effects or rebound effects and to document the dechallenge in the case of a previous AE. The delayed effect of fialuridine in producing lactic acidosis and liver failure will influence further decisions in this area, but the liver function tests did not presage the problem even just one or two weeks before the liver failure developed (McKenzie *et al.*, 1995).
- To repeat any abnormal laboratory tests.
- To repeat the laboratory screen while off the drug. Any minor pharmacological or toxicological changes can then be seen to have reversed and help to confirm or reject the hypothesis that the changes seen were drug related and not due to disease progression.
- If a laboratory investigation is used as an efficacy marker then it will be necessary as a proof of cure.

The Timing of Post-study Laboratory Testing

The timing of any post-drug laboratory tests will depend upon the stage of development of the drug. Little has been published on the timing of laboratory tests in drug development. The US Department of Health, Education and Welfare has published *Guidelines for Detection of Hepatotoxicity Due to Drugs and Chemicals* (Davidson *et al.*,) and in Chapter 7 under the heading 'Minimal guidelines for detection of hepatotoxicity in early clinical trials of new drugs (clinical pharmacology and clinical investigation)', it is suggested that the following testing is performed after administration of the drug (single dose and multiple dose trials) at 24 hours and 5–7 days, and that the first introduction of the drug into patients with the target condition (i.e. phase 2) examinations should be at 24 hours, 5–7 days and 4–6 weeks after the last dose.

In Chapter 8 under 'Guidelines for evaluation of potential hepatotoxicty of drugs in clinical trials (phase 3), it is suggested that for drugs used long term (lasting six months or more) the patient should be followed up off therapy for two years and that a subset should be followed up for 20 years! For drugs used for short term (less than six months) the follow-up should be for two months following cessation of therapy. Drugs for single administration should have an abbreviated laboratory screen at 24 hours, 72 hours and weekly intervals thereafter for one month.

A few drugs have a very long half-life (e.g. terolidine) and the follow-up visit should then be after total clearance of the drug from the body (Harkins, 1996).

Laboratory Adverse Event

A great deal of attention has been given to defining clinical ADRs in different body systems (Bénichou and Danan, 1989), but it has been difficult to define a laboratory adverse event. It has been suggested that the combination of the ULN (or LLN) and a measure of the spontaneous variation (variation threshold) would be suitable. The variation threshold can be compared with the 'reference change' and the 'delta limits' described earlier (see page 160). Using the two measures gave a high predictive value (Sibille *et al.*, 1997).

Analysis of Laboratory Data

Laboratory abnormalities due to drugs can be divided, in a similar way to clinical adverse events, into type A and type B effects.

Type A Effects

These are pharmacologically mediated events that are usually predictable and common and are usually not serious. First, let us look at those that are common and not serious. These will be small changes, mostly within the normal reference interval and best picked up by changes in the mean value. There will, of course, be other type A reactions where the changes will be larger and will be outside the reference interval, but the number doing so are likely to be fewer than those showing only a small change. Some type A reactions will be rarer due to different pharmacokinetics and tissue sensitivities and they may be too infrequent to be picked up by changes in the mean unless they are also large. If there are a few large changes then there may be some change in the mean, but it may be difficult to differentiate these from changes in the mean due to many small changes. In order to separate these two types it is necessary to count the number of patients with changes beyond certain threshold limits. There will, of course, be changes falling between these two extremes and these can be identified by counting the numbers going beyond a lower threshold limit.

Type A changes should show a dose–response effect, but this will depend upon how many volunteers and patients have received different doses and the range of doses used. If there are many abnormalities in the pre-treatment screen due to the indication for the drug many of the patients' parameters may have already exceeded the set threshold limits and therefore any adverse change will not be recognized if only those beyond the threshold set are counted. In these circumstances the count of the number of patients whose parameters show a percentage change from baseline should also be used. Two different percentage changes, one representing a serious clinical change and one indicating a more minor change may be required. The critical difference would be a suitable criterion for the minor change.

Type B Effects

These are the reactions that are bizarre and they are usually due to some form of hypersensitivity. They are not predictable from the drug's pharmacology and do not usually show any dose–response effect. They are relatively rare, but are likely to be serious. Although the change to abnormal will usually be large, type B effects are so rare that they are unlikely to affect the mean value to any extent. They will be represented in the number of values beyond certain threshold limits as well as being a large percentage change from baseline. These patients need to be identified for individual assessment.

Abnormalities in a single parameter have been considered, but other parameters in the same organ group are also likely to show changes (see flagging on page 175).

Summary of Changes to be Identified

To summarize there are four types of changes to be identified:

1. Small changes in many patients. Use changes in the means and/or medians.
2. Larger changes in fewer patients. Count the number of values going beyond certain threshold limits. This can be either in absolute terms or in percentage changes from baseline values (shift tables).
3. Serious changes in the occasional patient. These require individual assessment and are usually referred to by the FDA as 'individual marked abnormalities'.
4. Changes affecting more than one parameter in any one organ group.

These four methods and the various ways these data can be presented now need to be looked at in more detail:

Small Changes in many Patients

This is sometimes referred to as 'changes in central tendency' since it mostly concerns movement within the reference interval.

Difference between 'before' and 'after' means   The simplest version is where there is one before-treatment measurement and one immediately after the end of treatment. The difference between these two means can be compared for the study drug and its control and a 'p' value calculated. This is fine if only making the one comparison as using 'p' < 0.05 there is only a 1 in 20 chance of making a type 1 error; however, we will be repeating the statistical calculation on the comparison of the differences between the means of 25–36 different parameters and therefore there will be a strong likelihood that one or many differences will be found purely by chance. There is no easy answer to this problem, there are two alternative ways of dealing with it. The first is to quote the two means, but not to make a statistical comparison. The second is to adjust the 'p' value for the number of comparisons. (This is dealt with by Dunnett, C. and Goldsmith, C. in a chapter entitled 'When and how to do multiple comparisons' in *Statistics in the Pharmaceutical Industry*; ed. Buncher and Tsay, Marcel Dekker, 1981.) If, however, a statistical comparison is made without any adjustment, reference must be made to the number of comparisons. The simplest of these adjustments to the 'p' value is the Bonferroni method (Elashoff, 1981). This involves dividing the 'p' value by the number of comparisons, but it is only useful when $n < 40$. With any adjustment the likelihood of detecting a real difference is reduced.

Where there are also Intermediate Values   We have discussed comparing the differences between two means before and after treatment; but in many studies these measurements are made at more than two visits. One method is to plot the mean data with time along the x-axis and one line per treatment group; this will show the overall trend for each treatment (Davis, 1994). The Lilly approach is to use the minimum or maximum (depending upon which direction one is interested in)

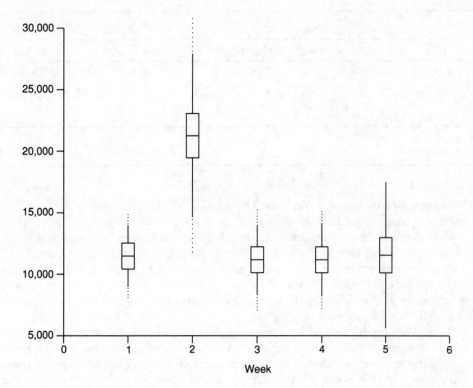

Figure 7   Box and whisker plots

value in the intervening measurements as well as the comparison between the base-line and the final measurement. An alternative is to plot the means of the test drug and its control over time either simply or more elaborately with a 'box and whisker' plot (Windhorst *et al.*, 1987) as shown in Figure 7. The top and bottom edges of the boxes represent the 25th and 75th percentiles of the sample. The horizontal line within the box represents the median and sometimes an asterisk is used to represent the mean. The whiskers extend to cover the 95 percentile range derived from fitting a normal distribution to the data and the asterisks at the extremities are the individual results outside the 95 percentile.

Comparison of Variables Across the Reference Interval   For each parameter at each time point the results are displayed in 12 columns. The first column gives the number of patients with results below the lower limit of the reference interval and the last column gives the number of those with results higher than the upper limit. The ten intermediate columns give the numbers of results for each 10% of the reference interval (Table 8).

A similar table can then be made for the comparator drug or placebo and the distribution of variables compared (Harkins, 1996).

Larger Changes in Fewer Patients
(a)   Numbers of values going beyond various threshold limits.
(b)   Numbers of values going beyond certain percentages of baseline.

Table 8

Visit	< LL	10%	20%	30%	40%	50%	60%	70%	80%	90%	100%	> UL
base line												
intermediate												
end of study												
post-study												

LL, lower limit of reference interval
UL, upper limit of reference interval

Numbers Going Beyond Various Threshold Levels The threshold limits are fixed at clinically significant levels regardless of the baseline level.

In its simplest terms, presuming all the values are normal at baseline, how many became abnormal? Here the reference interval is used for 'covering' the normal and with some parameters the interest is in movement in one direction (e.g. creatinine and liver function tests) whereas with others the interest is in movement in both directions (e.g. glucose and potassium). Graphically these movements can be shown as a shift table (Figure 8).

Values that are unchanged fall across the diagonal, while increases are to the right of the diagonal and decreases to the left. A statistical comparison can also be made comparing increases and decreases. When there have been several laboratory screens during the study the maximum value at any time can be used instead of using the last value on treatment.

The Lilly approach is to use five levels instead of three. Instead of just taking the middle 95% as in the normal reference interval they use the middle 98% as well (Thompson *et al.*, 1988) (Figure 9).

Syntex used four levels and for those where one is only interested in movement in one direction there are three different threshold levels (Rees, 1989) (Figure 10). They group similar tests by function, for example for creatinine:

Level 1—ULN to 30% above.
Level 2—30% above to 100% above.
Level 3—> 100% above or > 2 × ULN.

Other threshold levels besides Syntex's have been proposed by the FDA, WHO and others.

Figure 8   Standard shift table

		AFTER				
		<1%	<2.5%	Middle	>97.5%	>99%
BEFORE	<1%					
	<2.5%					
	Middle					
	>97.5%					
	>99%					

* The percentages are the levels of the reference interval

Figure 9   Lilly shift table

		AFTER				
	BASELINE	NORMAL	LEVEL 1	LEVEL 2	LEVEL 3
BEFORE	NORMAL				
	LOW				
	HIGH				
	MISSING				

Figure 10   Syntex shift table

FDA 'Clinically Significant Abnormals' (Food and Drug Administration, 1986)
These are:

- Liver enzymes, AST, ALT, AP, LDH $\geq$ three times ULN.
- Bilirubin (total) $\geq$ 2.0 mg/dl.
- BUN $\geq$ 30 mg/dl.
- Creatinine $\geq$ 2.0 mg/dl.
- Uric Acid (male) $\geq$ 10.5 mg/dl; (female) $\geq$ 8.5 mg/dl.
- Haematocrit (male) $\leq$ 37; (female) $\leq$ 32.
- Haemoglobin (male) $\leq$ 11.5 g/dl; (female) $\leq$ 9.5 g/dl.
- WBC $\leq$ 2800 mm^3 or $\geq$ 16 000 mm^3.
- Eosinophils $\geq$ 10%.
- Neutrophils $\leq$ 15%.
- Platelets $\leq$ 75 000 mm^3 or $\geq$ 700 000 mm^3.

In Reviewer Draft Guidance 'Conducting a clinical safety review of a new product application and preparing a report on the review', which was released for comment on November 22, 1996, by the FDA there was a list of 'potentially clinically significant changes' some of which are similar to the above FDA 'clinically significant abnormalities' as follows:

- Albumin—low (< 2.5 g/dl).
- AP—High (> 400 U/L).
- Bilirubin (total)—high (> 2 mg/dl).
- BUN—high (> 30 mg/dl).
- Creatine kinase—High (> 3 × ULN).
- Calcium—low (< 7 mg/dl); high (> 12 mg/dl).
- Cholesterol—high (> 300 mg/dl).
- Creatinine—high (> 2 mg/dl).
- GGT—high (> 3 × ULN).
- Glucose—low (< 50 mg/dl); High (> 250 mg/dl).
- LDH—high (> 3 × ULN).
- Phosphorus—low (< 2.0 mg/dl), high (> 5.0 mg/dl).
- Potassium—low (< 3.0 mmol/l), high (> 5.5 mmol/l).
- AST—high (> 3 × ULN).
- ALT—high (> 3 × ULN).
- Sodium—low (< 130 mmol/l), high (> 150 mmol/l).
- Triglycerides—high (> 300 mg/dl).
- Uric Acid (female)—high (> 8.0 mg/dl, (male)—high (> 10.0mg/dl).

WHO Recommendations for Grading Acute and Subacute Toxicities (cancer) An adaption to these (WHO, 1979) was made in 1981 (Miller *et al.*, 1981) and the clinical cooperative groups in the USA put forward their version in 1989 (US Co-operative Groups, 1989).

Liver 'Fogarty Conference' Guidelines (Davidson et al., 1979)

Pfizer criteria Pfizer used different criteria depending upon whether the baseline was normal or abnormal and the degree of homeostatic control of the particular parameter, so each parameter had the following four levels:

(a) When the baseline value was normal or missing—1. Clinically minimal abnormality (Insignificant); 2. Clinically important abnormality (marked).
(b) When baseline value was abnormal—1. Clinically minimal abnormality; 2. Clinically important abnormality.

The clinically minimal abnormalities vary from 5–25% above ULN and the important abnormalities from 10–50% above ULN.

Changes Greater than the Span of the Normal Range That is, greater than four standard deviations. This was put forward by Kershner of Stirling Laboratory at the 1990 DIA Conference Amsterdam (Kershner *et al.*, 1990).

Critical Limits Physicians need to be aware of potentially life-threatening conditions and a survey of American hospitals use of critical limits was performed in 1990. The resulting list of critical limits may be of use in some studies (Kost, 1990). A more refined form of the 'shift table' is the two-dimensional scatter plot, sometimes called

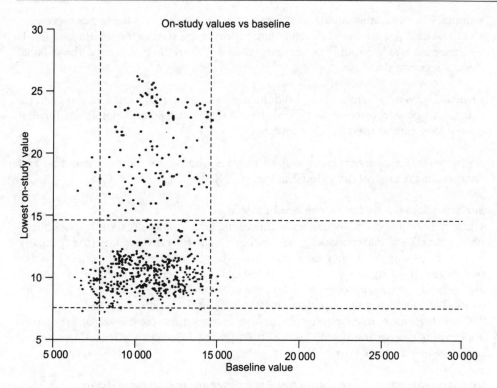

Figure 11   Two-dimensional scatter plot (x–y plot)

an X-Y plot. In this case instead of categorizing the values the actual values are plotted. Again unchanged values tend to fall on the diagonal, but each outlier is accounted for (Figure 11).

The asterisks represent the plots of results for individual patients. The vertical and horizontal lines represent the upper and lower limits of the reference interval, similar to the 'shift table'. If the individual results were unchanged they would fall on an imaginary 45° line bisecting the angle between the x and y axes.

Numbers Going Beyond Various Percentages of Baseline   Syntex use grades of change from baseline (percentage of the normal range)
These are:

Grade 1: > 33% of baseline.
Grade 2: > 67% of baseline.
Grade 3: > 100% of baseline.

If there is more than one follow-up value while on treatment the most extreme value in each direction is summarized regardless of time.

Lilly use 'Delta Limits'   Using a large number of values from patients in clinical trials ($n = 3556$) who have had two blood samples taken at an interval of one or two weeks Lilly defined the distribution of the differences between the first and second samples. The delta limits are those values that just exclude 1% of the largest decreases and those that just exclude 1% of the largest increases, so that for creatinine (μml/l) the decrease was −35 and the increase was +35. Lilly then validated these limits using a separate database.

Critical Differences   Since critical differences (see page 160) represent the changes that must occur from baseline before the change is considered significant for that patient they can be used in this context.

A histogram of the percentage changes   There is a histogram for the active drug and another for the control drug (Kershner *et al.*, 1990).

Serious Changes in the Occasional Patient
These require individual assessment. They must be identified as soon as possible as part of the clinical trial monitoring so that they can be fully investigated (the company may want to suggest further investigations). These cases can be identified by flags (see page 174) or by using one of the threshold levels mentioned earlier. In order to assess these cases a complete patient profile is required (see pages 174, 195). Another method of identifying these patients is dealt with in the next section below.

Guidelines have been published for the management of clinical or laboratory abnormalities occurring during clinical trials by the Pharmacovigilance Department of Roussel Uclaf, Paris (Bénichou *et al.*, 1988).

Changes Affecting more than One Parameter in any Organ Group

Flags   These changes may be identified by flags (see page 175)
Genie Score   This is a global score for a group of functionally related parameters and uses the normalized deviations from the normal range of a combination of related parameters (Sogliero-Gilbert *et al.*, 1986; Gilbert *et al.*, 1991).

Non-parametric approach to four groups of related tests   This is being explored by Lilly. The four groups of related tests assess liver, kidney, marrow and urine. The maximum (or minimum) test result for each parameter after starting treatment is identified. These maximum values for all patients are then ranked starting with number 1 as the highest (or the lowest.) Similarly the changes from baseline are also ranked. These ranks are then summed across all the parameters in an organ group, both for maximal value and for maximal change. These scores can be used for identifying patients for individual assessment, The differences between two treatment groups can be tested in two ways outlined in their paper.

Clinical trialists opinion   It is obviously important to collect the clinical trialist's opinion since he or she may well be able to say that any changes were due to the indication or other underlying disease. It is reasonable to ask the trialist to give one opinion on each organ group at a time rather than on individual parameters. The amount of weight given to the investigator's opinion must depend upon whether the trialist is knowledgeable about laboratory values and this may depend upon his or her specialty and experience. A review of his or her curriculum vitae may be valuable.

When to use the Different Techniques for Analysing Laboratory Data

Changes in the Mean

This method should always be used when there are likely to be small changes in most patients or when there is a very slow onset. This is likely to occur when changes are expected because of the pharmacological properties of the drug (type A adverse reactions)—for example potassium ions with with beta-2 agonists. When there have been several laboratory screens during the study changes over time are best shown using a 'box and whisker' plot (see Figure 7).

Numbers Going Beyond Certain Absolute Limits

This is best used when the baseline screens are expected to be normal and there are no expectations of a problem (i.e. no type A reactions). This method is then ideal for picking out patients who require individual assessment. This is best demonstrated using either a 'shift table' (see Figures 8–10) or a two-dimensional scatter plot (an X-Y plot) (see Figure 11). This is a good method for detecting and demonstrating type B reactions.

Numbers Going Beyond Certain Percentages from Baseline

This is best used when the baseline screens are not expected to be normal and no type A reactions are expected. A good display for these changes is a histogram of the various percentage changes for the drug and its control. This is well suited to picking up and demonstrating type B reactions (Davis, 1994).

Individual Assessment

This will be essential in all studies. All clinically significant changes will require individual assessment with a patient profile.

Aggregation of Data from all the Parameters in an Organ Group

The only essential method in this group is the use of the clinical trialist's opinion and it should be used in all types of studies.

Analysis of Sub-groups

The analyses described will be used across the whole study and all patients will be included, but changes may be confined to a subgroup and this will need to be looked at separately. The factors or variables defining these subgroups can be related to:

- The drug(s).
- The patient.
- The disease(s).

Drug variables are:

- Dose and/or blood level.
- Route of administration.
- Duration.
- Frequency of dosing.

- Concomitant therapy.
- Formulation.

  Patient variables are:

- Age.
- Sex.
- Weight.
- Alcohol intake/tobacco usage.
- Centre, race or country.
- Human leucocyte antigen (HLA) factor.
- Pharmacogenetics.

  Disease variables are:

- Subclasses of the indication and/or different degrees of severity.
- Concomitant diseases (e.g. renal failure).

It is obviously not possible to analyse all parameters for all variables and some sort of selection will have to be made. The first choice will be for any hypotheses developed from the analysis of all patients and any *a priori* hypotheses (e.g. all type A reactions) will have to be examined for a correlationship with dose. The FDA are interested in questions of safety in subgroups (gender, age, race and gender by age, etc.) (Harkins, 1996).

A limiting factor will be the size of the study, small studies (e.g. 20 patients will not warrant looking at more than two or three relationships). There will also be occasions where it will be necessary to correlate one laboratory parameter with another, for example haemoglobin against creatinine to indicate the anaemia of renal failure (an X–Y plot).

Presentation of Laboratory Data

Wherever possible graphic presentations should enliven tables. The possibilities are immense and it is worth scanning *Presentation of Clinical Data* by Bert Spilker and John Schoenfelder and published by Raven Press. Several of the papers already referred to have displays of graphics (Sogliero-Gilbert *et al.*, 1986; Weeks *et al.*, 1986; Thompson *et al.*, 1988; Gilbert *et al.*, 1991).

Another excellent paper, both for its graphics and its text, is Windhorst D. B., Pun E. F. C., Zubkoff I. A. (1987) 'Data on drugs and adverse experiences; moving from the specific to the general' in *Drug Information Journal*, **21**, 39–46. Finally one must consult the FDA *Guideline for the Format and Content of the Clinical and Statistical Sections of New Drug Applications*, US Department of Health and Human Services, 1988.

Investigation of an Hypothesis

If during the analysis an abnormality is found, it becomes necessary to look for data that either supports or refutes the hypothesis that the abnormality is due to the test

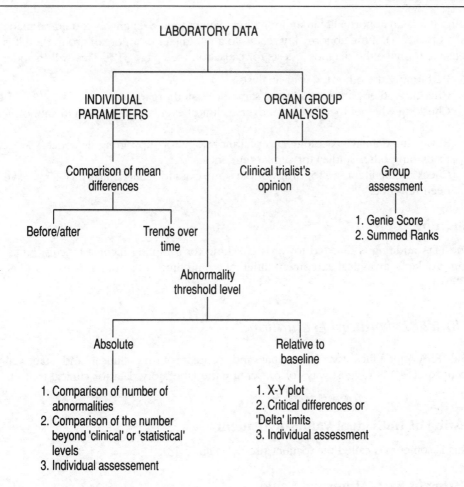

Figure 12   Laboratory data summary

Patient	Time	Age	Sex	Race	Weight	Dose	SGOT	SGPT	AP
1	0	70	M	W	65 kg	20 mg	v1	v2	v3
	1						v4	v5	v6
	2						v7	v8	v9
	3						v10	v11	v12
	4						v13	v14	v15
2	0	65	F	B	50 kg	10 mg	v16	v17	v18
	1						v19	v20	v21

Figure 13   The patient profile

drug. If it is an abnormality in an individual patient then a diagnosis should be made (see Chapter 4). If the abnormality relates to a parameter or an organ group then it is sensible to make the diagnostic tests for causation (see page 312). This will include:

- Performing the other types of analysis.
- Checking other parameters in the same or related organ group.
- Checking whether there are any adverse clinical events in those with the abnormalities.
- Reviewing animal toxicology and pharmacology for supporting evidence.
- Examining other studies for similar tendencies.
- Checking the literature for drugs of the same class to see if similar problems have been reported.

Auditing

The FDA auditing is directed towards checking for sampling inconsistencies, handling problems, analytical equipment differences and time of day differences (Harkins, 1996).

Clinical Laboratory Evaluation

The FDA guidelines for the format and content of the clinical and statistical sections of NDAs suggest ways of presenting the laboratory data for clinical trials as follows:

Listing of Individual Values by Patient

This is sometimes called the 'patient profile' (Figure 13).

Listing of Each Abnormal Value

This is a by-patient listing in a similar format to the above.

Evaluation of Each Laboratory Parameter

Mean values over time
This is the mean or median at each visit as well as the range of values and the number of patients with abnormal values or with abnormal values over a certain size.

Individual Patient Changes

(i) Shift tables
(ii) Change of predetermined size. This shows the number of patients who have a change in parameter of a predetermined size at selected time intervals.
(iii) X–Y plot.

Individual Marked Abnormalities
This should be in narrative form.

Chapter 7

The Pre-marketing Establishment of the Side-effect Profile of a New Drug

M. D. B. Stephens

'Drugs become top-sellers because of their side-effect profile rather than because of their efficacy profile' (Pratley quoting Refsum, 1996).

The safety monitor should be familiar with the notes for guidance on:

- Good clinical practice (CPMP/ICH/135/95) and guideline for good clinical practice—Feb 2, 1997 (419 KB).
- General considerations for clinical trials (CPMP/ICH/291/95).
- Good clinical safety data management; definition and standards for expedited reporting (CPMP/ICH/377/95).
- Population exposure: the extent of population exposure to assess clinical safety (CPMP/ICH/375/95).
- Clinical safety data management; data elements for transmission of individual case safety reports (CPMP/ICH/287/95).
- The particular clinical area for which the drug is intended (e.g. Alzheimer's disease).
- The more general document: The *Declaration of Helsinki* (Reproduced in Annas and Grodin, 1992).

Regulations and guidelines have to deal with principles that are generally applicable to a wide range of circumstances; as such they form the basis for clinical trials. There may be a tendency to assume that if the regulations and guidelines are followed nothing more should be done. Many of the suggestions in this chapter have to be seen as additions to this basic framework.

Pre-marketing Studies

The pre-marketing programme for the detection of new adverse drug reactions (ADRs) can be divided into two types:

1. The non-specific search for ADRs, which will aim to detect ADRs not previously foreseen.
2. The specific search for ADRs that may be foreseen for historical, toxicological, pharmacological or clinical reasons.

Non-specific Adverse Drug Reactions

This is the search for ADRs that is undertaken for all drugs and excludes the specific search for particular ADRs that might be foreseen from previous information. An ADR may manifest itself either by subjective symptoms or objective findings or a combination of both.

Subjective Symptoms

The phase 1 and early phase 2 studies should aim to pick up the minor events, which are fairly common (see Chapter 4). If a particular event is shown to be more common in the drug group than in the placebo group, the later phase 3 studies can be planned with this in mind.

Most minor events are described inadequately by clinicians (e.g. 'headache'), but if they are recognized early in the clinical trial programme, a specific questionnaire or form can be designed to obtain a full description as described on page 108. If the minor event has some special characteristics, then its drug relationship can be recognized once the drug is marketed and possibly the drug will not need to be stopped unnecessarily. The questionnaire or form must therefore try to identify the particular clinical characteristics of the event.

Second, the background characteristics of the patients suffering the event must be identified to see if a susceptible subgroup can be identified as being more at risk (e.g. the elderly, those with renal failure). Further investigation of these patients may also indicate the mechanism of action.

Rechallenge, when it is ethical and the patient has consented, is of vital importance in establishing the drug/event relationship and may be encouraged in the protocol.

Treating the event frequently confounds the effect of stopping the drug so the latter should precede treatment whenever possible. Minor events are usually completely reversible on stopping the drug, but it is helpful if the speed of reversibility can be ascertained.

Objective Findings

These are usually covered by the standard laboratory investigation scheme and the standard clinical investigations, but are of special importance when considering the effect of the drug on the course of any chronic diseases that may be present in addition to the primary disease. In these circumstances, it is important to measure the effect of the drug on the chronic disease and the parameters usually used for its diagnosis and prognosis.

Specific Adverse Drug Reactions

These may be predicted because of the known pharmacology of the drug, experience with drugs of the same class, animal toxicology or previous use in humans. Their discovery will be a function of the number of patients studied and the investigations undertaken.

Drug Development Phase I to Phase III

The goals of the various phases of drug development (phases I–III) from the point of view of safety and efficacy have been tabulated by D. M. Cocchetto and R. V. Nardi in a 1986 paper entitled 'Benefit–risk assessment of investigational drugs, current methodology, limitations, and alternative approaches'.

Phase 1 Studies (Volunteer Studies)

Czerwinski from New York wrote a very good introductory paper on phase 1 studies in 1974 (Czerwinski, 1974).

The purpose of Phase 1 studies is to obtain information on:

- Initial safety and tolerability.
- Pharmacokinetics and bioavailability.
- Initial efficacy.
- Drug metabolism.
- Drug interactions.

Certain physiological parameters that measure the function of an organ with limited power of repair and regeneration are ideally evaluated in Phase l. These include the special senses and the central and peripheral nervous system (i.e. ophthalmological screen, audiometry, etc.; (Goldberg *et al.*, 1975).

Volunteer studies seem to uncover the following types of ADR:

- Those masked or modified in patients by disease or concomitant medication.
- ADRs likely to be induced by higher doses of the study drug (i.e. in dose-ranging studies).
- ADRs that are extensions of the pharmacological action of the drug.
- ADRs related to interaction between drug and common events in normal life (i.e. alcohol. (Idänpään-Heikkilä, 1983).

Motivation of Volunteers

A survey of 28 young volunteers and 28 elderly volunteers showed the prime motive for taking part was money. Altruism played a part in the elderly continuing to take part in studies (Kirkpatrick, 1991). The results when volunteers were asked to indicate the importance in volunteering were as follows:

- Money 88.6%.
- Wanting to help people 51%.
- Curiosity regarding drug studies 35.4%.
- Assisting pharmaceutical development 15.5%.

Only 18.43% would participate without financial remuneration (Collins and Johnston, 1995).

Rarity of Serious ADRs in Volunteers

Serious ADRs are extremely rare in volunteers (Cardon *et al.*, 1976). In a survey in the USA there was only one drug-related sequel in one of 29 162 volunteers used over 12 years and only one clinically significant medical event occurring every 26.3 years of individual volunteer's participation (Zarafonetis *et al.*, 1978). Minor adverse reactions are not uncommon and help towards the detection of similar adverse reactions in the clinical trials by alerting the trial designer to potential problems. However, in 1985 there were two deaths. The first occurred in Dublin when, unbeknown to those in charge of the study, a volunteer had received a depot injection of flupenthixol the day before receiving an injection of the trial drug. The volunteer had not revealed that he was under a psychiatric clinic (Darragh *et al.*, 1985). The second death occurred in Cardiff and was due to aplastic anaemia nine months after taking part in the study of a new benzodiazepine. It was not possible to say whether the disease was due to the test drug (Leader, 1985). These two deaths resulted in a re-examination of the problems of research in healthy human volunteers. In March, 1996 a student died after a fit due to acute lidocaine toxicity following the use of a lidocaine spray for a bronchoscopy at the University of Rochester, USA (Sunday Telegraph, 13 July 1997).

The Association of the British Pharmaceutical Industry (ABPI) published the results of a 1984 survey of its member companies on their experience in this area including both in-house and external studies (Royle and Snell, 1986). The number of serious suspected reactions in in-house studies was 5 (0.27/1000 subjects exposed) and in external studies 8 (0.91/1000). A re-appraisal in 1986 from the USA cited a further death in a volunteer who had unbeknown to the investigator anorexia nervosa. The author of that paper therefore suggests that the investigator asks himself a series of questions prior to the study (Powell, 1986).

1. Do some studies pay subjects so much that they are willing to give inaccurate histories?
2. Are you so busy that you do not actually participate in screening subjects or in conducting the study?
3. Is the study conducted in an environment and with appropriate medical supervision to respond to a medical emergency?
4. Is the research question asked either trivial or predictable in outcome?
5. Should the research question be asked in the population for which the drug is intended?
6. Have you made adequate provision to cover medical expenses of the subject and liability expenses for yourself?

A survey among members of the British Pharmacological Society in 1987 showed that 69% of volunteers ($n = 8163$) had adverse effects. They were moderately severe in 0.55% and these, in order of frequency were postural hypotension, abdominal pain, nausea and vomiting, palpitations, bronchoconstriction, drowsiness and headache. There were three severe life-threatening effects: anaphylaxis, a perforated duodenal ulcer and a skin reaction, but all made a complete recovery. Professor

Orme suggested that general practitioners should be given exclusions for studies and thereby prevent those who match an exclusion criterion from entering the study (Orme *et al.*, 1989).

Another study from France in 430 volunteers had an overall incidence rate of 13.5% adverse effects (AEs), covering 69 different types of AE. Severe AEs accounted for only 0.36% of AEs. A total of nine deaths and life-threatening AEs have been reported in clinical research up to 1992 (Sibille *et al.*, 1992). The same group have updated this study with 1015 patients. The incidence rate for AEs with active drugs was 13.7% and for placebo 7.9% (Sibille *et al.*, 1998).

The ABPI have issued a booklet which summarizes the present situation. An update, *Medical Experiments in Non-patient Human Volunteers*, (ABPI, 1998) is due in late 1997. The Royal College of Physicians' report on research in healthy volunteers was published in 1986 (RCP Report, 1986).

The Place of Women in Phase I and II Studies

A study of the proportion of young women taking part in all phases of pre-marketing clinical trials for two drugs showed that they were under-represented in phase 1 and phase 2 studies and approximately equally represented in phase 3 studies when compared with their proportionate use after marketing (Kinney *et al.*, 1981). The reason for this was that the previous Food and Drug Administration (FDA) guidelines proscribed administering new drugs to pregnant women and also those who might become pregnant, and specifically stated that women of childbearing potential should be excluded from large-scale clinical trials until the *FDA Animal Reproduction Guidelines* had been completed (US Dept of Health, 1977). These guidelines were designed to protect the potential offspring of these women. All this changed in 1993 when the ban on women was lifted and the *FDA Guidelines for the Study and Evaluation of Gender Differences in the Clinical Evaluation of Drugs* were produced (FDA, 1993), but there was no regulatory basis for requiring routinely that women in general or women of childbearing potential should be included in particular trials such as initial human studies (Rarick, 1995). The guideline was designed to:

- Ensure that clinical trial programme participation is accessible to women of childbearing potential.
- Ensure early accumulation of information about responses to drugs in women that could be used for designing later trials.
- Improve the likelihood of making adjustments in larger clinical studies if gender-specific differences are noted in early trials.
- Remove the perception that men should be the primary focus of medicine and drug development.
- Encourage sponsors to develop initiatives to recruit women of childbearing potential into clinical trials (Johnson-Pratt and Bush, 1996).

Sponsors must now submit gender analyses for NDA filing (Federal Register, 1994).

At the same time, in 1993, the US National Institutes of Health (NIH) Revitalization Act was signed, which included guidelines for the inclusion of women and minorities in clinical research (Federal Register, 1994). It stated that "in the case of any clinical trial in which women or members of minority groups will be included as subjects the NIH shall ensure that the trial is designed and carried out in a manner sufficient to provide for valid analysis of whether the variables being studied in the trial affect women or minority groups differently than other subjects in the trial" and goes on to detail the circumstances when this does not apply (e.g. when there is evidence that there is no difference in the effects of the variables in women) (Freedman *et al.*, 1995).

Problems With Including Women

Before a Study It is not generally expected that reproductive toxicology studies will be completed before phase II studies. Therefore it is essential that adequate reproductive precautions are taken after counselling. Current reproductive toxicology information must be given to the participant. This should cover the risk–benefits of study participation, the importance of adequate contraception, lists of contraceptive choices with risk–benefit–drug interactions, information on teratology and the need to avoid pregnancy during drug exposure (Johnson-Pratt and Bush, 1996).

The new drug must not be shown to be an enzyme-inducing agent lest the volunteer/patient on the contraceptive pill should become pregnant while on the new drug or if this is not possible, then the contraceptive pill must be avoided. Normal contraceptive failure rates are high—condom 12–16%, the pill 3–7%, cap, sponge diaphragm 18–22% (Trussel *et al.*, 1990)—therefore females of childbearing potential should have a pregnancy test and a test for recent occurrence of ovulation before and at appropriate intervals during and at the end of the study (Larson *et al.*, 1982).

Legal Liability The problem of false negative pregnancy tests during the early periods of embryogenesis and organogenesis and the risk of liability suits if a fetus is damaged have not been resolved (Fox, 1995). Although a woman may not be able to claim damages because of signing a consent form there are still the rights of the child to consider and the increased cost of liability insurance (Ritrovato and Dinella, 1995). If a woman is able to prove causation then a consent form will not protect the company (Austrian, 1996).

A survey of 28 clinical pharmacology units showed that while 79% conducted clinical trials in women of childbearing potential only 86% did pregnancy tests routinely at screening and immediately before the first dose and only 18% at the post-study visit. Although 91% specified that volunteers should be using a reliable form of contraception only 9% on the oral contraceptive were asked if they had missed any pills, and of those using other methods only 36% were asked if they had used adequate contraception while on the study. The following recommendations were made:

- All female volunteers should have their menstrual history taken at screening
- All postmenopausal females should have their hormone levels checked at screening
- All women of childbearing potential should be tested for pregnancy at screening and this should be repeated at the beginning of each study session and again at the post-study visit (Higginbotham and Rolan, 1997).

Analysis Women in phase I studies have 2.3 times the frequency of AEs as men, with a higher percentage due to laboratory abnormalities (males: females, 15%:26%) (Vomvouras and Piergies, 1995). In addition the presence of women suffering from premenstrual tension could increase the background noise in the control and trial drug groups and if distributed unevenly between the two drug groups in controlled studies could produce misleading ADR data. This can be dealt with by stratifying the randomization by sex.

Since the 1993 guidelines two new products have been found to have gender effects (Sherman, 1996).

Difference Between Adverse Events in Volunteers and Patients

Adverse events occurring in volunteers need to be considered quite separately from those occurring in patients and should not be added to the ADR file for the following reasons:

- Due to absence of disease. The volunteer does not have the disease that the drug can correct. Therefore there may be an exaggerated pharmacological reaction in volunteers that would not occur in patients or would occur to a lesser extent, thus producing either objective or subjective effects e.g. hypertension (Hollister, 1972).
- Due to incorrect dosage. The dosage used may be outside the subsequent recommended therapeutic range due to differences between volunteers and patients (Lasagna and Von Felsinger, 1954; Azarnoff, 1972).
- Due to different formulation. Volunteers are often given a different formulation from that marketed later.
- Due to different age, intelligence and psychological make-up. Excluding the absence of disease, the volunteers are likely to differ from the patients who subsequently take the drug. In the UK, volunteers have often been either university students or staff from the pharmaceutical company and are likely to be of greater intelligence and younger than the patients, having a more scientific background and perhaps a different psychological make-up (Lasagna and Von Felsinger, 1954; Azarnoff, 1972). Volunteers have been assessed as more extrovert, flexible, tolerant, self-confident, content and optimistic than other students with lower levels of anxiety, higher general sensation seeking tendency, tendency to thrill and adventure seeking and disinhibition (Pieters *et al.*, 1990) and as having a type A behaviour pattern (i.e. competitive and aggressive) (Drici *et al.*, 1995). Italian volunteers recruited by word of mouth, being relatives or acquaintances of research staff, were tested with the Minnesota Multi-phasic Personality Inventory (Dahlstrom *et al.*, 1986) and were found to be substantially balanced, self-assured, reliable people motivated by extremely realistic objectives. Those between 56–80 years showed a higher capacity to internalize emotive answers together with lower self-evaluation and social adaptation (Berto *et al.*, 1996). Both this study and two others showed no prevalence of or trend towards an 'obsessional or schizoid personality' (Pieters *et al.*, 1992; Ball *et al.*, 1993).
- Due to a different relationship with the clinical trialist. The relationship between the volunteer and the person responsible is frequently that of a junior (the volunteer) to a senior (the clinical trialist) and this could affect the reporting of AEs.

Because of these differences between patients and volunteers, it has been advocated that volunteer patients should be used more often (Oates, 1972; Weissman, 1981).

Screening

The screening of new volunteers when they join the volunteer panel is obviously essential and will cover medical history of the volunteer, history of allergy, family medical history, smoking and drinking history. Inclusion criteria will cover age, weight, fluency or literacy in relevant language, absence of physical abnormality, laboratory examination for hepatitis and for drugs of abuse (TOXI-LAB drug screening system) plus the usual pre-study screen to include an endocrine screen (Jackson, 1990a and b), electrocardiogram (ECG), ophthalmological examination and chest X-ray examination. These are followed by exclusion criteria relating to abnormalities in the medical history, alcohol or drug abuse and current treatment, if any.

Drug Abuse Screening for drug abuse is essential. In the USA 7.7% of volunteers used illicit drugs, 5.8% cannaboids, 3.6% amphetamines, 1.2% barbiturates, 1.1% cocaine, 1.0% opiates and 0.3% benzodiazepines (De Vries *et al.*, 1991).

Electrocardiography The importance of ECGs was shown in a paper from Simbec Research Ltd where the use of 24-hour Holter monitoring in 57 healthy male volunteers aged 18–46 years revealed:

- Sinus bradycardia in 53.
- Sinus tachycardia in 54.
- Sinus arrhythmia in 30.
- Ventricular ectopics in 25.
- Atrial premature beats in 43.
- First degree block in 7.
- Pause of more than 2 s in 3.
- Second degree block in 5.
- Atrial bigeminy in 1.
- Two consecutive unifocal ventricular ectopics in 2.
- Three consecutive unifocal ventricular ectopics in 1.

The authors recommend 24-hour ambulatory monitoring before drug treatment with new chemical entities (NCE) (Barrington *et al.*, 1990).

Screening of 156 volunteers found that only 20 (13%) had normal sinus rhythm throughout, 83% had supraventricular ectopics, 11% had ventricular ectopics, 2% had unsustained ventricular tachycardia and 6.5% had sinus pauses. One volunteer was in atrial fibrillation throughout. The authors also gave some guidelines for the management of ambulatory cardiac monitoring in volunteers (Stinson *et al.*, 1995).

Hepatitis B Screening Serological tests for hepatitis B surface antigen (HBsAg) are required to exclude those with a positive test who may risk infecting others. Three volunteers had acute hepatitis B and another had positive serology following a trial where this screening was not done. One of the volunteers who was a carrier infected the other four, probably via contamination of the gloves worn by the staff (Mehlman *et al.*, 1994; Ward, 1995).

Human Immunodeficiency Virus Screening A survey of 74 clinical pharmacology units had a 93% response (42 commercial units and 27 academic units) and found that the majority did not believe that it was necessary to perform HIV testing with HIV antibody, but that six commercial units and three academic units did (Thompson *et al.*, 1993). It was recommended that all volunteers should be tested (Sanchez *et al.*, 1994; Vickers *et al.*, 1994). An academic unit reported that all of its 500 subjects tested negative for HIV1 and HIV2 antibodies despite drawing 41.8% of volunteers from South Africa (Jagathesan *et al.*, 1995). A well-reasoned letter from three commercial clinical pharmacology laboratories said that the negative aspects of testing outweighed the positive aspects. It was, however, important to take a careful history to elicit high-risk activities related to HIV infection (Harry *et al.*, 1995).

Exclusions
A request for information from the volunteer's general practitioner (GP) is essential. Of 831 applicants to take part in volunteer studies 14.4% were rejected after review of all applicants, 5.4% after history, examination and investigation, 5.3% after information from their GP (depressive illness, alcohol dependency, drug dependency, neurological disorders), and 3.7% for non-medical reasons (Watson and Wyld, 1992).

In Sweden in a similar study of 772 screenings 11.5% were excluded, 1.4% on history, 1% after examination, 3.9% because of abnormal investigations. There were no serious ADRs during the study period. Information from the GP was not requested (Nilsson, 1996).

In another series from Barcelona 14.2% were excluded on the basis of 'transient and slight clinical or analytical disturbances'. This series were screened by ECG, electroencephalography (EEG), psychological examination, serology for syphilis and hepatitis B Virus (HBV) and faecal blood loss, in addition to the standard clinical history, examination and laboratory screen. Of those excluded 20% were because of disturbances of cardiac conduction (Bartlett *et al.*, 1990).

A further series from Lyons, France, excluded 54% and of these 48% because of disease, 13% due to laboratory abnormalities, 10% because of social, psychiatric, drug addiction or age, 9% due to smoking, 10% because of height or weight, and 10% because of drug treatment (Sibille, 1990).

The exclusion of volunteers with laboratory test results outside the normal limits resulted in 25 of 29 healthy young male volunteers being excluded. The problem was discussed by Joubert, Riviera-Calimlim and Lasagna in *Clinical Pharmaceutics and Therapeutics*, **17(3)**, and they suggested eliminating meaningless lower limits from normal ranges in protocols and allowing a variation of 10% above or below the normal ranges if there is no other evidence of disease. Laboratory screening for volunteers is dealt with further in Chapter 6.

The medical examination may cover simple intelligence tests, a psychiatric questionnaire, audiometry, ophthalmological history and examination, and blood and urine examination. There has to be a limit to screening of volunteers just as there has to be within the National Health Service or any health service. If a hypothesis has been generated from the animal toxicology or pharmacology, previous studies in man or because of problems with drugs of the same class or because of the indication, then audiometry, EEGs, faecal blood loss and 24-hour Holter monitoring may be required, but not for the general non-specific screen unless the volunteer's personal or family history give rise to concern. The standard haematological, biochemical and urine tests, plus history and physical examination, should be repeated 1–2 weeks before a drug study unless there are special circumstances. The GP should be notified when the volunteer joins the volunteer panel and in multiple-dose studies the volunteer should carry a card identifying him or her as a volunteer and giving a contact telephone number in case of emergency.

Monitoring During the Study

The baseline for a single-dose study should entail a pre-study history and medical and laboratory screen plus a limited physical examination, two weeks before the start, repeat of laboratory tests. In single-dose studies on the start day there will be a baseline for heart rate, blood pressure and ECG, etc. and then after the drug has been given a repeat of cardiovascular and other dynamic variables at selected intervals for a given period (usually up to 8–12 hours). On the post-study day there will usually be a laboratory screen at 48 hours after administration of the drug and a further screen 1–2 weeks post-drug (Thomas, personal communication). Multiple-dose studies also require laboratory examination at four days, one week, end of study and post-study. Adverse event reporting during studies may consist of:

- Spontaneous reporting.
- A standard question.
- Stimulated reporting in controlled studies only (questionnaires).

Follow-up in the two weeks following any drug study is essential.

Possible Improvements in Adverse Event Collection from Volunteers

It is important that maximum use is made of the opportunity to collect AEs efficiently. This may be improved by:

- Use of an anonymous questionnaire in controlled studies on possible sexual effects. The questionnaire, identified only by a number, can be placed in an envelope to be given to a person outside the unit, who also has the randomization code. It has been suggested that a list of specific symptoms depending upon the pharmacology and toxicology—with a visual analogue scale (VAS)—should be used (Jackson, 1990). The use of a questionnaire so early in the clinical trial programme means that only predictable ADRs can be covered unless a very exhaustive questionnaire is used. There is always the concern that new minor AEs may not be mentioned when a questionnaire is used. The relationship in a phase 1 unit between staff and volunteers is usually such that minor AEs are mentioned with the use of a single standard question (Jackson, 1990).
- The use of a follow-up question 24 hours after a single dose study.
- The use of a standard question in all studies (i.e. 'Have you noticed any physical or mental changes during the study?'
- Rechallenge—the consideration of rechallenge using placebo and active drug in volunteers with non-serious type A symptoms only.
- An initial single-blind placebo period, which might reduce the number of placebo reactions while in the controlled part of the study. In a small study using an 'All Body Organs and Functions' (ABOF) questionnaire (see Chapter 4) there were 13 AEs in the initial placebo period and nine during the controlled part of the study (Nony *et al.*, 1994).

The reason for taking so much space with details of phase I studies is that the volunteers are the most closely monitored population, have repeated exposure to placebo-containing studies and do not have any disease that might make attribution to the drug difficult. These studies are a constant reminder of the normal variations of healthy people and put the AEs of patients in perspective.

Phase 2 Studies

The primary purpose of phase 2 studies is to test whether the new drug is effective for one or more clinical indications (Hollister *et al.*, 1975) and to determine doses for further study. These studies should only include patients with the target disease and with no other concomitant disease. The number of patients involved is relatively small, averaging about 200. These studies should detect the most frequent ADRs and may predict the target organ system for other ADRs found later in phase 3 studies, but they are seldom able to define any precise or comparative incidence of ADRs or discover ADRs that typically appear in a subgroup of patients (Idänpään-Heikkilä, 1983).

The monitoring of patients in phase 2 studies is similar, whenever possible, to that used in phase 1 studies. There should be two laboratory examinations before taking the new drug. The first should be 1–2 weeks before the study so that the results are available before the new drug is taken and patients can be excluded if necessary. The second is immediately before the drug is taken on day 1. The logic of reducing the background abnormalities was shown on page 179. The problems met in early clinical trials have been described in the Council for International Organization of Medical Sciences (CIOMS) review of safety issues in early clinical trials of drugs (CIOMS, 1983) and are:

- Collaboration between sponsor and investigator may be less interactive than is desirable.
- Potentially serious ADRs may be poorly documented and the relevant forms not properly completed.
- Patients may be admitted to trials who do not fulfil the selection criteria, making interpretation of potential AEs difficult.
- Pre-treatment assessment is inadequate and incomplete and therefore it is difficult to interpret AEs occurring during treatment.
- Appropriate actions that are needed to evaluate a potential ADR properly are often not instituted.
- Treatment may be instituted before appropriate safety assessments have been taken or the results received.
- Rechallenge after an AE may be undertaken without appropriate monitoring.
- Parochial attitudes may be adopted and the sponsoring organization and experts in the evaluation of ADRs may not be involved until very late.
- Occasionally ADRs are published without adequate investigation and may lead to problems in determining the true situation.
- Often there seems to be a lack of appreciation of the regulatory and legal implications of handling ADRs sensibly.

As is clear from the problems outlined by the CIOMS the protocol must lay down the exact procedures to be undertaken if there is an AE. This is especially important in phase 2 studies and must include a rigorous follow-up procedure for dropouts. A single serious AE in an early phase 2 study may abort an entire new drug programme if sufficient information is not collected and a proper assessment of causality made. Spilker covers the various safety parameters that can be measured in clinical studies covering laboratory tests, ophthalmological testing, psychological and performance tests in chapter 17 of his guide to clinical studies and developing protocols (Spilker, 1984).

The death of a clinical trial patient during the pre-marketing phase may be due to many reasons, but if due to the drug may be disproportionately catastrophic for the future of that compound. The steps to take in these unfortunate circumstances are dealt with by A. Cato and L. Cached in Chapter 10 'How to deal with a sudden, unexpected death in clinical studies?' in *Clinical Trials and Tribulations* (Ed. A. E. Cato, Marcel Dekker).

There is a requirement to have treated at least 100 patients for one year before a marketing application. A survey of 27 drugs showed that of the total serious AEs:

- 54% occurred during the first three months.
- 75% occurred during the first six months.
- 25% occurred during the last six months.

Of the total serious ADRs:

- 66% occurred during the first three months.
- 82% occurred during the first six months.
- 18% occurred during the last six months.

Only 4% (25 events) of first occurences appeared in the second six month period. Of these 25 ADRs there were 13 type A reactions; ADRs in this context being AEs possibly, probably or definitely due to the drug (Brown *et al.*, 1996). It is therefore sensible to try to recruit patients from phase 2 studies into long-term extension studies.

Phase 3 Studies

FDA Problems with Non-USA Data

In late 1985 a group of 30 scientists including FDA scientists, academic clinical pharmacologists and industrial scientists discussed the value of foreign data on new drugs in achieving FDA approval for a new drug application (NDA) (Lasagna, 1986). Their following conclusions are of great importance to non-USA companies:

- Foreign clinical trials can be useful, but often they are not.
- The problems include deficient protocol design, poor conduct of the trial (often because of poor monitoring) and inability of the FDA to verify data.
- The usefulness of foreign data as evidence of safety depends upon assurances of study quality.
- Proven performance in carrying out clinical trials is the relevant criterion not academic fame or lengthy bibliography.
- Some problems are remediable with reasonable facility:
    (a) Screening of protocols in advance by FDA for trials planned abroad.
    (b) Foreign protocols need to be as detailed as US ones.

(c) Details of case report forms could be improved.

(d) Use of English as routine as one of the languages of the record form.

(e) FDA could declare publicly that for certain purposes such as clinical trials, so-called 'ordinary practitioners' can provide acceptable data.

(f) Greater familiarity with the kinds of statistical analysis requested by the FDA.

● Other problems seem more difficult to solve:

(a) The number and type of statistical analyses plus the priorities given to the different analyses.

(b) Detailed monitoring of foreign clinical data by sponsors to assure the completeness of data.

In 1990 the problems that were found by the FDA were published in Scrip (1990) as:

● Not adhering to the protocol (i.e. enrolment of patients outside the inclusion criteria).

● Clinic appointments outside the scheduled visits.

● Missing laboratory data.

● Change in dosage not previously agreed with the sponsor.

● Concomitant therapy reporting.

● Lack of study accountability.

● Discrepancies between case report form and the raw data. The FDA conducts approximately 20 non-USA inspections of clinical trials per year. More than 80% revealed inadequate and/or inaccurate record keeping, protocol non-adherence in almost 67% of studies, consent problems in 45% and inadequate drug accountability in 40% of studies. Any study that is pivotal for an NDA will be inspected.

For foreign data to be accepted it must be:

● Applicable to the USA population.

● Performed by investigators of recognized competence.

● Available for FDA audit or evaluable through appropriate means (*Scrip*, 1989).

FDA Comment on NDAs

FDA comments concerning the pre-marketing programme and the resultant NDA (Temple, 1991a) were:

● Sponsors exclude patient populations deemed 'too sick' even when the drug is clearly going to be used in such populations.

● Some safety databases are not adequate enough to support the planned dose or the planned duration of use.

● Existing databases are not examined because doing so would require more time.

● Sometimes there is complete indifference to finding the right dose of the drug.

● There is a tendency to focus on the good effect of the drug and to forget that it may also have other less desirable effects that need study.

A subsequent review in 1995 of the 1993 cohort of new molecular entities approved by the FDA said that the FDA did not receive data analysed in the way it would like to have it. With 'nuisance' AEs there were seldom any subgroup summaries, by age, gender, race, or ethnicity and analyses seldom accounted for the length of exposure or dose. If the AE limits the dose or causes discontinuation that although reported it was seldom analysed statistically. There was also little assessment of the range of discomfort or the timing relative to the start of treatment or relative to the disease state.

With serious AEs there was usually no attempt to analyse them statistically and they were not discussed in relation to the patient's condition, demographics or pharmacokinetics. The time course of therapy and the AE were usually not systematically examined. As far as laboratory data were concerned movements within the normal range were generally ignored (Fairweather, 1996).

Medicines Control Agency Comment on UK Licence Applications
Dr Jenkins, who was with the UK Department of Health and Social Security (DHSS) at the time, outlined the problems with the reporting of AEs in the application for a UK product licence at a DIA workshop in December 1985 as:

● Failure to investigate the effect of dose and duration of treatment on incidence of ADRs.
● Failure to ask the question 'Is a particular group at risk?'
● Failure in trial design to test the new drug in the target population.
● Failure to investigate target organ toxicity identified in animal studies.
● Failure to update ADR experiences during the assessment of the application.
● Failure to translate ADR experiences into data sheet warnings.

There are several recurring issues in the rejection of an application on safety grounds (Jefferys *et al.*, 1991):

● An inadequately defined safe starting dose.
● An inadequate demonstration of long-term safety.
● An overall safety analysis is frequently missing.
● Trend analyses are lacking from some safety assessments.
● Failure to follow through target organ toxicity seen in the preclinical studies.
● Assessment of at-risk groups is often a source of difficulty.

The above issues still apply today (Jefferys, 1998).

Japanese Ministry of Health and Welfare Comment on Japanese Studies
In 1994 41 pharmaceutical companies, 26 national hospitals and 51 private hospitals were inspected by the MHW. The report points out a general inadequacy of reporting of serious adverse drug experiences (ADEs) in all clinical tests, failures to measure clinical test values, failures to take into account safety data from previous phases and protocol violations (Fukuhara *et al.*, 1997).

Pharmacokinetic Screening
Temple (1987) said 'Aim to identify subgroups which handle medication differently from volunteers. One or two blood samples taken at specific times from most patients enrolled in phase 3 studies'. This was countered by Colburn (1989).

The data sheet or product labelling will be based on the results of the phase 3 studies. The inclusion and exclusion criteria in phase 3 protocols should therefore

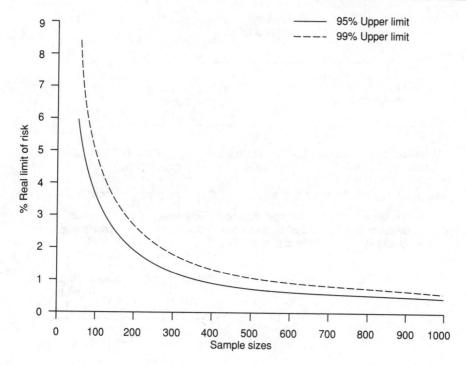

Figure 1   Confidence limits for a zero observation

reflect the intended labelling for the new drug. If all patients over 65 have been excluded from the pre-marketing trials then they should be excluded on the data sheet. The number of patients involved in phase 3 studies will usually be in excess of 1000 and for most drugs will be nearer 3000. At least two specific subsets of patients will require specific monitoring:

1.   Elderly patients.
2.   Patients in whom disease will modify absorption, distribution, metabolism or excretion of the drug, though these tend to be the very patients who are excluded by the protocol in randomized clinical trials (Riegelman, 1984).

If the drug is intended for chronic usage, a minimum of 100 patients should be followed up for one year (Jenkins, 1985). However, if a subgroup of 100 patients shows no serious AE, how certain can one be that no serious ADR will occur in that subgroup in subsequent use? With the information from the Geigy Scientific tables Venning (1984) drew the graph and it can be seen that for 100 patients and taking the 95% curve then the real limit of risk is 3.5% (Figure 1). The chance that this would detect a benoxaprofen type of problem is very small. It has been suggested that on the marketing of a new drug risks of 1% should be known (Anon, 1981a). If this is required then the minimum size of any subgroup should be 350. At a meeting of the German association of doctors in the pharmaceutical industry in early 1987, Dr L. Blumenbach of the Bundesgesundheitsamt (BGA) said he thought that the EEC directive specifying 100 patients over a year as enough to show ADRs was

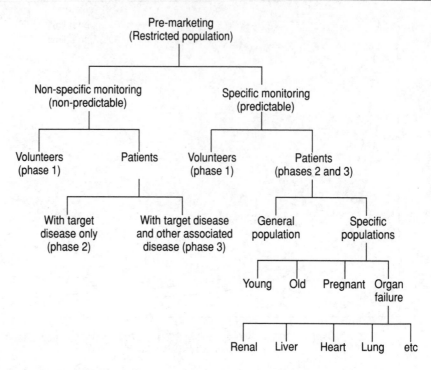

Figure 2   The establishment of the side-effect profile of a new drug.

inadequate since, for instance, a tenfold higher risk of developing an ulcer could not be demonstrated in 100 patients followed for one year: at least 300 patients were necessary (*Scrip*, 1987). There are the following simple rules for calculating the risk for different size subgroups:

- Rule 1—if none of n patients shows the AE we can be 95% confident that the chance of the event is at most 3 in n (i.e. 3/n). The two corollaries for this rule are:
- Rule 2—for 99% confidence interval the figure is 4.6 (i.e. 4.6/n).
- Rule 3—for 99.5% confidence interval the figure is 6.9.

The aptly entitled paper 'If nothing goes wrong is everything all right', which contains these rules is worth reading (Hanley and Lippman-Hand, 1983). There is a saying that the second 500 patients reveal nothing that was not known from the first 500. A glance at Venning's graph shows the truth of this saying. For any material change in risk discovery the increase in size of the denominator should be in the order of magnitudes (i.e. 1 000, 10 000, 100 000, etc.).

Idäpään-Heikkilä (1983) has said that phase 3 studies lasting two weeks or less uncover the most frequent and the acute ADR, but that for AEs with longer latent intervals these trials need to be extended to three months; there will still be some important ADRs, that will only be detected in studies lasting six months. All long-term studies are dogged with increasing numbers of dropouts and the protocol must make sufficient provision for a determined effort to find out their fate. The diminishing numbers can give a false impression of the incidence of ADRs with a long latent period and life table analysis should be used to cope with this situation (O'Neill, 1987). The advantages put forward for the method are the following:

- It permits estimation of the cumulative ADR rate over a specific time interval.
- It handles losses from observation adequately.
- It allows determination of whether a time-specific ADR is occurring at a constant, decreasing or increasing rate.
- It may allow combining safety data from more than one clinical trial. Severe and easily recognized ADRs will be as easily detected in uncontrolled as controlled studies (Idänpään-Heikkilä, 1983).

Controlled Trials

Protocol

The protocol needs to consider all aspects of the clinical trial and it is useful to run through a checklist (Clinical Trials Unit, Department of Pharmacology and Therapeutics, London Hospital Medical College, 1977; Spriet and Simon, 1977; Bulpitt, 1983) to make certain that all the essentials have been considered. The following are the questions concerning adverse reactions that should be considered when writing the protocol. A safety monitoring evaluation plan should be in place before the start of any clinical trial.

Aim Do the aims of the study accurately describe the purpose of the trial as far as adverse reactions are concerned? Can estimates of the expected incidence of death and serious AEs in the study population, based on the disease and/or concomitant medications used to treat the disease, be provided? Any deaths or serious AEs that exceed these estimates would presume a drug relatedness and require notification of the regulatory authorities; remember fialuridine (Nickas, 1997).

Patient Selection Does the selection of patients bias the study as far as adverse reactions are concerned as follows?

- Have patients who have previously had one of the trial drugs been excluded? If not, how will they be dealt with? There is more likely to be a problem in comparative controlled trials in chronic diseases where the alternative drugs are the new drug and the standard therapy. A patient who has already had the standard therapy without any problem is very unlikely to have an ADR in the study, whereas the patient who has developed an ADR while previously on the standard therapy will be excluded from the study. The statistical analysis of the trial results can weight the effect of previously having the standard against not having had it. Exclusion of these patients from the study could have a serious effect on trial recruitment. The record card must therefore have a space with the phrase 'Has the patient ever had any of the trial medications? If so, with what result?'
- Has the background noise been reduced to a reasonable level? (see page 182)?
- Does the choice of clinical trialist or hospital bias the selection of patients as far as type, severity or resistance to treatment of the target illness?

- If the target illness is chronic, will the clinical features and relevant laboratory investigations be shown to be stable before the study?
- Are the inclusion and exclusion criteria pitched at the right level so that the trial results can be extrapolated to a reasonable population of patients on the drug (i.e. females of childbearing age, etc.) (US Dept of Health, 1977).

Trial Design   Features to consider include the following:

- If the underlying disease is likely to produce AEs that might be confused with drug toxicity consider the use of a formal control group; remember fialuridine (Nickas, 1997).
- If the study is not double-blind, will the lack of blindness bias the production/collection of AEs in favour of one of the trial drugs?
- Will the known ADR of the trial drugs unblind the study? If so, how will this problem be overcome? Any controlled clinical trial where the type A ADR of the drugs might allow the patients to discover which drug they are taking should be assessed for maintenance of blindness. This should be done by the patient and the physician guessing the medication at the end of the study. If this indicates loss of blindness enquiry should be made as to whether this was due to efficacy or ADR. If due to ADR the importance of this loss of blinding should be related to the study findings (Moscucci, 1990). Unblinding is most likely in placebo-controlled studies due to lack of AEs and efficacy in the placebo group (Moscucci *et al.*, 1994). In a double-blind study where the patient and investigator were asked to guess which they were on of those patients on active drug (hydroxurea) 53% guessed probably active drug, 34% did not know and 13% thought probably placebo. Of those on placebo 35% thought it was the active drug and 28% placebo with 37% not knowing. Therefore patients on active drug were more accurate with their guess, while those on placebo were less accurate. The investigators guessed that of those on active treatment 54% were on active and 25% on placebo and did not know 21%. Of those on placebo they thought 23% were on active, 51% on placebo and did not know for 26%. Therefore the investigators were more accurate for both groups. Clinic staff and patients cited impressions of improvement or no change in clinical course for their guess (Barton *et al.*, 1996).

The protocol should say under what circumstances the code will be broken; usually this will be carried out for all serious unexpected ADRs by the sponsor for expedited reporting, but may be delegated to an Independent Data Monitoring Committee (IDMC) in large phase III studies. It is important that the biometric and clinical research staff are kept blind, so it should be the job of the pharmacovigilance (PV) staff to break the code when necessary. This will enable the pharmaceutical company to restrict reporting to a regulatory authority to an active comparator or the study drug and also allow them to update the investigator's brochure (IB). This approach is encouraged by the Medicines Control Agency (MCA).

- Does the consent form adequately represent the risks of the study?
- Does the protocol detail notification of serious AE to the trial ethics committee/institutional review board (IRB)?

Concurrent Therapy   Factors to consider include:

- What concurrent therapy should be permitted or forbidden?
- Is sufficient provision made for recording of concurrent therapy on the case record form (CRF)?
- With the ever increasing number of drugs changing from prescription only medicines (POM) to over-the-counter (OTC) drugs there should be special provision made to record all OTC drugs.

Adverse Events (Symptomatic)   Questions to ask include:

- Have the AEs to be collected been defined? (see page 100).
- How are the adverse events to be collected: (i) Diary card? (ii) Questionnaire with or without analogue scale? Has the questionnaire been validated (Offerhaus, 1979)? (iii) Checklist? (iv) Standard question? Is the wording in the protocol and CRF? (v) Other? Quality of life?
- Does the protocol require the clinical trialist to investigate fully all AEs, including seeking the aid of specialists where necessary? Almost inevitably there is a failure of companies to follow-up serious AEs sufficiently. This seems universal and it is rare to obtain all the data that must have been collected and would help decide on the cause of the AE.
- Does the protocol request the physician to make any interim diagnosis or drug attribution before breaking the drug code?
- Does the protocol allow for a sample of blood to be taken for drug levels in the case of all serious AEs?
- Does the protocol inform the clinical trialist that all serious AEs must be notified immediately to the company?
- Do the record forms allow sufficient space and require sufficient details for assessment of all types of AE (see page 218)?
- Does the protocol request full follow-up on patients who have stopped a trial drug due to an AE (i.e. dechallenge), or who have a laboratory abnormality or an AE at the last visit while on the drug?
- Does the protocol require full details of treatment of any AE to be recorded?
- Does the protocol request consideration of rechallenge where ethically justified?
- Is the frequency of trial visits adequate to pick up the AEs and is the timing of the post-study visit suitable considering the disease and the drug ?
- Who is to assess the causality of the AE: clinical trialist, company physicians, clinical pharmacologist, consultant specialist. All?
- How are the AEs to be analysed and compared? Clinically only? Statistically? If the latter, how? (see page 238).

Adverse Events (Asymptomatic)   Questions to ask are:

- Do the laboratory and other objective investigations cover the field of potential adverse reactions (ABPI Guidelines, 1977)?
- Is the frequency of sampling adequate and has a post-study sampling been agreed ?
- How is the handling of patients with asymptomatic abnormal laboratory investigation to be dealt with (Sackett and Gent, 1979; DeMets *et al.*, 1980)? (i) by

repeating tests? (ii) by further confirmatory tests? (iii) by clinical examination? (iv) by dechallenge? (v) by rechallenge?

- How are the laboratory examination results to be assessed (Cancer Research Campaign Working Party, 1980; May *et al.*, 1981; Fletcher and Bulpitt, 1986). (i) according to the normal laboratory range as normal or abnormal ? (ii) by the clinician and/or a company physician? (iii) clinically as well as statistically?
- Will the samples be analysed centrally in a multicentre trial? If analysed in the hospital where the trial takes place, has the pathologist been approached? Have the details of storage and transport been decided.

Drop-outs How are drop-outs to be investigated/followed up to make certain that the cause was not drug intolerance? Other questions to consider are:

- Is there a financial disincentive for the trialists to follow up dropouts (i.e. drop-outs not paid for)?
- Is there provision for following up patients who change GP or move, so that they can be contacted for long-term follow-up?
- If the study is in the UK and is long term, have arrangements been made with the NHS Central Register in Southport for patients to be flagged so that deaths will be identified? (Cancer Research Campaign Working Party, 1980).
- Is there a SOP for follow-up of drop-outs?

Third Party 'Interference' Have sufficient arrangements (e.g. provision of a letter to be held by the patient) been made to ensure cooperation with the management of the patient during the trial, but outside the confines of the trial? Relevant factors to consider are:

- Provision for notification of trial with request to GP for cooperation.
- Provision for possible emergency admission to another hospital.
- Recording of the use of OTC products by the patient. This is becoming much more important as governments try to shift the costs of drug to the patient by allowing them to become OTC products.
- Provision of a card for the patient giving details of the trial and a contact telephone number/address, requesting information from any doctor consulted.

General What is the possibility that the trial will fulfil its aim as to ADRs (i.e. what is the size of the type 2 error)? This involves considering:

- What incidence of adverse reactions (95% confidence limits) appearing with only one of the comparative drugs could be detected?
- What difference in incidence of AEs in the trial drug group compared with the control drug group, or the expected incidence of AEs from previous epidemio-logical studies, would the trial detect?
- Has it been agreed that adequate space will be given to the reporting of AEs in any subsequent papers (Laganière and Biron, 1979), including statements about the power of the study.
- Will all patients who have been randomized and taken even a single tablet be analysed and accounted for as far as AEs are concerned (May *et al.*, 1981).

- Since all pre-marketing studies have some risk to the patient all studies need to be monitored for any undue risk and in studies of any length the possibility of interim analyses must be considered. Guidelines should be listed in the protocol that clearly specify safety variable outcomes that could necessitate patient discontinuation from the study or complete study termination (Enas *et al.*, 1989).
- During the last few years there has been increasing use of clinical research organizations (CROs) for carrying out part of the development of a drug and also an increase in the licensing out of products to other manufacturers. Inadequate preparation for these multiple sources of AE data can result in chaos when finally it is all put together for a license application. Some form of template is necessary to develop a detailed agreement covering AE collection, processing, distribution and reporting (Fieldstad *et al.*, 1996; The Society of Pharmaceutical Medicine Pharmacovigilance Group Working Party, 1998).

Uncontrolled Studies

These may vary from the use of the drug by a physician in a single patient resistant to other therapy to relatively large-scale dose-titration studies. All these studies should be governed by a protocol. All patients must be accounted for and detailed records kept (as for controlled studies).

Difficulties in Attribution

From the point of view of ADRs, uncontrolled studies pose several problems not found in controlled studies:

- Without a control group the AEs that are symptoms alone and can occur in normal persons without drugs often cannot be attributed to the drug.
- Since the type of patient admitted to the study may not be tightly controlled by a protocol, patients are entered having diseases or complications other than the target disease, giving rise to the difficulty in deciding whether an AE is due to the natural course of the concurrent disease (or a complication) or to the drug.
- Concurrent therapy is often permitted in these uncontrolled studies and therefore attribution of AEs to the trial drug may be difficult.
- The consent form, if it lists potential ADRs, may well bias reporting of AEs (Levine, 1987; Myers *et al.*, 1987), but the patient's package insert does not 'suggest' ADRs yet increases the chance that a patient will attribute AEs to the drug (Morris and Kanouse, 1982).

Regulation of Uncontrolled Studies

An unaccountable fatal outcome occurring in an early uncontrolled study may, quite unjustly, be attributed to the drug and all further studies stopped or delayed. The practice of allowing physicians involved in controlled studies to use the drug in a parallel uncontrolled study must be strictly limited and the physician must be prepared to monitor the patients as strictly as if in a formal controlled study. All adverse medical events, no matter how trivial, must be documented and the pharmaceutical company notified without delay of any serious reaction. This can be done using either a specifically designed record card, which is returned at regular intervals, or by the use of a standard AE form, which is returnable immediately after the event has occurred. The latter has the advantage that the event report is not delayed until the main trial form is returned.

Recording Adverse Events in Clinical Trials

From the point of view of recording AEs the essential division is into serious or non-serious AEs according to the International Conference on Harmonization (ICH) guidelines. It is unusual that non-serious AEs or symptoms can be causally related to the drug on an individual basis; however, they can be grouped together and their incidence compared statistically in the two drug groups. Clinicians are only likely to supply very limited information concerning non-serious events, and a full AE form may be inappropriate. A delay until the main record card is returned may be important for non-serious events if they have caused the drug to be stopped and there is a possibility that they are causally related to the drug. They will need to be assessed individually for causality and more detailed information will be required. There are unlikely to be many similar serious events in the two drug groups and they will therefore not be suitable for statistical comparison. The dropouts possibly due to the drug should probably be notified to the company when they occur and therefore before the patient finishes the study. They will require subsequent follow-up.

Non-serious Adverse Events

These are AEs that do not satisfy the ICH definition of serious (see page 35). These can be recorded on a special events form or on the laboratory investigation sheet, and the date of onset, duration, frequency, severity (mild, moderate or severe) and outcome should be noted. These will be assessed when the CRF is returned to the company. The clinician must be encouraged to give full descriptions of these events as a single word is not sufficient. Where the event comrpises one or more symptoms with little objective data to back it up it becomes very important for the trialist to record the patient's own words on the record form. The diagnosis that the doctor makes should be recorded in the doctor's own words. Eli Lilly, USA ask the clinical trialist to select a preferred term using Codification of Standard Terminology for Adverse Reaction Terms (COSTART) only after recording the diagnosis in his or her terms. This has the advantage that the selected term should be the most appropriate (Zerbe, 1989). For the rheumatic patient a daily diary card appears to be the most successful method of assessing minor AEs and has proved particularly reliable in practice (Bird *et al.*, 1985).

Serious Adverse Events

These are all AEs that satisfy the ICH definition of serious (see page 35).

Serious AEs should be recorded on a serious AE form, and a copy despatched immediately to the trial sponsor. The clinical trialist will record all AEs regardless of causality, but should be asked to make a causality judgement while blind to the actual treatment. For serious events the seriousness and courses of action open may demand that the code be broken and the initial causality judgement may need to be changed once the results of all tests are known. These cases must be followed up by the company. The latter must be emphasized because otherwise the clinician may delay sending the form until he has more information and there is always a difficulty in deciding whether to notify a possible ADR as soon as the possibility arises or wait until all the data are available and thus establish a causal relationship (Boisseau *et al.*, 1980; Dangoumau *et al.*, 1978). The follow-up may need to be repeated on several occasions if the results of dechallenge and rechallenge are to be collected. In many studies the single criterion of 'warranting the stopping of the drug' can be used to decide between a case that needs to be notified to the sponsor straightaway or await the end of the study. In the USA the Upjohn Company has used a two-form approach. The Form B for serious events was based on the FD 1639 and was despatched as soon as possible after the event, serious being defined as a significant hazard or threat to life or general health of the patient in this study. The form for non-serious events (Form A) was part of the clinical record form and contained pre-printed events as well as 'other' events, and had space for multiple events. For each event the following were required:

- Date started and stopped.
- Number of episodes (if applicable).
- Intensity (mild, moderate or severe).
- Course (1, persisted without intervention; 2, disappeared without intervention; 3, required intervention; 4, other; the latter two require further comment).
- Relation (1, probably due to drug; 2, possibly due to drug; 3, probably not due to drug. The rationale to be given in the comments box).

If the event occurred during the use of concomitant therapy an entry was made on a special form. The form also asked 'In general were the events observed? volunteered? or prompted?'

The use of the forms has been 97% with Form A (non-serious) and only 3% with Form B (serious). The company has made certain of the acceptability of the forms by extensive field testing (Mohberg, 1987).

The Stirling Company uses a form in which the first page is for non-serious events and a second page is added for serious events. The non-serious page has space for two concurrent events. A very explicit set of instructions accompanies the forms and the monitors and investigators are trained to use them. The first page deals with the following information: study; patient; brief description of event; dates and dosage of treatment; action taken; whether it is a single occurrence or after most doses; date and time of onset; duration in days, hours, minutes, seconds; severity (mild, moderate, severe); outcome—five alternatives. The second page covers drug blood levels, with time of last dose, relevant patient history, ECG and autopsy results, space for further tests and four concurrent drugs, and outcome data (Rosenberg, 1985).

Roussel-Uclaf have, several specific forms for different types of AE as well as a standard form. These can be found in the back of the book *Adverse Drug Reactions, A practical Guide to Diagnosis and Management.* (Bénichou, 1994) (see Bibliography).

Why Include Dropouts Due to Adverse Events as a Reason for Notification Before the End of a Trial?

One can question the advantages using solely the serious criterion as a reason for immediate notification. Drug withdrawals due to AEs may indicate too high a dosage regimen and need further investigation. Of drugs approved in the USA since 1979 20% required dose reduction after approval (Bagshaw, 1992). The same point has been emphasized in the UK. The reasons put forward were:

- The dose is commonly fixed at the level that has been shown to be effective in 90% of the population *provided that the unwanted effects at this dosage are considered acceptable.* In 25% of patients a smaller dose will be effective.
- Digit preference (e.g. a correct dose of over 50 mg may be rounded up to 100 mg).
- To avoid dose titration (not loved by marketing departments!) (Herxheimer, 1991; Venning, 1991).
- Once phase III studies have started at the wrong dose repeating the studies atthecorrect dose would produce an unacceptable delay in the application date.
- 'The common practice of selecting the highest possible dose for use in large trials may result in an unacceptable incidence of unwanted and potentially serious adverse outcomes' (e.g. Hirudin) (Conrad, 1995).

If type A adverse reactions due to an incorrect dose for an individual patient cause a patient to drop out from a phase II study their notification at the end of the study may be too late for a change in dose for phase III studies. This may be particularly relevant to indications requiring long-term therapy. Similarly notification during phase III studies would allow studies at the correct dose to run in parallel so that early in the post-marketing phase a lower dose would be available. It would also be sensible to take blood for drug levels in any patients complaining of type A events during phase I and phase II studies.

Dropouts due to adverse medical events may be for several reasons:

(a) The patient or physician may have thought the AE to be due to the drug.
(b) The patient or physician may have thought the AE was not due to the drug, but that the AE made continuing with the drug undesirable (e.g. if the AE was renal failure from natural causes treatment with a renally excreted drug may be inappropriate).
(c) The physician may not know the cause of the event and has therefore stopped all drugs
(d) The patient might have had several different signs and symptoms, but only one of these might be the actual reason for stopping the drug.
(d) The drug may have been ineffective.

Follow-up is vital in order to obtain:

(a) Causality assessment.
(b) Response to dechallenge and possibly to rechallenge.
(c) Further investigations that would help in causality assessment, but may not be required for the patient's clinical management.

Follow-up may also allow the trial monitor to help the clinician by giving previous experience with the event or suggesting reduction of dosage rather than stoppage for type A reactions.

Special Areas of Concern

There are two areas which come under the heading of non-specific ADR search, which are of particular concern in chronic usage of drugs:

1. Damage to the eye.
2. Effect of drugs on skilled performance.

Damage to the Eye

In the *General Consideration for the Clinical Evaluation of Drugs*, published by the US Department of Health, Education and Welfare Public Health Service, FDA in 1977, it is stated that for chronically administered drugs that are known to be absorbed, complete ophthalmological examination (pre- and post-drug) should be performed in a representative number of patients followed for six months or preferably longer. For drugs that are administered for shorter periods in clinical trials eye examination should be performed at the end of drug administration.

Effect of Drugs on Skilled Performance

All new drugs should be tested for effects on the CNS at some stage (Jackson, 1990). The danger of drugs affecting car driving ability has attracted more attention in recent years. The estimated drug use related to road accidents per year has been given in the form of 50 000 hospital admissions, 15 000 non-fatal injuries and a cost to the European Union of over 7 billion ECU (De Gier, 1997). In 1984 the first international symposium on prescription drugs and driving performance was held in Holland and the proceedings were published as *Drugs and Driving*, edited by J. F. O'Hanlon and J. J. de Gier, and published by Taylor and Francis in 1986. A great deal of discussion revolved round the tests required to discover any impairment. Speakers from the industry suggested that the present physiological tests are adequate while others thought that driving simulator tests were required. All drug applications in the EEC must now be accompanied by a 'Summary of Product Characteristics', which includes a statement on the effects of the product on the ability to drive and operate machinery (Isaacs, 1988).

In a chapter entitled 'Performance studies and the manufacturers of CNS active drugs', J. Haller, J. Ward and R. Amrein listed the tests used in assessing performance impairment of drugs (Table 1). A later paper (Druce, 1990) listed the objective measurements of CNS function used for antihistamines: after the two reaction times, digit symbol substitution, critical flicker fusion as mentioned in Table 1 he adds dynamic visual acuity, pupillary light responses and latency of P3–evoked EEG potential. A new test for the measurement of daytime sleepiness and alertness, the multiple sleep latency test (MSLT) is discussed. The use of psychomotor tests has been assessed in the elderly using the Automated Psychomotor Test Battery (Kalra *et al.*, 1993) and with benzodiazepines (Kunsman *et al.*, 1992).

The subject has also been dealt with by A. N. Nicholson in a chapter entitled 'Impaired performance' in the book *Iatrogenic Disease* (see Bibliography). (Nicholson, 1986) (see Bibliography).

The categories for ascribing effect in the summary of product characteristics (SPC) on activities relevant to driving are:

Table 1   Tests used in assessing performance impairment of drugs

Pharmaco-EEG
Evoked potentials
Critical flicker fusion
Pupillometry
Choice reaction time (Vienna reaction time apparatus)
Reaction time (Vienna reaction time apparatus)
Complex reaction time (stress reaction tester)
Neurological examination
Sleep laboratory studies including residual effects
Saccadic eye movements
Tracing test (Oswald and Roth)
Purdue pegboard tasks
Platform balance skill
Digit symbol substitution test
Symbol copying
Digit span
Free recall (10 nonsense syllables)
Number and colour test
Letter cancellation test D2
Eigenschaftwörteliste (EWL)
Subject's self-assessment (sedation, muscle relaxation, concentration capacity)
Investigator's subjective assessment on subject's wakefulness and ability to concentrate

- Presumed to be safe or unlikely to produce an effect.
- Likely to produce minor or moderate AEs.
- Likely to produce severe AEs or presumed to be potentially dangerous.

For the latter two categories special precautions relevant to the category should be mentioned. 'In the past it has been unusual to test a medicine directly on driving ability pre-marketing' (Price, 1997). The prescriber will be informed via the data sheet or SPC and the patient via the package insert. Despite these warnings, research into the possible effect of new drugs on driving and operating machinery is sadly lacking. How often do prescribers mention the subject to patients? Of patients who took drugs in Spain regularly 76.5% had never been warned (Carmen Del Rio and Alvarez, 1996). How often are patients who are involved in driving accidents interrogated about medication? In a French study of victims of road traffic accidents (RTAs) 23.6% admitted having taken medication five days before the accident (Montastruc et al., 1988; Carmen Del Rio and Alvarez, 1996). It has been estimated that at least 10% of all people killed or injured in RTAs have been using some kind of psychotropic medication that could be considered as a contributory factor (Carmen Del Rio and Alvarez, 1996).

Two studies have been undertaken using large databases on drugs and traffic accidents:

- Benzodiazepines in Canada (Neutel, 1995).
- Psychoactive medications in the USA (Leveille et al., 1994).

These both showed an increased risk in users, but the latter study was in elderly patients and the effect was only seen in those on antidepressants and opiates, but not in those on antihistamines or benzodiazepines. Suggested further reading is *Medicines and the Road Traffic Safety*, Editors: D. Burley, and T. Silverstone, Clinical Neuroscience, London, 1988.

In June 1983 Dr J. Idänpään-Heikkilä from Finland published the results of a study he undertook while on a year's sabbatical leave in the USA. This consisted of a review of safety information obtained in phases 1, 2 and 3 clinical investigations of 16 drugs. He concluded that phase 1 studies seem to uncover certain adverse reactions that are difficult to find in phase 2 and 3 studies (see page 197). Phase 2 studies detect the most frequent adverse reactions and may predict target organ systems for other adverse reactions subsequently discovered in phase 3 studies. Lack of numbers restricts the possibility of discovering adverse reactions limited to small subgroups and makes it difficult to give accurate incidence figures. Idänpään-Heikkilä suggested that phase 2 studies could be extended in time to collect long-term safety data.

Phase 3 studies lasting less than two weeks reveal the most frequent and acute adverse reactions and controlled studies demonstrate the actual incidences. Increasing the numbers of patients in these studies from a few hundred to over 1000 does not often lead to the detection of the rarer adverse reactions (with the exception of antibiotics). It is better to extend the duration of these studies rather than to increase the number of patients since many adverse reactions have long latent periods (i.e. 3–6 months). Idänpään-Heikkilä also emphasizes the importance of following up dropouts in long-term studies and that the dropout reduces the number of patients available to suffer adverse reactions with long latent periods. Application of the life table method enables a more accurate estimate of the incidence of these adverse reactions over a period of time. A separate author, Dr R. T. O'Neill, gives a good account of the life table method in the appendix of (Idänpään-Heikklilä (1983).

Specific Populations

At this stage, if not before, consideration should be given to the special groups (see Figure 2).

Paediatrics

There are EC guidelines for clinical investigation of medicinal products in children (CPMP/EWP/462/95), which came into operation in September 1997. In the USA the guidelines for the ethical conduct of studies to evaluate drugs in paediatric populations were put forward by The Committee on Drugs/AAP in *Pediatrics*, 1995, **95**, 286–294.

The four age groups are:

- Pre-term newborn infants (born at < 36 weeks' gestation).
- Term newborn infants (age 0–27 days).
- Infants and toddlers (age 28 days to 23 months).
- Children (age 2–11 years).
- Adolescents (age 12–17 years).

The four groups of medicinal products are:

- To treat diseases in adults and children for which treatment exists.
- To treat diseases in adults and children that have no current treatment.
- To treat diseases that mainly affect children or are of particular gravity in children or have a different natural history in children.
- For diseases only affecting children.

These groupings come from the EC guidelines (CPMP/EWP/462/95). The first grouping is worded differently in the *Guidelines for Industry. The Content and Format for Pediatric Use Supplements* (May 1996; 59 FR 64242) as follows:

- Neonates—birth up to one month.
- Infants—one month to two years.
- Children—2–12 years.
- Adolescents—12–16 years.

On the whole, the adult experience of dose/effect relationships will provide a framework for dose titration and ADR monitoring. In other circumstances the medicinal product should be contraindicated for children until further data are available after initial marketing authorization (Jefferys, 1995).

A survey of new molecular entities approved by the FDA from 1984–1989 showed that 80% had no information regarding paediatric use (Roberts, 1996) and this continued until as late as 1992 (Kearns, 1996). A UK paediatrician has been reported as saying that 25% of drug administration in children is off-label or unlicensed use and that this is associated with a high frequency of ADR, the percentage of off-label use rising in neonates and preterms (Nunn, 1997). Drug for use in children may be accompanied by problems not seen in adults or cause ADRs that are more frequent than in adults, for example antibiotic toxicity in neonates (sulphonamides, chloramphenicol), hepatoxicity with sodium valproate and Reye's syndrome with aspirin use for viral infections.

The metabolism of drugs differs in young children. The activity of many P450 enzymes is reduced in the neonatal period and the variation in maturation of different enzymes makes it difficult to predict dosage requirements accurately at different ages. Glucuronidation is a major process of drug elimination in adults, but is significantly reduced in neonates (e.g. paracetamol and morphine). Renal excretion is impaired in full term neonates in the first few days of life, but in preterm infants it remains impaired in the first few weeks of life. After the neonatal period renal function is normal (Choonara *et al.*, 1996).

Suggested further reading is as follows:

- Leary P. M. (1991). Adverse reactions in children, special considerations in prevention and management. *Drug Safety*, **6**(3), 171–182.
- (1996). Drug development for infants and children: Rescuing the therapeutic orphan. Keams, I. (1996). *Drug Inform. J.* **30**, 1121–1186.
- ABPI/British Paediatric Association (1996) *Licensing Medicines for Children*, ISBN 09500491 74.

Geriatrics

Patients over 65 years of age comprise about 14% of the population in most industrialized countries and consume nearly 35% of the drugs (Avorn, 1997). The EC/ICH guidelines are provided in *Note for Guidance on Studies in Support of Special Populations: Geriatrics* (CPMP/ ICH/379.95). The usual definition of elderly is over 65 years of age, but the FDA definition is over 60 years. There is a threefold increase in the incidence of ADRs in patients over 60 years compared with patients under 30, and one in ten hospital admissions of older patients are for ADRs (Swafford, 1997).

The healthy old person does not seem to be more susceptible to ADRs compared with the young (see page 11) but as a group the elderly have many factors predisposing them to ADRs.

Concomitant Disease   Increased morbidity means the elderly are often taking several drugs. Drug expenditure for the elderly accounts for 40% of UK drug expenditure (O'Brien, 1995). There is also a parallel increase in the use of OTC drugs, resulting in an increased chance of drug interactions. The elderly are also targeted by manufacturers of alternative medicines.

Altered Pharmacokinetics   Although drug absorption does not change, the drug distribution depends on the lean/adipose body mass ratio and this declines with age. Protein-bound drugs are distributed differently due to a reduced serum albumin concentration. Drugs excreted via the kidneys tend to have a lower clearance rate due to a decline in renal function. The hepatic blood flow and liver mass decline with age and oxidative metabolism may be impaired (CYP4502D6 does not appear to change with age alone, (see chapter 2)).

Altered Pharmacodynamics   Beta blockers have less clinical effect for a given concentration in the elderly, but the elderly are more susceptible to the sedative effects of benzodiazepines. Anticoagulants are more likely to cause bleeding. In general the elderly have less effective homeostatic mechanisms (e.g. temperature and blood pressure control) (Beard, 1991; Pollock, 1996).

Poorer Compliance   This may be partly due to polypharmacy, poor sight or failing memory. After discharge from hospital 50% of patients were making medication errors when visited ten days later (Parkin *et al.*, 1976). Age is not itself a factor in poor compliance, which are as follows:

- Altered physiology
- Cerebral factors. The cerebral blood flow decreases. Cerebral autoregulation is impaired and there is increased permeability of the blood–brain barrier.
- Cardiovascular factors, including poor homeostatic mechanism; impaired control and vascular reactivity; deterioration of the conducting system; loss of vessel elasticity and distensibility (a 90% decrease between the ages of 20 and 80 years); decreased baroreceptor sensitivity; attenuated β adrenergic response; blunted postural reflexes and decreased body water.
- Renal factors. Decrease in glomerular filtration rate (GFR) by 25% and renal blood flow by 50% at 80 years of age; tubular function decreases by 7% per decade (Kitler, 1989).

If a product is likely to be used by the elderly then studies need to be performed, especially if the following factors are present:

- A low therapeutic index.
- The drug is excreted renally.
- A possibility of interactions.
- Problems with drugs of the same class.
- Deterioration in organ function, which may affect pharmacokinetics or pharmacodynamics (O'Brien, 1995).

Interaction studies are usually recommended with the following groups of drugs:

- Digoxin and oral anticoagulants.
- Hepatic enzyme inducers.
- Drugs metabolized by cytochrome P450 enzymes.
- Other drugs likely to be used with the test drug.

These details are from an excellent paper entitled 'Licensing of drugs for the elderly' (O'Brien, 1995).

Inclusion of Elderly Patients in Clinical Trials

- Any drug likely to be used by elderly people should be included in pre-marketing studies with an age distribution comparable to that expected when the drug is in routine use.
- Pre-marketing evaluation should include assessing whether important age-related differences exist in efficacy and toxicity.
- Since unexpected differences may emerge in effectiveness or side effects when a drug is used by large numbers of elderly patients, especially those too frail to be included in trials, plans for post-marketing surveillance (PMS) should be required at the time a drug is approved (Avorn, 1997).

Suggested further reading is 'The elderly in clinical trials: regulatory concerns' (Kitler, 1989).

Pregnancy

Approximately 35% of pregnant women in the UK take some drug during pregnancy and this includes about 9% who take OTC products (Rubin, 1995). The total figure for the USA in 1993 was 68% (Rubin *et al.*, 1993), for Italy 80% in 1995 (Maggini *et al.*, 1997), and for Brazil in 1996 94.6% (Fonseca *et al.*, 1997). The animal toxicology will probably be the only evidence for or against teratogenicity until the drug is on the market and from then on the evidence will be anecdotal unless large-scale epidemiological studies are undertaken. In the UK the background incidence of major malformations is about 2.3% at birth rising to 4.5% by five years of age. The incidence of spontaneous abortions in clinically recognized pregnancies is 10–20% (Lack *et al.*, 1968). Drugs and chemicals together are thought to account for only about 4–6% of malformations with 65–70% unknown (Wilson, 1977). All drugs given to the mother except high molecular weight compounds such as insulin and heparin can cross the placenta.

Many physiological changes that may affect drug levels occur during pregnancy and include:

- Increased plasma, extracellular fluid, and fat stores.
- Increased hydroxylation capacity by steroids, which may alter metabolism.

- Albumin binding and binding to specific receptors may be altered.
- The 40–50% increase in GFR, which may affect drug excretion.
- Gastrointestinal absorption of oral preparations may be impaired (Redmond, 1985).

The risks of drug use in pregnancy have been classified differently by several countries:

- Sweden—four categories A–D.
- USA—five categories A–D (different from the above) and X.
- Australia—five categories A, B (B1, B2, B3), C, D, X.
- Netherlands—five categories; same as Swedish, but with an extra X.
- Germany—seven categories A–G.
- Denmark—five standardized phrases (Sannerstedt *et al.*, 1996).

This would seem to be another area for the attention of CIOMS or a similar group. The increased number of women suggested in clinical trials may result in some pregnancies in the early stages of a drug's development. Since there is a 3% chance of major abnormalities in live births (DeLap *et al.*, 1996) or 40 / 1000 overall (Shaw *et al.*, 1986) there will be the possibility that mothers with babies with abnormalities will sue the drug company.

During the pre-marketing period a decision will have to be made concerning PMS studies. The possibilities are:

- Case–control studies.
- Cohort studies—prescription event monitoring (UK), which will pick up any pregnancies in the first six months; medication events monitoring organization (MEMO) database in Scotland; general practice research database (GPRD) database (see appendix 4).
- Specific registries—national birth defect registries (Schardein, 1993); UK National Teratology Information Service, which is part of the European network of teratology information services (Bateman and McElhatton, 1997); International Clearing House for Birth Defects Monitoring Systems (see Bibliography— Teratogenesis, Pregnancy and Lactation), which covers Australia, France, Israel, Italy, Japan and South America, is referred to as the MADRE project (malformation drug exposure surveillance), and has been collecting cases since 1990; the Pegasus project—all pregnancies in Munich—14 000 births per year and 85% of women used at least one drug during pregnancy (Hasford, 1996; Cornelia *et al.*, 1997).

Pregnancy Registry   The criteria for selecting agents for a registry are:

- Issues arising from conduct of animal studies.
- Expectation of AEs during pregnancy based on structure-activity relationships.
- Findings of concern from case reports in the literature or identified from PMS.
- Expectation of high use pattern in women of childbearing age.
- Treatment needed for conditions associated with high morbidity or mortality; inability to discontinue treatment ethically during pregnancy (Manson, 1997) (e.g. new drugs in epilepsy where there is a 2–3 times greater incidence of malformations, mostly due to older drugs; Craig and Morrow, 1997) and the fluoxetine registry (Goldstein *et al.*, 1997).

Suggested further reading is 'Special considerations in studies of drug-induced birth defects', by A. A. Mitchell, Chapter 38, 595–609, Pharmacoepidemiology, Ed. B. L. Strom, Wiley, Chichester, 1996.

Multi-ethnic Populations

There is a *Note for Guidance on Ethnic Factors in the Acceptability of Foreign Clinical Data* (CPMP/ICH/289/95/step 3). The majority of clinical trial subjects in the USA and Western Europe are Caucasian males, but 80% of the world's population live outside this area. Even in the USA 25% of the population have ethnic minority backgrounds (Lin *et al.*, 1994). The ICH 3 meeting in December 1995 of the Efficacy 5 Working Party discussed the ethnic factors in the acceptability of foreign data and proposed limiting inter-regional approval to three groups; Asian, Caucasian and Black.

Ethnic differences can be divided into:

- Intrinsic factors (e.g. metabolic genetic polymorphism, receptor sensitivity, sex, height, race, age and liver/kidney function).
- Extrinsic factors (e.g. culture, diet, medical practice, language, compliance).

Intrinsic Factors   Metabolic genetic polymorphism can be divided into:

(a)   Cytochrome P-450 systems.
(b)   Selective protein transport systems.

Cytochrome P-450 Systems   The cytochrome P-450 enzymes have been studied extensively. The activities of metabolizing enzymes are bimodally or trimodally distributed so that there are extensive metabolizers (EM), poor metabolizers (PM) and slow metabolizers (SM), and the percentages of PMs and SMs vary between ethnic groups. Examples are:

(i)   Debrisoquine hydroxylase (CYP 2D6): PM—Canadian Chinese 32%; US 7%, Japanese 0.5%. Affected drugs include chlorpromazine, amitriptyline, nortriptyline, imipramine, desipramine, clomipramine, paroxetine, brofaromine, beta blockers, propanolol, haloperidol, codeine, metoprolol, perphenazine, fluphenazine, phenazine, risperidone, dextromethorphan, some antiarrhythmics and anticancer drugs (Pollock, 1996).
(ii)   Mephenytoin hydroxylase (CYP_{mp}): PM—Japanese 18–22%; US/Europe 3–5%. Affected drugs include mephobarbital, diazepam, omeprazole, hexobarbital and imipramine.
(iii)   N-acetyl transferase (NAT-2). Most Asians, especially Japanese, are fast acetylators (88–93%), other fast acetylators are Caucasians and Blacks (50%), and eskimos (almost 100%). Affected drugs include isoniazid, sulphonamides, clonazepam, hydralazine, procainamide and nitrazepam. Isoniazid hepatitis risk is greater in fast acetylators, whereas the risk of drug-induced systemic lupus erythematosus (SLE) and hypersensitivity reaction is greater in slow acetylators.
(iv)   Aldehyde dehydrogenase (ALDH). 50% of Asians have an 'antabuse' effect with alcohol.

(v) Alcohol dehydrogenase (ADH). The percentage of PMs varies widely between ALDH and ADH and also between African-Americans, African Blacks, American Indians, Caucasians and Hispanics (Lin *et al.*, 1994; Flicker, 1995).

Selective Protein Transport High levels of α-1 acid glycoprotein are found in 44% of the Swiss, USA Caucasians and Blacks, but in only 15–27% of the Japanese (Flicker, 1995).

There are also pharmacodynamic differences, for example mydriasis with cocaine (Caucasians > Chinese > Blacks); sensitivity to beta blockade with propanolol (Chinese > Caucasians); sensitivity to neuroleptic agents (Chinese > Caucasians). The difficulties in ascribing ethnic background is exemplified with Ashkenazi Jews and the risk of agranulocytosis with clozapine, which is 20%, but only 1% in the general schizophrenic population (Flicker, 1995).

Extrinsic Factors The general reporting rates for AEs in different countries vary:

High – Australia, Canada, Sweden and UK – rates > 50%.
Medium – Denmark, Finland, France, Hong Kong, the Netherlands and Norway – rates between 35% and 45%.
Low – Belgium, Germany and Italy – rates below 30%.

The reporting rates for serious AEs are different:

High – Australia and the Netherlands – rates about 20%.
Medium – Canada, Denmark, Finland, France, Germany, Norway and Sweden – rates between 6% and 12%.
Low – Belgium, Hong Kong, Italy and the UK – rates between 1% and 3%.

The types of AE also differ from country to country (Joelson *et al.*, 1997).

A comparison of AEs with non-steroidal anti-inflammatory drugs (NSAIDs) between the USA, EC and Japan showed that the incidence was always higher in Japan than in the USA or EC. Vomiting and skin rash were only seen in the phase III and open studies in Japan, but not in the USA or EC (Homma *et al.*, 1994). The ICH guideline should define the requirements for foreign data for Product Licence Applications (PLAs).

Table 2 **Characteristics of ethnically**	
Sensitive compounds	Insensitive compounds
Steep pharmacodynamic (PD) curve	Flat effect–concentration (PD) curve
Narrow therapeutic range	Broad therapeutic range
Highly metabolized	Little metabolism
Non-linear pharmacokinetics	Linear pharmacokinetics
Limited bioavailability	Very high bioavailability
Use in a setting of polypharmacy (Flicker, 1995)	Local sites of activity

Specific Adverse Drug Reactions Search

A particular ADR that might be foreseen because of:

- Historical reasons—previous similar compounds have been associated with a specific ADR (e.g. practolol and a subsequent beta adrenoceptor antagonist).
- Toxicological reasons—animal studies have identified an area of possible danger.
- Pharmacological reasons—the pharmacology of the drug predicts specific ADRs (type A reactions).
- Clinical reasons—ADRs have occurred in phase 1 or early phase 2 studies and are therefore foreseen in subsequent polypharmacy studies. Although it is possible to consider the problems of the non-specific ADR search in clinical trials in general terms, the search for a special ADR based on previous information must be tailored according to the known facts: the drug, the disease it will be used for, the possible duration of treatment and investigational techniques available. Professor E. Weber, Clinical Pharmacologist at Heidelberg University Hospital, Germany when discussing the documentation of clinical trials said that she found that the factors selected in trial protocols for monitoring did not reflect the findings in pre-clinical testing, even where the variations have been marked (*Scrip*, 1987).

The special studies may be either:

- In special subgroups of patients with other diseases. It is not usually possible to examine the effect of the drug on the complications of the additional illness or on the more severe cases, and this sometimes remains a gap in the knowledge of the drug until spontaneous reporting in the post-marketing period identifies the problem.
- In patients with the target disease only, but in whom special investigations are arranged to measure any effect the drug might have on a particular organ or function. This is a difficult area since the additional investigations are not really in these patients' interest and if they entail additional clinic visits or unpleasant investigation, are unlikely to be successful. Although all the patients' additional expenses will be refunded, they may still decline to take part. The special investigations usually involve a different discipline to that of the clinical trialist and sometimes a different hospital, all of which adds to the difficulties.

Historical Reasons

Literature searches on the ADR profile of standard therapies will pinpoint important relevant areas. Protocol exclusions frequently reduce the number of patients who might be susceptible to ADRs. For each protocol exclusion the decision should be made either to examine the exclusion in a special study before marketing or to make it a contraindication in the data sheet. The publicity given to benoxaprofen should ensure that in future differences in drug handling by subsets of patients (i.e. the elderly) will be more fully investigated before marketing.

Toxicological Reasons

Before the new drug goes into humans, discussion with toxicologists will indicate areas that require special attention in man. Differences in absorption curve, metabolism, distribution and excretion between the animals tested and man should be given special attention.

Pharmacological Reasons

Animal toxicology and pharmacology should give advance warning of type A ADRs and where objective signs are to be found, but minor ADRs with symptoms only will not be found until the drug is used in humans.

Clinical Reasons

Early in the use of a new drug, either in volunteers or patients, a possible side effect may appear that has not been foreseen for any of the reasons previously mentioned. This possible adverse reaction will then need special attention in subsequent clinical trials. Two factors need to be considered in searching for an anticipated adverse reaction:

1. The expected frequency of the adverse reaction.
2. Any predictive factors.

If the anticipated adverse reaction is likely to be common, then it can be sought in clinical trials, but if it is rare, it may need a large scale multicentre study. However, if it is known that certain factors predetermine the patients who will experience the adverse reaction, then special studies can be set up requiring relatively small numbers. 'Monitored release studies' or large-scale studies in general practice tend to produce the symptoms of adverse reactions rather than diagnoses confirmed by objective data, and as such do not produce data of the quality one can expect from well-conducted multicentre hospital studies.

Investigator's Brochure

Under the Code of Federal Regulations on Food and Drugs, Title 21, part 312.55 it is a requirement that all investigators are given an investigator's brochure (IB) (Federal register, 1991). The ICH *Guideline for Good Clinical Practice* (GCP) E6, 1996 defines the IB as "A compilation of the clinical and non-clinical data on the investigational product(s) which is relevant to the study of the investigational product(s) in human subjects". In the safety section of the IB "Tabular summaries of ADR for all the clinical trials would be useful. Important differences in ADR patterns/incidences across indications or sub-groups should be discussed" (ICH, 1996). There is no mention of AEs. "Guidance should be provided on the recognition and treatment of possible overdose and ADR that is based on previous human experience and on the pharmacology of the investigational product".

The IB should provide a description of the possible risks and ADRs to be anticipated on the basis of previous experiences with the product under investigation and with related products.

Updating

The IB should be updated at least annually, but the frequency will depend upon whether there is any relevant new information (ICH, 1996). There have been some cases where the IB has not been updated during clinical studies (Mikail, 1993). The question on how often the IB should be updated is difficult. It is easy to say whenever there is any relevant new data. In between regular updates a letter can be sent to all investigators and the ethical committees announcing any serious AEs etc. (Mikhail, 1993). Since the term 'expected' refers to its mention in the IB some companies take the view that the more AEs that are put in the IB the less they will need to report. The ICH recommend that the IB is kept current (e.g. through amendments/attachments) particularly for medically important safety data (ICH, 1996). The aim should be to have a single IB for use in all countries and since there are no regulations other than those of the FDA, updates should contain details of all IND reports as well as anything relevant from new animal studies.

Monitoring During Clinical Trials

A new procedure for overcoming the problem of reporting deaths in large-scale pre-marketing double-blind clinical trials where the underlying disease has a high mortality was described in September 1986 at a Paris conference. The UK Department of Health (DoH) has agreed that an independent statistical monitor who is independent of the DoH and the company will receive the reports of deaths and serious AEs as they occur, and will break the trial code and enter the information into a statistical trend analysis that is performed at regular intervals (*Scrip*, 1986).

The MCA now suggest that in high morbidity and/or high mortality disease states a Safety Data Monitoring Committee (SDMC, or DSMC in the USA) is appointed, which decodes trialists' reports, constructs the group sequential analysis and reports direct to the MCA at agreed time intervals, usually three months. There should be either an Institutional Review Board (IRB) or an Independent Ethics Committee (IEC), details of which are in the ICH GCP guideline. Their purpose is to safeguard the rights, safety and wellbeing of all trial subjects. They will be informed of all serious unexpected ADRs. The ICH GCP guideline does not envisage that they will break the randomization code for serious AEs, but it does mention the possibility of establishing an independent data-monitoring committee (IDMC) to assess the safety data and progress of a study and to recommend whether to continue, modify, or stop a trial. The IDMC is a further development of the statistical monitor mentioned above.

The unblinding of serious unexpected AEs must take place before notification to a regulatory authority (MCA), before updating the IB or informing an IRB/IEC, but it is important that the biometric and clinical research staff stay blinded. The unblinding should be performed by the safety department or the IDMC. The place for an IDMC is in large phase III studies. The composition and function of the IDMC were discussed at a Drug Information Association (DIA) meeting in 1994 (Ellenberg, 1994).

Unblinding

The advantages of maintaining blindness as to the study drug is that it maintains the integrity of the study and this approach is often emphasized by the statistician. However ICH (see page 335) advises that blinding should be broken for serious, unexpected AEs but not for serious expected AEs. The problem with this approach is that the frequency of the ADR in a large study might reach proportions that require further rapid action. The advantages of unblinding are:

- Allows ongoing safety evaluation of the product in development.
- Facilitates updating of the investigator's brochure.
- Avoids need to update safety database.
- Avoids expedited reporting of placebo/comparator cases.
- Meets regulatory requirements (Simmons, 1998).

In Germany the ICH ruling is interpreted as reporting obligations before registration:

- Serious unexpected ADRs within 15 days after code break.
- Serious expected ADRs: code break might be at the end of the study, only then does the deadline for 15-day report start (Pfeiffer, 1998).

End of Clinical Study Reports

These are governed by the *Structure and Content of Clinical Study Reports* (ICH E3, December 1995) and CPMP guidelines *Note for Guidance on Structure and Content of Clinical Study Reports* (CPMP/ICH/137/95) (see chapter 13).

The safety evaluation is considered at three levels:

- The extent of exposure (dose, duration and number of patients).
- The more common AEs.
- Serious AEs and other significant AEs.

Three kinds of analysis and display are called for:

- Summarized data using tables and graphical presentations.
- Listing of patient data.
- Narrative statements of events of particular interest.

Large studies will require detailed analysis of subgroups, almost approaching the 'integrated safety summary level' whereas small studies may only require minimal analysis. The study report is best written by the person who has been dealing with the AEs during the clinical trial and is familiar with the protocol and the data.

Reporting of Clinical Trials

The final purpose of a clinical trial is to influence opinion, and the three groups to be influenced are the originating pharmaceutical company, the regulatory authorities and the prescribing doctors.

Publication of Clinical Trial Results

The published reports of drug safety in clinical trials are more often than not inadequate.

A survey of 23 papers published by a reputable medical journal found that 65% of the papers could not be relied upon for specificity, 52% may have been insensitive in their methodology, 88% did not quantify the symptoms observed, 95% failed to characterize susceptible patients and 52% contained no information on dosage in affected patients (Feinstein, 1987). Similar criticisms have been made concerning the French medical press (Laganière and Biron, 1979).

A survey of studies of diclofenac and simvastatin in the USA and Japan made the following points:

1. The Japanese literature was mostly (95%) made up of primary reports whereas in the USA there were more secondary reports and reviews (70%), and only the primary reports gave sufficient information to understand the design of the studies and the procedures for identifying AEs. Secondary reports were defined as data whose source was not described or 'on file' with a company.
2. Japanese studies were mostly comparisons with active drugs while the USA studies were mostly placebo controlled.
3. In reports from the USA and Japan it was not common to give information sufficient to interpret the reported frequency of AEs.
4. Only the Japanese reports gave the full results of laboratory tests.
5. Neither country's reports provided any detail about the methods used for detection of AEs during the trials.
6. The Japanese authorities recommend publication of trials before the NDA is approved whereas this is not so in the USA. On the other hand the reports in the USA had more overview and interpretation than the Japanese reports.

The authors recommended either:

(a) All AEs to be recorded according to a protocol that involves active observation, standard physical examination, standard laboratory testing and both closed and open-ended questions. AEs should be classified according to type, frequency, severity and attribution.
(b) A minimalist course. Only fatal and life-threatening reactions to be recorded and refrain from tabulation of casual, not reproducible and possibly biased reports arising from ill-defined surveillance (Hayashi and Walker, 1996).

Marketing Authorization Applications

The safety monitor should be familiar with:

*   The *FDA Guidelines for the Format and Content of the Clinical and Statistical Sections of the New Drug Applications* (1988) (integrated summary of safety).
*   *Reviewer Guidance, Conducting a Clinical Study Review of a New Product Application and Preparing a Report on the Review* (US Department of Health and Human Services, draft version Nov. 1996).
*   *Notice to Applicants for Marketing Authorisation for Medicinal Products for Human Use* in European Community (111/5944/94) December, 1994.

Pooling of Safety Data

Many clinical trials are too small to reveal differences in AE rates between the active drug and control and even the larger studies are unlikely to be large enough to show differences in subgroups of patients. Pooling of safety data is required to maximize the usefulness of the total exposure to a new drug. The most thorough analysis is required by the FDA while the European regulatory authorities seem to be satisfied with a relatively superficial approach; however, some European countries are now demanding a more thorough analysis. Anyone dealing with pooling of data should be familiar with the *Guidelines for the Format and Content of the Clinical and Statistical Sections of New Drug Applications* from the Centre for Drug Evaluation and Research, Food and Drug Administration Department of Health Sciences, dated July 1988. The relevant section is 'Integrated summary of safety information', pages 32–46 and the safety section for an individual clinical study on pages 71–82. A recent paper also deals with the subject (Skinner, 1991). The separate headings are:

1. Overview.
2. Format/content.
   (a) Table of all studies.
   (b) Overall extent of exposure.
      (i) Number and duration.
      (ii) Number and doses.
   (c) Demographic and other characteristics of study population.
   (d) Adverse experiences in clinical trials.
      (i) Overall narrative.
      (ii) Display of AE and occurrence rates.
      Grouping of studies.
      Grouping of events.
      (iii) Analysis of AE rates.
      (iv) Display and analysis of deaths, dropouts due to AEs and other serious or potentially serious AEs.
   (e) Clinical laboratory evaluation in clinical trials.
   (f) AEs, including laboratory abnormalities, from sources other than clinical trials.
   (g) Animal data.
   (h) Analysis of AE dose–response information.
   (i) Drug–drug interactions.
   (j) Drug–demographic and drug–disease interactions.
   (k) Other pharmacological properties.
   (l) Long-term AEs.
   (m) Withdrawal effects.
3. Update of safety information.

Before writing an integrated safety summary it is useful to read a series of three papers published in the *Drug Information Journal* (Garvey, 1991; Lineberry, 1991; Temple, 1991b).

The aim of pooling data is:

- To evaluate serious AEs too rare to be seen in each individual study.
- To discover if any particular subgroup is more susceptible to an AE.

Analysis of subgroups which had not been defined prior to the study (so called 'data dredging') should not be performed as a part of efficacy analysis but is essential as far as safety analysis is concerned. However when 'subgroups defined by the data are generated by the study results; often an effect is so suggested and then confirmed with statistical significance on the same data set' (Scott & Campbell, 1998). Ideally any 'subgroup ADRs' found by this method should be confirmed by a subsequent study as well as by 'group causation' methods (see page 317).

The first aim is subject to the total number of patients taking the drug while the second depends upon looking at those subgroups of patients by variables. These may be patient, drug or trial variables.

Patient Variables

These are:

1. Age.
2. Sex.
3. Weight.
4. Race, country or centre.
5. Concomitant disease (e.g. renal failure).
6. Indication and severity.
7. Alcohol intake and smoking.

Drug Variables

These are:

1. Dose.
2. Formulation.
3. Frequency of administration.
4. Route.
5. Duration.
6. Comparative therapy.
7. Concomitant therapy.
8. Blood/plasma level.

Trial Variables

These are:

1. Type of study—controlled, uncontrolled or named patients.
2. Method of collection of AEs—diary card, checklist, questionnaire, general question or spontaneous reporting.

Approaches

All patients who have had one or more doses of the new drug (any formulation) must be included in the safety analysis.

There are three approaches to the examination of the pool by variables.

All Studies Pooled

This is only suitable if the variables that one wishes to examine are similarly represented in all studies (e.g. age, sex) and the studies are similar in design (a rarity). With this approach the effect of small subgroups may be swamped by the majority of the patients.

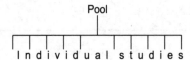

Figure 3   Individual studies

Hierarchical Approach

If some studies have a common characteristic then they form a subgroup, which may have a different ADR pattern from the remainder of the studies. The first step is to look at the drug and indication concerned and then to list the variables starting with those that are likely to have the greatest effect down to those not expected to have an effect. The former should be at the top of the hierarchical tree and the latter at the bottom. For example, one might expect more AEs in trials against an active drug rather than one against placebo since only mild disease cases are likely to be in the latter and uncontrolled studies may contain patients not acceptable to controlled studies due to their stricter inclusion and exclusion criteria. Groups with a concentration of one variable that may show differences could be, for example:

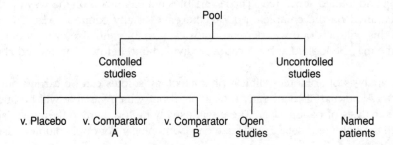

Figure 4   Pooling of Hierarchy

- Patient—Race or country (Joelsen *et al.*, 1997); concomitant disease (e.g. renal failure with a drug excreted renally); indication; drug; dose/blood level; duration; route.
- Trial—collection of AEs by questionnaire/checklist (these should always be analysed separately).

This is only an example and whether or not a variable has a little or great effect will change from drug to drug. A further example is given in Figure 5.

Using the above example as an illustration, the process of combining the studies starts at the roots of the hierarchical tree. If there is more than one placebo study then the incidence rates and the types of AEs are compared and if similar they can be combined. If they differ the trials are examined to see if there is another variable that might be responsible for the difference (e.g. one study, unknown to the sponsors, had used a questionnaire and had thereby increased the incidence rate of all ADRs). If no explanation is forthcoming then the data are combined and a note made of the discrepancy. It may be that a similar discrepancy will be noted in other studies and point to a variable not previously considered. This process of comparing and then

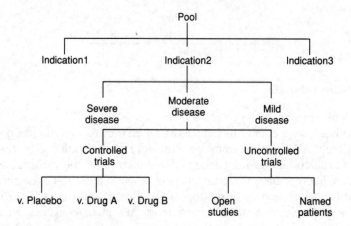

Figure 5   An example of pooling safety data

combining is continued to the top of the tree. When a definite difference is spotted and the responsible variable identified then this group may be left out of the final pooling and treated separately. Those variables not examined on the way up the tree are examined on the complete pool of the data for any common AEs. The way in which this will be done will depend upon the variable and size of the pooled data (e.g. age may be looked at by decades or divided into below 65 years and above 65 years).

The analysis of volunteer clinical pharmacology studies can be carried out in the same way and may give an early indication about which variable will be important for the analysis of patient data. There will usually be too many differing variables to pool all the volunteer data. For the same reason one cannot pool volunteer data with patient data.

The advantages of the hierarchical approach are:

- Analysis can frequently be started earlier (i.e. when a subgroup is complete rather than waiting for the whole database to be available.
- The effect of variables not apparent from analysis of just the whole database may be discovered.
- The incidence rates are likely to be more accurate since variation due to a known subgroup will be excluded.

When comparing incidence rates of AEs one is comparing them directly or indir-ectly with the placebo rate (or if there are no placebo-controlled trials, with a standard treatment in a controlled trial) (see figure 6).

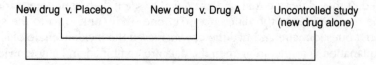

Figure 6   Comparison of incidence rates of adverse events

During this analysis it is likely that differences will be seen between incidence rates and the question about whether these represent ADRs will arise. Further help can be found in two ways:

(i) Statistical. The pros and cons of the use of statistics in multiple comparisons is considered in Chapter 9. In the UK only a minimum amount of statistics seems to be required for safety data. This may be related to the fact that there have been only three statisticians employed by the MCA.

(ii) Individual ADR pattern.

- Is the possible ADR seen in other studies (i.e. is there consistency)?
- Is there a dose–response relationship?
- Is the time to onset consistent with an ADR?
- Was it predictable or does it fit with the drug's known pharmacology?
- Was there a positive dechallenge?
- Is the description specific?
- Is there any support from the laboratory tests?
- What was the clinical trialist's opinion?

FDA Groupings to Consider (see page 237)
- Those with available case report forms and those without.
- All controlled trials or subsets, such as placebo-controlled trials, trials with any positive control, trials with a particular positive control, trials with a particular indication.
- All trials, excluding short-term studies in normals and usually in patients.
- All trials of the same duration.
- Trials where AEs have been collected by means other than spontaneous reporting and those using spontaneous reporting only.
- Foreign trials; domestic trials (USA trials).

Grouping of ADRs

Adverse reactions are grouped by body system using an AE dictionary. There are usually four levels of grouping:

- Body system.
- High-level term.
- Preferred term.
- Original wording of the trialist, which in the case of symptoms may be the original words of the patient (verbatim).

All these levels should be used in individual study reports, but only the first three levels in the pooling of studies.

Serious Adverse Events, Dropouts and Deaths

Dr R. J. Temple has put forward the hypothesis that previously unrecognized ADRs, will be found in the deaths and dropouts if they occur in the database (Temple, 1991b).

Serious Adverse Events

Due to the small size of the pool of patients treated before application for a product licence, serious AEs are likely to be rare and even with a database of 4000 patients there are only likely to be a few AEs of this nature. Therefore a meaningful comparison with a control group will probably not be possible. This generalization does not apply to very toxic drugs such as cancer chemotherapy and will of course depend upon the background noise from the disease being treated. If AEs are type B events then the denominator must only include those patients who have taken the drug for a sufficient length of time, usually more than five days.

Dropouts

All dropouts should be listed with their cause. Those due to adverse effects of treatment should be treated similarly to the serious events; this includes those withdrawn due to abnormal laboratory tests.

Deaths

All deaths should be listed and assessed as for serious events, and compared to the number of deaths expected in the study population. They should be examined for any common variable.

Clinical Laboratory Tests in Clinical Studies

Again a hierarchical tree can be used, but it may need to be a different tree to that used for clinical events since the effect of the variables may be different. Also, whereas clinical adverse non-drug events will tend to vary directly with the duration of treatment, the number of chance abnormal laboratory tests will vary directly with the number of samplings.

Whereas in individual studies the laboratory results will (hopefully) be related to a single laboratory range, this is unlikely to hold for the whole database. The problem of different laboratory ranges is dealt with on page 170.

Certain categories of laboratory changes are mentioned in the guidelines (page 187) as possibly worthy of further investigation and these are the origins of some of the flags mentioned on page 175:

- Any clinically significant abnormality (Flag 6b).
- Smaller deviation of the above parameter (Flag 6a).
- Relationship between laboratory tests (abnormal parameters in the same organ group) (Flag 4).
- Specified abnormality on more than one occasion (Flag 3).
- Associated with adverse clinical events (Flag 5).
- Comparison with patient's baseline (Flags 7a and 7b).

Any apparent drug-related abnormalities should be analysed for the variables, as mentioned under clinical events, on page 236.

Type A laboratory abnormalities will usually be found by changes in the mean (or median). Both types A and B will be represented by shifts from normal, but the effect of type A will probably predominate due to the rarity of type B events. Type B events will be picked up by analysis of individual marked events (i.e. Flag 6b).

The 'minimal' analysis would be to look at means for predictable abnormalities and shifts from the normal range and clinically significant abnormalities across all groups. If there are many abnormal laboratory parameters at baseline it is better to substitute percentage changes from baseline in place of shifts from normal.

Any of the above flags can be used to help confirm any suspicions. Again any suspicious changes can be examined for an individual ADR pattern.

Issues Involved in Product Licensing Application Rejections in the UK

The clinical safety issues raised in the rejection of 64 applications were given by Dr Jefferys in 1995 (Jefferys, 1995):

- Specific ADR 34.
- Overall safety analysis 27.
- Potential or actual interactions 23.
- Target organ monitoring 19.
- Safety in the elderly 19.
- Safety when there is impaired renal function 15.
- Long-term safety 6.

Incidence Rates in the Pre-marketing Period

Type A ADRs are predictable because the factors underlying their occurrence are known. If all of the factors are present then the patient will have the ADR (i.e. the incidence rate will be 100%). Dose, or to be exact, drug tissue level is a primary factor for the majority of type A ADRs. The drug tissue level depends upon the absorption, distribution, metabolism and excretion of the drug as well as the dose, and each of these will have factors influencing them, ranging from diet and concurrent drugs to renal function.

The crude incidence rate is the number of people with the ADR, divided by the number of persons exposed to the drug. In pre-marketing clinical trials the numerator is assessed by the collection of adverse medical events and the number of each AE on the test drug is compared with the number on placebo to get the relative risk compared with placebo. Note, however, that it is the relative risk of that AE, not adverse reaction. This will be dealt with further later, but first it is necessary to look at the problems collecting the numerator, the AEs.

The Numerator

Collection
The incidence rate of AEs will depend upon the method used for their collection. Presuming that an AE occurs to a patient while on the drug or placebo there are numerous factors that will influence whether or not it is analysed at the end of the clinical trial, for example:

1. The patient experiencing an AE may not remember it, depending upon its severity; or may presume that it is nothing to do with the drug and therefore not report it, or may be too embarrassed to report it if it concerns a 'taboo' area; or if it is severe and the patient thinks that it is due to the drug the patient may stop the drug and not report back to the doctor, thereby becoming a 'dropout'.
2. The doctor may not allow a patient to report the AE if he is hurried or has a brusque manner. The doctor may not record the AE if he or she does not think that it is due to the drug despite the protocol's exhortations.

So far we have considered only spontaneous reporting and some of its failings. Other methods of collecting AEs are:

(a) Diary card. The patient records all the AEs that have occurred during each day. This will include many non-drug related AEs.
(b) Response to a standard question, sometimes referred to as an open question (e.g. 'Have you had any medical problems since your last visit?').
(c) Checklist, (sometimes referred to as a closed question). The doctor reads and/or interprets a short list of possible AEs and notes the reply.
(d) Self-answering questionnaire, sometimes referred to as a closed question. This tends to collect a rich harvest of AEs.

Each of these methods collects a different slice of the AEs that actually occurred to the patient and it is therefore not possible to mix them together to calculate an incidence rate. These methods are dealt with more fully in Chapter 4.

Let us presume that all of the AEs are collected by spontaneous reporting and a standard question and that the AE we are concerned with is 'headache'. A decision must be made about whether it is better to calculate the numerator as the number of patients complaining of headache during the trial or whether the number of head-aches per patient or both is needed (Cato *et al.*, 1983). Looking first at the 'Number of patients complaining of headache'. Unfortunately patients on placebo may 'catch' the same type of AE as the patient on active drug and this will distort the analysis by artificially reducing the incidence rate. Presuming that the headache has occurred as part of flu and has been reported then the doctor may record it as headache, or as headaches, fever and general aches, or as headaches, fever, general aches: diagnosis flu or just flu or 'viral infection'. So the same patient may have different words recorded depending upon the attending doctor as follows:

1. Headache.
2. Headache, fever and general muscular aches.
3. Flu or virus infection.

When it comes to analysis of the AEs the method of counting them is important. In the USA there is a tendency to count all symptoms, whether the symptom is an isolated symptom or part of a symptom complex or part of a diagnosis. Grouping of symptoms when they have different mechanisms or aetiologies is wrong in the first instance. A drug-related effect may be drowned by unrelated events with different mechanisms. The other end of the scale where the AEs are split into very small groups using the patient's actual words is too far in the other direction (e.g. *reductio ad absurdum*—counting separately right- and left-sided headaches). These processes are sometimes referred to as 'lumping and splitting'. The degree of grouping must make clinical sense, having the same mechanism or pathology (i.e events that probably represent the same phenomena). This is best done by scanning all of the events to see if there is a natural clinical grouping. The same symptom complex in many cases may represent a new ADR and should be counted separately from those cases with just a single symptom. So there may be headaches occurring in three categories:

1. Headaches alone.
2. Headaches with other symptoms.
3. Headaches as part of a diagnosis.

This makes it important that the trialist is told to group concurrent signs and symptoms together and give a diagnosis where possible. There is nothing to prevent grouping the first two categories together if separately they are equally represented in both the active drug group and the control group. The next hurdle is the classification of the AE using a dictionary; if different staff classify the same event under different terms then the incidence rates will of course be incorrect. The bigger the study, the bigger the problem.

In large-scale placebo-controlled studies there is a problem with the number of different types of AEs since they can easily be over 100 different types of events. When these are compared statistically between the active drug and its control group using $p < 0.05$ there are likely to be several statistically different results purely by chance. One of the solutions to this problem of multiple comparisons has been to adjust the p value required for each comparison so that the overall value remains at $p < 0.05$ (e.g. Bonferroni inequality) (Dunnett and Goldsmith, 1981). This sacrifices some sensitivity for specificity. Another approach is to use $p < 0.05$ for each comparison, realising that there will be 1 in 20 false positives, but using it to generate hypotheses rather than test them (Enas, 1991). Further examination of the clinical details may then provide data to prove or rebut the hypothesis.

So far there is the presumption that the unit of time for the event to occur has been short and constant (i.e. the same number finished the study as started). In this circumstance the crude incidence rate is satisfactory, but in longer studies there are likely to be dropouts and this will alter the denominator and perhaps the numerator. If it is presumed that satisfactory statistical significance has been shown between the incidence rate in the active drug group compared with the control group then the attributable incidence rate for the drug-related event should not be arrived at solely by subtracting the placebo rate from that of the active group, but should be given with confidence intervals. If specific ADRs have a negligible background incidence with objective data then it is possible to calculate an ADR incidence rate, but these are extremely rare.

The Denominator

Incidence rates with confidence intervals only apply to the group of patients tested and it may not be possible to extrapolate to the general population or to a subsection of that population. Pre-marketing clinical trials are 'notorious' for their exclusion criteria, often excluding the very old, the very young, those who are pregnant, those with concomitant disease and those with abnormal laboratory tests.

The last problem to face is, having established that the active drug has a certain incidence rate of AEs (with confidence intervals), that within the trial groups there may be subgroups with very large differences in incidence rates varying from 0%–100%. These must therefore be looked at as well as the factors that govern them. Many factors or variables need consideration, not all being relevant for all studies. These include:

1. Patient factors—age, sex, weight, race, country or centre, concomitant disease, indication, severity, alcohol and/or tobacco usage.
2. Drug factors—dose or blood level, formulation, route of administration, duration, comparator therapy and concomitant therapy.

The number of patients in each subgroup may be so small that the power of the study is insufficient to show any differences and therefore it will be necessary to pool the experience from as many of the pre-marketing trials as possible; but that may still leave many subgroups inadequately represented.

During the pre-marketing studies serious AEs will have been notified rapidly by telephone while the minor AEs will accumulate slowly as the studies progress and the CRFs are returned to the sponsor. At any one time the numerator for the serious AEs will be known accurately, but there will be only a hazy idea of the total denominator (Guess, 1991).

As already mentioned many subgroups will not have been exposed to the drug by the time of marketing and life table analysis will be required for exposures of different durations. The time to onset of a type A ADR depends upon the pharmacokinetics of the drug. If the various factors in the pharmacokinetic equation remain equal all the patients who are going to have a particular reaction should have had it by the time that the steady state has been reached for a particular tissue, the incidence rate after that time becoming extremely low. However, for type B ADRs depending upon hypersensitivity, the chance of hypersensitivity occurring before five days of treatment at the first exposure to a drug must be near zero and then increases after the first week. These ADRs with a varying hazard rate use the number of patients exposed for a sufficient length of time that if they were going to have the ADR it would have occurred as a denominator. On the other hand there are other ADRs with an almost constant hazard rate (e.g. thromboembolism with the oral contraceptive), and under this circumstance the denominator is patient-weeks/months. Dr O'Neill deals with this problem in his chapter 'Assessment of safety' in *Biopharmaceutical Statistics for Drug Development*, editor: K. Peace, Marcel Dekker, 1988. Another useful text on the subject is Summarization, analysis and monitoring of adverse experiences by S. Edwards, G. G. Koch and W. A. Sollecito, in Statistical Issues in Drug Research and Development, editor K. E. Peace, Marcel Dekker, 19–170, 1990.

Patient compliance, or lack of it, has been cited as a cause for efficacy figures that are too low in clinical trials, but it also affects the denominator in the ADR incidence equation.

Methods for the display of incidence rates are covered in an article in the *Drug Information Journal* (Huster, 1991). The correct statistical approach to ADRs is given in Chapter 9.

Although an incidence rate for common type A AEs can be given for the study drug and possibly for placebo or standard drug from the clinical trial data, rare type A or B

ADRs may be absent or only present in ones or twos in the whole trial programme. In this case the small denominators for placebo and/or comparative drug will not allow a valid comparison and a cohort study of historical controls will often be necessary to establish the background incidence in the population (Guess, 1991, 1996).

Data Sheets or Summary of Product Characteristics

A 'core data sheet' is defined as a document prepared by the pharmaceutical man-ufacturer that contains, among other things, all relevant safety information, such as ADRs, which the manufacturer requires to be listed for the drug in all countries where the drug is marketed. It is the reference document by which 'labelled' and 'unla-belled' are determined (CIOMS, 1995).

The 'summary of product characteristics' (SPC) is the term used by the European Union, approved by the CPMP, as part of the marketing authorization and its purpose is to set out the agreed position of the product. It is the definitive statement between the competent authority and the company and the common basis of communication between the competent authorities of all member states (document III/9163/90–EN from CPMP).

The core safety information (CSI) is a collective term covering ADRs (undesirable effects), warnings, precautions and contraindications and such pharmacodynamic and pharmacokinetic information that has important bearing on the safe use of medicines. It is the CIOMS term and it is hoped it will form part of the core data sheet. Individual countries may require additional safety information for their national data sheets.

The UK 'data sheet' is a document relating to medicinal products of a particular description. It is prepared by or on behalf of the holder of a product licence applicable to medicinal products and:

- Complies with such requirements as to dimensions and form, as to the particulars to be contained in it, and as to the matter (whether in respect of type, size, colour or disposition of lettering or otherwise) in which any such particulars are to be contained, as may be prescribed for the purposes of this subsection, (Medicines Act, 1968).
- Does not contain information relating to medicinal products of that description except the particulars so prescribed (Medicines Act, 1968).

The UK *Medicines Act Leaflet (MAL) 25 Notes on Data Sheets* (May 1984) refers to 'main side effects and adverse reactions likely to be associated with the product'. 'Labeling' is the term used in the USA and is defined in the April 1993 edition of the *US Code of Federal Regulations* under 21 CFR chapter 1, §201.56 and §201.57. The decision whether to include adverse events in labelling often rests with legal staff who are anxious to avoid product liability suits. Courts in the USA have said that an ADR must be placed in a data sheet "when a reasonable and prudent expert in the field would do so" while the FDA say if the ADRs is "reasonably associated with the use of the drug" even if unpredictable in occurrence. This is obviously a question of judgement (Young and Rave, 1993). Dr. Rashmi Shah from the MCA has been reported as saying that the companies tend to want too much information in the pharmacodynamic and clinical sections and too little on the safety sections while the authorities wish to see a lot of information on the safety and less on the clinical and pharmacodynamic sections (Shah, 1997).

We owe a considerable debt to the CIOMS working group who produced the *Guidelines for Preparing Core Clinical Safety Information on Drugs* (CIOMS, 1995). They suggest that "The decision to include safety information in the CSI must in all instances be determined by the usefulness of that information in enabling health professionals to balance risks of harm against benefits in making good therapeutic decisions", but to exclude "events, especially minor events, that have had no well-established relationship to therapy". Elsewhere it is stated "Safety information will cross the 'threshold' for inclusion if it is judged that it will influence physicians' decisions on therapy".

The CIOMS also advises on the contents of the initial core CSI and states that there may be some value in including a table of adverse events (usually 1% or greater) from pivotal studies where there are controls such as placebo or an active drug.

The next step is for the guidelines to be adopted. There will be many problems during the process of trying to harmonize data sheets across the world (Graham, 1993). The areas of the data sheet that may involve the pharmacovigilance (PV) staff are:

- Contraindications.
- Warnings.
- General precautions.
- Laboratory tests.
- Drug interactions.
- Carcinogenicity.
- Mutagenicity.
- Impairment of fertility.
- Pregnancy and nursing.
- Pediatric and geriatric use and use by other subpopulations.
- Ability to drive and use machinery.
- Adverse reactions.
- Overdose.
- Drug abuse (Gans *et al.*, 1996).

There are arguments for and against putting all known ADRs in the data sheet. Arguments for are as follows:

- Avoids potential legal liability. This applies more to the USA than elsewhere and many AEs are added when the evidence is very poor. Comments that the incidence of a particular AE is equal in the active and placebo groups are just a waste of time.
- Provides full disclosure. If the information might alter the physician's prescribing then it should be in the data sheet.
- Lack of certainty shared with the prescriber. This is not a very good excuse. If the company with all its resources cannot decide whether on the balance of probabilities the event is more likely due to the drug than other possible causes then it should not be included.

Arguments against are:

- Long 'laundry list' may blunt the understanding of drug-related AEs. This is obviously true if AEs that are not ADRs are included.
- Marketing disadvantage. This unfortunately still plays an important part in the thinking of some companies. It is quite dishonest to allow a marketing department to play any part in the composition of a data sheet.
- Unfair shifting of the burden to the prescriber for deciding drug relationship. As argued above this is a company responsibility and should not be avoided. These headings come from an article in the *Drug Information Journal* (Newman, 1995).

It is important not to use high-level terms inappropriately. Phrases such as 'visual disturbances', and 'arrhythmias', are sometimes used to hide more specific ADRs, which can be more serious than the high-level term would suggest. They may also prevent a prescriber from reporting an AE since they may believe that it has already been covered by the high-level term (see comments on the investigator's brochure).

It has been said that only 25% of UK doctors use the *ABPI Data Sheet Compendium* (see Bibliography—Reference Books) and that only 35% find it useful, whereas in the USA the average doctor consults the *Physician's Desk Reference* (see Bibiliography—Reference books) ten times a week (Medawar, 1993).

A survey of 120 pharmaceutical companies produced only 46 replies to the question about whether they could report side effects as a frequency. Only one company could provide the information. Most of the others said that the denominator was not known and that ADRs were underreported. (Bracchi, 1996; St George, 1996). Let us hope that following the CIOMS III report that frequencies will be given in the form suggested.

Conclusions

As far as adverse reactions are concerned, the clinical trial programme for a new drug, needs to be based on the known problems found with similar drugs and the results of investigations in animals. The results of the studies in volunteers need to be assessed carefully for potential adverse reactions and then interpreted with previous findings from the animal studies. Each clinical trial will contribute information concerning the adverse reaction profile of the drug and each protocol should be examined carefully in order to make the most of the drug exposure. The overall trial plan must be balanced such that questionnaires and checklists are used at the right stage with sufficient numbers of patients in order to have a reasonable chance to distinguish between the active drug and its control.

The early clinical trials will, whenever possible, try to distinguish the adverse reactions of the new drug from those of placebo-treated patients, while later clinical trials will concentrate on comparisons with its potential competitors. Certain of the clinical trials may be allotted the task of monitoring for specific adverse reactions. All clinical trial records need to be viewed by intelligent eyes before being put on computer if the opportunity to respond to a potential problem is not to be missed.

All patients in clinical trials should be asked a standard open question at each visit and given the opportunity to reply. Adverse symptoms should be followed up by clinical examination and/or investigations to search for objective confirmation. In those cases where the drug is withdrawn, the results of the dechallenge should be observed, preferably without addition of other treatment either in substitution for the original drug or for treatment of the adverse reactions. Any investigations found to be abnormal at the time of the event should be repeated. Uncontrolled studies before to marketing should be restricted and should be documented and monitored as closely as the normal double-blind randomised clinical trials.

Whoever is responsible for the analysis of safety data should be able to check the protocols and have an input into their design with future safety analysis in mind. This is often difficult where individual clinical trial monitors want to stamp their protocols with their own personality. There will be many reasons why the clinical trials cannot be completely standardized, but there should be a 'by default' standard trial protocol that can be altered when necessary. The aim should be not to have completely standardized protocols, but to have them consistent: that is using standard safety modules where possible, and where this is not possible making certain that the analysis will not be made more difficult. This is especially true of uncontrolled trials where a standard protocol can often be used for all uncontrolled studies. Similarly named patients can still follow a standard protocol designed solely for that purpose. Uncontrolled studies should not be an opportunity for investigators to follow their own whims.

Biologicals

There is a *Note for Guidance on Safety Studies for Biotechnological Products* (CPMP/ICH/303/95).

Vaccines and some other biological drugs have been available a long time, (see Chapter 1) but since 1982 there has been a rapid increase with the arrival of recombinant DNA products. There are some differences in the handling of the safety of biological drugs when compared with normal pharmaceutical drugs.

Vaccines

Since vaccines are generally given to healthy people, frequently babies and children, minimal risk is essential, for example the risk with the Sabin polio vaccine for paralysis is approximately 1 in 2 000 000 recipients, the absolute risk of idiopathic thrombocytopenia with the mumps, measles and rubella (MMR) vaccine is 1 in 24 000 doses, anaphylaxis with MMR, 1 in 100 000 (Salisbury and Begg, 1996), Guillain-Barré syndrome after swine flu vaccine < 1 in 100 000 doses (Singleton *et al.*, 1995).

The absence of concomitant illness at the time of vaccination means that the diagnosis of an ADR is not hampered by any underlying disease. However, there is a growing use of vaccines in patients with underlying disease and these special risk cases are asthmatics; people with congenital heart disease, Down's syndrome, HIV infection; splenectomized patients; haemodialysis patients and the elderly. Although a quiescent period in the disease is usually chosen, the risk of confounding factors will be more likely. The ADRs in the immediate post-vaccination period are usually self-limiting (syncope, fever, rash and injection site reactions) with the exception of anaphylaxis, which may occur up to 72 hours later. Serious suspected reactions are reported at a rate of approximately 1 in 100 000 doses of vaccine. Those thought to be causally related are Guillain-Barré syndrome, anaphylaxis and acute encephalopathy—diphtheria/tetanus/pertussis (DTP), MMR, diphtheria/tetanus (DT) and oral polio (OPV).

In collecting AE data, in addition to the type of data collected for ordinary drugs, the following need special attention:

- Site of injection—even 'sore arms' need precise description since there may be litigation several years later.
- Batch numbers—there may be clustering of problems related to particular batches.
- Previous vaccination history.
- GP's name and address—reports often originate from clinics other than those run by GPs.
- History of illness and intercurrent disease—immunocompromise by drugs or illness is very important.
- Family history—especially epilepsy.
- Storage and transit conditions.
- Cross referencing with other cases—with live vaccines, relatives of the vaccinee may be infected, groups of cases from a single clinic or clustering in time due to a school vaccination programme and linking batch results.

Clinical Trials

Phase I
Usually 10–50 people, but recruitment of adults who are still susceptible may be difficult.

Phase II–III
Usually require 100–200 per group. Increasing use of multiple vaccines makes it difficult to isolate the AE of an individual vaccine (Singleton *et al.*, 1995). When a placebo group is unethical a two-week pretreatment period has been used instead. In the post-marketing period a modified cohort method has been used (Farrington *et al.*, 1996). The very rare ADRs are best detected using a case-control design. Record linkage studies where the district health authority vaccination records are linked with hospital admissions has been successful (Farrington *et al.*, 1995). Despite the rapid increase in deoxyribonucleic acid (DNA) vaccine research the vaccines are not yet clinically available and two safety questions remain to be answered. The first is whether they create cancer-causing mutations and the second whether they generate lupus like anti-DNA autoimmune disease (McCarthy, 1996).

In the USA there has been a separate reporting system for vaccines since 1990, the *Vaccines Adverse Event Reporting System* (VAERS). Plotting the proportional morbidity as histograms enables the safety profiles of vaccines to be compared (Chen and Haber, 1995).

Suggested further reading is:

- Begg, N. and Miller, E. (1990). Role of epidemiology in vaccine policy. *Vaccine*, **8**, 180–189.
- Salisbury, D. M. and Begg, N. T. (1996). *Immunisation Against Infectious Disease*. HMSO Publications Centre.
- Chen, R. T. (1996). Special methodological issues in pharmacoepidemiology studies of vaccine safety. *Pharmacoepidemiology*, Chapter 37, 581–595. Ed. B. L. Strom, Wiley, Chichester.
- Freed, G. L., Katz, S. L. and Clark, S. J. (1996). Safety of Vaccines, *JAMA*: **276**, 1869–1972.

Cytokines and Recombinant DNA Products

Whereas vaccines are generally given to basically healthy patients, the underlying diseases treated by recombinant products are usually serious (e.g. cancer, chemotherapy ADRs, AIDS, chronic hepatitis, sepsis). Therefore the diagnoses of ADR are much more difficult, with a large number of AEs caused by the indication, intercurrent diseases and concomitant therapy. Some of the ADRs themselves may be different from those found with normal pharmaceuticals.

Examples of ADRs

- Multi-organ failure. This is usually the final stage of fulminant sepsis.
- The flu-like syndrome (fever, chills, myalgias, headache, arthralgia, and sweating) has an onset of usually 2–4 hours and lasting 4–8 hours.
- Capillary leak syndrome. This is seen with interleukin 2 and in severe sepsis (Zbinden, 1990; Gauci, 1991).
- Bone pain with onset within 15 minutes and lasting for 2–3 days (GM-CSF) and 12 hours (G-CSF). It is probably due to myelopoietic stimulation with GM-CSF and G-CSF (Decoster *et al.*, 1994).
- Interferon transaminase 'flare'. This usually occurs after 7–9 weeks and may reach 10–20 times the upper limit of normal of the reference range (Dusheiko *et al.*, 1985; Perrillo, 1989).
- Autoimmune diseases. Thyroiditis with interferon α, interleukin 2 and GM-CSF (Hoekman *et al.*, 1991).

The ADRs found in HIV-positive patients have been covered by Bénichou *et al.*, (1995).

Biotechnical companies differ from normal pharmaceutical companies in several ways that will affect the pharmacovigilance department. They are small, highly academic companies producing novel molecules so there are usually no comparator products. Their management is very much by consensus with frequent brainstorming sessions. They may also have inexperience regarding the varied clinical settings where the product will be used (Evens *et al.*, 1996). The basis of the company may be the academic scientists involved in the original research and they may have little allegiance to the pharmaceutical industry and its experience with pharmacovigilance. There needs to be a two way learning process whereby the scientists become familiar with imprecise clinical AE data, while pharmacovigilance staff, trained in the industry, need to educate themselves in the complex world of biotechnology and its unusual ambience.

Phase 1 clinical trials will usually be in patients rather than healthy volunteers. Phase 4 clinical studies will predominate in the early post marketing phase.

Suggested further reading is 'Meeting summary report: biotechnology and drug development' (Gauci, 1991).

Gene Therapy

This is at a very early stage and only 68 patients have been involved in single gene disorders and 78 patients in cancer related projects. So far no major ADRs have been discovered (Nevin, 1998). 'It is conceivable that these may be dose-dependent where the gene expression is excessive or dose-independent usually due to immunological response leading to allergic reaction'. The latter response may be to the expressed gene product or protein but could also be to the vector (Caulfield and Cafferkey, 1998).

Chapter 8

Pharmacoepidemiology in the Pharmaceutical Industry

H. Tilson

Senior Medical Adviser for Health Affairs, GlaxoWellcome, Clinical Professor, Epidemiology and Health Policy, School of Public Health, University of North Carolina, USA

Pharmacoepidemiology is the scientific contribution of the public health methods of observation to our understanding of medicines and related medical interventions: biologicals, devices, interventive diagnostics and, by extension, non-pharmacologic interventions against which the impact of medicines might be compared. Complementing the activities of the surveillance offices and those of the clinical trialists, the epidemiologist brings an important set of skills, approaches and products to the pharmaceutical table; filling in, often proactively, the gaps left by the partner disciplines.

Epidemiology, a public health science, is not defined by a singular concept or set of words. In schools of Public Health and Hygiene, the field may be taught by teams involving statisticians, computer scientists, academic/research epidemiology specialists, and clinicians. The curriculum may often embrace good analytic and study design methodology, including the skills and approaches of the clinical trialist. Epidemiological curricula certainly embrace the approaches of the epidemiological intelligence field, generally reflected in the pharmaceutical industry by the pharmacovigilance specialty. More recently, epidemiologists have been central in advancing the specialties of 'evidence-based medicine', leading to the development and application of medical practice guidelines; often considered the domain of the 'disease management' movement within pharmaceutical groups. Further, a fundamental component of the approach to understanding the value of medicines, pharmacoeconomics, includes an understanding of the burden of illness, the natural history of disease with or without treatments, and the use of modelling and simulation methods; also part of the basic curriculum of academic epidemiologists. Indeed, a whole 'new' field has been created in the wake of the cost-containment revolution, the so-called 'outcomes research' world. Outcomes research analyses the 'outcomes' of interventions, including pharmaceutical treatments. These analyses are most usually at the population level and use observational techniques; under these circumstances, the field becomes coterminous with pharmacoepidemiology. Needless to say, epidemiology also involves extensive use of automation, information technology (IT) and education of other health professionals in the area. The development of complicated statistical techniques to define, model, project and understand population phenomena and trends is part of the basic curriculum.

Thus, in the pharmaceutical industry it is not unusual to see people with formal epidemiological training contributing to or even leading the efforts of any of the fields mentioned above and the subject of separate chapters in this book. However, in addition, over the past two decades, a substantial body of experience that uniquely relies on the training and approach of the epidemiologist has developed to complement these activities. It is this special application that has become commonly understood as 'Pharmacoepidemiology' and this forms the fabric of this chapter.

In its most generally accepted form, pharmacoepidemiology applies the non-experimental, observational methods of the epidemiologist to the population-level impact of pharmaceuticals. Most generally, the focus of the discipline has been upon the safety in post-approval use of drugs, the so-called post-marketing surveillance (PMS). The term PMS has fallen somewhat into disuse, if not disrepute, since it includes the non-formal epidemiological intelligence work of PV, the more structured formal observational research approaches of the pharmacoepidemiologist, and some less structured and perhaps less scientifically rigorous surveys variously used to stimulate early commercial uptake.

Pharmacoepidemiology. The Why?

The quick answer to the question: 'Why pharmacoepidemiology?' is that the other ways of learning about drug safety are too limited to provide society with the levels of assurance and certainty that it demands. Here, the 'driver' is that no chemically active drug is without its side effects or adverse drug reactions (ADRs). Some of these are serious; some are frequent (frequent enough to have been detected during the early development of a new drug and often the cause of an early termination of a drug development programme). The extent to which we accept such ADRs is a function of the extent to which the drug contributes to our wellbeing, its benefit. Often expressed as a benefit-to-risk ratio, the science of defining the balance of ADRs to positive effects is roughly understood as the product of the pre-approval process of drug development, initially through animal models and testing in normal volunteers, then progressively through programmes of clinical trials involving larger groups of selected patients. At the time of general release for marketing, through the extensive process of regulatory approvals described elsewhere in this book, it is likely that the drug will have been tested in relatively small numbers of patients, perhaps only several hundred or several thousand. Even these people, the 'subjects' of a pre-approval experimental programmes, are unique; chosen to demonstrate, as is the purpose of pre-approval drug study, whether a drug is efficacious.

Because of the ethics of experimentation, the high costs and great complexity of such an endeavour, programmes of pre-approval drug development are by necessity kept as small and focused as possible. In the process, the most frequent of the ADRs will probably be discovered and well characterized and will be portrayed to potential prescribers as part of the approved product prescribing information (in the US called 'Labeling'). However, rarer, particularly unpredictable, side effects cannot have been uncovered in such a process. It is to the post-marketing environment and our on-going activities of surveillance and continuing research that these tasks must be left.

Likewise, our efforts at understanding such events through the use of surveillance/pharmacovigilance techniques, described thoroughly in Chapter 12, are not completely effective. ADRs occurring in the post-marketing environment are flagged for regulators and sponsors variably and variously in differing contexts, generally through a spontaneous appearance in the practice of a careful and observant practitioner who takes the trouble to report, voluntarily in most nations, to manufacturers or regulators or both, or in the *Lancet!* Taken together, such vigilance activities constitute the Spontaneous Adverse Drug Reaction Reporting Systems (SADRRS) of most of the mature national markets.

The contributions of such spontaneous reports are many, providing, as they do, a powerful signalling generator through the detective work and observational powers of the entire prescribing force. However, the limits of this system are also well understood, particularly by the strongest advocates of the system. ADRs may be difficult to differentiate from undesirable events occurring as part of disease progression, or coincidentally occurring problems. The more the ADRs resembles a problem that occurs independently in the population (e.g. coronary event or fevers), and the further such events are removed from the prescribing activity (e.g. late occurring immunological or malignant events) or removed from the prescriber (e.g. birth defects in association with a non-pregnancy treatment), the more elusive such ADRs are from the vigilance of even the most vigilant and diligent of treaters.

The SADRRS is also affected by the system problems of any system that relies on the voluntary offices of busy clinicians whose primary focus is, quite properly, the health of their individual patients. Thus under- and possibly overreporting and under- and possibly misattribution are serious problems faced by even the most extensive and effective programmes of pharmacovigilance. Such systems are excellent for 'signal generation'; generating possible evidence of problems from the entire 'denominator' of the national treated population. However, because of their unreliability and the unknown extent of ascertainment and attribution, they cannot be used to define the exposed denominator or the 'true' numerator and thus must 'never' be used to calculate the true rate at which an ADR is occurring in the population in question.

The case has therefore been made, repeatedly, for a more structured, systematic, comprehensive and proactive way to follow the evolving drug experience in large populations: to permit true identification and quantification of the 'denominator'; the entire and precise number, dose and duration of population-based exposure from which the ADR experience is drawn; and the 'numerator', the entire inventory of ADRs occurring in association with drug exposure in a population. Likewise, a fundamental concept in all drug development and experience monitoring is the appropriate comparator. Here again, undesirable experiences are a part of life. They are known to occur apropos of no drug exposure, hence the insistence in modern drug development on randomization, masking and proper controlling of trials, lest one be 'fooled' by a biased estimate or a placebo effect. Similarly, in spontaneous reporting, misattribution can be a recurring problem. *Post-hoc ergo propter hoc* reasoning is the bane of existence for those who try to make individual attributions on individual cases in a pharmacovigilance system, often leading surveillance officers to the unhappy conclusion that the only firm rule of attribution is 'if it happened before the drug was given, the drug probably didn't cause it!'.

A key part of the rationale for structured pharmacoepidemiological approaches is the basic nature of medical treatment itself. Each patient represents a unique set of experiences, with non-standard dosages, durations, combinations with other treatments and individual characteristics, often involving multiple diseases and treatments and always involving the vagaries of variable adherence to recommended regimens: so-called non-compliance. The 'hothouse' effect of the experimental situation, the randomized controlled trial (RCT), while excellent for showing whether a drug 'could' work cannot show its effectiveness and actual safety in the real world. This is a job well suited to the observational world of pharmacoepidemiology. These are the reasons for efforts to assemble whole populations of treated and untreated persons and look for excesses in the rates of AEs among those taking the drugs under study over those occurring among appropriate comparison populations.

There are some additional answers to the 'Why Pharmacoepidemiology' question. One involves the costs of experimental medicine, which have become prohibitively high for all but the most focused of programmes. Thus, monitoring of large populations to ascertain the frequency and nature of relatively rare events must be undertaken with an approach that spreads the ascertainment net broadly but not too deeply. Additionally, the non-experimental rigorous research approach allows one to learn from actual experience without intervening or altering the circumstances of therapy, without the risks inherent in the experimental situation, allowing comparison with actual appropriate marketplace choices, again without the artefact of the experimentally driven protocol or its costs.

Finally, the ethics of experimentation on vulnerable populations are important to consider, avoiding unnecessary exposure to experimental risk in the very young, very old, the very vulnerable and the fetus. Yet such populations are going to be treated in the marketplace and an extensive network of population-based pharmacoepidemiological studies can capture and learn from these treatment experiences and pass on such learnings to subsequently treated similar populations.

Of course, an equally appropriate question might be 'Why not pharmacoepidemiology?' The limitations of the field, and the need to target its use where it might contribute uniquely will be explored later, after some of the details of the science have been covered.

Pharmacoepidemiology—the 'How'?

The epidemiologist approaches this and all such challenges of discovering and quantifying the association between exposure and outcome as a population problem. The tools of the epidemiologist involve observing outcomes/outputs/events (the 'numerator') and placing them into perspective by clarifying the population, which

includes all those at risk of that outcome (the 'denominator'). A fundamental requirement of the epidemiological risk fraction is that it must not be possible to become
counted as an event in the numerator unless the person is assured to be included in
the reference population denominator.

A population with a shared experience is termed, in epidemiology, a 'cohort'.
Generally, such populations are characterized according to the type of experience,
and invariably time-and-place defined (e.g. the cohort taking drug X in 1950 in
Birmingham or in Health Plan A). In a cohort study, the experience of such a
population is compared with one or more comparative (or control) cohorts, for
example the cohort taking drug Y, and the cohort with the same underlying diseases,
but taking no drugs in 1950 in Birmingham, or, for that matter, the 'entire' population
from which the treated population is drawn, (i.e. the 'population-expected rates').
This is particularly the case when the object of the epidemiological study is the search
for rare but important events, which are expected to occur rarely, if at all, in the city
of Birmingham, where even non-concurrent controls are appropriate.

Every attempt is made to examine the populations under study to characterize
any unique features that may make their subsequent experience likely to be different,
the so-called selection biases, or any subtle attributes that might co-vary with the
intervention under study and cause misattribution to the intervention rather than the
other attribute, a so-called 'confounder'. For example, if a drug is thought to be
particularly safe for persons with heart diseases because of a cardiac effect-free
pharmacologic profile, it is likely that the drug will be prescribed more frequently
than other drugs for people with underlying heart disease. Thus a higher risk of
subsequent cardiac events might be expected in such a population, the *so*-called
'confounding by indication'. Every effort is made in the cohort study to guard against
such influences, which may cause differences other than the intervention being
studied (i.e. by limiting a follow-up cohort to those patients who appear similar or
by subsequent creations of segments with similar risks, the so-called stratified analyses).

Against these denominators of otherwise essentially similar populations, differing
only because they received differing interventions for similar conditions, the rates of
the various outcomes under study are computed and compared. If undesirable outcomes are occurring in one exposed cohort at rates in excess of those in the others,
and if there is no other apparent explanation for such excesses, such studies can raise
concerns about the possibility that the drug may be 'causing' the excess.

A specific technique useful in pharmacoepidemiology when searching for especially rare but unacceptable toxicities or drug-idiosyncratic events (e.g. Lyell's syndrome) is the so-called 'follow-up study', in which the comparator is the historical
rate in the population under study. Another cohort technique is the 'exposure-
specific registry'. In contrast to the techniques of pharmacovigilance, in which the
outcomes (ie AEs) are 'registered' (a retrospective approach to be considered later in
this chapter), the prospective epidemiological registry attempts to select and follow-
up patients who have experienced an exposure, but not yet any 'outcome'. Classic
epidemiological registration techniques have been used to follow the populations of
Hiroshima and Chernobyl following nuclear radiation exposure.

A particularly useful experience for pharmacoepidemiology has been the 'pregnancy registry' approach. This involves registering all patients possible following an

unintentional (or, of course, intentional) first trimester exposure to a drug to detect any unique pattern or excess in frequency of birth defect in the exposed cohort subsequently followed through birth.

For efficiency, epidemiologists often use a conceptual strategy, which examines the same population experience retrospectively, the so-called 'case–control method'. In this approach, the same population-based experience can be explored by starting with a collection of a sample of those who experience the undesired event—'cases' of the problem under study. Using an exactly similar approach to the same population under study, one then finds people who are identical in every way to the 'cases' except that they do not have the problem under study— for example, the same sex, the same age, the person next door (neighbourhood controls) or in the next bed (hospital controls): Assuming there is no unusual characteristic of such people (e.g. "we don't put very sick persons next to those with terminal states in our hospital"), such 'cases' and 'controls' can then be characterized by their previous drug exposure experience. If drug X is 'causing' a problem, it is more likely than comparators (e.g. drug Y or a medical procedure) to be mentioned in association with cases than with controls, and the extent to which such mentions are more frequent becomes an epidemiological expression of risk; in this case the risk ratio also reflects the relative likelihood, of the adverse event in persons with drug X over drug Y. Such population-based observations, which permit expressions of drug risk, are, of course, extremely valuable in understanding the actual experience in the post-marketing environment. With precise denominators and complete ascertainment of the numerator, an actual population-based statement of frequency, nature, duration and outcome can be derived.

Epidemiology and the Safety of Pharmaceuticals—the When?

Epidemiological considerations are critical throughout public health, wherever and whenever precision is required in the quantification of population-based phenomena—the 'epidemics'. With medications, these public health considerations are no less appropriate. A new drug is marketed on the basis of very limited data, with an apparently 'acceptable risk' of serious adverse experiences compared to other drugs in the class and an apparently 'acceptable uncertainty' that the very rare but potentially very serious adverse experiences, inevitably associated with any active medication, are likely to occur with such rarity that they will not materially compromise the apparent benefit to risk ratio. It remains for the pharmacoepidemiologist, in tandem with the pharmacovigilance team, to help society be sure that it is correct in its assumptions.

A programme of PMS of any new pharmacological entity will, perforce, include a strong approach to pharmacovigilance; the more finely tuned and focused the more such rare problems would be of major consequence (i.e. the less 'acceptable' the residual uncertainty is). Coupled with such pharmacovigilance, the responsible pharmaceutical company is increasingly considering a proactive programme of more structured pharmacoepidemiology studies.

Of course, an epidemiological study can be undertaken at any time. However, it is most often thought of when a potential 'signal' of a safety problem emerges from spontaneous reports and further quantification of the signal is needed. How frequently does it really occur? How much in excess is it occurring over the 'population-expected rate' among untreated patients? In other words, how much is the excess risk, and does it exceed the 'acceptable risk' for drugs in this class? The problem with this approach is that once a potential signal is detected among spontaneous reports, it is already 'too late' to be launching a new study of side effects. Regulatory action may be under consideration; media pressures may emerge; the crisis may be building. While epidemiological studies are much less costly per patient studied and may be launched much more rapidly than clinical trials of comparable size and scope, nevertheless they also take time and money to launch. Thus, if it is likely that the answers from a programme of structured pharmacoepidemiological studies may be needed, such a programme should be launched 'before' a signal prompts one to ask the pressing question!

There are many reasons for adding one or more structured cohort or follow-up studies to the proactive PV activity, but they rest on the premise that if a 'signal' emerges from the spontaneous voluntary adverse reaction reporting system, it is too late to begin to contemplate doing a structured epidemiological study. The best way to handle a crisis that involves a safety signal is to have anticipated it and launched a proactive programme of complementary epidemiological studies in advance of the emergence of a problem.

The circumstances of early drug experience may dictate such a programme. There may have been suggestions, either from animal studies or from early clinical studies, of possible troublesome adverse effects, that in actual experience in more general use following marketing, such serious ADRs would be more probable than with other agents. Being attuned to this risk and building a system to monitor relatively large populations using epidemiological methods then makes good sense. The less 'serious' the underlying problem being treated, the less society tolerates serious ADRs, even very rarely, the more useful it may be to have a database of population-based actual use experience in hand.

In general, structured programmes of pharmacoepidemiological studies are desireable when a drug is going to be used rather more commonly and/or chronically, in healthier and/or younger patients.

Conditions Conducive of Proactive Post-marketing Surveillance Programmes

These are:

- Drug to be used in healthy patients.
- Drug for chronic conditions.
- Drug with many others in the same class.
- Others in the same class known to have serious/frequent ADRs.
- Residual 'concerns' from actual clinical or preclinical experience.
- 'Special' populations likely to be treated without RCT experience (e.g. children, the very old, women of childbearing age).

Resources for Pharmacoepidemiology

Expertise

Critical to the field is a shortage of well-trained, experienced pharmacoepidemiologists to ensure that the complexities of study design, conduct, analysis, and reporting are properly addressed; a process that is central to any scholarly discipline. Training programmes in pharmacoepidemiology or in general epidemiology, with special emphases on those issues specific to and unique with pharmaceuticals, are remarkably few, and structured curricula are only now being developed in those few centres of excellence in the field.

The pharmacoepidemiologist must be trained in the skills and disciplines of all epidemiologists, the methodologies and approaches of non-experimental research and the appropriate statistical tools for analysis, computer skills, interview and survey methodology, and an understanding of research method. In addition, to conduct pharmacoepidemiological research, the investigator requires a grounding in the disciplines requisite for the pharmaceutical sector. Epidemiology may be involved in understanding the population dynamics of treated and untreated populations for drug development decision making, in supporting a broader understanding of unmet need (and potential market) and in assessing the population impacts needed to pinpoint effectiveness (to support programmes of pharmacoeconomics). In this case a thorough grounding in clinical pharmacology and the public health research disciplines of outcomes research, health services research, policy analysis and economics is needed.

Centres offering the researcher assistance or leadership in programmes in pharmacoepidemiological research tend to be co-located, with such teaching efforts at major university centres in the USA, Europe, and Japan. The major university centres in which pharmacoepidemiological research is being conducted today have grown in number and quality over the past 20 years from a handful (Boston, Oxford and Bern) to over a dozen, including prominently Harvard, Johns Hopkins, Vanderbilt, University of Washington, University of North Carolina in the USA, McGill and McMaster in Canada and Basle, Southampton and Potsdam in Europe.

Systems for Pharmacoepidemiological Research

The basic tool of pharmacoepidemiology, as it is for all drug research, is the ad hoc study, protocol driven and designed to fit the specific circumstance. Such a traditional, hands-on approach is time-tested and may be the only satisfactory way to answer a question at the population level. However, such a hands-on approach is also labour and resource intensive and may take too much time to organize and complete to permit it to be useful in much pharmacoepidemiological decision-making.

Several more structured systematic approaches have been developed as an aide to the sector to more economically and broadly approach population-level pharmaceutical epidemiological research. The oldest and best known of these resources, the Boston Collaborative Drug Surveillance Program (BCDSP), placed nurse monitors in strategic medical centres in the USA and Europe and monitored all hospitalizations on appropriate medical services by interviewing all patients regarding their anteced-ent medication use and then abstracting medical charts to monitor prescriptions within hospital. This permitted calculation of rates of major medical events in association with exposures to major outpatient and inpatient drugs and recognition of excess morbidity among certain exposed groups.

The successor of the BCDSP, the Slone Epidemiology Unit continues in this tradition to this day, particularly collecting all cases of certain drug-important cancers and birth defects from selected hospitals and permitting systematic study of relatively commonly used drugs in a system termed 'case–control surveillance'.

Another useful systematic approach—'prescription event monitoring' (PEM) was launched in the prior decade by Professor William Inman. In this systematic approach, all prescriptions for all newly marketed drugs are retrieved from the British Prescription Pricing Authority, entered into an automated database, which generates letter queries of the prescribing physicians (Inman's now well-known 'green card'), now carried forward by Dr Ron Mann (see Appendix 4).

In the UK, the 'Oxford Record Linkage Scheme' was created to link together medical and health records from multiple sources for the entire reference population, that of the Health District around Oxford University. The intention was to be able to associate data from one resource (e.g. prescribing files) with others (e.g. the paper medical records from the University Medical Centre). This permitted a multipurpose comprehensive data set, which could be queried to look for associations between various exposures, including drug exposures, and their related serious medical events, including hospitalizations. This linkage permitted calculation of the rates (*viz* risks) of serious problems with exposures, such as drugs under surveillance, and compare them with those experienced with various comparators.

All of these systematic approaches share the advantages of size, comprehensive-ness, and multipurposefulness of their resultant databases. However, they are also 'hands-on' approaches, themselves requiring extensive (and often expensive) data collection, patient interviews with attendant recall biases and/or physician question-naires with resulting non-response and other biases.

Harnessing the New Technology for Pharmacoepidemiology—the Automated Record Linkage Schemes

One of the great challenges for pharmacoepidemiology has been to develop com-prehensive systems that permit rapid affordable searches of large linked population experiences whenever the need should arise in response to a 'signal' or proactively under circumstances suggesting that such anticipatory PMS would be useful.

By the end of the 1980s in North America, quite unrelated to the evolving expecta-tions of the pharmaceutical sector for modernized and more extensive epidemiolo-gical approaches, several large automated databases had been created for medical management purposes. Agents responsible for these data sets included the large third party insurers, particularly the government insurers, such as the Medicaid programmes of several large states and the health plans for the province of Saskatchewan, automating their large numbers of billing/payment transactions for administrative efficiency. Several of the major medical care organizations, notably health maintenance organizations, were also automating many of their medical care management systems, particularly the membership files, pharmacy files and hospital accounts, to permit more accurate actuarial calculations and programme evaluations.

In this context, several of these databases were recognized by sector leaders early in the evolution of their administrative use as potentially powerful tools for record linkage. The key to such linkages is the 'link', generally a single patient identification number, which is used to identify the individual in each database. When the same number is used for each encounter, then longitudinal patient-specific experience can be created (i.e. a full year's worth of prescription data for a given patient). When the same number is used in 'each' database, then linkages across the databases can be accomplished. Using the power of the computer, such patient identifiers can be used for cross-database linkage. Such identifying numbers can be readily encrypted so that research can be done at the population level, erecting profiles of individually characterized patients, while insulating the patient from individual identification and protecting the vital pledge of confidentiality.

The prescription databases, with date, dose, duration, and drug can be linked with a single patient identity so that drug use studies become relatively straightforward, and quite rapid. Cohorts of prescription recipients can be constructed through routine computer searching. Similar, comprehensive medical experience can be erected over time for each patient, recording every hospitalization with, usually, an ICD9-coded set of discharge diagnoses and procedures. Membership files containing vital statistics, demographics, family size and other characterizing data are generally also available in such systems. Linking them together, cohorts can be characterized demographically and all subsequent medical events determined. Then, if there are excesses of serious events occurring in the drug-exposed population the requirements of the epidemiological approach can be satisfied, and population experience documented.

Among the major advantages of these approaches perhaps the greatest is that the cohort accumulates for administrative reasons independent of any epidemiological study and is therefore available for study if and when the need should arise. Often there is a confusion of terminology emerging from this situation. Since the data are available and comprise a historical information set, such studies are occasionally termed 'retrospective'. However, one of the great advantages of these data sets is that they can be analysed historically using 'prospective' (i.e. cohort) methods. Of course, such data can also be viewed using case–control ('retrospective') methodology.

The published literature is now replete with examples of useful information that has been gleaned from such automated record linkage studies over the past two decades. Perhaps the most powerful of these resources is the General Practice Research Database (GPRD) of the UK, formerly known as valve-added medical products (VAMP) (see Appendix 4). Having been in effect for over seven years, this data set contains automated medical record information on a population in excess of seven million British subjects, with over four million 'currently active' files among over 400 active general practitioner practices. In the hands of Hershel Jick (perhaps the first true pioneer of the effective use of such record linkage approaches using automated data sets) and his collaborators at the BCDSP, it has provided useful population-based information to clarify the safety debates regarding virtually every major suspect drug safety problem faced by the sector in the past decade. These have ranged from exact rates of significant gastrointestinal bleeding with the various non-steroidal anti-inflammatory drugs (NSAIDS) to a comprehensive understanding of the rates of gynaecological cancers among users of various formulations of hormone replacement therapy and oral contraception.

Similar productivity has been gained from the databases of the major medical care programmes in the USA, particularly from Group Health Cooperative of Puget Sound (Jick/Stergachis); Kaiser Permanente (Johnson/MacFarland); Medicaid (Ray/Strom); Harvard Community Health Plan/Harvard Pilgrim (Platt); and several others (particularly in the hands of Walker), to name but a few of the most active and productive of the pharmacoepidemiologists working with these valuable resources. The complexity of dealing with the automated databases, however, cannot be underestimated. Such work requires highly trained, scrupulously careful methodologists, teams including skilled analysts and computer programmers and, of course, close medical professional links with the practitioners providing actual patient care. It is to these practitioners that one must turn for validation of possible findings from the computer and more extensive primary data from the patient and patient medical record to elucidate possible computer linkage findings.

Pharmacoepidemiology—the 'Why Not'

What . . . with all this promise and contribution you mean there are also limitations? Absolutely! Pharmacoepidemiologists find themselves instantly fending off unrealistic demands for answers for which the epidemiological method is less than ideally suited. The scientific approach, which developed the randomized, blinded, controlled clinical trial methodology that now forms the backbone of the drug development process did so because of the limitations of other less rigorous approaches, such as the observational approaches so useful to epidemiology. Randomization is necessary to be absolutely sure that the groups being compared are truly essentially the same with the exception of the differences in exposure under study (and even then of course, such absolute certainty is not guaranteed!). Blinding is a vital tool to protect against the biases of the observers with pre-existing excesses in optimism (or the contrary) or simply greater efforts at detection of problems when they know a new compound is being used. Simultaneous controls ensure that the findings are due to the intervention, and not some hidden concurrent environmental or epidemic force. Thus, when looking for 'proof of efficacy', the RCT is by far the preferable vehicle and pundits have argued that the objective of the research epidemiologist is to render the observational study as much like an RCT as possible!

On the other side of the equation, however, it is 'not' always necessary to develop absolute or precise population estimates. When there is no epidemic of Guillain-Barré syndrome in the community and yet within the first year of marketing, four or five people receiving a new antidepressant (Zimeldine) are reported to the manufacturer/regulator as experiencing an ascending paralysis syndrome, then precise population rates are probably unnecessary for the appropriate regulatory actions to be undertaken. The same could be said for an 'epidemic' of phocomelia, the result of thalidomide.

It is in the vast middle ground where epidemiology finds its unique contribution in the pharmaceutical world, where the RCT is not appropriate or not affordable; where the vigilance system is inadequately precise or quantitative; where time is of the essence. Even then, let the buyer beware! Epidemiology is a very tricky business and it is easy to be fooled by finding associations between apparent exposures and outcomes caused by subtle differences in the exposed population that cannot be detected from the data available. It is possible not to find associations that are actually there because of assumptions about diagnoses or exposures, which cannot be clearly defined because of limitations of the data or questions one forgot to ask. It is not possible to develop certainties beyond the numbers available within the relatively limited resources currently available. To be relatively certain of detecting a doubling of a rare but unacceptable side effect (e.g. from 1 in 10 000 to 2 in 10 000 person/ years) many tens of thousands of persons taking the medicine must be studied. This is not an easy challenge, even within the current constraints of automated population data, and virtually impossible to afford for all but the most widely used medicines (e.g. vaccine field trials).

Organizing for Epidemiology Within the Pharmaceutical Company

Three parallel movements have occurred over the past 20 years. As findings from epidemiological studies have proven to be more and more useful, they have been more in demand. As understanding of their usefulness has grown, more and more of the agents responsible for assuring society of necessary health protections have turned to them. As perhaps the *primus inter pares* for such responsibility, pharmaceutical companies have added staff specializing in the use of non-experimental methods to oversee professional contract relationships with major academic centres for the conduct of such PMS studies and to undertake some such epidemiological efforts in house.

Depending upon a drug company's strategic approach, the staffing of pharmacoepidemiological units has varied from the hiring of one or two people trained in epidemiology, to work in the statistics group or with the pharmacovigilance team, to the creation of fully staffed, free-standing departments of medical epidemiology, to undertake the full spectrum of epidemiologic activity needed to support drug development, drug safety, economics analysis and disease management. At the core of any drug company's strategy, however organized, is the consideration, product by product, of what the package of epidemiological research should comprise.

Epidemiology in the Drug Development Decision

When deciding whether and how aggressively to advance a compound into and through full product development, most companies consider the potential size of the marketplace as one of the 'drivers' for the decision. Marketing estimates are notoriously inaccurate for reasons outside the scope of this chapter. Suffice it to say, pharmaceutical firms are increasingly calling on their epidemiological colleagues, within companies, in universities, and in most modern marketing research firms, to develop estimates of population burdens of illness; the classic estimates of morbidity and mortality for which epidemiology is perhaps at its best!

Epidemiology During Drug Development

As a product progresses through phases I and II, and into phase III, epidemiology contributes in several ways. In some disease areas, the clinical endpoints under study may be 'fresh' (i.e. with no established baseline). An epidemiological study of the actual clinical experience with the condition can tell the investigator exactly how many days, on average, elapse between first and second hospitalization for the same condition and even develop estimates stratified by demographics or severity/duration of first episode. This further refines the process of protocol development and power calculations for clinical trials.

Programmes of pharmacoeconomics research now rely heavily on their epidemiological colleagues to provide the 'effectiveness' indicators from actual practice to support the models necessary to extend from the findings of RCTs. When an RCT programme comes across a serious and unexpected side effect or set of adverse events, it may be important and useful to have the epidemiologist help with estimates of the 'true' population-expected rates for these problems. This is particularly helpful in studies in which the 'control arm' is much smaller than the active drug arm because of the severity of the underlying condition, with resultant morbidity lag among the controls.

The outcomes research movement has occasioned a major shift in the relationship between pharmaceutical companies and their health care delivery system 'customers'. Perhaps most prominently in the USA, with its major transition toward integrated health care systems and Health Maintenance Organizations, (HMOs), but certainly now with great emphasis throughout Europe as well, the managers of these integrated health care systems are looking towards epidemiology to provide the management support data to document that the interventions applied in the specific settings are having the desired impact on population morbidity and mortality indicators, the 'outcomes', as expected. The favourite example providing the impetus for such a broadcast use of epidemiology is the otherwise inexplicable difference in caesarean section rates across the regions of America with no apparent difference in the associated rates of perinatal morbidity and mortality.

The extent to which pharmaceutical companies depend upon their epidemiological staff for support in these areas often dictates 'where' the epidemiological group is to be found within the organization and the numbers and credentials of the epidemiologists involved.

Organizing for Epidemiology Within the Pharmaceutical Sector

Irrespective of how such groups are organized within individual drug companies, the realities of the next century will certainly be that they 'will' be organized and functioning. Thus, the opportunity will also emerge for cooperative cross-company efforts, where the interests of the common good, the public health side of pharmacoepidemiology, outweigh the commercial competitive issues. Within the pharmaceutical industry in the USA, for example, in addition to the usual pharmacovigilance and pharmacoeconomics committees (and, of course, working closely with them) at the industry association, the Pharmaceutical Research and Manufacturers of America (PhRMA), a working group has been organized to focus upon the issues of pharmacoepidemiology. Among issues of common interest on their table at the turn of the twenty-first century are:

- Capacity-building—there is a need for additional centres of excellence within the university and research communities, with whom pharmaceutical companies can collaborate.
- Fellowships, traineeships and building the expertise—within such centres, in addition to the need for quality researchers, is the need to generate the next wave of trained scholars in the area. Any company trying to build its programme of pharmacoepidemiology has encountered a 'very' limited marketplace of well-trained scientists available to do this critical work. Pharmaceutical companies are therefore developing approaches to staff development, which include provision of financing for postgraduate training in pharmacoepidemiology.
- Database development—as the above argument has shown (one would hope), the large, automated, population-based multipurpose database is a very powerful tool for pharmacoepidemiological research. When problem signals emerge, it is important to be able to turn to such populations and get the rapid, affordable answers that can enlighten public policy decision making by companies, clinicians, and regulators alike. But these resources are far from fully matured, even those that are currently widely in use; and often their financing, particularly the components of greatest use for the pharmacoepidemiological community, may be less than stable. For example, the ongoing funding of the highly valuable GPRD in the UK has been an ongoing source of concern among many in the pharmacoepidemiology community, relying as it does on a system of licenses among researchers who must themselves then lay out large sums of cash and hope for the best in the way of revenue from potential researchers. This is scarcely the way to assure continuous flow of critical public information! For every population currently available for pharmacoepidemiological monitoring, there are several more needed. For example, such data resources in each of the countries of Europe would be the best assurance to the citizens of those countries that problems emerging from use of drugs in their communities could be detected, quantified and well-understood (or that 'false alarms' or clinical practice-dependent findings from other countries could be properly investigated at 'home'). Finally, as society begins to learn how to make decisions around 'firmer' population-based epidemiological estimates of actual experience, the need for greater precision and earlier results will become clear and these will be demanded. This will, in turn, require larger and more populations for whom such automated data are available.
- Human rights and data privacy—critical to the integrity of any research process is an organized effort to ensure that the rights of the patients and populations from

whom the data are recovered are protected at all times, particularly against misrepresentations, manipulations and invasions of privacy. These are problematic less for observational research, involving as it does less intervention and by definition generally no experimentation. However, there are ethical issues which have long received and continue to warrant concerted attention by the profession:

— The methods best to assure that the privacy of individuals will not be compromised by searches at the population level for trends and associations.
— The rules for maintaining data on individuals when the information is collected at sites other than the clinic (e.g. in population-based surveys and registries).
— The circumstances and best forms under which protocols and programmes should receive ethical review (where the traditional institutional review board may be unnecessary or even inappropriate) (e.g. at the population level, where there is no 'institution' per se).

Other National Level Organizations include the following:

— Under the umbrella of a far-sighted initiative started by Ciba-Geigy in Europe, the Risk Assessment, Detection And Response (RADAR) initiative, similar national-level organizations have been formed in many of the nations of Europe; and the Clinical Safety Surveillance Committee (CSSC) of the PhRMA functioned as the RADAR council for the USA. While these councils have largely been superseded by international efforts, their legacy is visible throughout the sector.
— The International Society for Pharmacoepidemiology (ISPE). Internationally, this helps to steer and encourage the development of good science and the infrastructure to move the field forward. It is a multisector, multidisciplinary membership organization. Following several very successful international conferences on pharmacoepidemiology in the early 1980s, the organizers of those conferences under the persistent leadership of Professor Stanley Edlavitch, helped to create a more formal context in which the conferences could be coordinated and the sector could communicate and help to move the science forward, and the ISPE was officially formed in 1987. The annual meetings of the ISPE permit the scholarly presentation of research and policy papers. The volume and quality of these have increased yearly and the meetings are now among the most stimulating and challenging of professional meetings in any field. In addition, the epidemiology community converges on many of the policy issues just described, and organizes around working parties to help move the sector-building agendas forward. The legacy of the national RADAR councils includes the caucuses of ISPE, including the industry caucus, which meets annually to survey evolving industry concerns and plan for concerted contribution to move the sector forward.

The Way Forward

What lies ahead for pharmacoepidemiology in the twenty-first century? The trend lines seems unambiguous. Progressively, as the field generates more and more scholarly work, which is understood by more research partners and policy makers as useful to them for their work, the demand will inexorably and dramatically grow. The sector does not wish to broadcast preventable risks of undesired and undesirable side effects as part of its innovations in medicine; it wishes, along with society's demands, to prevent unnecessary exposures and excessive risks as much as possible. As epidemiology shows itself to be the powerful tool for detecting, defining, and quantifying such risks, society will demand such protections and the sector will respond by providing them. As the large databases develop and emerge as the powerful and useful tools they have already proven to be, society and the sector will increasingly turn to them and help them to mature in directions to support the needs to know actual experiences and outcomes even faster, with even greater precision (and power) and with even stronger supporting data to permit even more sophisticated: and reliable analyses.

The result will be even greater demands on our academic institutions to perform the requisite research, train the required next generation of scholars and build the evidence base and new and more sophisticated techniques.

Challenging? Yes, indeed. Exciting? Yes, indeed. Vital to the future of the pharmaceutical enterprise? Absolutely!

The reader will have noted that this chapter addresses a rapidly developing field in which the capacity—building efforts of those concerned about more rigorous and structured approaches to study the population effects of medicines are beginning to bear fruit.

As such, the chapter refers to the rapidly evolving experiences of several of the leading scientists/scholars in the field and the academic/organizational bases from which they serve the sector. The chapter similarly refers to the perhaps even more rapidly evolving capacity to conduct epidemiological monitoring of drug experiences—the population based databases and monitoring systems, which permit assembly of large cohorts and the performance of cohort and case–control analyses on aggregated population data

Therefore, perhaps more useful than the traditional 'scholarly' array of publications, the author proposes (and the editors have accepted) the following approach. Each of the systems and the chief scholar responsible for/experienced with using it has been listed in Table 1. The reader is urged to contact these people for the most current listing of the scholarly works produced by these groups.

In doing this, we run several risks:

- First, there will be the omissions; apologies to friends and colleagues who wish I had listed them. Please do not take it personally! (And remember that is what next printings are for!)
- Second, much of the work and output and bibliographies from these units are conducted and generated by members of the staff, who are not listed here. Many of these have become close personal as well as professional friends, and I apologise to you, as well for the shorthand!
- Third, as emphasized in the body of the chapter, an evolving approach in this sector is for multidisciplinary research, which involves industry collaboration. In any cases . . . increasingly (a very good trend!). . . . the industry partners are included in bibliographies; increasingly data sets are being made available to industry collaborators for independent scholarly work. Thus friends and colleagues at

Table 1

Active scientist/ scientific group	Major resource
Jerry Avorn, MD Harvard Medical School USA	US Medicaid (state level)
Ulf Bergman MD, PhD Karolinska Institute Sweden	Swedish drug and disease database
Winanne Downey, BSP Saskatchewan Health	Saskatchewan pharmacy and medical data
Nancy A. Dreyer, MPH, PhD Epidemiology Resources Inc.	United healthCare/multiple databases
Gary Friedman, MD Northern Carolina Kaiser Permanente	Kaiser Permanente Database
Hershel Jick, MD Boston Collaborative Drug Surveillance Program USA	BCDSP Hospital Database, Group Health Cooperative of Puget Sound, General Practice Research Database (see Appendix 4)
Judith K. Jones, MD, PhD The Degge Group Ltd	Various Medicaid and hospital discharge databases
Thomas M. MacDonald, MD	MEMO/ Ninewells database (see Appendix 4)
Bentson MacFarland, MD, PhD Kaiser Permanente Northwest	Kaiser Permanente Northwest Group Health Cooperative
Ronald D. Mann, MD Drug Safety Research Unit	Prescription Event Monitoring (see Appendix 4)
Salvatore Mannino, MD, MSc National Research Council CNR	NRC/Northern Italy database
Richard D. Moore, MD Johns Hopkins University	Maryland HIV database
Wayne Ray, PhD Vanderbilt University	Tennessee Medicaid
Kenneth Rothman Epidemiology Resources, Inc.	United Health Care/multiple databases
Sidney Shapiro, MD Slone Epidemiology unit	Case–control Surveillance Cancer and Births Defects Database
Andy Stergachis, PhD University of Washington	Group Health Co-operative and others
Brian Strom, MD, PHM University of Pennsylvania	Computerized On-Line Medicaid Pharmaceutic Analysis and Surveillance System (COMPASS)/various State Medicaid
Samy Suissa, PhD McGill University	Saskatchewan/and other Canadian databases
Alexander Walker, MD, Dr PH Harvard School of Public Health	Fallon Clinic, several New England databases

Some of the basic papers describing these databases are asterisked in the reference section.

Merck, Ciba-Geigy/Novartis, Roche, SmithKline Beecham, Berlex, BMS, HMR, Lilly and many others, and, of course Glaxo Wellcome, will recognize their absence from this inventory. I hope I may be forgiven equally for this. These scholarly works indeed contribute greatly to the evolution of the field. The names and addresses of the active pharmacoepidemiology units within the pharmaceutical industry may be obtained from the relevant national industry association. The International Society for Pharmacoepidemiology maintains a current mailing list of epidemiological resources in industry, current research organizations and the academic units listed in this inventory. The reader should contact The International Society of Pharmacoepidemiology, c/o TEAM Management, 2000 L Steet NW Suite 200, Washington DC 20036, USA; tel: 202–416–1647; fax: 202–833–3843.

A relatively complete annotated bibliography is included in the third edition of the textbook '*Pharmacoepidemiology: An Introduction*' by A. Hartzema, M. Porta and H. Tilson, Harvey Whitney Publishers, Cincinatti, Ohio, USA, forthcoming around July 1998.

A project to develop a comprehensive inventory of databases and researchers worldwide has been conducted under the auspices of RADAR, the International Medical Benefit-risk Foundation, by Dr Judith Jones, President, The Degge Group, Suite 1430, 1616 North Fort Myer Drive, Arlington, Virginia 22209–0067, USA. It is currently undergoing update.

Chapter 9

Statistics for Safety Data

Christy Chuang-Stein

Director, Clinical Biostatistics I, 9162–227–400, Pharmacia and Upjohn Company, Kalamazoo, MI 49001, USA

Introduction

The importance of the safety profile of a pharmaceutical product is evidenced by its prominent position in the product's package insert/summary of product characteristics (SPC). Understanding the product's major adverse reactions is also essential to conducting benefit–risk assessment; however, despite the consensus on the role of adverse events (AE) data in product licensing, many questions concerning the collection and reporting of AEs remain (Finney, 1996). (In this chapter, adverse events include adverse reactions to the treatment under investigation.) These questions range from the basic issue such as 'how to define an AE or a treatment-emergent AE', to more complicated questions concerning 'how to define expected *versus* unexpected', 'whether to report syndromes or/and symptoms', 'whether to use checklist solicitation or open-ended style to obtain AE information'. Many researchers have tried to address these questions (Bénichou and Danan, 1989; Alexander, 1991; Newman, 1995; Nickas, 1995; Northington, 1996; Scherer and Wiltse, 1996). Recently, the International Conference on Harmonization (ICH) of Technical Requirements for Registration of Pharmaceuticals for Human Use made a serious attempt to standardize definitions and procedures for clinical safety data management (ICH, 1994). Similar efforts to manage post-marketing safety data have been undertaken by the Council for International Organizations of Medical Sciences (CIOMS) (CIOMS Working Group, 1990; CIOMS Working Group II, 1992). The latter efforts led to recommendations on standards similar to those recommended by the ICH.

The adequacy of the safety data to support a product licence or marketing approval needs to be examined in the context of total patient exposure to the product, the duration of the exposure, findings from laboratory testings and the available dose–response information regarding the occurrence of AEs. Even if a product ultimately receives a licence or approval based on benefit–risk consideration, serious safety problems identified during the development process need to be mitigated by cautionary statements in the labelling such as limitations of use, special monitoring, product contraindication and at times boxed warning—Food and Drug Administration (FDA).

This chapter, will focus on the analysis and presentation of safety data. Safety data include clinical signs and symptoms, safety laboratory assays, vital signs and physiological tests such as electrocardiography (ECG) and chest radiography. Since all 'abnormal' or 'unusual' findings and observations are typically recorded as AEs, the term AE will be used to denote any negative event that a patient or subject experiences while taking or shortly after stopping a pharmaceutical product. The summarization of such data in both the context of clinical trials and the post-marketing spontaneous report systems, with emphasis on the former because of the more rigorous data collection process, will be discussed. It is assumed that AEs have been collected in a uniform and consistent fashion. In other words, assuming that within a reporting environment (clinical trials or post-marketing report systems) decisions about the fundamental questions mentioned above have been adequately dealt with so that the collection and reporting of these data are not subject to differential reporting practices. In addition, it is also assumed that an appropriate coding thesaurus have been used to assign preferred terms to investigators' verbatims. The latter characterization is important for appropriately quantifying the occurrence of AEs.

Measures to summarize adverse events in general are discussed, in the next part of this chapter and then ways to present laboratory data are examined. This is followed by a discussion of the special issues and challenges concerning safety assessment and data presentation, and this chapter concludes with some further discussion and comments.

Measures to Summarize Adverse Events

There are various opinions on the role of inferential procedures (i.e. procedures that allow one to pass from sample data to generalizations or hypothesis testing) in the analysis of safety data (Peace, 1987). Although some people support the use of inferential statistical methodology (Enas, 1991), others prefer the descriptive techniques (Huster, 1991). Many statisticians take the middle ground, applying the inferential methodology, but interpreting the results (i.e. p values) descriptively (Abt, 1987, 1990). This position is understandable since the applications of inferential procedures to safety data are plagued with multiplicity and data-driven issues. Besides, the sensitivity of the inferential procedures to detect clinically important differences for rare events is often limited (O'Neill, 1988). Furthermore, the emphasis on safety data analysis is directed more towards the few cases of serious adverse reactions than the average population response. This difference between safety and efficacy evaluations often renders the inferential procedures, which focus on the central tendency, less useful in analysing safety data.

In this chapter, the middle ground is taken, focusing on exploration and estimation techniques. Even though reference is made to inferential statistical methodologies from time to time, p values produced by the identified inferential procedures are only meant to give some ideas on the significance of the comparisons. The focus of discussion is estimation instead of hypothesis testing. Two good references for the discussion in this section are O'Neill (1988) and Tremmel (1996).

Crude Rate

The simplest measure to summarize the occurrence of an AE associated with a pharmaceutical product is the crude rate obtained as the number of patients with the event divided by the number of patients 'at risk'. The patients 'at risk' are those who took the product under discussion and are at risk for developing the AE. For example, if 23 patients (among 520) experienced pancreatic toxicity upon receiving an antiretroviral product, then the crude rate is 4% (23/520). Because of its simplicity, the crude rate is by far the most common measure for the occurrence of an AE and is used almost exclusively in product labellings. Similarly, one can estimate the crude rate for a set of pre-specified AEs, or the crude rate for any event.

Normal approximation can be used to construct a 95% confidence interval for the true (but unknown) crude rate when there are at least five subjects with the event of interest. In the example above, a 95% confidence interval is (2.6%, 6.2%). A rule that is commonly used to construct one-sided confidence limits is the rule of 3. The rule of 3 suggests that if one observes no events of a given type in $3n$ patients exposed, then the one-sided 95% upper confidence limit for the crude rate is $1/n$.

The biggest drawback of the crude rate is that it does not take product exposure time into consideration. As a result, the rate obtained from a short-term trial (< *six* months) for AEs that tend to occur after a relatively long period of exposure (e.g. six months), can be very misleading.

Events Per Unit Time of Exposure

To avoid confusion, we assume that the event under discussion is an absorbing event, (i.e. a permanent or irreversible condition, such as death). The measure 'event per unit time of exposure' is the ratio of the number of subjects with the event divided by the total period of patient exposure until the time of the event or censoring (censoring occurs when the endpoint of interest is not observed either because a subject is lost to follow-up or because the follow-up is interrupted for data analysis). In other words, this measure focuses on 'time at risk' instead of 'people at risk'. An example for the 'unit of exposure' is 'patient year'. If the total number of patients at risk in the calculation of the crude rate is replaced by the total time of exposure given in the time unit of interest, for example person days or person years (PY), the incidence rate per unit time of exposure is obtained. For example, if 510 PY were followed among 2322 patients, of whom 12 died, then the incidence rate for death per 1000 PY is (12/510) × 1000 = 23.5. On the other hand, the crude death rate is (12/2322) × 1000 = 5.2 deaths per 1000 patients. As demonstrated by this example, exposure duration (person time) is frequently the greatest confounder in estimating the occurrence of an AE.

For events reported through post-marketing spontaneous reporting systems, the summarization of spontaneous AEs is often hampered by the sparsity of data as well as the lack of a clearly-defined denominator to calculate the incidence rate. A common practice is to use the total number of prescriptions as a surrogate for the total exposure time. Under this practice, a measure for the incidence of an absorbing event is the number of events per 1000 prescriptions.

The calculation of events per unit of exposure assumes a constant risk for the AE over time for all patients. If this assumption is not valid for the product under examination, this measure does not have much meaning. Furthermore, this measure can only be interpreted from the epidemiological perspective. It has no meaning for individual patients.

Using Hazard Function to Describe Risk Over Time

When the risk of an AE is not constant, a measure that is often used to describe the varying risk is the hazard function. Hazard functions can help address questions concerning how 'quickly' and how 'frequently' the AEs develop. Assume, for the time being, that the concern is an absorbing event and that the time duration can be roughly divided into intervals such that the risk within an interval is approximately constant. Under these assumptions, the hazard rate at time t can be expressed as:

$$h(t) = \frac{\text{Number of events within the interval containing } t}{\text{Total patient-time units within the interval containing } t} \quad (1)$$

This is often referred to as the life table estimate of the hazard (Abt *et al.*, 1989). In addition to providing estimated risk for the AE at different time points, the estimated rate h(t) can also be used to determine the need and/or frequency of monitoring. For example, Salsburg posed the following question from the perspective of a treating physician — "If I have treated the patient for x months and the adverse event has not appeared, can I relax my vigilance? How long must I be vigilant?" Salsburg argued that for managing a patient, it would be helpful for the physician to know the general shape of the hazard function along with a rough estimate of time to specific endpoint such as the occurrence of a serious event (Salsburg, 1993).

Other Measures

Occasionally, one needs to estimate the number of distinct episodes of a recurrent event per unit time to address such questions as "How many times can I expect to experience the event within a certain time frame?" Assuming the event is of a relatively short duration, a measure to address this issue can be calculated as:

$$\frac{\text{Total number of recurrent events}}{\text{Total number of patients exposed}} \quad (2)$$

where the total patient exposure in the denominator is appropriately scaled to reflect the exposure unit of interest. This measure assumes a constant risk for the event over time within a subject as well as across subjects. When this assumption does not hold, a better estimate for the expected frequency of the event can be obtained from the hazard function as pointed out by Tremmel (1996).

Tremmel also discussed measures of risk for events with a longer duration. A measure called the prevalence rate and familiar to epidemiologists can be applied here. The prevalence rate is defined as the 'proportion of a population that is affected by disease at a given point in time' (Rothman, 1986). An estimate for the prevalence rate can be calculated as the ratio of the total patient-time affected by the event divided by the total patient-time with patient-time appropriately scaled to reflect the time unit of interest. The estimated proportion of time affected by the event is similar to the expected number of events per unit of patient exposure except that the former calculation includes the time period where the event is present. A better measure, argued by Tremmel, is to use a Markov model and estimate the prevalence based on the transition probabilities to start and to exit the event under discussion (Tremmel, 1996).

Presentation of Laboratory Data

Laboratory testing is frequently used to ensure that patients are not experiencing any untoward systemic toxicities on receiving a new treatment. Even though laboratory toxicity can be treated as an AE and summarized qualitatively as described in the previous section, the numeric nature of laboratory data provides opportunities to summarize these data in a more quantitative fashion.

In the USA, laboratory data summarization has been greatly influenced by the FDA *Guideline for the Format and Content of the Clinical and Statistical Sections of New Drug Applications* (1988). A routine laboratory data summary includes tables giving the percentage of patients with each type of laboratory abnormality. Laboratory abnormality is typically determined with the use of a set of reference ranges in conjunction with some predetermined rules regarding the grade (extent) of abnormality. Tables that provide the frequencies of subjects experiencing a change from normal to abnormal status or from abnormal to normal for each selected laboratory parameter are also helpful. A slight variation is to give the frequencies of subjects who experienced a change (or no change) from their pre-treatment laboratory toxicity grade (not just normal or abnormal) to the maximum toxicity or the toxicity grade at the end of the trial. Another routine practice is to provide summary statistics on the amount of change such as the mean (median) change or percentage change. Recently, graphic displays of laboratory data have received increasing attention because of their ability to present a large amount of data in a very informative way (Thompson *et al.*, 1988; Levine and Szarfman, 1996).

Beyond the routine summarization of laboratory data, the analysis of laboratory data faces some unique challenges (Chuang-Stein, 1992). Some of them are discussed here. First, while the importance of interpreting laboratory data using a set of reference ranges is realized, these ranges are often affected by many factors that make their usefulness in the clinical trial setting questionable (Oliver and Chuang-Stein, 1993). In addition, summarizing the amount of change when specimens are assayed in different laboratories presents some serious challenges. Even though Chuang-Stein proposed two procedures to normalize laboratory data from different laboratories, there has not been an agreed methodology to combine data from different laboratories in a quantitative manner (Chuang-Stein, 1992).

Second, the usual laboratory data summarization does not take into account the multivariate nature of laboratory parameters. While everyone would agree that an increase in both amylase and lipase carries more diagnostic value than an increase in only one, our current analysis of laboratory data does not routinely combine information from different assays. Instead, it remains largely a 'one-parameter-at-a-time' procedure. Some limited efforts to combine laboratory data in a multivariate fashion have been given by Brown *et al.*, 1979; Sogliero-Gilbert *et al.*, 1986 and Gilbert *et al.*, 1991.

Third, protocols for clinical trials often contain inclusion and exclusion criteria. In terms of laboratory parameters, this means that patients are often required to have 'normal' or 'clinically normal' laboratory values at screening to be eligible for a study. This selection creates the regression to the mean phenomenon and results in a general tendency for certain biochemistry parameters such as aspartate aminotransferase (AST), also known as serum glutamic oxaloacetic transaminase (SGOT), and alanine aminotransferase (ALT), also known as serum glutamic pyruvic transaminase (SGPT) to increase even though the intervention has no effect on these parameters. The extent of the regression effect can be substantial as demonstrated by McDonald *et al.*, 1983, 1989 and Senn, 1988. The impact and implication of regression to the mean on the design and analysis of medical investigations was discussed in some detail by Chuang-Stein (1993), and Chuang-Stein and Tong (1997). The regression effect is something that one should watch for in the clinical trial setting.

There have been some recent efforts to model the response distribution as a mixture distribution with some individuals affected by a new investigational treatment while others are not affected at all. For example, one can hypothesize that the response distribution to a new investigational treatment G(x) can be written as:

$$G(x) = pF(x) + (1 - p) F((x - \Delta)/\sigma) \qquad (3)$$

where F(x) is the response distribution for the control group and Δ and σ represent a location and a scale parameter, respectively. One aspect of the analysis is to estimate the mixture proportion p. Some procedures to test the hypothesis of $p = 1$ (i.e. $G = F$) were given by Cherng *et al.*, 1996, who applied the tests proposed by Conover and Salsburg, 1988 and O'Brien, 1988. A similar discussion of mixture survival models was given by Greenhouse and Silliman, 1996.

Another noteworthy effort in the summarization of laboratory data is the use of tolerance limits to construct an interval that contains a desirable portion of the population (e.g. 90%) with a certain confidence level (e.g. 95%). In addition to advocating the use of tolerance limits in place of reference ranges, Nickens, 1998, applied the tolerance limit concept to change in the laboratory value to characterize the range of change. Furthermore, tolerance limits can be used to determine the sample size of a study so that, for example, the limits given by the second smallest and the fifth largest observations contain a specified portion of the population values with a pre-specified confidence level (Sachs, 1984). The latter is important for trials designed from the safety perspective.

When summarizing laboratory data, one needs to be aware of the many potential sources of variability associated with the process that generated the data. Such sources include:

- Variations due to the patients.
- Short-term and long-term biological variations.
- Variations due to specimen handling (e.g. site of venepuncture, interferences and altered states, possible contamination, specimen evaporation and transportation) and analytical variations (operational bias and staff factor).

One should learn as much as possible about a laboratory before using it to process the specimens. Including spontaneously reported laboratory results when calculating group summary statistics should be avoided. Most important, using multiple laboratories in a trial for safety assessment should be avoided as much as possible (Trost, 1996).

Special Issues Concerning Safety Assessment

The biggest challenge in summarizing safety data is the need to consolidate the massive amount of safety data into a manageable format. Chuang-Stein *et al.*, 1992, proposed to do this by grouping the safety data into K classes characterized by body systems and determined in conjunction with the underlying disease as well as the treatments involved. Within each class, they proposed to assign to each patient an overall intensity grade based on all relevant information. The intensity grade reflects the extent and degree of safety concerns for the corresponding body function when all things are considered. The analysis of such organized data should focus on comparing the overall safety profiles between different treatments using multivariate procedures. This process of consolidating the safety information follows the process a treating physician typically uses when sorting through test results and clinical observations to decide upon the safety experience of a patient to a treatment. It would be helpful to automate this process so that the algorithm-generated conclusions could closely mimic those reached by the treating physicians, but in a more consistent manner. This systems-oriented evaluation can greatly facilitate the preparation of product labellings because it focuses on organ toxicity in a comprehensive manner.

One of the steps necessary in crafting the package insert is to pool AEs from different studies. According to the 1988 US FDA clinical and statistical guideline, pooling data from different studies allows examination of differences among population subsets not possible with the relatively small numbers of patients in individual studies (*Guideline for the Format and Content of the Clinical and Statistical Sections of New Drug Applications*, 1988). In this regard, pooling data is simply a summation of data from individual studies. Subgroups that are typically of interest are paediatric patients, geriatric patients, patients with impaired organ functions, patients receiving common concomitant medications, or patients with specific comorbidity.

It is generally agreed that if studies are similar in terms of study design, extent of exposure, and target population, pooling is not a problem. Pooling in this case is especially helpful for rare events. However, if studies are not comparable, pooling across studies by summing data directly can be misleading. In the latter case, meta-analysis is a preferred way for combining information from different studies (Koch *et al.*, 1993). Meta-analysis such as the Cochran-Mantel-Haenszel procedure (Mantel and Haenszel, 1959), logistic regression and survival analysis, typically uses factors to adjust for potential study differences. A different type of meta-analysis was proposed by Laird and DerSimonian (1986) who used a Bayesian approach to combine results from different studies.

When it is known that a pharmaceutical product causes serious AEs, it is essential to find out who has a greater risk for these untoward events. Factors often considered in this context are age, gender, race, prognostic factors at baseline such as target and comorbid illness, genetic and environmental factors, and concomitant medications etc. While simple subgroup analysis can help identify the important risk factors in a univariate manner, modelling approaches such as logistic regression and survival analysis can be more productive in evaluating the joint effect of multiple factors. Benefits of the modelling approaches can be substantial when the serious events under consideration are rare.

Any decision on the approval of a pharmaceutical product comes down to the assessment of benefit to risk of the product. Failure to adequately address the benefit–risk issue can delay the review of a new drug application (NDA), and therefore the product's subsequent approval (Miller, 1992). Yet, despite the need to conduct benefit–risk assessment, efficacy and safety data are routinely summarized separately without much effort to bring these two concepts together into a single endpoint. Although some efforts have been made towards this end, more work is necessary (Payne and Loken, 1975; Chang and Fineberg, 1983; Hilden, 1987; Chuang-Stein *et al.*, 1991; Chuang-Stein, 1994; Herson, 1996).

For certain pharmaceutical products that produce high intersubject variability in terms of plasma drug concentration, it is important to determine whether the observed serious or important AEs occurred at high plasma drug concentrations. If this is the case, it might be desirable to recommend therapeutic drug monitoring. Hale proposed an exploratory procedure to study the relationship between a binary outcome (presence or absence of an AE) and pharmacokinetic parameters such as area under the plasma drug concentration against time curve (AUC) and the maximum plasma drug concentration (C_{max}) using the receiver operating characteristic (ROC) analysis (Hale, 1996).

Comments

Clinical safety assessment is necessary for all pharmaceutical products both before and after marketing approval. Although one would hope that standardization and automation have been or are being implemented so that the majority of the safety assessment can be conducted in an efficient way, leaving most of the energy and effort to handle product-specific issues, this goal has unfortunately not yet been achieved. Standardization and automation can only be achieved through worldwide agreement among regulatory agencies and sponsors on a standardized approach to defining, evaluating, recording, and summarizing AEs. With all the efforts towards harmonization, there is hope that even with the increased surveillance following the Fialuridine issue by the FDA in the USA, standardization and automation are possible in the near future (Nickas, 1997).

Chuang-Stein (1992) questioned whether too much or not enough is being done when it comes to safety assessment. Whatever the answer is, statistics for safety data are only meaningful when the data are of good quality. Compared to efficacy endpoints, adverse clinical signs and symptoms are much less rigorously defined and are therefore subject to the interpretation and judgement of individual investigators.

Therefore, orienting the investigators who will be participating in a trial to record clinical observations in a uniform fashion is probably one of the greatest challenges for the trial sponsor.

Challenges abound in any post-marketing surveillance (PMS) programme where AEs reported for marketed pharmaceutical products are 'informally' acquired and 'spontaneously' submitted to regulatory authorities. Rawlins (1995) gave a recent survey of the problems faced by the pharmacoepidemiologists. Finney recently reviewed the 'Yellow Card' system established by the British Committee on Safety of Drugs in 1963 and concluded that the time has arrived for renewed efforts to test alternative methods of data acquisition and hoped that the latter would improve our ability to acquire better measures for drug safety (Finney, 1996). While PMS programmes have provided vital information that has led to the removal of products from the marketplace, spontaneous reports in most cases remain a challenge to the PV specialists who need, among many challenges, to assess the causal relationship between the reports and a product.

Dropouts often complicate the analysis of efficacy endpoints in clinical trials. This is also the case with safety assessment. While lack-of-efficacy dropouts can be viewed as a treatment failure from the efficacy perspective, the lack of AEs for some of these patients might simply be a result of not being exposed to the treatment long enough. The impact of this should be considered carefully since the crude rate is based on all patients who received the treatment regardless of the duration or amount. If there is an excessive premature dropout, the crude rate for an AE can be greatly underestimated.

As pointed out earlier, safety assessment should focus on estimation instead of hypothesis testing with confidence intervals being the preferred approach. Even if p values are used descriptively, one needs to be aware of the great number of p values that can be produced for the safety parameters. Thus, the false positive rate can be extremely high. In this regard, the approach proposed by Chuang-Stein *et al.*, (1992) with an emphasis on body systems has the advantage of looking at a higher level of functionality instead of individual events or test items.

The primary purpose for summarizing the AEs data across studies is to prepare the package insert so that physicians can be educated on how to use a product. Unfortunately, current package inserts seem to have fallen short of this expectation. It appears that many physicians are relying on pharmaceutical companies' sales representatives for vital information concerning a product's usage while the corresponding package insert is viewed as a legal document by these physicians. Whether this is a desirable trend is beyond the scope of the current chapter. However, unless the presentation of the data in the patient package insert (PPI) or patient information leaflet (PIL) is such that physicians find the information easy to use and useful, this trend will continue. Therefore, it is vital that statisticians work closely with their physician colleagues to find ways to better summarize and present AE data. Furthermore, with patients becoming more involved in determining their own treatment regimens in the current health care environment, PILs and PPIs have become the primary source of information for patients. Thus, it remains crucial that the passage of adverse experience from bedside to package insert is treated in a scientific manner with due diligence.

Chapter 10

Management of Adverse Drug Reaction and Adverse Event Data through Collection, Storage and Retrieval

V. Pinkston[1] and E. J. Swain[2]

[1] *North American Product Surveillance, Glaxo Wellcome Inc., 5 Moore Drive, Research Triangle Park, NC 27709, USA*
[2] *Worldwide Clinical Safety Quality Management Group, SmithKline Beecham Pharmaceuticals, New Frontiers Science Park, Third Avenue, Harlow, Essex, CM19 5AW, UK.*

Introduction

This chapter is based on that previously written Mrs E. J. Swain and Dr L. J. West and we are grateful to Dr West for allowing us to update some of her material. All sections have been updated and considerably revised in the light of fast progress in this area. Topics covered include methods of data collection, electronic storage and retrieval of information on adverse drug reactions (ADRs). As part of data collection, the sources of material and limitations of these data have been evaluated. Information to help the decision to build or purchase an adverse event (AE) database are also provided. System design and case handling procedures must reflect the requirements of the business, balancing easy input with effective retrieval.

In monitoring the safety of products, pharmaceutical companies need to comply with worldwide regulations as well as the primary requirement of helping doctors to prescribe safely. It is not intended to provide a comprehensive review in this chapter, but to provide an insight into the methods of managing ADR data. When seriously considering setting up a new or enhanced computer system, we recommend talking to colleagues with experience in different types of systems or organizations mentioned later in this chapter. The opinions expressed are personal ones and not necessarily those of Glaxo Wellcome or SmithKline Beecham.

Data Collection

Sources of Data

There can be an enormous variation in the nature and quality of data depending upon the source, and this must be considered when the data is processed, computerized and analysed. Safety data may come from any of the sources described below.

Clinical Trials

In phase I studies, good documentation and additional investigations should be standard practice. Serious reactions are very unusual in these studies, which will detect only very common ADRs, in particular those that are pharmacologically mediated (e.g. bradycardia with beta adrenergic receptor antagonists).

Good documentation and follow-up should be possible in phase II studies, but rare reactions will not be identified due to the small numbers of patients involved. The larger numbers in phase III trials can pose problems, but these can be minimized by careful choice of investigators, good case report form design and procedures for follow-up. Phase IV studies are designed to test the efficacy and safety of the drug in clinical practice and often share the same constraints in patient numbers as pre-marketing trials.

Post-marketing Surveillance Studies

Any surveillance of safety of a drug after marketing is post-marketing surveillance (PMS) (now often referred to as a post-authorization safety study). In practice, the distinction between phase IV studies and PMS is blurred (e.g. German drug experience studies).

In the past, company PMS studies only made a limited contribution to the assessment of drug safety, mainly due to weak study designs and difficulties in recruitment (Waller *et al.*, 1992). As a result the SAMM (Safety Assessment of Marketed Medicines) guidelines were issued in the UK (see Appendix 6). As computerization increases so does the linkage of data from different systems enabling use as PMS data. There are now numerous databases available for research ranging from general practitioner (GP)-linked (e.g. MEDIPLUS) to large multipurpose (e.g. MEDICAID) databases. Issues for consideration include data quality and ensuring that the system in question has the data content required for a particular study (see Chapter 8).

Spontaneous Reports

Spontaneous reports are the most effective means of identifying rare, serious adverse reactions (usually idiosyncratic or type B) after marketing despite the under-reporting that exists. Spontaneous reports are an unsolicited communication to a company, regulatory authority or other organization that describes an AE in a patient given one or more medical products. These reports do not originate from a study or from any organized data collection scheme. Unless indicated otherwise by the reporter, all spontaneous AEs are assumed to be possible ADRs. The quality and completeness of spontaneous reports is often inadequate. Pharmaceutical companies or regulatory authorities can only achieve good case documentation through effective data collection, detailed follow-up and use of field workers for complex cases. The quality of spontaneous reports also varies from country to country. Some countries do not have a regulatory reporting form for ADRs. There are differences among countries in publicity of drug safety issues and drug regulations differ regarding the format, content and submission timeframes for ADR reporting.

Reports received by companies via regulatory authorities are often edited and poorly documented, but they cannot be ignored and should be handled alongside reports received directly. The FDA implemented the Medical Products Reporting Program (Medwatch) in 1993, which encourages health care providers to regard reporting as a fundamental professional and public health responsibility and submit serious AE reports directly to the FDA on the FDA3500A form (Kessler, 1993). The FDA forwards these reports to the manufacturer, who is obliged to follow up with the reporter and submit any relevant information obtained to the FDA and other regulatory agencies worldwide as required.

Literature

The publication of case reports in medical and scientific journals is an important primary source of information on ADRs. Many ADRs are noted in medical and scientific journals before they become well-known. For example, the association of thalidomide with birth defects was first noted in a letter to the *Lancet* (Distillers Company, 1961). The quality of ADR reports in the published literature can be variable and has been the subject of much criticism and correspondence. Some guidelines have been given to authors of case reports and some journals have raised their standards for acceptance of such articles (see Information required for reports later in this chapter).

Despite the anecdotal nature and sometimes poor documentation, publication of case reports in journals remains one of the most useful primary sources of information on ADRs. ADR reports in the literature can be identified in several different ways. Pre-publication manuscripts describing a spontaneous case report or an event from a clinical trial are sometimes provided by authors to the manufacturer of the drug and the regulatory authority in that country. Pharmaceutical companies and some regulatory authorities undertake routine screening of the literature. This can take the form of scanning journals and abstracting services. Some companies also run routine searches of on-line databases, called selective dissemination of information (SDI) while other companies rely solely on SDI.

Searching for ADRs in the Literature   With the increasing number of scientific and biomedical journals there are more sources of ADR data on many drugs. Conversely, for some drugs, particularly those recently marketed, there is a scarcity of clinical publications and frequently there is an inadequate account of the adverse reaction profile. Searching for ADRs in the literature may be assisted by on-line databases such as MEDLINE (Index Medicus), EMBASE (Excerpta Medica) and secondary sources such as SEDBASE (Meyler's side effects of drugs) and ADIS on-line services such as REACTIONS. Many journals contain relevant information, but some specific ADR-related journals may assist in the search for information. Increasingly, the use of high-capacity storage systems such as compact disks (CD-ROM) has lead to stand-alone systems for storage and search of the literature rather than on-line systems. Integrated dictionaries have allowed the development of user-friendly literature searching. The Internet is also an important source of potential ADR information; however, due to the anecdotal nature of these reports, pharmaceutical companies should have a clear policy on how to handle them.

Information Required for Reports

In order to draw a conclusion about the possible relationship between a drug and an AE certain minimal information elements are required. Points considered essential for literature reports have been proposed (Jones, 1982) and some journals issue guidelines or checklists for potential authors. These can be adapted as a potential checklist for information that should be included in any ADR report as follows:

- Patient demography—age, sex, body weight, height, race, pregnancy.
- Medical history—previous medical history and concurrent conditions, known allergies (including ADRs with similar drugs, previous experience with drug).
- Timing—duration of treatment with the suspect drug before AE.
- Concurrent medications—details of other drugs including formulation, dose and duration.
- Dechallenge—action taken with the suspect drug (stopped, continued, dose reduction).
- Outcome—outcomes of the AEs.
- Alternative causes—what other factors could have accounted for the AE (diet, occupational exposure) and which were excluded?
- Rechallenge—was the patient rechallenged and if so, what was the result?
- Relevant additional data—blood levels, laboratory data, biopsy data and where relevant, postmortem findings.

Adverse Drug Reaction Forms and Form Design

Many forms are used by different organizations to collect ADR information. Most regulatory authorities have their own form (see appendix 5 for examples—Medicines Control Agency (MCA) yellow card and the Food and Drug Administration (FDA) 3500A). Although the content of these forms is similar, little attempt has been made to standardize the design other than Council for International Organization of Medical Sciences (CIOMS). An example of this form is given in Appendix 5. In addition, each pharmaceutical company usually has its own form or forms.

In order to design the best form for their needs, users must first define what data they wish to collect and which factors are of the greatest importance. In addition, all the usual factors in form design need to be considered, (e.g. size, layout, colour, print type, spacing, flow of questions, boxes, language and instructions). A pilot to test the form should be carried out before formal introduction and use.

Consideration should be given to what happens to the form once it is returned. Form design will be affected depending upon whether it is intended to serve as a direct entry document (i.e. the data elements closely match the data entry screens), or whether a transcription document will be used.

The key factor in ADR form design is the compatibility with other forms required for output, most importantly regulatory authority forms. The FDA, for example, require ADR reports to be submitted on an FDA3500A. If the pharmaceutical company does not wish to collect data on an FDA3500A but must submit reports to the FDA, it will need to design a form that collects the same information. Adverse event report forms generally collect the basic data elements outlined below:

- Patient demography.
- Relevant medical history and allergies.
- Suspect and concurrent drugs, route, indication.
- AE(s).
- Treatment and management of AE.
- Dechallenge, rechallenge, outcome.
- Relevant laboratory data.
- Reporter's opinion of causality.
- Report source of information.

The form can be printed as a folding postage pre-paid envelope for domestic use to encourage a reply. The pharmaceutical company must be able to demonstrate due diligence in seeking relevant follow-up information on each AE report.

Within the next two years, several key regulatory authorities including the MCA and FDA will require electronic data submission by companies for both expedited and non-expedited case reports. The compatibility between the company's and the regulatory authority's databases with regard to content and format of the key data elements for transmission is a critical factor to success of these initiatives. The adoption of internationally sanctioned standards such as a dictionary of medical terms, various code lists (e.g. countries, routes, units), file formats and periodic safety update reports are essential to enable efficient and accurate transmission. The International Conference on Harmonization (ICH) guideline (ICH E2B) defines data elements for transmission of individual case safety reports. The guideline aims to standardize the data elements for all individual case safety reports regardless of source and destination and covers reports for both pre-approval and post-approval periods. It also defines the minimum information for a report and the requirements for proper processing of the report. The medium for electronic submissions will be Electronic Data Interchange (EDI)-encrypted transmissions over the Internet.

Storage

Computer Systems

The following section looks at computer systems available for drug safety monitoring. Methods of data collection, input and verification are outlined. Useful dictionaries to input and output medical and drug terms are described. The use of computers as expert systems, in computer-aided evaluation and in assessment of the cause of an ADR are not covered here.

Computer systems used in monitoring drug safety can be bought off the shelf. Examples of current vendor products are:

- ALERT (DLB Systems, Cambridge, UK).
- ARIS (Clinarium Inc., Philadelphia, USA).
- Clintrace (Domain Software Solutions [formerly BBN], Cambridge, Massachusetts, USA).
- EventNet (Net Force Inc., San Francisco, USA).
- Argus Safety System (Relsys International Inc., Irvine, California, USA).

The decision that each customer (pharmaceutical company) has to make will depend upon business needs, budget, time scales and availability of in-house system support. After a review of potential options, companies either buy, buy and customize, or build their own system. Irrespective of whether an 'off the shelf' or in-house system is chosen, careful analysis of business and user requirements is needed before any decision can be made. Consideration should also be given to the technical architecture and the degree to which interfaces with other systems are required.

Computerization of Drug Safety Data

Data Collection and Input

'Rubbish in, rubbish out' applies to safety data as to any other computerized data. The enforced control of terms at entry can be linked to checking of data, which should form part of the quality control procedures. Such controls should be driven by the business so that clinical trial data, free from all errors and needed for statistical analysis, will probably involve double data entry whereas single data entry is generally considered adequate for AE databases used for signal generation and regulatory reporting.

Data are still generally typed into a database rather than electronically loaded from other systems. The first step of any data entry process should involve a check for duplicate cases. The need for decision making at the data entry stage will depend upon the type of database design. In all cases, there should be clear rules on how data should be entered into each field to ensure consistency and aid subsequent searching and outputting. This is particularly important when there are multiple users distributed over a number of international sites. Use of electronically available field specific lists of values and well-defined coding conventions will help with this.

In the future, data will increasingly be captured electronically. Image processing and developments in optical character recognition are already proving useful. Electronic data capture (using FAX or pen-based methods) is used to collect data in some clinical trials.

With the increase in licensing agreements between pharmaceutical companies, safety data frequently needs to be exchanged between one or more parties. If the case volume is sufficient, it is worth considering electronic data exchange between the databases involved. In addition to preventing rekeying of data, this minimizes discrepancies between the data sets. With the adoption of proposed ICH standards in the future, this will become a much simpler process.

Medical and Drug Terminology

Medical and drug terminology is at the heart of ADR systems. Accurate and consistent input of terms is critical for retrieval and analysis of ADR information. An integrated dictionary allows the capture of original text, which is autoencoded against the dictionary to retrieve the correct code for that piece of text. Coded information allows easy retrieval and analysis. The dictionary structure should allow different ways of grouping and analysing data encompassing body systems at the highest level to specific reporter's wording at the lowest level.

A coding dictionary should meet the following needs:

- Acceptable to all users of the system.
- New terms can be easily added.
- No loss of medical integrity by adding new terms.
- Specificity of the reported term preserved.
- Hierarchical structure to group terms at various levels of specificity.
- Logical groupings so similar terms are not scattered.
- A default grouping for each term.
- Unambiguous to enable autoencoding on input.

Dictionaries

This section compares commonly used dictionaries in monitoring drug safety. As electronic exchange of ADR data between industry and regulatory authorities in different countries increases, so does the need for standardization of terminology (Danan and Benichou, 1990; Benichou *et al.*, 1991). MedDRA (Medical Dictionary for Drug Regulatory Affairs) is currently in development and will become the global industry standard for ADR reporting. MedDRA is described in detail on page 289.

Medical Term Coding Dictionaries   It is logical to deal with AEs, indications, diseases, surgeries and procedures using one system for the following reasons:

- ADRs frequently mimic spontaneously occurring diseases, hence the same diagnosis or symptom could appear as an AE or disease.
- In the identification of new ADRs, it is important not to separate a possible side effect from a disease.
- Separate classifications can lead to confusion and add a layer of complexity when developing ADR systems.

Meaningful codes may or may not be needed for modern dictionaries. For example, the new Adverse Drug Reactions On-Line Information Tracking (ADROIT) dictionaries do not use meaningful codes, but rely on linkage of related terms and effective text processing. Where codes are considered necessary, they should be as short as possible (Westland, 1991). Whenever a system is used for AEs from the literature, spontaneous reports, clinical trials or a combination of these, the needs of the users of the system will influence the selection of the dictionary.

Rather than give a comprehensive review of all available dictionaries, six types are described below.

ADROIT Medical Dictionary   This was developed at the MCA by a team of physicians supported by information scientists. It is well suited for ADR autoencoding and output. The dictionary allows a multiaxial link to different body systems and group terms. Surgical terms and procedures are included. The lowest level is the reporter's term, which is linked to the preferred term used for outputting. Preferred terms can be linked straight to a system organ class (SOC), into a special search category or to a high-level term. The high-level term can be linked directly to a SOC or to a group term, which must link to a SOC. This classification was based on the Shepherd morbidity dictionary which retains some of its origins in the International Classification of Disease, 9th Revision (ICD9) and can map to World Health Organization (WHO) and Coding Symbols for a Theasurus of Adverse Reaction Terms (COSTART) terms. There is no meaningful code in this system, which may be considered an advantage or disadvantage depending upon business needs and user perspective. The ADROIT dictionary was reviewed and modified to produce the first version of MedDRA.

COSTART   (COSTART Coding Symbols for a Thesaurus of Adverse Reaction Terms) uses abbreviated phrases up to 24 characters as preferred term coding symbols to describe AEs. The dictionary holds approximately 1200 terms. There is also a body system classification and terms can be linked to more than one body system. Coding symbols may be translated into full text and body system descriptions automatically. Specific reporter's terms are lost on encoding with COSTART. An electronic version of COSTART is available from the FDA. COSTART is maintained by the FDA and revisions occur about once a year. An active COSTART user group exists internationally. Lilly implemented pure COSTART after having used a 'home-grown' COSTART with interesting results (Matsumoto, 1991). There is an expanded COSTART dictionary called HARTS (Hoechst Adverse Reaction Terminology) available in English, French, German and Japanese. Also, there is a translation between COSTART and WHO called WHO-Adverse Reaction Terminology (WHO-ART). COSTART is currently used by the FDA, but the FDA plan to move to MedDRA in 1998

WHO-ART   The WHO WHO-ART consists of preferred terms up to 33 characters long. Each preferred term is associated with a number of synonyms (included terms). There are 30 system organ classes designated by a four digit code. There is some degree of hierarchy with a higher level group term between the preferred term and SOC, but these are of limited value. The dictionary is available electronically and in different languages. There is an active WHO-ART user group.

ICD-9, ICD-9-Clinical Modification (CM), ICD-10   The ICD dictionaries are morbidity and mortality coding systems developed by the WHO and WHO centres assist with problems in classification. They are highly structured with a hierarchy based primarily on body systems with other major categories (e.g. infectious and parasitic diseases). Discrete ranges of three digits incorporate a body system. The first three digits form a subclass, such as 070 for viral hepatitis and a fourth digit gives specific conditions. For example, 070.2 corresponds to 'viral hepatitis B with hepatic coma'.

There is a dual classification for some terms (e.g. 573.1 'Hepatitis in viral diseases classified elsewhere'), but this is not extensive. The dictionaries are very comprehensive with the exception of symptoms, which tend to be scattered. They have been widely used in coding patient histories and hospital charts.

ICD-9 CM is a clinical modification of ICD-9 and offers some advantages, particularly the inclusion of synonyms, but is constrained by systems that have used the older versions of ICD-9. ICD-10 is more comprehensive than any ICD revision to date (see Websites). It extends well beyond the traditional causes of death and causes of hospitalization. The content has been expanded to include symptoms, signs, abnormal findings, factors related to lifestyle and other factors causing contact with health services.

SNOMED International SNOMED (Systemized Nomenclature of Human and Veterinary Medicine) is a comprehensive, multiaxial nomenclature used for indexing the entire medical record including signs, symptoms, diagnoses and procedures. Like the ICD dictionaries, SNOMED is primarily used in coding patient histories and medical records (see Websites). A meaningful code is used to enhance data retrieval. The dictionary is maintained by the College of American Pathologists, which issues updates at least twice a year. It contains more than 144 000 separate terms in 11 separate modules.

MedDRA (Medical Dictionary for Regulatory Activities) MedDRA is a medical dictionary encompassing terms relevant to pre- and post-marketing phases of the regulatory process. It was developed by the MCA to support its information systems and has subsequently been further developed by the MedDRA working party and the ICH Medical Terminology Working Group. The objective is to harmonize on standards for electronic submissions among regulatory authorities, between authorities and industry within and across regions. The aims of the dictionary are:

- To address pre- and post-marketing AE reporting.
- To cover multiple medical product areas.
- To be available in multiple languages.
- To be available in multiple formats and platforms.
- To be well maintained.

The guiding principles are:

- To build from existing terminologies to maximize compatibility.
- To focus on the international community need rather than optimizing on individual countries.
- To ensure worldwide use through collaboration and participation in development.
- To ensure mechanisms and structures are in place for translation into many languages.
- To ensure long-term maintenance.

The scope of MedDRA is as follows:

- Diseases.
- Diagnoses.

- Signs and symptoms.
- Therapeutic indications.
- Investigation names and qualitative results.
- Medical and surgical procedures.
- Medical, social, and family history.
- Terms from COSTART, WHO-ART, ICD-9-CM, HARTS, J-ART.

The current structure of MedDRA is defined in Table 1.

There will be a central maintenance organization responsible for development, user support, implementation and communication as well as an international user group. A management board will oversee the activities of the central maintenance organization with direction provided by the ICH Steering Committee. A standard medical dictionary will facilitate electronic data exchange between industry and regulatory authorities worldwide, as recommended by the ICH.

In-house Dictionary Development   Dictionary design may be viewed as a process of resolving conflicts between system objectives and the practicalities of implementation (Gillum, 1990). In the authors' views, the best advice to anyone wishing to construct such an in-house dictionary is 'don't'. The needs of the users should be balanced against available dictionaries to see if any fulfil their mandatory requirements.

If development of an in-house dictionary is considered essential, it is vital that all potential users are represented in structuring the dictionary. The first step is to determine the concepts to be included and the method of grouping the terms together. It is important that physicians are closely involved with development of

Table 1   MedDRA Structure

Level of hierarchy	Approximate number of terms	Definition	Example
System organ class	26	Broadest collection of concepts for retrieval; grouped by anatomy or physiology	Cardiac disorders
High-level group term	334	Broad concepts for linking clinically related terms; can be linked to one or more SOCs	Cardiac rhythm disorders
High-level term	1663	Groups of preferred terms related by anatomy, pathology, physiology, aetiology or function; can be linked to one or more high-level group terms or SOCs	Tachyarrhythmia
Preferred term	11 193	International level of information exchange; single, unambiguous clinical concept	Ventricular tachycardia
Lowest level term	46 258	Synonyms and quasi synonyms; help define scope of preferred terms	Paroxysmal ventricular tachycardia

the dictionary. After working out the practicalities of what software and hardware are needed and how to input and link data, a pilot study to test the dictionary is advised. It is essential to map existing dictionaries to the new dictionary if other systems will continue to use the old dictionaries. Working practices and maintenance of the dictionary must be carefully defined.

Dictionaries of Drug and Therapy Terms   In addition to the drug under evaluation in a clinical trial or the drug that is the subject of an AE report, patients are frequently receiving other therapies. In many cases, these could be alternative causes of the ADR or a possible drug interaction. All concurrent drugs must be recorded on the clinical trial record forms and ADR forms and the information coded and processed. There are a number of coding dictionaries for drugs available. Users must decide which system best meets their needs.

There are several different ways of approaching the task. Classification can be based on chemical structures (e.g. benzodiazepines), pharmacological action (e.g. anxiolytics), or therapeutic use (e.g. minor tranquillizers). Some drugs, which have the same pharmacological action (e.g. beta adrenergic receptor antagonists), may have many different indications such as angina, hypertension, cardiac arrhythmias, prevention of myocardial reinfarction and migraine prophylaxis. Not all members of the class, however, have the same indications. If the user wanted to identify all patients receiving a beta adrenergic receptor antagonist, this would not be possible if a therapeutic use classification only had been used. Alternatively, the user may want to identify all patients receiving antihypertensives in which case several pharmacological groups would have to be used although this does not necessarily mean that the patient was taking the drug for hypertension. This problem could be overcome by using two or more different classifications and putting the drug into several therapeutic categories. Before doing this, the complexity of the system and the time needed to develop it should be considered. In practice, most users only need a simple system. As with coding systems for medical terms there is no one ideal system and the choice must be that which best meets the user's needs.

Four coding systems considered by the authors to be the most useful are as follows.

Aberdeen/Dundee Medicines Codes   This system was developed in 1972 by the Medicines Evaluation and Monitoring section of the Department of Community Medicine in the University of Aberdeen and the Pharmacy Department in the Aberdeen Royal Infirmary, UK. The code consists of five digits, the first two indicating a therapeutic group and the last three identifying individual drugs. Drug names appear as both approved and proprietary, together with non-standard names and common misspellings, but all have the same five-digit code. As each drug has a unique number, it can only be entered in one therapeutic area and drugs have been assigned to the area considered most important. An additional pharmacological classification consisting of a further two digits was later added at the request of the Dundee group. The dictionary is available electronically and is comprehensive for UK-marketed drugs though lacking for non-UK products. It can be taken and added to by pharmaceutical companies.

British National Formulary The British National Formulary (BNF) classifies drugs and preparations under therapeutic categories, which are then subdivided. It is updated every six months. Drugs may appear in more than one therapeutic group as appropriate. It can be used as a coding system for groups of drugs or serve as the basis of an in-house system where unique drug codes would be developed. Several hospital pharmacies and the prescription pricing authority in the UK use a coding dictionary based on the BNF system. It does not include non-prescription drugs, investigational drugs and non-UK drugs.

ATC The Nordic ATC (anatomical, therapeutic, chemical) classification was developed by the Nordic Council of Medicines as a common classification system for all medicines in the Nordic countries. It is a logical chemical and therapeutic classification system and is available in published form and electronically. It is updated regularly by a professional drug committee within the Nordic community. There are four levels of classification, which allow a drug to be included in one or more therapeutic, chemical and pharmacological groups. Drugs include primarily those on the Nordic market.

ADROIT Drug Dictionary (Wood, 1989) This was developed in-house at the MCA using the Swedish drug substance dictionary and the Nordic ATC classification for the pharmacological classification. It consists of the ATC classification and sections representing the ways product and drug information is provided on ADR reports (e.g. as a named product or drug substance and chemical variant or drug synonym). Drugs can exist in more than one pharmacological classification. It is very comprehensive, including herbal remedies and over-the-counter (OTC) medicines.

Other Systems Other systems that could be considered include MIMS (Monthly Index of Medical Specialties), which has similar advantages and disadvantages to the BNF; the WHO Drug Reference list, which is a cross index of drugs available from the WHO Monitoring Program of Adverse Reactions to Drugs and includes all drugs that have appeared on the ADR reports reviewed; an in-house system. The previous comments on the development of an in-house coding system for medical terms also applies to drugs except that it is useful to involve pharmacists in the design rather than physicians.

Data Retrieval

The data are the core of any drug safety monitoring scheme, providing signals of possible ADRs. Depending upon the purpose and destination of the output, the data tabulations and analyses are likely to vary. The user must decide upon the most effective search strategy and associated outputs for the task at hand. As mentioned earlier in the chapter, the way data is stored effects data retrieval and output. Data retrieval and analysis is a specialized skill, requiring knowledge of the search and analysis tools as well as knowledge of how the data are stored in the database. A broad range of output requirements should be considered when designing a database. The following section suggests some ideas and points out pitfalls from the authors' experiences.

Searching

In order to respond to queries, output data tabulations and produce reports, it is necessary to search the database to obtain the required data set. It is essential to fully understand the question or task and understand the way data are stored in the database before development of a search strategy. The way the data have been captured and coded will affect the way the user is able to retrieve them. If AE coding has been done at a very specific level in order to retain verbatim the reporter's wording and there are no function to group terms, a very large number of codes may need to be entered in order to retrieve all the data on one ADR.

Different types of software lead to different approaches in search strategy. For example, relational databases are typically designed for ease of data input, not output. Time should be spent on the development of standard queries and reports linking commonly asked questions with predetermined output, along with ad hoc query functionality for the less common but necessary searches. Several vendor products are designed specifically for ad hoc data retrieval and reporting from relational databases (e.g. Brio Query, Business Objects, Cognos, Impromptu and Powerplay).

The following examples illustrate some of the problems encountered when searching using dictionary terminology. There are several methods of solving these problems depending upon the way ADR data are structured:

- Neonatal disorders—if just the specific disease code is stored (e.g. bradycardia), it will not be possible to retrieve neonatal bradycardia separately. If a code of neonatal bradycardia is used, it may not be possible to pull out all the bradycardias together. One solution is to code neonatal disorder and bradycardia, thus allowing all possible search requirements to be covered, particularly if combined with a search on age of patient.
- Administration errors—enquiries sometimes require the user to identify all cases where a drug has been given by the wrong route. This is difficult to achieve unless a code for administration error has been included.
- Allergic reactions, bleeding disorders, congenital abnormalities, etc.—many terms are included in various body systems. Use of groupings via a core code should be considered.
- Drug interactions—cases may not be coded as drug interactions. It is important to search on all suspect and concurrent drugs to capture all potential drug interactions.
- Pregnancy cases—in order to analyse all pregnancy cases, both prospective and retrospective cases should be retrieved.

Reports and Outputs

A number of standard forms, bulletins, reports and tables are likely to be required from the database.

Individual Regulatory Report

Computer generation of the reporting forms required by regulatory authorities is standard practice in pharmaceutical companies. This has the advantage of enabling production of high-quality forms from one data set rather than having to type them individually. If a worldwide database is used, the forms can be output in the country where they are required to be submitted using data entered elsewhere. This can greatly speed up reporting timeframes. Computer production of the forms does have an impact on data storage. It is important to ensure that the data are compatible with all of the various types of regulatory reporting forms as outlined below:

- FDA3500A (Medwatch form)—mandatory for reporting individual cases to the FDA.
- Yellow card—mandatory for reporting UK cases to the MCA.
- CIOMS I—mandatory for reporting individual foreign cases to many countries.

Periodic Reports

Many regulatory authorities require detailed summary reports on groups of cases on a regular basis. The FDA requires annual progress reports for investigational compounds and periodic reports for marketed drugs either quarterly or annually depending upon the length of time the product has been on the USA market. CIOMS II guidelines recommend submission of line listings of serious, unlabelled, attributable clinical study cases and all serious and non-serious, unlabelled spontaneous cases in conjunction with a summary of the drug safety profile on a six-monthly basis. These reports are well defined in format, content and submission timeframe. Most major pharmaceutical companies produce them electronically.

The regulatory requirements, particularly regarding frequency of submission and content, differ in the three regions (Europe, Japan and USA). In order to avoid duplication of effort and to ensure that important data are submitted with consistency to regulatory authorities worldwide, the ICH3 Topic E2C Guideline on the Format and Content for Comprehensive Periodic Safety Update Reports (PSUR) (1996) of marketed medicinal products has been developed. The general principles of this guideline include:

- One report is submitted for one active substance. All dosage forms as well as indications for a given active substance should be covered in one PSUR.
- The focus is on ADRs, which include all spontaneous reports and all drug-related clinical trial and literature reports.
- An international birthdate and frequency of review and reporting is defined. The international birthdate is the date of the first marketing authorization for the product granted to any company in any country in the world. Preparation of PSURs should be based on data sets of six months or multiples thereof. The PSUR should be submitted within 60 days of the data lock point.
- The reference safety information is the company core data sheet to determine whether an ADR is listed or unlisted.
- ADR data are presented in line listings and/or summary tabulations.

Other Reports

In addition, regular reviews of drug safety data are needed for changes to the product labelling, to respond to regulatory enquiries, for new product applications and a host of other activities. The database must be flexible enough for users to produce ad hoc queries and reports. Bulletins of new cases received in a specified timeframe are often used internally within a pharmaceutical company to inform interested parties of drug safety issues.

Electronic Submission to Regulatory Authorities

Electronic submission of periodic and expedited reports to the FDA via the Internet will soon become mandatory. Data standards such as MedDRA and encryption standards are being developed to facilitate this process. This initiative will eventually lead to a two-way electronic data exchange between all major regulatory authorities and pharmaceutical companies. Several major companies are involved in an FDA electronic submission pilot to perfect the process before mandating its use.

EudraNet/EudraWatch is a project started in January 1996. The purpose is to improve communication and facilitate collaboration in pharmacovigilance between the EC, the European Medicines Evaluation Agency (EMEA) and the national competent authorities within the framework of the new system for supervision of medical products. The specific objective is to develop tools to process and exchange ADR notifications electronically.

Analysis

Many software systems are capable of straightforward numerical outputs. The more sophisticated systems can also present data in tabular or graphical format to facilitate identification of risk factors for the ADR such as age, sex, other drugs and underlying disease. Some are able to perform further numerical and statistical analyses on the data. Alternatively, data may be output to a separate graphics or statistical package (e.g. Lotus 1 2 3, Freelance or SAS) for further manipulation.

Analysis of ADRs from clinical trial data is a complex subject, which is represented in textbooks on this subject (Spilker and Schoenfelder, 1990). No attempt is made here to go into the detail. However, problems to look out for are standardization of safety data collected across trials, how serious AE data are captured for rapid reporting to worldwide authorities, subsequent analysis of data contained in multiple databases, and integration issues if pharmaceutical companies attempt to integrate clinical trial and post-marketing ADR systems.

Conclusions

This chapter has outlined the sources of ADR data, their differences and some of their limitations. As mentioned throughout, the choice of computer hardware and software depends upon many factors, but essentially user requirements. The characteristics, advantages and disadvantages of some coding dictionaries have been described, but again selection will be based on user needs and preference. Methods of data retrieval and some of the problems encountered are discussed. It is essential to consider output requirements when designing a new computer system. Finally, it is important to ensure a high degree of flexibility in a system as requirements and regulations change with time.

Acknowledgements

The authors wish to thank their colleagues who provided constructive advice and comment on this chapter.

Chapter 11

Causality Assessment and Signal Recognition

M. D. B. Stephens

Decisions have to be made by pharmaceutical companies and regulatory authorities about whether a drug can cause a particular adverse event (AE) so that an appropriate action can be taken. What does 'can cause' mean? Does it imply certainty? In many cases to wait for 'certainty' before taking action would entail many patients suffering unnecessarily. The degree of certainty or 'probability' required will vary according to the situation.

There are, nearly always, many factors other than the administration of a drug, that can cause an AE and will determine whether the AE will occur in a particular patient (see Chapter 1, page 11). The drug may be 'the last straw that broke the camel's back'. If an AE would not have occurred as and when it did but for the drug then the drug 'caused' the AE (Hutchinson, 1992). So with an adverse drug interaction both drugs 'caused' the AE. Using this definition the drug may only be a minor factor.

Certainty is rarely obtainable; perhaps an AE with a positive rechallenge where there is objective evidence and an absence of confounders in an individual case would be considered as certainly due to the drug. In the majority of cases action is needed before there is absolute certainty that a drug can cause an AE. This lack of certainty in individual cases has been described using rather vague terms such as 'almost certain', 'probable', 'possible', 'unlikely', etc. These terms have also been defined, but each author has a slightly different definition (Venulet *et al.*, 1982; Stephens, 1987). Some of the various alternatives used in clinical trials are shown in Chapter 4, page 127.

It has been suggested in CIOMS III that one should 'avoid including in the core safety information AEs that have had no well-established relationship to therapy'. This implies that drugs are innocent of causing an ADR until proven guilty. The meaning of 'well-established' is arguable (CIOMS Working Group III, 1995).

Again in epidemiological studies or clinical trials there is nearly always a degree of uncertainty due to bias, chance and confounders. In these studies uncertainty is measured in terms of p values, odds ratios, and relative risks etc. (see Chapter 9).

The differential diagnosis of AEs associated with a drug or drug(s) is an everyday part of a practising clinician's life; however, the term 'causality assessment' is reserved for a similar process performed at one or more stages removed from the patient and with some important differences. Clinicians do not necessarily need to find out whether a drug caused an AE in order to satisfy themselves and their patients. They will be more interested in resolving the event as quickly as possible. If there is a possibility that the event might be an ADR, it may be resolved by either reducing the dose or stopping the drug or by treating the ADR while waiting for tolerance to develop, or it may resolve if any of the underlying factors are altered. The resolution of the AE might be because the event has been caused by the drug or it may have been a transient natural occurrence: either way the patient and doctor will welcome its disappearance. If, however, the doctor is interested in knowing whether it was an ADR further investigations can be undertaken, as long as the patient is willing, until it is established or refuted.

When causality assessment is undertaken by a regulatory authority or a scientist/physician in industry, it is unlikely that the full details known to the clinician treating the patient will be reported, even after further inquiry is made. The only way to obtain all available data is usually by visiting the physician and, with permission, reading the notes and discussing the case with him or her.

Aims of causality assessment   Classification of AEs, To decide on the nature of further inquiries, To satisfy regulatory requirements, To decide whether the drug can cause an ADR, To aid signal recognition, To provide the basis for a label change.

Aims of Causality Assessment

Classification of Adverse Events

Of the many similar events on an AE database only a few have sufficient and relevant data to enable the assessor to decide that the AE was more likely caused by the drug than by any other cause or vice versa. A preliminary assessment (sometimes referred to as 'triage') can be made by placing the event into a category (e.g. probable, possible or unlikely, or using the EEC classification of A, B or O) (Meyboom and Royer, 1992). This will enable the company to extract the probable cases at regular intervals in order to consider whether there is a 'signal'. The possible and unlikely cases will probably not contribute much to this signal.

This preliminary assessment will need to be updated as and when further information becomes available. It should err on the side of sensitivity rather than specificity so that a borderline possible/probable case is classified as probable rather than possible to make certain that the case is not lost when at a later stage the probable cases are picked out as a signal. A full assessment when all the information is available can then rectify any misclassifications.

To Decide on the Nature of Further Inquiries

Until one has read the AE report and considered the possibility of a drug relationship, it is not possible to decide on exactly what other inquiries are necessary. It is important that if further questions are to be sent to the reporter that they are focussed, specific and essential. Frequently this will require input from a physician about what would be both helpful and is available.

To Satisfy Regulatory Requirements

Some authorities require an assessment to be made. The French regulatory authorities require the use of the French method and the Germans require an assessment, but do not stipulate a method. Other authorities—for example the Food and Drug Administration (FDA), want (IND) safety reports of '(A) Any adverse experience associated with the use of the drug that is both serious and unexpected'. Elsewhere (Federal Register, 1997) it says 'associated with the use of the drug' means 'There is a reasonable possibility that the experience may have been caused by the drug'. It would be reasonable to assume that this includes the following assessments: 'certain', 'probable' and 'possible', but excludes 'unlikely' and 'definitely not due to the drug'. However, IND safety reports (written) are required within 15 calendar days (page 52245). ... in clinical investigation cases, if 'there is a reasonable suspected causal relationship between the investigational product and the adverse event (i.e. the causal relationship cannot be ruled out)'. This implies that all the above assessments plus 'unlikely' need to be reported and only if it is 'definitely not due to the drug' can it not be reported. The latter are so rare that nearly all AEs would need reporting if, as is usual, the investigator's assessment is taken. This anomaly needs to be addressed.

To Decide whether a Drug can cause an Adverse Drug Reaction

If further information is received reassessment will be necessary.

- investigational new drug

The event will need a final full assessment once no more information is obtainable. All factors have to be considered.

To Aid Signal Recognition

This can be achieved by reviewing just those cases that have been assessed as probable or almost certain, as mentioned above, but if causality assessment is not the company's policy there are several other means for detecting signals.

To Provide the Basis for a Label Change

When a signal has been generated by several 'probable' cases, all cases will need to be assessed as a group and this group assessment will require additional factors to be considered over and above those required for an individual case. Even if a pharmaceutical company does not assess individual cases it will need to perform some sort of group assessment. The results from group assessment will often be the basis for a labelling committee judgement about whether the ADR is mentioned in the data sheet.

When to do an Assessment

The first assessment needs to be performed within the first few days. Initially a decision has to be made concerning reporting to the regulatory authorities and this is usually done immediately on receipt of the report. It is also a convenient time to make a preliminary assessment for causality and decide what further information should be requested. This means that there will be a chance that the reporter has not forgotten all about the case by the time he or she receives the request for more details. If the report is from a hospital clinical trial then there is the possibility of further investigations before the patient is discharged.

When no further information is expected, a full assessment should be performed preferably by a physician within the pharmacovigilance department. Some methods of assessment are suitable for the preliminary assessment and others for the full assessment and these will be dealt with later.

All companies need to have a monitoring programme to pick up signals throughout the life of a drug. These monitoring screens are likely to be fairly frequent during the pre-marketing phase, becoming more infrequent with the passage of time. As soon as a signal has been identified, a group assessment needs to be performed.

Type of Assessment

The type of assessment will vary depending upon whether there is an individual case or a group of cases, whether the report is from a clinical trial or is a spontaneous report, whether it is pre-marketing or post-marketing and whether a type A or type B mechanism is likely.

Individual Cases

Clinical Trials and Cohort Studies
The protocol will have stipulated that AEs must be collected and usually the investigator will be asked to give an opinion concerning causality on the AE form. It is important that the assessment is balanced between the probability that the study drug caused the event and the probability that there was an alternative cause; that is on 'the balance of probabilities', which is similar to a case in civil law. There is sometimes evidence from the wording that a clinical trialist uses the equivalent of criminal law; that is that the drug is 'innocent until proved guilty'. This can be avoided by a suitably worded paragraph in the protocol.

Spontaneous Reports

These are post-marketing reports where the reporter suspects that the drug is a possible cause of an AE. One could argue that in the UK, for a black triangle drug (a new drug still under special surveillance), all AEs that 'could conceivably be attributed to the drug will be reported'. Nevertheless all these AEs should be considered as possibly related to the drug until evidence pushes the assessment one way or the other. In other words there is a prior possibility that they are suspected ADRs. Under these circumstances the reporting doctor is under no obligation to give further information, so any request for further information must be carefully worded and only deal with essential items so as to ensure their cooperation.

Pre-marketing Reports

During the clinical trial development programme the clinical trialists are paid to provide data and it is essential that they provide any information that the company considers necessary for assessment (as long as it is in the patient's interest). Too frequently the trial monitors seem unable to obtain all the required data. This may be due to a breakdown in communication between the pharmacovigilance department and the clinical trial monitor or a reluctance on the part of the monitor to pester the trialist. The licensing of a drug worldwide is, at the moment, a gradual procedure and the early countries to licence a new drug will be receiving spontaneous reports while others are still in the pre-marketing phase. This is a very difficult period because frequently the total number of patients worldwide who have received the drug is relatively small and serious type B spontaneous reports with little data create hypotheses that cannot be confirmed or refuted.

Type A or Type B Adverse Events

Although type A and type B are usually used for referring to ADRs, AEs can often be considered as potential type A or type B (e.g. any reports of headache without any qualifying details are usually type A AE whereas a suspected immunological disease would be a type B AE). Headaches reported as AEs in clinical trials are usually counted and statistical analysis applied. In most cases individual causality assessment is inappropriate. The rare type B event, on the other hand, can usually only be assessed individually due to its rarity. In very large studies with thousands of patients there may, however, be a sufficient number of serious type B events to warrant statistical analysis.

Important Factors to Consider in Assessment

Previous Adverse Drug Reaction History of the Drugs Involved

If one or more of the drugs in use at the time of the AE has a history of causing the AE in question then this increases the likelihood that that drug is a factor in this AE. The sources of information are:

- *MIMS* (Monthly Index of Medical Specialties)—since this is published monthly it may contain ADRs not mentioned in the yearly edition of the Association of the

British Pharmaceutical Industry (ABPI) compendium, but not all ADRs are mentioned.

- *British National Formulary* (BNF)—this is published twice yearly and has some ADRs not mentioned in the data sheets.
- *ABPI Data Sheet Compendium*—although not as up-to-date as MIMS it contains much more detail and is more specific.
- Other national drug compendia, for example, Vidal, Physician's Desk Reference (PDR)—see Bibliography for details.
- *Reactions Weekly*—this surveys the world literature and publishes details of both new and old ADRs. *Reactions* three-monthly, six-monthly and annually are indexes of *Reactions Weekly*. At the back of each edition there is a list of drug-induced diseases with the drugs that have caused them in the period covered.
- *Meyler's Side Effects of Drugs*—this is published every few years and deals with drugs by therapeutic/pharmacological groups. It is authoritative with different experts writing the sections.
- *Meyler's Side Effects of Drugs Annuals*—by the same publishers as the above, but contains only the new ADRs since the last edition.

Factors to consider in assessment   Previous ADR history of the drugs involved, The event, Time to onset, Dechallenge, Rechallenge, Investigations, Alternative causes

---

The Event

The proportion of an AE due to drugs compared with that due to natural causes varies greatly. Some serious events are renowned for the high proportion of drug-induced AEs, (for example toxic epidermal necrolysis (TEN). When this type of AE is seen the likelihood of drug involvement is increased.

Adverse events commonly caused by drugs   Toxic epidermal necrolysis, Torsades de pointe, Stevens-Johnson syndrome, Agranulocytosis, Aplastic anaemia, Guillain-Barré syndrome, Pseudomembranous colitis, Tardive dyskinesia, Neuroleptic malignant syndrome, Anaphylaxis, Anaphylactoid reactions, Angioedema

---

Time to Onset

This is the time from the first dose of the drug until the onset of the AE. Very little research has been done on this topic. The figures available have usually been the opinion of experts in the field rather than the result of cases. The time to onset will vary according to pharmacokinetic parameters for type A reactions. Type B reactions will depend upon the type of hypersensitivity, which in many cases is unknown.

Type A

Many ADRs are caused by the same mechanism as the primary efficacy and therefore might appear at the same time, but since the side effects often appear at a higher tissue level than efficacy they tend to appear a little later. There are some ADRs where the pharmacological action might be fairly immediate, but the resulting ADRs take longer to appear or be noticed (e.g. constipation, osteoporosis). The 'confusion' that can occur with H_2 antagonists takes about three days to appear and there is a suggestion that this occurs in the elderly and the ill due to passage through a leaky blood–brain barrier. With some ADRs the first sign is a change in a laboratory value and in this situation the AE obviously occurred before the test, but the time cannot be pinpointed. It is only when the action of the drug is turned into an immediate symptom (e.g. flushing with a vasodilator) that an accurate time can be given. For the most part only knowledge of the physiological mechanism of an ADR can give an indication of the period between the drug's action and the endpoint, for example indigestion from a non-steroidal anti-inflammatory drug (NSAID) may be almost immediate, but the consequent anaemia may not be apparent for some months. Remember that some drugs have a very long half-life and their effects may be delayed (e.g. terodiline has a mean half-life of 189 hours, SD 135 hours, range 69–485 hours—time to total removal from the body can be 14.5 weeks) (Malone-Lee and Wiseman, 1991).

Type B

Drug hypersensitivity has been divided into four classes according to the Gell and Coombs classification (Coombs and Gell, 1968). Although it is useful for the type one reactions, antigen and antibody of the IgE immunoglobulin class in anaphylaxis, urticaria etc., the other three classes are much more difficult to allocate to different type B ADRs. The Van Arsdel classification for allergic reactions is more helpful dividing them into:

1. Mast cell mediated.
2. T-lymphocyte mediated.
3. Photodermatitis (systemic).
4. Other cutaneous reactions (mechanism uncertain).
5. Drug fever
6. Systemic lupus erythematosus (SLE) and other autoimmune reactions.
7. Organ system groups—haematological, hepatic, pulmonary, renal and cardiac (Van Arsdel, 1986).

See Appendix 2 for details of times to onset and offset.

Long Latency Adverse Drug Reaction

This has been defined by Fletcher and Griffin (1991) as apparent six months or more after initial exposure. This may be:

(a) Via offspring—thalidomide and phocomelia (McBride, 1961); diethylstilboestrol and adenocarcinoma of the vagina (Herbst, 1971).
(b) Carcinogenesis—hepatocellular carcinoma with C^{17} substituted testosterones (Sherlock, 1979).
(c) Type A—osteoporosis due to corticosteroids.

(d) Type B—NSAID renal papillary necrosis (Nanra *et al.*, 1978); neuroleptic tardive dyskinesia (Crane, 1968; Lane and Routledge, 1983); practolol oculomucocutaneous syndrome (Wright, 1974); benoxaprofen hepatorenal syndrome (Taggart and Alderdice, 1982).

Dechallenge

This simply means stopping the drug. Subsequent disappearance of the AE is referred to as a positive dechallenge while negative dechallenge infers that the AE continues. Several variations need to be considered.

Dechallenge—factors to consider Time to improvement or resolution, Partial reversibility or complete irreversibility, Tolerance or desensitization, Confounding ADR treatment, Replacement therapy, Reasonable time to offset, Delayed or latent ADR, Multiple dechallenge, Drug withdrawal or rebound effect, Placebo dechallenge, Drug stopped or dosage reduced.

Time to Improvement or Resolution
The time to improvement is often far shorter than the time to resolution and is more critical; so usually this time should be used.

Irreversibility
Some ADRs are due to a change in function of a tissue triggering an event that is identical to a naturally occurring disease (e.g. Guillain-Barré syndrome). The time to resolution or improvement becomes that of the naturally occurring disease. Neurological tissue is very unforgiving of drug insults and neurological ADRs are frequently irreversible or partially irreversible.

Tolerance or Desensitization
Physiological homeostatic mechanisms will tend to reverse any situation that is detrimental to the normal body functions (i.e. tachyphylaxis or tolerance will occur). Cholestatic jaundice due to chlorpromazine may resolve even though the drug is continued (Paton, 1976). It is also possible to desensitize patients who are allergic to penicillin by starting with a very small dose and then slowly increasing it. Both of these mechanisms can act to cause resolution of the AE while still continuing on the guilty drug.

Confounding Treatment of the Adverse Event
Frequently allergic reactions are treated with a corticosteroid so the subsequent resolution may be due either to the dechallenge or the steroid.

Replacement Therapy
After dechallenge the patient may still require further treatment and often this is with a similar drug of the same class in the hope that the second drug will not produce the same reaction. Sometimes this hope is misplaced and the reaction returns or continues, for example angiotensin-converting enzyme (ACE) inhibitor cough.

Delayed or Latent Adverse Drug Reaction

From what has already been said some ADRs can occur after dechallenge and hence the dechallenge itself becomes meaningless.

Dechallenge of Two or More Drugs Simultaneously

Life-threatening type B reactions in a patient who is taking many drugs, any of which could cause the ADR, frequently results in simultaneously stopping all but the most essential drugs. The dechallenge under these circumstances means that it does not help to differentiate the responsible drug.

Withdrawal Reactions

An ADR can be caused by suddenly stopping a drug (i.e. the signs and symptoms occurring after stoppage of the drug). These are called drug withdrawal or rebound reactions. The latter infers a greater severity of symptoms due to the underlying disease and is caused by the same mechanism (e.g. myocardial infarction on withdrawal of a beta blocker given for angina). Withdrawal reactions are considered in Chapter 1.

Placebo Dechallenge

Since a placebo can cause an ADR, stopping a placebo can cause a false positive dechallenge. If a patient has been 'infected' (see Chapter 1) with an ADR then it is likely to resolve on stopping the drug—a false positive dechallenge.

Delayed Dechallenge

After a positive rechallenge the subsequent dechallenge may be delayed for longer than on the first occasion and in some circumstances may be irreversible.

Drug Stopped or Dosage Reduced

The dechallenge for a type A reaction is usually brought about by reducing the dosage of the drug so that the tissue drug level falls below the threshold for a reaction. This is then a partial positive dechallenge. With a type B reaction it is necessary to stop the drug.

Rechallenge

This means reintroduction of a drug that has been associated with an AE. A positive rechallenge infers reproduction of the same AE. There are again several variations.

Rechallenge—variations Multiple rechallenge, Protopathic bias, Interaction, Different route or dose, Desensitization

---

Multiple Positive Rechallenges

This can occur when the reaction comes on soon after ingestion and resolves before the next dose is due. Patients usually say that they get the reaction after every tablet. This is usually confined to type A reactions. Girard (1987) points out that for a proper rechallenge the discontinuation before the rechallenge should be until all drug has left the tissue (i.e. at least five half-lives).

Protopathic Bias

If, when looked at retrospectively, the drug has been given for the early symptoms of what turns out to be a severe AE it may seem that the drug caused the AE when it was a naturally occurring event (e.g. a patient has epigastric pain and is given a H_2 antagonist and the symptoms of pancreatitis develop so the drug is stopped, only to be given again for further epigastric pain with the resulting second attack of pancreatitis). This gives a false positive rechallenge.

Interactions

If both drug X and drug Y are necessary for a reaction then stopping one drug, say X, will cause resolution of the ADR and it is likely to be blamed as the sole factor in the ADR. It is only when drug Y is stopped, after a rechallenge with both drugs, that it will be apparent that drug X is not the sole factor (e.g. serotonin syndrome) (Sporer, 1995).

Different Route or Dose

With serious type B reactions, if rechallenge is ethical, the reintroduction may be by a different route (e.g. patch test or by the same route but at a much lower dose). The latter may then cause a different reaction to the original reaction (e.g. raised liver function tests rather than a full-blown hepatitis). This will count as a positive rechallenge. Girard (1987), in his excellent paper, says this should count only as 'suggestive' rather than 'positive'.

Desensitization

Of patients who had had an allergic reaction to penicillin only 21% had a positive skin test at a later date and only 1% had an immediate reaction on rechallenge (Rocklin, 1978). Sensitization can therefore take place between a reaction and a rechallenge and in these circumstances a negative rechallenge does not mean that the first reaction was not due to the drug.

Investigations

The ultimate decision as to causality will depend upon judgement as to whether the probability of drug involvement is greater than the probability of an alternative cause. In theory the clinician in charge of the patient will exclude alternative causes by continuing to examine and investigate the patient until he or she reaches a decision. However, in practice, the clinician often stops a suspected drug and if the reaction disappears no further investigations are considered necessary. On investigating hepatocellular liver reactions it is common to find that all the tests required to exclude a viral cause have not been performed. Hydralazine-induced SLE is more probable if the patient is female, a slow acetylator and has an HLA factor DR4 (Batchelor *et al.*, 1980). Although drug-induced SLE patients usually have positive deoxyribonucleic acid (DNA) antibodies they do not have them to double-stranded DNA, which is usually present in the natural disease. Also drug-induced SLE does not usually affect the kidney or central nervous system.

These types of investigation may help in a difficult case. The number of possibly helpful investigations across the whole gamut of ADRs is legion and help must be found in the large medical textbooks. In addition to the range of clinical investigations there are the more specific immunological tests referred to in Chapter 2.

Methods of Causality Assessment

There are many different methods as follows:

1. Clinical differential diagnosis.
2. Irey's method—six factors, definitions (Irey, 1972).
3. Karch and Lasagna's method—three decision tables, seven questions (Karch and Lasagna, 1977).
4. The French method—ten questions, binary format (Dangoumau *et al.*, 1978); updated (Bégaud, 1984).
5. Blanc *et al.*'s method—decision table, 11 questions (Blanc *et al.*, 1979).
6. Kramer *et al.*'s method—six main axes, 56 questions, binary format with weightings (Hutchinson *et al.*, 1979; Kramer *et al.*, 1979; Leventhal *et al.*, 1979).
7. Naranjo *et al.*'s method—ten questions, yes, no, don't know (Naranjo *et al.*, 1981).
8. Lagier *et al.*'s method—balanced assessment, 16 factors plus analogue scale (Lagier *et al.*, 1983).
9. FDA (Jones') method—six questions, binary format (Jones, 1982).
10. Ruskin's variation of the above method—seven questions, binary format (Stephens, 1988).
11. Australian probability rating—definitions, 1978 (Mashford, 1984).
12. Swedish criteria—seven different criteria (Wiholm, 1984).
13. Committee for the safety of Medicines (CSM) (Weber's) method—ten questions, binary format (Weber, 1980).
14. Venulet *et al.*'s method—27 questions, analogue scale, weightings (Venulet *et al.*, 1980); updated (Venulet *et al.*, 1986).
15. Emanueli and Sacchetti's method—eight questions (Emanueli and Sacchetti, 1978 and 1982).
16. Cornelli's method—five headings, 21 questions (Cornelli, 1984).
17. Farina *et al.*'s methods modified Karch and Lasagna method—six questions (Farina *et al.*, 1978).
18. Stephens' personal scoring method—72 questions, weightings (Stephens, 1984).
19. Maistrello *et al.*'s method—depressed patients, Hamilton rating scale, binary format, weightings (Maistrello *et al.*, 1983).
20. Stricker and Spoelstra's method—liver events, diagnostic decision tree, weightings (Stricker and Spoelstra, 1985).
21. Ruskin's method, drug-associated death—eight questions, binary format, 1985 (Stephens, 1988).
22. Loupi *et al.*'s method, teratogenic effect—three main questions, binary format (Loupi *et al.*, 1986).

23. ADRIAN (Adverse Drug Reaction Interactive Advice Network) Educational—15 factors (Castle, 1991).
24. Jain's triage method—seven questions (Jain, 1995).
25. Jannsen Research Foundation's method—15 questions integrated methods 4, 7 and 8, 1992 (Vervaet and Amery, 1992).
26. Benichou and Danan's method. 7 criteria, weightings, organ oriented (Danan and Bénichou, 1993).
27. EEC definitions, A, B and O categories (Meyboom and Royer, 1992).
28. Kitaguchi's method—six questions (Kitaguchi *et al.*, 1983).
29. Spain's method—four headings each with 4–7 alternatives, weightings (Meyboom and Royer, 1992).
30. Variations on definitions from Belgium, Greece, Italy, Netherlands and Portugal (Meyboom and Royer, 1992).
31. WHO method, index cases are defined (not really a causality method) (Edwards *et al.*, 1990).
32. Bayesian Adverse Reaction Diagnostic Instrument (BARDI) method—a Bayesian method (Auriche, 1985; Lane, 1984; Naranjo 1986).
33. Computer-based decision support algorithm (Hoskins and Mannino, 1992).
34. TAIWAN (Triage Application for Imputologists Without An Interesting Name)—see appendix 3.
35. Hsu-Stoll method—seven questions in a algorithmic format (Hsu and Stoll, 1993b).
36. Fuzzy reasoning (Lanctôt *et al.*, 1996).

There is a large literature on these various methods. Methods 1–22 have been outlined in a review (Stephens, 1987). Further details are available from the Active Permanent Workshop of Imputology (APWI) (contact Professor Bégaud at the Université Victor Segalen—Bordeaux 2; see page 319).

Two of these methods require more discussion.

Clinical Differential Diagnosis

This is sometimes referred to as 'global introspection'. It is the normal diagnostic process with any illness associated with a drug. When the same cases have been assessed by different physicians there has been a wide divergence in their opinions (Dangoumau *et al.*, 1980). Complete agreement between three clinical pharmacologists and the treating physician occurred in 47% of cases (Karch *et al.*, 1976). In a further study three clinical pharmacologists judged only 21% of the AEs reported by the treating physician as due to drug (Dangoumau *et al.*, 1980). It was as a result of these disagreements that many of the algorithms mentioned above were produced. In 1986 Lane and Hutchinson wrote a paper discussing the merits and faults of many of the methods and gave six criteria by which causality methods should be judged (Lane and Hutchinson, 1986). This paper is not easily obtainable, but the essence was distilled in a paper by one of the authors (Hutchinson, 1986) and this is more readily available. The six criteria used are:

1. Repeatability—given the same information different assessors should reach the same conclusion.

2. Explicitness—The method should require its user to make explicit his 'state of information' and to state their degree of uncertainty about each element of information.
3. Explanatory capability—from the information users must be able to explain how they reached their conclusion.
4. Completeness—the user must be able to incorporate any fact, theory or opinion that can affect the assessment.
5. Biological balancing—the probability that the suspect drug caused the AE must be weighed against the probability that an alternative candidate caused it. It is not sufficient to consider whether the evidence is for or against the suspect drug without weighing up the evidence in favour of another cause.
6. No a priori constraints on the effects of any factor—that is, no score or specific weighting given before the assessment.

If a test for the drug relatedness of an AE had a 100% sensitivity and 100% specificity the fact that it was positive should outweigh any other factor. It is a great pity that such a test does not exist.

Examination of 'clinical differential diagnosis' is necessary to see why there is such disagreement. The amount of knowledge of fact and experience will differ from physician to physician and in the papers referred to their state of information was not made explicit, and there was no attempt to explain how they reached their conclusion. We cannot tell whether they meet the criteria of completeness or no a priori constraints. When the algorithms were examined by the same criteria none of the methods were found to be satisfactory. The algorithms will give greater concordance, but that is due to the reduced number of facts they use. The fewer the questions the more likely is agreement. If only one question is asked 'Are you 100% certain that the drug caused the AE?' there should be almost complete agreement—'No!'. The only method that meets all the criteria is the use of Bayes' theorem.

Criteria for assessing causality methods Repeatability, Explicitness, Explanatory capacity, Completeness, Biological balancing, No a priori constraints

---

Bayes' Theorem

"The theorem expresses the relation that should exist between the probability of a proposition evaluated before and after the acquisition of new data" (Lane *et al.*, 1987). The prior probability is based on the information available before the case(s) under assessment arose. The 'likelihood' is the probability of observing the new data given that the proposition is true. The posterior probability is the probability of the proposal after the new data—present case(s)—are considered. It is usually expressed in an odds form (i.e. the ratio of the probability that the proposition is true to the position that it is not true):

$$\text{Posterior odds} = \text{Prior odds} \times \text{likelihood ratio} \qquad (1)$$

The posterior odds is expressed as **P**robability (**D**rug caused the **E**vent given the **B**ackground information and the **C**ase information), written:

$$P(D \Rightarrow E/B.C) \tag{2}$$

While the opposite is written:

$$P(A \Rightarrow E/B.C.) \tag{3}$$

where A stands for alternative causes:

$$\frac{P(D \Rightarrow E/B.C.)}{P(A \Rightarrow E/B.C.)} \tag{4}$$

$$\text{The prior odds} = \frac{P(D \Rightarrow E/B)}{P(A \Rightarrow E/B)} \tag{5}$$

$$\text{The likelihood ratio} = \frac{P(C/D \Rightarrow E, B)}{P(C/A \Rightarrow E, B)} \tag{6}$$

So

$$\frac{P(D \Rightarrow E/B.C)}{P(A \Rightarrow E/B.C)} = \frac{P(D \Rightarrow E/B)}{P(A \Rightarrow E/B)} \times \frac{P(C/D \Rightarrow E/B)}{P(C/A \Rightarrow E/B)} \tag{7}$$

In the likelihood ratio (LR) the case information is broken down into its constituents of history (Hi), timing (Ti), characteristics of the event (Ch), dechallenge (De) and rechallenge (Re).

$$LR = LR(Hi) \times LR(Ti) \times LR(Ch) \times LR(De) \times LR(Re) \tag{8}$$

Each constituent is therefore calculated conditionally on the case information that precedes it, and expressed as the odds ratio:

$$LR(Ti) = \frac{P(Ti/D \Rightarrow E, B, Hi)}{P(Ti/A \Rightarrow E, B, Hi)} \tag{9}$$

Each drug has to be evaluated separately.

There are now many papers on this subject, but the essential paper is that of Lane *et al.*, (1987). This is really a subject where one needs 'to drink deep or taste not the Pierean stream'. Considerable ongoing experience using this method is necessary and it is unlikely that those in industry or the regulatory authorities would have sufficient number of cases to warrant using it.

The Bayes' theorem meets all the criteria mentioned, but does have some problems. The prior odds usually involves a meta-analysis of previous clinical trials or epidemiological studies to establish the previous incidence of the event in the correct subgroup. The LR needs an expert(s) in the field of the AE to judge the timings and uncertainties. All this takes time and access to databases and experts. It should be considered when the possibility of an ADR is of considerable importance to the company and patients. The two centres with a great deal of experience are Professor C. Naranjo, Psychopharmacology Research Program, University of Toronto, Canada (Lanctôt *et al.*, 1995) and Dr J. Jones, The Degge Group Ltd, 1616 Northfort Myer Drive, Suite 1430, Arlington VA 22209, USA.

Use in Clinical Trials

Most clinical trial AE report forms have space for the investigator's opinion as to the causality. For reasons expressed above some regulatory authorities place little credence on investigators' opinions. An analysis of six studies showed that the investigators' assessments were consistent with conventional causality expectations and that all the known factors which were treatment and dose-related had been used (Hsu and Stoll, 1993a).

Summary

Normal clinical diagnosis is probably the fastest and most practical method if used by an experienced clinician both for classification and for full assessment. Algorithms are suitable for triage by non-medically qualified staff. Bayes' theorem is best considered for particularly important ADR issues.

Signal Recognition

The purpose of signal recognition is to recognize when one or more AEs represent a probable ADR requiring some sort of action by the pharmacovigilance (PV) department. This usually involves searching the database at certain times as well as having an observant member of staff viewing the data as they are received.

There is a wide variation in the frequency with which companies examine their databases for signals. A survey of 25 major companies around the world showed that seven did ad hoc examinations of the database and 23 did them regularly so some did ad hoc examinations as well as a regular search. These regular searches again varied widely: three made weekly checks, one fortnightly, three monthly, six three-monthly, eleven six-monthly and two annually (Stephens, 1997). Different kinds of AE need different approaches and the individual companies' responses were as follows:

1. Unlabelled serious were dealt with monthly and unlabelled six-monthly.
2. Every six months for the first two years after launch and then yearly.
3. New products monthly (weekly scan) and old products six-monthly to yearly.
4. Frequency three-monthly and new reactions weekly.
5. Marketed products three-monthly and all drugs in depth annually. Phase I and II watched very closely, phase III monitored by special clinical trial physician group
6. As a minimum annually, but more frequently if needed.
7. All serious unlabelled cases and all 'alert' terms monthly, three-monthly, six-monthly and annually.
8. Every month a physician and an epidemiologist follow an SOP (i.e in a detailed and formal way), the computer giving a monthly listing on all drugs for all AEs in the last month, the previous month, the month before that, the total for the year, the last year, the year before that and the total on the database. There is a total cross reference to each case.
9. Automated signal recognition. This gives for each AE the number of cases so far, the number of cases as a percentage of the total number of AEs, the average

causality for all the cases of that event and the number of probable and almost certain cases so far. This is printed out monthly. Previously case by case review at time of receipt.

10. Takeda Tracks, Reports, Alerts and Communication (TRAC) system (Sakurai *et al.*, 1995).
11. A monthly reviewing of listings and an annual review at the time of the FDA annual report preparation.
12. At variable times. When a manager has seen a number of cases, at the time of quarterly reports (all compounds in development and marketed drugs), at the time of *ad hoc* searches.
13. During the writing of CIOMS reports (six-monthly), following requests for information (random), following 'interesting' reports.
14. At regular intervals (e.g. before starting a periodic safety update).
15. As cases come in—two-weekly, plus formal at six-monthly update.
16. Every six months as well as on an ad hoc basis.
17. At least monthly. Interval count of each event per drug compared to previous quarters plus ad hoc in each instance where newly received information arouses suspicion of 'something interesting'.
18. Rules for triggering labelling review for particular AE.
19. Ad hoc and at safety update occasions.
20. Regularly.
21. Weekly review of all serious unlabelled, semi-annual review of all unlabelled (according to USA data sheet).
22. About every six months as required by the Committee for Proprietary Medicinal Products (CPMP) guidelines.
23. The database is frequently searched in response to internal and external queries. Monthly compilations are made and analysed for each project/product.
24. At the time of periodic reports lists of labelled versus non-labelled events are generated and the need for label changes considered.
25. When CIOMS II reports are prepared (every six months) or ad hoc.

The next problem is deciding what represents a signal. The World Health Organization (WHO) uses three 'index' cases (Edwards *et al.*, 1990). An 'index' case is one that contains information on all eleven major items and the absence of any confounding variables. The major items are:

- Information of source of the case.
- Identification of the case.
- Description of the reaction.
- Name of the drug.
- Treatment dates.
- Reaction date.
- Age.
- Sex.
- All drugs with doses and dates.
- Indication for treatment/underlying disease.
- Outcome.

If the first six items are present it is called a 'feasible' case. If the last five items are present it is called a 'substantial' case. An index case is equivalent to two 'substantial' cases or four 'feasible' cases. It is suggested that before publishing that there should be three 'index' cases or their equivalent, but there should be at least one 'index' case (Edwards *et al.*, 1990). A 'signal' will depend also upon the unexpectedness of an AE and this can be calculated from:

1. The background incidence of the disease in the considered population.
2. The number of patients treated by the drug under study.
3. The duration of the follow-up.

Using this method on the basis of 300 000 patients treated the probability of observing at least three cases was calculated for four diseases (Table 1).

The conclusion was that three cases constituted a strong signal requiring *ad hoc* investigation (Bégaud *et al.*, 1995).

However, the strength of signal required will depend upon what action follows from the signal. The pharmaceutical industry does not publish details about ADRs and so usually the use of signals is for internal action such as prompting a data sheet change by the company or, during clinical development, deciding on further action. Within the pharmacovigilance department one should be looking for 'straws in the wind' so that the responsible person can be on the lookout for similar cases. To quote Dr J. Johnson from the FDA "Generating the initial signal is probably as much an art as it is a science, and requires natural curiosity and a thorough pharmacologic background" (Johnson *et al.*, 1993). Of 25 companies surveyed, 11 had no definition for what comprised a signal and of the remaining 14, six used increased frequency and nine used unexpected cases. The approaches used by the companies were:

(a) One or more ADRs not yet described in the data sheet.
(b) Serious new event very likely to be causally related or increased frequency of serious known event.
(c) Any significant change in frequency of known ADR or appearance of unexpected ADR.
(d) All serious unlabelled cases are always reviewed and previous cases in the same rubric listed.
(e) New reactions or increased frequency of known reaction.
(f) Seven new reports since the last review or positive rechallenge or any other suspicion by reviewer.

Table 1 The probability of 3 cases occurring in 4 other drug-alerted diseases

	One month Expected No.	Probability of three cases	One year Expected No.	Probability of three cases
Agranulocytosis	0.150	0.0005	1.800	0.27
Toxic epidermal necrolysis	0.030	0.000004	0.360	0.006
Guillain-Barré syndrome	0.625	0.026	7.500	0.98
Creutzfeldt-Jakob syndrome	0.025	0.000003	0.300	0.0036

(g)   Logic system grades AE either 'AA' or 'A' for serious unexpected cases and 'BB' or 'B' for unlabelled AEs.

(h)   Varies by therapeutic area, increased frequency in general, many rules apply.

(i)   Unexpected (according to company core data sheet) or WHO critical term.

(j)   Increased frequency or seriousness, a 'particular AE' has occurred.

(k)   Any new finding that could modify risk–benefit assessment (nature, severity, frequency of events).

(l)   Pattern in spontaneous reporting suggestive of possible previously unknown causal association.

(m)   Unexpectedness or change in frequency.

(n)   No definition, but consider any cases that may lead to a labelling change or mention in the investigator's brochure; unexpectedness or change in frequency are important.

(o)   It is a matter of medical judgement and subjective feeling.

(p)   Subjective perceptions of trends, increased incidences etc.

(q)   An indication from drug safety surveillance that a particular AE or AEs have occurred or that their frequency of occurrence or severity is increased. They are generally unlabelled and may or may not be serious and may or may not be caused by the drug.

(r)   New reports since last review or positive rechallenge triggers consideration or any other suspicion by reviewer.

(s)   Signals are detected by means of 'medical judgement'.

From these approaches used by the 25 companies we can distil a list of factors that they considered:

(i)   Probability that the event is an ADR, reviewing only those cases that are probable or almost certain as a signal.

(ii)   The type of AE. Increased monitoring for serious cases rather than non-serious. Creating a hypothesis on very few cases of certain AEs that are frequently caused by drugs (e.g. TEN). Common type A AEs are usually best counted and use an increased frequency formula.

(iii)   Pre- or post-marketing. Those drugs still in clinical development will need monitoring on a daily basis. During the first two years of post-marketing closer monitoring is needed than after two years.

(iv)   Labelled or unlabelled. Labelled ADRs probably do not need a causality assessment, but will need to be monitored for a change in frequency. Unlabelled AEs need a more frequent search for signals than labelled ADR.

(v)   Amount of data. Some reports have too little data to allow individual assessment and can only be counted.

(vi)   Type of drug. Different drugs or therapeutic areas will often need a different monitoring regimen.

(vii)   Background disease. Those diseases with a high morbidity or/and mortality may require the counting of AEs rather than individual assessments (e.g. myocardial infarctions in an angina trial).

(viii)   Subjective judgement. This is probably one of the most important factors and, if possible, the same person should see all the AEs for a particular drug.

On the output side:

(ix)   Regulatory reports are an obvious time for searches of the database for signals.

(x)   Internal and external queries will prompt inspection of some areas.

(xi)   Computerized output. Several of the methods depend upon a routine output of specific events.

> **Important factors in signal recognition** Probability of an ADR, Type of AE, Type of drug, Labelled or unlabelled, Serious or non-serious, Amount of data, Subjective judgement, Background disease(s), Periodic regulatory reports, Change in frequency or severity, Computerized programmes

Conclusions

It is clear that each pharmaceutical company needs to consider its own requirements over and above those required by the regulations. Regulatory authorities cannot calculate a figure since, as it has been seen, the degree of underreporting is difficult to calculate for a specific AE (see pages 4–8). The WHO figure of three or its equivalent has little scientific justification, but seems a 'reasonable' figure for the WHO to use. It relies basically on causality assessment and adequate information. If the methods for calculating a figure for underreporting and the expected figure for specific diseases are extended the regulatory authorities would require more staff.

The MCA have devised a useful tool for helping in signal recognition called the Proportional Reporting Ratio (PRR), which compares the proportion of reactions to a drug, which are of a particular type, with the analogous proportion for all drugs forming a 2 × 2 table.

	Drug of interest	All other drugs
Reaction of interest	A	B
All other reactions	C	D

The PRR is A × D/B × C.

The screening is according to defined criteria. These might be

$$A\ Signal = (PRR > 3) + (Chi\text{-}squared > 5) + (Number\ of\ cases > 3)$$

One is reminded that this is only one aspect of causality assessment and that the PRRs are still subject to the usual biases inherent in spontaneous reporting (Waller, 1998). A similar approach is also used by the Drug Research Safety Unit, Southampton.

The 'Signal Cascade'

So far the various pharmaceutical company practices have been described and conclusions have been drawn from them. The signals and the subsequent actions can also be considered as a continuum of signals of increasing strength or actions of increasing importance. It is important that the actions taken following a signal are appropriate and proportionate to the strength of the signal. The first signal may be two or three similar cases that strike one as unusual; these are the 'straws in the wind'. An appropriate action would be to follow-up the cases and make certain that any information that would help identify their cause is obtained. If this information confirms a likely relationship to the drug the signal is strengthened and the next appropriate action is to search the drug database for any similar cases. If further cases are discovered either in the database or are subsequently reported in the course of time other factors will come into play depending upon the type of cases etc. Subsequent actions (Figure 1) may include:

- Creating a special questionnaire or form for collecting additional information on an ongoing basis.
- Adding further investigations to subsequent clinical trials.
- Setting up a special clinical trial, toxological study or epidemiological study to help solve the problem.
- Setting up a panel of experts from within and without the company to debate the problem.
- Adding the AE to the investigator's brochure or data sheet.
- Stopping the clinical trial programme.

As the signal is strengthened (or weakened) by each successive action, another action (or inaction) becomes appropriate. Actions taken will depend upon the following factors:

- The seriousness of the AE.
- The incidence rate of the AE in the drug-treated population.
- The incidence of the AE in a control population.

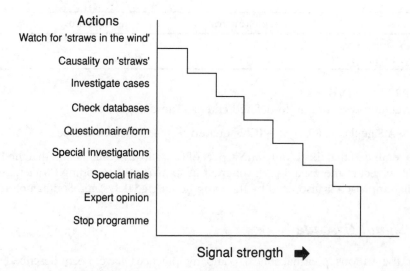

Figure 1   The strength of the signal must be reflected by an appropriate action

- The probability that the signal cases are due to the drug rather than to other causes.
- Whether the incidence of the AEs can be restricted by defining a susceptible subgroup.
- The seriousness of the indication.
- The risk–benefit of the drug before the signal.
- The risk–benefit of alternative drugs for treatment of the same indication.
- The cost in time, labour and money of any possible actions.
- Whether the pharmaceutical company's pharmacovigilance department is proactive or reactive. 'Reactive' means how quickly the company responds to a recognized signal. Some companies, although they have recognized a signal, take no action to change their data sheet until told to do so by a regulatory authority.

It should be clear that the strength of each of these factors may be different and no formula or algorithm can cope with the almost infinite variations. The appropriate action is therefore a matter of judgement when all available information has been collected.

Group Assessment

When a signal arises each of the probable cases needs reappraisal and, if necessary, further information is sought and a full assessment made of each of these cases both separately and combined. The latter assessment needs to consider some additional factors over and above those required for individual assessment. These factors used for judging studies are:

- Strength—refers to how significant the difference is between the active drug group and the placebo group in any studies performed to date. Unfortunately the type B ADRs are often too rare for this to be of help, but a few of the large simple studies now recommended for marketed drugs have tackled this problem (Castle *et al.*, 1993; Mitchell and Lesko, 1995).
- Dose-response of an ADR—this may be noticeable in a group of cases when compared with the average dose used before the assessment.
- Temporality—this is not a problem with spontaneous reports or clinical trials, but can be in case–control studies.
- Consistency—this implies that the AE has been seen in different studies, groups, and countries rather that in a single centre or group.
- Specificity of an ADR—this is rare since they normally mimic a naturally occurring event, but 'scalp tingling' with labetalol is a good example.
- Plausibility—in the sense of making biological sense this is very helpful, but the mechanism of a new or bizarre ADR may not be discovered until long after it is acknowledged as an ADR (e.g. tendon rupture with the fluoroquinolone antibiotics).
- Reversibility on stopping the drug—this applies equally to group assessment.

Four references each cover this subject—Sackett *et al.*, (1985), Stolley, (1990), Levine (1992), Glynn, (1993).

It is wise to imagine that every causality assessment made will be challenged by an experienced barrister in a court of law. This practice will help prepare you for explaining the situation to the marketing director.

Association or causation   Strength, Dose–response, Temporality, Consistency, Specificity, Plausibility, Reversibility

---

Terms

The product of causality assessment is a phrase indicating the likelihood that the drug caused the event and there are numerous variations. The more alternatives there are the narrower each term becomes. The terms 'certain', 'definitely related' and 'definite' and their opposites should be avoided because certainty is not a characteristic of causality assessments, so 'not related' should be reserved for those occasions when the drug was not given or given after the event. It should not be a judgemental term. The essential terms are the equivalent of the EEC grades 'A', 'B', 'O' (i.e. 'probable', 'possible', 'unlikely' or 'unassessable' (Meyboom and Royer, 1992). The topic was fully explored in Professor Venulet's book *Assessing Causes of ADR* (see Bibliography).

Many of the causality methods mentioned have their own range of terms. A novel approach was taken in the Serevent study of leaving out 'possible' so that there were four terms—'definitely related', 'probably related', 'probably unrelated', or 'definitely unrelated' (Castle *et al.*, 1993). The two extreme terms should be avoided, while the absence of 'possible' may force someone who genuinely believes that the probabilities are equal, to hazard a guess. This will probably result in more 'probably unrelateds' than 'probably relateds' due to a subconscious opinion that a drug is innocent until proven guilty.

A yes/no answer is possible if the question is "Is there a reasonable possibility that the event may have been caused by the trial therapy?" This has the advantage in that it answers the question asked by the regulatory authorities. There are concerns that an opinion given by an individual assessor will leave pharmaceutical companies more open to legal liability suits. This is more understandable if the extreme terms, already mentioned, are used, but the very vagueness of the words, 'probable', 'possible' and 'unlikely' help to express the uncertainty of clinical judgement and must surely make them easier to defend in a law court. An excellent paper by Dr J. Jones reviewed the subject in *Pharmacoepidemiology and Drug Safety* (Jones, 1992). Bayes' theorem results in an odds ratio rather that a vague word.

Each pharmaceutical company has different needs and philosophies concerning assessments and signal recognition. Signals come in different strengths and at first these may only be 'straws in the wind' or a hunch. The response to a signal will depend upon its strength. The weaker signals probably only warrant trying to obtain more information about the signal cases. Stronger signals may warrant searching the whole of that product's database. The strongest signals may justify looking at other databases worldwide (post-marketing) or starting new studies with a definite hypothesis. Each signal will need an individual response.

Suggested further reading is 'A reader's guide to the evaluation of causation'. (Podrebarac *et al.*, 1996) and 'Principles of signal detection in pharmacovigilance' (Meyboom *et al.*, 1997).

Chapter 12

Pharmacovigilance Centres

Nicholas Moore, Bernard Bégaud

Department of Pharmacology, Université Victor Segalen—Bordeaux 2, 33076 Bordeaux, France

National and International Pharmacovigilance Centres and Processes

Spontaneous reporting is the mainstay of the regulatory surveillance of adverse drug reactions (ADRs). Most countries have set up the structures necessary to receive, process and analyse these reports. These structures and processes are usually defined by law. In the European Union (EU), these are described in national laws, but also in Community directive 75/319 and regulation 2309/93.

Reporting Pathways

Typically, a health professional observing an adverse event (AE) possibly related to the use of a drug (ADR), should report it. In some countries, notably the EU, only reports by health professionals will be considered, in others lay persons may also report. In certain countries (e.g. France), reporting is mandatory, though it is not certain whether this obligation has any impact on the reporting rates. Other countries insist on reporting of all reactions to recently marketed drugs (e.g. the 'black triangle' drugs in the UK), or of serious reactions, or of reactions that are not mentionned in the summary of product characteristics (i.e. unlabelled or 'unexpected' reactions) (Moore *et al.*, 1994).

Cases may also be reported to the pharmaceutical company—holder of marketing authorization (HMA) or marketing authorization holder (MAH)—to a professional organization, or to an officially empowered structure, which may be part of the regulatory process or act as an advisory resource, and may be centralized or regionally distributed.

The relative share of reporting to these different instances varies from country to country. For example, in the UK or Spain, most reports are sent to the national authorities—Medicines Control Agency (MCA) in the UK, regional centres in Spain—

whereas in Germany, most of the reports are intially sent to the HMA, and in France the reporting is about equally distributed between the HMA and regional centres. In Germany, some of the reporting is also to the physicians' professional organization. In the Netherlands, regional centres are managed by a non-profit foundation, Landelijke Registiratie Evaluatie Bijwerkingen (LAREB), under contract to the National authority.

Reports are then forwarded from the HMA, professional bodies, and regional centres, to the national authority. The forwarding periodicity may vary from country to country. Under European regulations, serious reports (i.e. fatal, life-threatening, causing or prolonging hospitalization, or disabling or incapacitating) must be forwarded by the HMA to national authorities within 15 days. In turn, and with the same delay national authorities must forward such reports to the HMA concerned. Non-serious reports to HMA are included in periodic safety updates, the periodicity depending upon the concerned drug's market age. Some national authorities insist that all reports worldwide are sent; others insist only on national reports, with summaries for other reports.

Beyond the individual national authorities, adverse reaction reports may be forwarded to supranational bodies, essentially the World Health Organization (WHO) and the European Medicines Evaluation Agency (EMEA).

The EMEA receives all reports of serious ADRs associated with centrally approved drugs occuring within the member states of the European Union, and is informed of reports concerning drugs approved according to the mutual recognition procedure. Reports are received within the 15-day time frame mentioned above, from the national centres. It has regulatory authority. (The EMEA can be found at http://www.eudra.org/home.html, with a list of links to other regulatory authorities.) In contrast the WHO Collaborating Centre for International Drug Monitoring, in Uppsala, Sweden, has no regulatory authority. It receives reports from all countries participating in the programme, including both serious and non-serious reports. Its main objectives are to analyse these data, providing alert as necessary if problems are identified. It also works on new ways and methods for analysing the data (see http://www.who.pharmasoft.se).

Analysing the Reports: Generating and Responding to Alerts

Reports are input to a database situated within the regulatory authority, though some subcontract database administration to the Uppsala centre. Data input may be more or less exhaustive, including for example for the UK, images of the actual reports.

Reports may be analyzed manually before input or the database may be analyzed automatically at given intervals or when each report is entered. This screening can look for new drug–reaction pairs, or 'critical terms' for reactions or for specific outcomes (fatal cases, fetal abnormalities). The alert may be triggered when a pre-determined number of reports has been reached (e.g. three reports) (Tubert *et al.*, 1991), or when the frequency of the reaction reported exceeds a predetermined threshold, often in comparison with the rest of the database (Edwards *et al.*, 1990; Meyboom *et al.*, 1997).

The analysis can be done by the central regulatory authority, even in those countries with regional centres (e.g. in Spain analysis is done by Instituto de Salud

Carlos III, which acts as advisor to the Ministry of Health), or by the regional centres as in France.

The results of these alert generating analyses are usually discussed by boards or committees, such as the Pharmacovigilance Technical Committee in France, which decides whether a formal alert procedure should be started. If this is the case, the relevant reaction reports will be further analyzed and compared to sales or prescription figures. An alert report will be produced and discussed by an advisory committee—Committee for the Safety of Medicines (CSM) in the UK, Pharmacovigilance Commission in France—and/or appropriate experts, which give recommendations for adapted measures to prevent further risk. These measures are finally decided upon by the Minister of Health or the Director of the National Agency. Within the EU, the emergence of an alert within a country will give rise to a 'rapid alert' procedure whereby the country identifying the alert informs the Committee for Proprietary Medicinal Products (CPMP) at the EMEA, and all other member states, if possible before making a decision. These in turn evaluate the alert in their countries and report back to the originating state, which compiles all answers and reports to the CPMP. The CPMP then makes a decision, recommendation or opinion, which gives guidance on the management of the alert, which may be binding. The results of this process are then sent back to the HMA (which has an opportunity to comment and give further information at various stages in this process), to the member states, and finally to the medical and general public.

If and as necessary, of course, these authorities also rely on further information beyond the spontaneous reports such as experimental studies, clinical trials, pharmacoepidemiological studies and drug utilization studies, to arrive at a decision. Differences between countries related to differing drug usage and medical culture may in some instances make a common decision difficult. However, when the decision has been made to remove a drug from the market or severely restrict its use, this usually applies to all countries where the drug is marketed, through either common decisions by the regulatory authorities, or through a worldwide decision by the product manufacturer (Edwards, 1993).

Harmonization

The data needed to make a report valid, the way the report can be sent from the HMA to the drug regulatory authority and back, the content of the regular safety update reports and the terminology to be used have been the object of ongoing harmonization for a number of years. The premier in this field was the CIOMS (Council for the International Organization of Medical Sciences), a group of experts that gave recommendations on a number of subjects, the first of which (in the field of pharmacovigilance) was a common format for the international reporting of ADRs (Royer and Bénichou, 1991). Other CIOMS initiatives have covered regular safety updates, use of terminology and evaluation of the risk–benefit ratio (Bénichou, 1990; CIOMS, 1990; Royer and Bénichou, 1991).

These harmonization endeavours have been complemented by others. For instance, European guidelines have been produced by the CPMP for the proper conduct of pharmacovigilance, by the HMA (the 'Notice to Applicants'), and by the regulatory authorities.

The ultimate harmonization body, the International Conference for Harmonization (ICH), which includes representatives from regulatory authorities and professional bodies from Europe, USA and Japan, has picked up and forwarded a number of these harmonization processes, including data elements for individual case reports (topic E2b), for regular safety updates (E2c), for terminology (M1), and other topics (see http://www.ifpma.org/ich1.html for an overview of the ICH process and the guidelines). In time ICH guidelines are worked into the national laws.

Research

In addition to the ongoing evolution of methods for the evaluation of drug-induced risk, generated at each alert, there are some research initiatives, both methodological and applied, funded by public sources such as the European Community's BIOMED program or national programs, or by private grants. Examples of such research teams could be, for Europe, the European Pharmacovigilance Research Group (EPRG), or the Eurohepatox group, which look into applied research concerning, for example, reporting patterns across the EU, or the setting up of registries of rare, often drug-induced, diseases (e.g. agranulocytosis, toxic epidermal necrolysis) (the Euronet project within the EPRG), or the mechanisms of drug-induced hepatotoxicity. Others are more methodological, such as the Association pour la Recherche Méthologique en Pharmacovigilance (ARME-P) in Bordeaux, or a recent Cochrane Collaboration methods working group on the evaluation of safety.

Regional Pharmacovigilance Centres

Some national pharmacovigilance systems, such as the French, Spanish, Dutch and Swedish systems, and possibly others in the future (German, Polish, Italian) are based on a network of regional centres, whose activities and roles are essentially similar. These centres are coordinated by a national agency or ministry, with some differences in the relative responsibilities of regional and national centres in data processing and analysis. The description below applies to the French regional pharmacovigilance centres, but it can also, with minor modifications, be adapted to other countries. As a broad rule of thumb, the structure of the French regionalized system can be viewed by analogy to the European structure (Figure 1).

The typical centre is part of a department of pharmacology, clinical pharmacology, or clinical toxicology. Its staff is composed of full or part-time physicians or pharmacists, of varying seniority. In addition to the core personnel dedicated to the day-to-day functions of the centre (between one and two full-time equivalents, mostly medically qualified), other personnel, mainly academic, but also PhD or postdoctoral fellows, interns, etc., participate in specific activities such as teaching or research within the larger department of which the centre is a part (Moore *et al.*, 1985; Royer, 1990; Bégaud *et al.*, 1994).

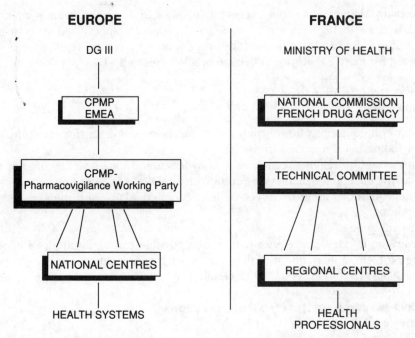

Figure 1 The European and French regionalized Pharmacovigilance Systems

Missions of Regional Pharmacovigilance Centres

These are defined by legal requirements, as set down in the decree of July 30, 1982 (revised March 13, 1995), and the Good Pharmacovigilance Practices (which can be obtained from the French Medicines Agency) (Anon, 1995).

Collect Adverse Drug Reaction Reports from Health Professionals

The ADR reports are to be:

- Assessed for completeness, follow-up.
- Classified for seriousness/novelty.
- Subjected to causality assessment.
- Assessed for alert value.
- Input into the national pharmacovigilance database.

Causality assessment means studying the temporal and semiological (signs and symptoms) association of the reaction with all possibly involved drugs, including those recently discontinued, independently from the reporter's opinion, using a predetermined method or algorithm. The systematic use of causality assessment on all cases also serves to control completeness of the case, identify essential missing data, and harmonize case management across different centres.

Alert value generally applies to serious, previously unknown or rarely described reactions with high causality scores to new drugs, or to special high-risk situations (e.g. pregnancy, children, preventive medicines). This implies ready access to a case report database and to the literature.

Receiving ADR reports is not necessarily passive. In a regional setting, where the centre is close to hospital wards, these, and especially specialized units such as haematology, dermatology, hepatology and nephrology can be regularly visited or contacted for more exhaustive collection of all or selected ADRs.

Serve as Drug Information Centres

This involves:

- Answering questions from health professionals regarding any aspect of drug use (including but not limited to ADRs).
- Promoting the regional centre as a knowledge and expertise resource in drug therapy, including management of individual ADRs, and their prevention.
- Using questions as leads for possible unreported ADRs, and thereby promote reporting.
- Recording questions.
- Assessing information request patterns for possible early indications of impending problem or alert, and for indication of teaching/educational need (Trechot *et al.*, 1990; Haramburu *et al.*, 1993; Graille *et al.*, 1994; Norsdkvist *et al.*, 1997).

Conduct Research on Adverse Drug Reactions

This involves:

- Researching ADR mechanisms, including experimental exploration of possible mechanisms (pharmacological, pharmacogenetic, interaction), individual (n of one) trials, pharmacokinetic exploration, clinical pharmacology.
- Researching ADR epidemiology, including pharmacoepidemiological studies, drug use.
- Research on methodology of ADR assessment, including epidemiological or statistical methods, causality, use of pre-marketing or pre-clinical data, etc.

This places the regional centre in the midst of a web of cooperations with other research resources including:

- Other parts of the pharmacology department (experimental pharmacology, pharmacokinetics, clinical pharmacology).
- Other fundamental research teams (e.g. for pharmacogenetics or molecular biology).
- Fundamental statistical or epidemiology units for methods research and modelling.
- The clinical specialist units.
- Networks of health professionals (general practitioners, pharmacists) for field studies.
- The pharmaceutical industry.

Teaching Pharmacovigilance

This is discussed on page 326.

Participation in Decision-making Processes

This involves participation:

- Locally—drug selection boards in hospitals (formulary committees), institutional review boards (ethics committees).
- Nationally—Pharmacovigilance Technical Committee, National Commission, Licensing Board.
- Internationally—serving as a national expert resource pool in international settings (CPMP, ICH, CIOMS).

Communication in Pharmacovigilance

Communication with regional centres can be envisioned as 'upwards' with national regulatory administration and through it, with the EMEA, WHO, other national drug regulatory authorities (DRAs), 'sideways' with other regional centres, and pharmaceutical industry HMAs, and 'downwards', with health professionals in the region covered by the centre (Figure 2).

With National Drug Regulatory Authority
The regional centres send:

- Individual ADR reports—directly input to a common database or sent using electronic report forms (ICH E2b / M2). These will then be retransmitted according to national and European regulations to the EMEA, the HMA, other DRAs, the WHO.
- Reports on national enquiries. These can be investigations into suspected or confirmed alerts. The source of the alert may be within the system (regional, national) or from the EMEA or other countries ('rapid alert' procedure). Alternatively they may be systematic investigations of selected new chemical entities, post-marketing. These investigations always include a review of all cases reported in the country to the regional centres or to the HMA, with the person responsible for pharmacovigilance of the HMA and experts. A report is generated, which is

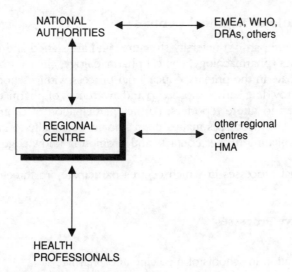

Figure 2   Communication in Pharmacovigilance

validated by national processes (technical committee, national commission), then send by the DRA to other DRAs, the EMEA and the CPMP.

The centres receive:

- Instructions on alerts to process and investigations to pursue, as discussed at technical committee meetings or received from the EMEA, CPMP, or other sources and despatched by the DRA.
- Results of decisional processes (national commission, CPMP).

With Other Centres, the Holder of the Marketing Authorization
Centres exchange:

- Case reports for evaluation in management of alert procedure.
- Help in managing questions or cases (according to individual expertise of different centres).
- Evaluation reports (other regional centres, HMA involved) for discussion.

With Health Professionals
Centres receive:

- ADR case reports and further information (e.g. on outcome).
- Information requests (questions).

Centres send out:

- Evaluation of case reports and requests for further information on individual cases.
- Answers to questions.
- Results of analysis of alerts by national commission, CPMP (decisions, opinions).
- Local drug bulletin.

Centres also provide teaching (see below).

Educational Role of Regional Centres

Regional centres are part of university structures and are staffed and/or managed by medical academics (pharmacology, clinical pharmacology, clinical toxicology). They therefore participate in the primary educational process within schools of medicine and pharmacy, providing early exposure to and awareness of pharmacovigilance and the need to report to future reporters. Further participation of centre personnel in continuing education processes makes them known personally to attending health professionals, facilitating further contacts and promoting knowledge of the centre's activity.

The educational processes in which centres participate are threefold as outlined below.

Formal Educative Processes
These include:

- Primary education in schools of medicine and pharmacy.
- Continuing medical and pharmaceutical education.

- Specialized diplomas in clinical pharmacology, pharmacovigilance and pharmacoepidemiology at a regional, national or international level.

Practical Educative Processes

These include:

- One on one education in answering questions.
- Educative function of drug bulletin and participation in local committees.

Informal Educative Processes

These include:

- Evaluation of drug alerts, explanation of methodologies of drug alert processing to junior centre personnel and to involved clinicians and experts.
- Publication of research results.

Role of the Regional Centres in Prevention of Adverse Drug Reactions

The general objectives of the centres' activities are prevention of:

- Type A reactions, (which are common, a public health burden and costly) by promoting better knowledge and use of pharmacology for the rational use of drugs and the management of drug therapy.
- Type B reactions by promoting early reporting and careful evaluation of such reactions, so that the appropriate regulatory measures can be taken in a timely manner.

Suggested further reading is *National Pharmacovigilance Systems*, ed. Dr Sten Olsson, Th3 Uppsala Monitoring Centre (WHO Collaborating Centre for Drug Monitoring) Box 26, S-751 03 Uppsala, Sweden, tel: +46 (18) 17 48 50; fax: +46 (18) 507840.

Chapter 13

Pharmacovigilance Regulations and Guidelines and the International Conference on Harmonization

John Talbot

Director, Pharmacovigilance
Astra Charnwood, Bakewell Road, Loughborough, Leicestershire LE11 5RH, UK

Introduction

Regulations and guidelines concerning pharmacovigilance have been in a continuous state of change and development in recent years. This makes the topic rather unsuitable for inclusion in a textbook, hence, unlike in previous editions, this chapter will not describe the current requirements for each country in great detail. This has been done in August 1997 by a *Scrip* report (PJB Publications) entitled *Global ADR Reporting Requirements* written by Dr Barry Arnold of Zeneca. This is an excellent and comprehensive report, but to remain useful in the longer term will require regular updating.

The major change over the past few years has been a significant attempt to harmonize regulations under the aegis of the International Conference of Harmonization (ICH) and this is covered in some depth below. The latest response to the ICH in its three participating regions (Europe, USA and Japan) is also described together with an update on the current UK regulations. The ICH potentially offers real advantages to the pharmaceutical industry, but the process takes time and countries have adopted and implemented the guidance in slightly different ways and at different times. National regulations and guidelines are therefore bound to change in the near future as each country embraces the ICH.

The International Conference on Harmonization

The ICH of Technical Requirements for Registration of Pharmaceuticals for Human Use brings together as equal partners the regulatory authorities of Europe, Japan and the USA and experts from the pharmaceutical industry in these regions to discuss scientific and technical aspects of product registration (Table 1). The World Health Organization (WHO), European Free Trade Area (EFTA) and Canada are observers, and the International Federation of Pharmaceutical Manufacturers Association (IFPMA) ensures contact with the research based industry outside the ICH regions.

The aim of the ICH is to achieve greater harmonization in the interpretation and application of technical guidelines and requirements for product registration and reduce or eliminate duplicate testing. This should result in better use of resources and eliminate unnecessary delay in the global development and availability of new medicines while maintaining safeguards on quality, safety and efficacy.

The terms of reference for the ICH are:

- To provide a forum for a constructive dialogue between regulatory authorities and the pharmaceutical industry on the real and perceived differences in the technical requirements for product registration in the EU, USA and Japan.
- To identify areas where modifications in technical requirements or greater mutual acceptance of research and development procedures could lead to more economical use of human, animal and material resources without compromising safety.
- To make recommendations on practical ways to achieve greater harmonization in the interpretation and application of technical guidelines and requirements for registration.

There are four broad topic areas within the ICH:

S—safety (animal toxicology and pharmacology).
Q—quality (pharmaceutical and analytical).
E—efficacy (clinical).
M—multidisciplinary topics.

Only selected E and M topics will be considered here as shown in Table 2, which describes the status of the E and M guidelines. The ICH Expert Working Groups (EWGs) are joint regulatory/industry groups for which experts are nominated from the six co-sponsors. The working groups deal with individual harmonization topics and each nominates a topic leader for the subject under discussion. There is a

---

Table 1   The regulatory and industry parties in different regions

ICH region	Regulatory party	Industry party
Europe	European Commission	European Federation of Pharmaceutical Industries Associations (EFPIA)
USA	Food and Drug Administration (FDA)	Pharmaceutical Research and Manufacturers of America (PhRMA)
Japan	Ministry of Health and Welfare (MHW)	Japan Pharmaceutical Manufacturers Association (JPMA)

Table 2 Status of ICH topics

Topic number		Title	Status
Efficacy (clinical)			
E1*	Extent of population exposure to assess clinical safety	Step 5	Final
E2A*	Clinical safety data management: definitions and standards for expedited reporting	Step 5	Final
E2B*	Clinical safety data management: data elements for transmission of ADR reports	Step 4	Final
E2C*	Clinical safety data management: periodic safety update reports for marketed drugs	Step 4	Final
E3*	Clinical study reports: structure and content	Step 5	Final
E4	Dose–response information to support drug registration	Step 5	Final
E5	Ethnic factors in the acceptability of foreign clinical data	Step 3	Draft
E6*	Good Clinical Practice (GCP) consolidated guideline	Step 5	Final
E7	Clinical trials in special populations: geriatrics	Step 5	Final
E8	General considerations for clinical trials	Step 3	Draft
E9	Statistical considerations in the design of clinical trials	Step 4	Final
E10	Choice of control group in clinical trials	Step 1	Draft
Multidisciplinary topics			
M1*	Medical terminology	Step 5	Final
M2	Electronic standards for the transfer of regulatory information and data	Step 4	Final
M3	Timing of pre-clinical studies in relation to clinical trials	Step 4	Final
M4	Common technical document	Pre-step 1	Feasibility study

* Described in some detail below.

stepwise ICH process for monitoring the progress of the harmonization work and identifying the action needed to reach a defined endpoint. The process is as follows:

Step 1

A six-party EWG is appointed for the topic and one of the topic leaders is designated as the rapporteur. Preliminary discussions of the topic are held between EWG members and a first draft is prepared by the rapporteur. This may be a draft guideline, policy statement, recommendation or 'points to consider' document. The draft is reviewed and revised by the experts and successive drafts are prepared until consensus is reached. It is then forwarded to the steering committee.

Step 2

The draft is 'signed off' by the six co-sponsors in the steering committee and is transmitted to the three regional regulatory agencies for formal consultation in the EU, Japan and the USA. This regulatory consultation may include organizations and associations outside the ICH process. The comment period should normally be six months, except when there are special circumstances to take into account.

Step 3

A regulatory rapporteur is designated from the EU, MHW or FDA. Comments are collected by the regulatory agencies in the three regions and exchanged with the other regulatory bodies. The regulatory rapporteur, in consultation with other regulatory experts, analyses the comments and amends the 'step 2' draft. When significant changes result from the consultation process, such that the original consensus is not maintained, one or more regulatory authorities may recirculate the amended parts of the draft. The regulatory rapporteur prepares a final draft and agrees this with the regulatory experts from the other parties. The final draft is referred to the ICH EWG and 'signed off' by the experts designated by the regulatory parties before being referred to the ICH steering committee for adoption.

Step 4

The final draft is discussed within the steering committee and 'signed off' by the three regulatory parties to the ICH. It is then recommended for adoption to the three regulatory bodies.

Step 5

The process is complete when the full recommendations are incorporated into the domestic regulations or other appropriate administrative measures, according to national/regional internal procedures.

Conferences

The ICH process was initiated in 1990 and since then there have been four ICH conferences:

- ICH 1 1991—Brussels.
- ICH 2 1993—Orlando.
- ICH 3 1995—Yokohama.
- ICH 4 1997—Brussels.

Key parts of the selected topics relating to pharmacovigilance are described below, but it is strongly recommended that the full documents are consulted. ICH guidelines are not in themselves regulatory requirements; only when they have been adopted and incorporated into local legislation do they have such status. This particularly applies to requirements for safety reporting.

Information on the ICH and copies of ICH documents are available from the ICH Home Page—http://www.pharmweb.net/pwmirror/pw9/ifpma/ich1.html.

ICH E1A Population Exposure: The Extent of Population Exposure to Assess Clinical Safety (CPMP/ICH/375/95)

This guideline presents a set of principles for the safety evaluation of drugs intended for long-term treatment (more than six months) of non-life-threatening diseases. Some of the key principles are:

- Standards for the safety evaluation of drugs should be based on previous experience with the occurrence and detection of ADRs and statistical and practical considerations.
- Adverse events are most frequent in the first few months of treatment. The number of exposed subjects should be large enough to observe whether the more frequent events (0.5–5%) increase or decrease over time (300–600 patients should be adequate).
- Some patients should be treated for 12 months; 100 patients exposed for a minimum of one year is considered acceptable.
- The total number of individuals treated, including short-term exposure will be about 1500.

There are exceptions to these general standards, for instance where there is:

- Concern from clinical studies, other similar drugs or pharmacokinetic or pharmacodynamic properties of late onset ADRs.
- Expected, low-frequency serious ADRs.
- Only a small benefit from the drug.
- Concern that the drug may add to a significant background morbidity or mortality.

ICH E2A Clinical Safety Data Management: Definitions and Standards for Expedited Reporting (CPMP/ICH/377/95)

This guideline covers the handling of clinical safety information for drugs under development and provides definitions and standards for reporting. The sections below are taken directly from the guideline without revision.

Definitions

Adverse Event (or Adverse Experience)
Any untoward medical occurrence in a patient or clinical investigation subject administered a pharmaceutical product and which does not necessarily have to have a causal relationship with this treatment.

Adverse Drug Reaction (ADR)
In the pre-approval clinical experience with a new medicinal product or its new usages, particularly as the therapeutic dose(s) may not be established "all noxious and unintended responses to a medicinal product related to any dose should be considered adverse drug reactions".

Unexpected Adverse Drug Reaction
An adverse reaction, the nature or severity of which is not consistent with the applicable product information (e.g. investigator's brochure for an unapproved investigational medicinal product).

Serious Adverse Event
A serious adverse event (experience) or reaction is any untoward medical occurrence that at any dose:

- Results in death.
- Is life-threatening.
- Requires inpatient hospitalization or prolongation of existing hospitalization.
- Results in persistent or significant disability/incapacity.
- Is a congenital anomaly/birth defect.

Note that the term 'life-threatening' in the definition of 'serious' refers to an event in which the patient was at risk of death at the time of the event; it does not refer to an event which hypothetically might have caused death if it were more severe.

Medical and scientific judgement should be exercised in deciding whether expedited reporting is appropriate in other situations, such as important medical events that may not be immediately life-threatening or result in death or hospitalization, but may jeopardize the patient or may require intervention to prevent one of the other outcomes listed in the definition above. These should also usually be considered to be serious.

Examples of such events are intensive treatment in an emergency room or at home for allergic bronchospasm; blood dyscrasias or convulsions that do not result in hospitalization; or development of drug dependency or drug abuse.

What Should be Reported?

Single cases of Serious, Unexpected adverse drug reactions

All ADRs that are both serious and unexpected are subject to expedited reporting. This applies to reports from spontaneous sources and from any type of clinical or epidemiological investigation, independent of design or purpose. It also applies to cases not reported directly to a sponsor or manufacturer (e.g. those found in regulatory authority-generated ADR registries or in publications). The source of a report (investigation, spontaneous, other) should always be specified.

Expedited reporting of reactions that are serious but expected will ordinarily be inappropriate. Expedited reporting is also inappropriate for serious events from clinical investigations that are considered to be *not* related to the study product, whether the event is expected or not.

Other Observations

There are situations in addition to single case reports of 'serious' adverse events or reactions that may necessitate rapid communication to regulatory authorities; appropriate medical and scientific judgement should be applied for each situation. In general, information that might materially influence the benefit–risk assessment of a medicinal product or that would be sufficient to consider changes in medicinal product administration or in the overall conduct of a clinical investigation represents such situations. Examples include:

- For an 'expected' serious ADR, an increase in the rate of occurrence that is judged to be clinically important.
- A significant hazard to the patient population, such as lack of efficacy with a medicinal product used in treating life-threatening disease.
- A major safety finding from a newly completed animal study (such as carcinogenicity).

Reporting Time Frames

Fatal or Life-Threatening Unexpected adverse drug reactions

Certain ADRs may be sufficiently alarming so as to require very rapid notification to regulators in countries where the medicinal product or indication, formulation or population for the medicinal product are still not approved for marketing because such reports may lead to consideration of suspension of, or other limitations to, a clinical investigations programme. Fatal or life-threatening, unexpected ADRs occurring in clinical investigations qualify for very rapid reporting. Regulatory agencies should be notified (e.g. by telephone, facsimile transmission or in writing) as soon as possible, but no later than seven calendar days after first knowledge by the sponsor that a case qualifies, followed by a report that is as complete as possible within eight additional calendar days. This report must include an assessment of the importance and implication of the findings, including relevant previous experience with the same or similar medicinal products.

All Other Serious, Unexpected adverse drug reactions

Serious, unexpected ADRs that are not fatal or life-threatening must be filed as soon as possible, but no later than 15 calendar days after first knowledge by the sponsor that the case meets the minimum criteria for expedited reporting.

Managing Blinded Therapy Cases

When the sponsor and investigator are blinded to individual patient treatment (as in a double-blind study), the occurrence of a serious event requires a decision on whether to open (break) the code for the specific patient. If the investigator breaks the blind, then it is assumed that the sponsor will also know the assigned treatment for that patient. Although it is advantageous to retain the blind for all patients prior to final study analysis, when a serious adverse reaction is judged reportable on an expedited basis, it is recommended that the blind be broken only for that specific patient by the sponsor even if the investigator has not broken the blind. It is also recommended that when possible and appropriate, the blind be maintained for those persons such as biometrics personnel responsible for analysis and interpretation of results at the study's conclusion.

There are several disadvantages to maintaining the blind under the circumstances described that outweigh the advantages. By retaining the blind, placebo and comparator (usually a marketed product) cases are filed unnecessarily. When the blind is eventually opened, which may be many weeks or months after reporting to regulators, it must be ensured that company and regulatory databases are revised. If the event is serious, new, and possibly related to the medicinal product, then if the investigator's brochure is updated, notifying relevant parties of the new information in a blinded fashion is inappropriate and possibly misleading. Moreover, breaking the blind for a single patient usually has little or no significant implications for the conduct of the clinical investigation or on the analysis of the final clinical investigation data.

However, when a fatal or other 'serious' outcome is the primary efficacy endpoint in a clinical investigation, the integrity of the clinical investigation may be compromised if the blind is broken. Under these and similar circumstances, it may be appropriate to reach agreement with regulatory authorities in advance concerning serious events that would be treated as disease-related and not subject to routine expedited reporting.

ICH E2B Clinical Safety Data Management: Data Elements for Transmission of Individual Case Safety Reports

This document, which was finalized in July 1997, defines the relevant data elements and provides notes on the format for the transmission of individual case reports. The data elements are comprehensive and not every data element will be available for every transmission. It provides the framework for transmission of cases between regulatory authorities, within and between companies (e.g. licensing situations) and between companies and authorities. It has already formed the basis for an ongoing pilot project involving the FDA and a small number of companies in the USA. Some authorities are already encouraging electronic reporting of cases and more will in the future; it could in due course become a requirement.

ICH E2C Clinical Safety Data Management: Periodic Safety Update Reports for Marketed Drugs (CPMP/ICH/288/95)

Although the main objective of the ICH is to harmonize requirements for marketing authorization, new products are introduced at different times in different markets and a product marketed in some, may still be under development in others. Hence, clinical safety information should be regarded as part of a continuum. It was also recognized that the regulatory requirements for the content and frequency of submission of periodic safety update reports (PSURs) were diverse.

The aims of the PSUR are to:

- Report all the relevant new safety information from appropriate sources.
- Relate these data to patient exposure.
- Summarize the market authorization status in different countries and any significant variations related to safety.
- Create periodically the opportunity for an overall safety re-evaluation.
- Indicate whether changes should be made to the product information in order to optimize the use of the product.

General principles regarding the scope of information, international birth date—the date of the first marketing authorization (MA) granted—presentation of data etc. are described. Features of note are that all dosage forms, formulations and indications for a given drug should be covered in one PSUR and each MA holder (MAH) is responsible for submitting PSURs even if other companies market the same product. Reporting frequency is six-monthly or in multiples of six months with submission within 60 days of the data lockpoint.

Sources of data to be included are:

- Spontaneous reports from health care professionals.
- Spontaneous reports from non-health care professionals.
- MAH-sponsored clinical studies and named patients.
- Literature.
- Reports from regulatory authorities.
- Reports exchanged between contractual partners.
- Data in special registries.
- Reports from poison control centres.
- Epidemiological databases.

Cases should be presented as line listings or summary tabulations. A model PSUR is provided and the contents of each section described. The sections, which are a mix of clinical and regulatory information, are:

- Introduction.
- Worldwide market authorization status.
- Update of regulatory authority or MAH actions taken for safety reasons.
- Changes to reference safety information.
- Patient exposure.
- Presentation of individual case histories.
- Studies.
- Other information.
- Overall safety evaluation.
- Conclusion.

The company core data sheet in effect at the beginning of the period covered should be included as an Appendix. Examples of how to present the worldwide MA status, individual case histories and number of reports by term are given.

ICH E3 Clinical Study Reports: Structure and Content

Although not relevant to the regulatory reporting of individual cases or PSURs, this comprehensive document provides valuable information on the production of clinical study reports. There is a substantial section on 'safety evaluation', which includes presentation and analysis of adverse events, case narratives, review of deaths, other serious adverse events and other significant adverse events, evaluation of laboratory data etc. This is essential reading for company pharmacovigilance staff who are involved in the analysis and presentation of safety data from clinical trials.

ICH E6 Good Clinical Practice (GCP): Consolidated Guideline (CPMP/ICH/135/95)

This is another excellent ICH document that describes the scientific quality standard for designing, conducting, recording and reporting clinical trials. It contains a glossary, which includes the definition of serious etc. and many other terms in addition.

There are sections on the responsibilities of institutional review boards/independent ethics committees (IRB/IEC), investigators and study sponsors. There are also guidelines on clinical trial protocols and protocol amendments and investigator brochures. There are numerous references to adverse events/ADRs including reporting by investigators to sponsors and by sponsors to regulatory authorities, investigators and IRB/IECs. The section on the investigator's brochure provides guidance on what safety information, and its implications, should be included.

ICH M1 Medical Terminology

Pharmaceutical companies and regulatory authorities use a variety of dictionaries to code adverse events and diseases and in the past there has been no single accepted terminology. In 1994, the ICH agreed to oversee the development of a single standard medical terminology that could be used globally for regulatory purposes. The M1 EWG first met in 1995 and supported the development of a new medical terminology based on MedDRA version 1.0, (formerly Medical Dictionary for Drug Regulatory Affairs). For a description of MedDRA see Chapter 10.

At the time of writing, MedDRA version 2.0 looks as if it will be the future standard for industry and regulatory authorities. However, a maintenance and support organization has not yet been appointed, hence MedDRA will not be available in a form that can be readily used until probably sometime in late 1998.

The Future of the ICH

ICH 4 marked the completion of the first phase of ICH activities and the six-party structure will continue as the operational basis for harmonizing technical requirements for new medicine development and registration. ICH activities will thus move into a second phase with the following revised terms of reference:

- To maintain a forum for a constructive dialogue between regulatory authorities and the pharmaceutical industry on the real and perceived differences in the technical requirements for product registration in the EU, USA and Japan in order to ensure a more timely introduction of new medicinal products and their availability to patients:
- To monitor and update harmonized technical requirements leading to a greater mutual acceptance of research and development data.
- To avoid divergent future requirements through harmonization of selected topics needed as a result of therapeutic advances and the development of new technologies for the production of medicinal products.
- To facilitate the adoption of new or improved technical research and development approaches that update or replace current practices where these permit a more economical use of human, animal and material resources without compromising safety
- To facilitate the dissemination and communication of information on harmonized guidelines and their use such as to encourage the implementation and integration of common standards.

The European Union

Background

The regulatory framework for reporting ADRs to authorities within the EU is a complex mix of Community legislation, national laws and various guidelines, and for marketed products, depends upon whether they were approved through the centralized, mutual recognition or national procedure.

In 1993 the Council of the EU adopted three Directives and a Regulation that formed the legal basis of the new European system for the authorization of medicinal products and this came into effect in January 1995. Those relating to pharmacovigilance are:

- Council Regulation 2309/93.
- Council Directive 75/319/EEC (amended by Council Directive 93/39/EEC).

The European Medicines Evaluation Agency (EMEA) began its work in 1995. It has a specific role with medicinal products authorized under the centralized procedure (see below). It has two scientific committees responsible for the EMEA's opinion on any question relating to the evaluation of human or veterinary products, namely the Committee for Proprietary Medicinal Products (CPMP) and its veterinary counterpart, CVMP. The CPMP has produced a series of guidelines on ADR reporting for investigational drugs and marketed products.

Investigational Drug Products

The regulatory requirements for the reporting of ADRs from clinical trials with investigational drugs are currently less developed than those for marketed products. ICH E2A (Clinical Safety Data Management: Definitions and Standards for Expedited Reporting) has been implemented by the EU (CPMP/377/95), but at the time of writing it had been formally adopted by only three member states—the UK (see below), Denmark and Sweden. The EC is also preparing a GCP/Clinical Trials Directive, which will govern the conduct of clinical trials in the future, including the reporting of ADRs. This is likely to be implemented in the year 2000 or 2001.

Marketed Drug Products

Council Regulation 2309/93 applies to products that have been approved under the centralized procedure and was immediately binding throughout the EU. However, the majority of marketed products have been approved through national procedures or under mutual recognition. These are covered by Council Directive 75/319/EEC and require endorsement through national legislation. There are, however, deficiencies and inconsistencies between the Regulation and the Directive, (see Chapter 14).

The draft *Notice to Applicants* (5944/94) Chapter V, 'Pharmacovigilance of medicinal products for human use', effective 1st January 1995, provided guidance on the implementation and practical procedures. At the time of writing, this guideline is under review by the CPMP Pharmacovigilance Working Party. It will probably be published in 1998 and should be a stand-alone document on the conduct of pharmacovigilance by companies.

Centrally Authorized Products

The CPMP has issued guidance on the conduct of pharmacovigilance for centrally authorised products (CPMP/183/97), adopted April 1997. This document outlines the legal framework, principles, functions and procedures for centralized products. The role and responsibilities of all parties involved are summarized below:

Those of the MAH are:

- To establish and maintain a system, accessible at a single point in the EU, to collect, collate, and evaluate pharmacovigilance data.
- To meet legal obligations for reporting suspected ADRs.
- To meet legal obligations regarding the preparation and submission of PSURs.
- To respond fully to requests from authorities for additional information necessary for the evaluation of the benefits and risks of a medicinal product.
- To ensure the MA is maintained and reflects the latest information.

The role and responsibilities of the member states are:

- To have national pharmacovigilance systems in place.
- To inform the European Commission, the CPMP, the EMEA, the member states and the MAHs of any relevant actions.
- To collect and collate risk–benefit data.
- To provide serious ADRs received in its territory to the EMEA and the relevant MAH within 15 days of receipt.
- To identify and evaluate drug safety alerts and conduct risk–benefit evaluations.
- To provide representation on the CPMP, Pharmacovigilance Working Party, rapporteurs/co-rapporteurs.
- To implement Commission decisions.
- In case of urgent action to protect public health, suspend the use of the product in the member state's territory and inform, in accordance with the legislation, the EMEA and the European Commission of the basis for action.

The role and responsibilities of the EMEA Secretariat are:

- Co-ordination of the centralized pharmacovigilance system.
- To monitor the legal obligations of the MAHs.
- Receipt of serious ADRs and provision to the member states and the rapporteur.
- In agreement with the rapporteur, identification of signals of possible unexpected hazards or changes in expected adverse effects.
- In agreement with the rapporteur, to inform all involved parties of any safety hazard concern.
- Co-ordination of the evaluation of data by the rapporteurs and consideration by the CPMP to reach opinions.
- Communication of opinions to the European Commission.
- Communication with the MAH on all relevant issues in consultation with the rapporteur.
- Maintenance of the crisis management system for centrally authorized products.

The roles and responsibilities of the rapporteur are:

- To evaluate all risk–benefit issues for centrally authorized products.

- To evaluate regularly ADRs and other risk–benefit data on receipt, PSURs, company reports and variation applications to agreed timetables, obtaining additional information from the MAH and the member states as necessary.
- To provide risk–benefit assessment reports to agreed timetables for consideration by the Pharmacovigilance Working Party and CPMP as necessary, with proposals on appropriate remedial action.

The role and responsibilities of the Pharmacovigilance Working Party are:

- To regularly review drug monitor of safety issues for centrally authorized products.
- To discuss emerging drug safety issues at the request of the rapporteur.
- To discuss PSURs at the request of the rapporteur.
- To make recommendations to the CPMP on risk–benefit evaluations and actions necessary to minimize risk and maximize benefit.

The role and responsibilities of the CPMP are:

- Discussion of the risk–benefit on the basis of the rapporteur's assessment report.
- Formulation of opinions.

The role and responsibilities of the European Commission are:

- Competent authority for centrally authorized products.
- Formulation of decisions.
- Enforcement of legislative requirements and enforcement of the implementation of decisions by member states and MAHs.

The United Kingdom

The legal basis for pharmacovigilance in the UK is the *Medicines Act* of 1968 under which the Secretaries of State for Health in England, Wales and Scotland have the power to make regulations using statutory instruments (SIs). The *Medicines for Human Use Regulations* 1994 (SI 1994/3144) superseded the previous SIs and implements the European Regulations concerning expedited reporting and PSURs. The *Medicines (Exemption from Licences) (Clinical Trials) Order* 1995 (SI 1995/2808) and the *Medicines (Exemption from Licences and Certificates) (Clinical Trials) Order* 1995 (SI 1995/2809) implements the European Regulations concerning reporting from clinical trials with investigational drugs. Medicines Act information leaflets (MAILs) published by the MCA offer general guidance on the interpretation of the regulations and updates on various issues.

Reporting for Investigational Drugs

The guidance for ADR reporting with investigational drugs is best described in the MCA publication *Medicines Act 1968—Guidance Notes on Applications for Clinical Trial Exemptions and Clinical Trial Certificates* (revised December 1995) (ISBN 1 900731 00 2) pages 94–99. This implements ICH E2A and the definitions and reporting timeframes given above. Companies are required to report only serious unexpected reactions occurring inside or outside the UK using a form similar to the yellow card (see Appendix 5). All cases judged by either the reporting health care professional or the sponsor as having a 'reasonable' suspected causal relationship to the medicinal product qualify as ADRs. Treatment codes should always be broken before reporting.

From July 1997 companies should submit such reports to the Adverse Drug Reactions On-Line Information Tracking (ADROIT) Unit, Department of Health, The Medicines Control Agency, Room 1001, Market Towers, 1 Nine Elms Lane, London SW8 5NQ (MAIL 100) instead of the Clinical Trials Unit. Clinical trial reports will thus be scanned into the computer and classified onto the ADROIT database in a similar way to spontaneous reports.

Companies are expected to monitor and keep records of each adverse event or reaction that occurs during a trial. Non-serious and serious ADRs that are expected should be reported in a brief summary either at the conclusion of the study or at the renewal of the clinical trial exemption certificate (CTX) if they occurred in the UK or with the MA if they occurred elsewhere.

For studies in high morbidity/high mortality disease states, companies are encouraged to appoint a safety data monitoring committee to decode trialists reports, construct the group sequential analysis and report directly to the MCA at agreed time intervals. An example of a suitable line listing format is provided in the MCA guidance notes and procedures can be discussed with the Clinical Trials Unit.

Reporting for Marketed Products

The guidance for ADR reporting with marketed products is best described in MAIL 87, January / February 1995. For spontaneous reports, this is summarized in Table 3.

The reporting format is the yellow form (see Appendix 5) and companies are obliged to submit reports received from all health professionals, doctors, dentists, coroners, pharmacists and nurses. Special reporting for new products designated by the black triangle symbol (▼) is no longer required, but the symbol is retained to alert doctors about reporting all suspected reactions with new medicines.

The format and content of PSURs is described in the draft *Notice to Applicants*.

Table 3   Summary of spontaneous adverse drug reaction reporting requirements

Timing	UK	Other EC Member States	Outside EC
Within 15 days (as individual reports) and with periodic safety updates**	Serious	Serious*	Serious and unexpected
Periodic safety updates only**	Non-serious	Non-serious and unexpected	Non-serious and unexpected

* Only if authorized nationally, either through mutual recognition or purely national procedure.
** Include as line-listing only.

The timing of PSURs is:

- Six monthly for the first two years.
- Annually for the next three years.
- For medicines that have been licensed for more than five years, a report covering the previous five years should be submitted at the time of license renewal.

To harmonize safety update reports internationally there is some flexibility regarding data lockpoints according to the international birth date. However, for products authorized through the centralized and decentralized systems the timing of submission is not flexible and should relate to the EC birth date.

Safety Assessment of Marketed Medicines (SAMM) Guidelines

The SAMM guidelines apply to the conduct of all company sponsored studies that evaluate the safety of marketed products in the UK. They were issued in late 1993 and replaced the so called 'Quadripartite' guidelines—Joint Committee of the Association of the British Pharamaceutical Industry, (ABPI), 'British Medical Association (BMA), Committee on Safety of Medicines (CSM) and Royal College of General Practice (RCGP) Guidelines on post-marketing surveillance (PMS), (1988). A fifth party, the MCA, was involved in the drafting, which aimed to address the limitations of the previous guidelines as identified by Waller *et al.*, (1992). The SAMM guidelines are reproduced in full in Appendix 6 and have also been published in the *British Journal of Clinical Pharmacology* (1994); and *Pharmacoepidemiology & Drug Safety* (1994).

In the author's opinion the SAMM guidelines initially caused a decrease in the number of new PMS studies conducted in the UK, but have probably improved their design and quality.

The guidelines also appeared almost word for word in Chapter V of the draft *Notice to Applicants*, under the heading 'Company-sponsored post-authorisation studies'. The SAMM guidelines themselves are unlikely to be revised, but the European guidance is currently under revision.

Pregnancy Reports

MAIL 100 (March/April 1997), page 6, provides guidance on the reporting of pregnancy outcomes. Individual adverse outcomes suspected by a health professional to be drug related should be reported as follows:

- Serious, suspected adverse reactions as expedited (15-day) reports.
- Non-serious suspected adverse reactions within PSURs.
- Pregnancy before the outcome is known should not be reported except when unintended pregnancy is suspected to be an ADR.

With regard to prospective registries of pregnant patients, the MCA should also be made promptly aware of any cluster of cases representing a possible signal of an adverse effect on pregnancy outcome which is not in the Summary of Product Characteristics (SPC). Aggregated data including the cumulative total experience of exposure should also be reviewed at the time of the PSUR.

The USA

Within the USA, the FDA is responsible for issuing rules and regulations governing new drug approvals and reporting of ADRs with both investigational and marketed drug products. The final rules, published in the *Federal Register* are legal
requirements and failure to comply with them is a federal criminal offence. The
regulations are complex, detailed and have been considerably amended over the past
ten years; they are also supplemented by guidelines, see *Federal Register 27 October
1994, Volume 59, Number 207, pages 54046–54064* http://www.access.gpo.gov/su
docs/aces/aces140.html.

For new chemical entities (NCEs), new indications or new formulations companies
must file an investigational new drug application (IND), which must be approved by
the FDA before a drug can be used in humans. The requirements for ADR reporting
for investigational drugs are thus known as the IND regulations. Before a new
product can be marketed, companies must file a new drug application (NDA) and
have it approved by the FDA. The requirements for ADR reporting after marketing
are thus known as the NDA Regulations. Both sets of regulations can apply to a drug
at the same time; for instance the NDA regulations apply to any marketed forms, but
the IND regulations apply to a new indication or formulation. At the time of writing,
the current regulations are in Title 21 of the *Code of Federal Regulations* (21 CFR) as
follows:

- 21 CFR 312.32 Safety reports for investigational products subject to an IND
  application (published 1987).
- 21 CFR 314.80 Post-marketing reporting of ADEs (NDA) (published 1985).
- 21 CFR 600.80 Post-marketing reporting of adverse experiences for licensed
  biological products (includes vaccines)(published 1994).

See also CFR web site: http://www.access.gpo.gov/nara/cfr/index.html.

An August 1997 guideline (Post-marketing adverse experience reporting for human
drug and licensed biological products: Clarification of what to report) defined the
minimum data relevant for a safety report as:

- An identifiable patient.
- An identifiable reporter.
- A suspect drug or biological product.
- An adverse event or fatal outcome.

If any of these items remain unknown after being actively sought, a report should
not be submitted to the FDA. The guideline also clarifies that adverse experiences
derived during planned contacts and active solicitation of information from patients
(e.g. company sponsored patient support programmes, disease management programmes) should be handled as safety information from a post-marketing study (i.e.
for expedited reporting, events must be serious, unexpected and a reasonable
possibility that the drug caused the event).

Other guidelines are not included here as they will be superseded by new ones
(see below). See also Center for Drug Evaluation and Research CDER guidance page
http://www.fda.gov/cder/guidance/index.htm.

These regulations and the guidelines have recently been extensively indexed in two publications in the *Drug Information Journal*—Curran and Engle (1997) and Curran and Sills (1997).

In the *Federal Register* of 27th October 1994, the FDA published a proposed rule to amend the regulations to provide consistency with certain standardized definitions, procedures and formats developed by the ICH and CIOMS. The FDA received many comments on these proposals and finally published detailed amended expedited safety reporting regulations, implementing ICH in October 1997 (*Federal Register, 7 October, 1997, Volume 62, Number 194, pages 52237–52253*). A revision of the associated guideline has also been proposed by the FDA, but was not available at the time of writing.

These new regulations for expedited reporting are effective 180 days later on 6th April 1998, but companies may comply with the provisions of this final rule before its effective date. Key points from the new regulations are described below. The amendments to the periodic post-marketing safety reporting regulations are delayed awaiting further consideration of the ICH E2C guideline and were not available for inclusion in this chapter.

IND Regulations

In 1994, the FDA proposed to amend requirements for clinical study design, conduct and annual sponsor reporting in the IND regulations as a result of events with fialuridine. In the light of comments received, the FDA withdrew the proposed amendments and will develop a guidance document with recommendations on study design and monitoring of investigational drugs used to treat serious and potentially fatal illnesses, with particular attention to detection of adverse events similar to those caused by underlying disease.

Increased Frequency Reports

The requirement for increased frequency reports for serious expected ADRs with marketed products is revoked. This was also published in the *Federal Register* of 25th June 1997 (Volume 62, Number 122, pages 34166–34168). The rationale for this was that despite receiving many such reports, only a small number of drug safety problems were identified.

Reporting Forms

FDA form 3500/3500A (see Appendix 5) is the standard form for notifying expedited reports and can also be used by companies to submit IND safety reports. Foreign cases may be reported on the CIOMS I form.

Definitions

The definition of 'serious' has been revised to make it consistent with ICH E2A and is the same for INDs and NDAs (see above).

The definition of 'unexpected' for IND reporting is "Any adverse drug experience, the specificity or severity of which is not consistent with the current investigator brochure; or if an investigator brochure is not required or available, the specificity or severity of which is not consistent with the risk information described in the general investigational plan or elsewhere in the current application, as amended. For example, under this definition, hepatic necrosis would be unexpected (by virtue of greater severity) if the investigator brochure only referred to elevated hepatic enzymes or hepatitis. Similarly, cerebral thromboembolism and cerebral vasculitis would be unexpected (by virtue of greater specificity) if the investigator brochure only listed cerebral vascular accidents. 'Unexpected', as used in this definition, refers to an adverse drug experience that has not been previously observed (e.g. included in the investigator brochure) rather than from the perspective of such experience not being anticipated from the pharmacological properties of the pharmaceutical product".

For NDA reporting, the following sentence has been added to the existing definition of unexpected: " 'unexpected' as used in this definition, refers to an adverse drug experience that has not been previously observed (i.e. included in the labelling) rather than from the perspective of such experience not being anticipated from the pharmacological properties of the pharmaceutical product."

Time Frames

The time period for submitting written IND safety reports reports has been revised from ten working days to 15 calendar days. For telephone reports (fatal and life-threatening unexpected reactions), it has been revised from three working days to seven calendar days. Such reports can also be made by fax. Telephone reporting was previously restricted to clinical studies conducted under the IND, but under the new rule, telephone reporting within seven calendar days applies to any unexpected fatal or life-threatening reaction from any source.

The time period for submitting NDA alert reports (serious and unexpected) has been revised from 15 working days to 15 calendar days.

Japan

The Japanese requirements, including the standards for the conduct of good post-marketing surveillance practice (GPMSP), have recently undergone review by the Ministry of Health and Welfare (MHW) and the new regulations came into force on 1st April 1997. The MHW had already implemented ICH E2A and ICH E2C, but in recent years there have been a number of issues including the contamination of blood products with human immunodeficiency virus (HIV) and deaths associated with Sorivudine drug interactions (see page 4). The relevant documents are:

- 1997 Ministerial Ordinance No. 10 of the MHW concerning the standard of GPMSP.
- 1997 Ministerial Ordinance No. 29 amending part of the Enforcement Regulations of the Pharmaceutical Affairs Law.
- Pharmaceutical Affairs Bureau Notification No. 421 (March 27th, 1997) Enforcement of the Law related to Partial Amendments to Pharmaceutical Affairs Law.

Definitions and time frames are generally in accordance with the ICH, but the regulations specify a number of other requirements such as the preparation and compliance with relevant SOPs, a responsible person for drug safety and a PMS department with sufficient qualified persons and independent of other departments such as marketing. A more proactive approach from companies is expected by the MHW.

All expedited and periodic reports must be submitted in Japanese, even for foreign cases. Companies developing or marketing products in Japan will almost certainly have to prepare their own reports containing Japanese and foreign data in Japan hence local expertise is essential.

Chapter 14

Legal Aspects of Pharmacovigilance

Christine Bendall, Partner, Cameron McKenna

Mitre House, 160 Aldersgate Street, London EC1A 4DD, UK

Introduction

Chapter 13 has already addressed the requirements currently applying in various different jurisdictions to pharmacovigilance activities and adverse event reporting. Requirements enshrined in legislation or powers provided generally in legislation and exercised administratively by regulators, form the legal basis for recording and reporting obligations and for enforcement by regulatory authorities. Often, legislation itself is broadly worded, dealing in concepts and principles, while the detail of how the obligations are, or may be, satisfied is left to guidelines and/or administrative provision made by regulators. For example, in the UK, before the revision of the Medicines Act in 1994, marketing authorization (MA) holders were required by standard provisions attaching to the MA; to report in accordance with requirements laid down by the licensing authority. These were set out and amended in MAIL editions (Medicines Act Information Letters) issued by the Medicines Control Agency. Provisions in the USA are relatively detailed for Investigational New Drug Authorizations (IND) and new drug applications (NDAs). Reporting serious adverse events relating to biologics is also subject to *Federal Register* notices e.g. (on the forms to be used and their completion).

In legal terms, this raises several issues, in particular:

- The proper interpretation of legal texts where they are broadly written.
- The extent to which any guidelines assist interpretation.
- The status of guidelines and the extent to which guidelines are themselves enforceable.

Laws are clearly made in an effort to regularize and control an activity in a range of situations, but in order to achieve a high level of compliance, the rules need to be clear, coherent and comprehensive and there must be 'certainty' about the nature and scope of the requirements. This is a goal that, in fact, relatively few pieces of legislation ever fully attain.

The legal status of guidance documentation depends upon whether it is incorporated/referenced in the legislation. In some cases, specific cross-reference to a document or documents may be made, together with a requirement for compliance, so incorporating the contents into the legislation. In general, however, guidance is merely guidance, and therefore, not legally enforceable. Non-compliance with such guidance is not a breach of the legal requirements, or subject to legal penalty. However, guidelines are, at least, a strong indication of the competent regulatory authorities' approach to interpreting and applying the law and in practice, guidance will play an important part in determining an authorization holder's policy and practice. Moreover, adopted guidance texts can have legal significance in the context of determining 'civil' liability. In cases where negligence is alleged, guidelines, especially those written by, or with the support of, regulatory authorities, provide a benchmark against which the civil Courts would tend to judge the 'reasonableness' of a defendant company's systems and the conduct of its business activities.

Although it is not intended to revisit the detail of relevant regulations and guidelines in this chapter, the issue of the adequacy of written requirements for the purposes of compliance and enforcement will be briefly addressed. Otherwise, the focus of this chapter will be to look at legal responsibility for compliance and the legal consequences in terms of both procedures and liability (civil and criminal) of failures in the practice of pharmacovigilance in relation to marketed products. This discussion will concentrate on the European Union (EU) with occasional comparative reference to the USA.

Legal Responsibility for Pharmacovigilance and Contracting (Licensing) In/Out

Under European Community (EC) rules, pharmacovigilance is one of several legal obligations of the product marketing authorization holder (MAH). The duty attaches whether or not the MAH intends itself to perform the obligation, or to invest in third party services. The legislation does not prohibit such contractual arrangements for buying in services for the purposes of achieving compliance, but the responsibility for compliance, as a matter of law, continues to rest with the MAH. Regulatory authorities are rarely, if ever, interested in excuses for regulatory reporting failures based upon the breach of some contractual obligation by someone other than the responsible MAH. There is, therefore, always a risk to contracting in services that are crucial to regulatory compliance, especially where a breach may give rise to criminal or other administrative sanctions. It is a commercial risk many companies take, and in many circumstances, they have little choice. Smaller entities may simply not possess the infrastructure to set up and run a 'full service' drug safety unit. Foreign companies establishing a presence in new markets may also not possess the necessary experience of the local regime to undertake pharmacovigilance (or other MAH obligations) without external help. This is a common reason for the commercial licensing out of products by smaller developer/niche companies.

Careful contractual drafting is essential in these circumstances. A high level of trust is placed by the MAH in a third party whose incompetence, should it occur, may have significant consequences for the MAH. In the more complex commercial arrangements, it is generally more practical and therefore preferable, to impose only the basic obligations in the contract itself and to incorporate by cross reference, a detailed operating procedure, a standard operating procedure (SOP) (ideally developed for the particular contractual relationship), which must thereafter be regularly reviewed, updated and amended in line with changes in the legal requirements and developments in good practice. This avoids producing a turgid, lengthy contract and facilitates subsequent amendment of the working document as necessary. Care with the accuracy and clarity of cross-reference is important. In some jurisdictions, the courts will look critically at the circumstances of inclusion (e.g. Sweden where the party agreeing to comply must have had sight of and understand the content of the reference document at or before signing). Such contractual safeguards, involving the detailed spelling out of the third party's obligations, are essential and offer the MAH a degree of protection, but cannot however, guarantee a total indemnity for all losses consequent upon a breach, or compensation for any criminal liability that could arise where failure nonetheless occurs.

These concerns arise irrespective of the jurisdiction to which the MAH is subject. The precise penalties for failure to comply will, however, differ from country to country, and whether there is individual, or merely corporate, exposure to them will also depend upon local law (see below).

In product liability terms, the basic issues to which the MAH must give thought are again common to most jurisdictions, although the precise principles and approach will depend upon local product liability provisions. In certain countries for example, the burden of proof in claims for product-related personal injury is 'relaxed' in favour of the claimant and the courts are quick to find that the burden has been satisfied (e.g. in the Netherlands). In others, there may be special provision made for pharmaceutical product claims through insurance pools, which pay out (usually at levels less than those obtainable through court proceedings) on proof of causation alone; there are such schemes in Sweden and Finland.

Clearly, the potential consequences of a breach of pharmacovigilance requirements are not only regulatory (e.g. action against the authorization and/or MAH and/or others by the regulatory authorities, and the imposition of penalties), but civil, where they may arise in the context of claims for personal injury based upon allegations of negligence and/or the supply of a defective product causing injury. In such a case, the claims might be expected to be framed in terms that a failure or delay in relation to the collection, analysis, periodic review and/or reporting of adverse drug reactions (ADRs) has meant that a significant safety issue was either not identified at all, identified too late, or was insufficiently characterized for proper action to have been taken to place limitations upon the availability and/or use and administration of a product. This would, for example, include failure in relation to implementing labelling changes or product withdrawal where, at the time, with proper attention, one or other would have been the appropriate course to have taken to safeguard patient health.

In claims based on negligence, a plaintiff might seek to establish that:

- The MAH knew or ought to have known through appropriate pharmacovigilance activities, of the risk posed by the product.
- The MAH should have acted or should have acted sooner or more expansively.

- The system was (still is) generally below reasonable operational standards compared against prevailing legal requirements and/or industry practice. The evidence for this type of pleading often arises from papers examined under the court rules for 'discovery' (i.e. disclosure of all relevant documents by each party to proceedings to the other).
- If the claimant can then show, on the balance of probabilities that the deficiency identified was 'causative' of the injury suffered, the claim will be established and damages obtained.

In strict liability cases, there is no need to show fault as in negligence claims. The mere fact of some inadequacy in pharmacovigilance practice having occurred where it has led to the product being less safe than persons would generally be entitled to expect (i.e. 'defective') will be sufficient (e.g. because the labelling fails to present the full side effects, warnings or precautions for the product accurately), providing that causation is established. The majority of defences made available by statute in strict liability cases will not apply. Again, the basic principles of strict liability are common to the European and USA jurisdictions. More detail will be set out below.

Contracting with a third party to perform a regulatory function for and on behalf of the MAH will not isolate the MAH from suit or a finding of liability, but the MAH may be able to recover at least part of any damages and costs awarded against it from the service provider under the contract. Clearly defined obligations and indemnities in the contract are of central importance to such recovery.

Interpreting Legal Provisions

Table 1 lists the relevant legal texts in which the EC has set out the pharmacovigilance requirements applicable in all member states. These provisions are 'over layered' or supplemented in several member states by provisions of local law, leading to a level of complexity in terms of compliance (regarding nationally authorized and Mutual Recognition (MR) products), which could, and in future should, be further reduced by EU harmonization initiatives without compromising public safety.

In looking at EC Law, (i.e. law passed by EC institutions) the approach to interpretation is 'purposive'. This means that the exact wording of the provisions is less important than the intention underlying the legislation. It would be normal practice, therefore, in considering EC legal provisions to look closely at the recitals set out, often in great detail, at the beginning of EC directives and regulations. The aim is to

Table 1	EC legislation for pharmacovigilance
Product	Legislation
Centrally authorized medicinal products	Regulation 2309/93 Regulation 540/95
Mutually recognized (MR) authorized medicinal products	Directive 75/319/EEC (as amended) plus local provisions
Nationally authorised medicinal products	Directive 75/319/EEC (as amended) plus local provisions

a

encourage interpretation in line with the objects that the legislation is stated to be intended to achieve.

In relation to pharmacovigilance, Regulation 2309/93 states "Where as it is also necessary to make provision for the supervision of medicinal products which have been authorised by the Community and, in particular, for the intensive monitoring of adverse reactions... in order to ensure the rapid withdrawal from the market of any medicinal product which presents an unacceptable risk under normal conditions of use".

Directive 75/319/EEC (as amended) states that it is "desirable to codify and improve the co-operation and exchange of information between member states relating to the supervision of medicinal products and in particular the monitoring of adverse reactions under practical conditions of use through national pharmacovigilance systems".

Furthermore, EC legislation must also be considered in the context of fundamental European legal principles, including:

- Respect for natural justice (e.g. the right to equal treatment in the EU, the right to be heard).
- 'Transparency' of requirements imposed and in respect of procedures applied.
- The protection of public health and the facilitation of free movement of goods within the EU.

The EC legal provisions for pharmacovigilance are 'supplemented' by guidance (listed in Table 2) issued by the CPMP and the Commission, although a significant proportion of this has been only available in draft form following the introduction of changes to legislation brought about by the introduction of the 'New Systems' for registration. This was evidently not ideal, given that provisions of the legislation can be relatively vague and are limited in scope. The authorities' considered approach to interpretation is therefore not yet formally set out in any adopted documentation. Chapter V of the *Notice to Applicants*, part IIA contained in the December 1994 draft (5944/94) is under revision and therefore of minimal current value. The replacement text is due to be published separately as *Volume IX of the Rules Governing Medicinal Products in the EU* during 1998.

The legislation does make cross-reference to the existence of guidelines to be adopted by the Commission: "The Commission in consultation with the Agency, Member States and interested parties shall draw up guidance on the collection, verification and presentation of adverse reaction reports". But the reference is oblique and while 'guidance' remains in draft, its status is doubly uncertain. This said, when the guidance does appear in final form, it will clearly constitute an important source of reference for MAHs.

There are also other difficulties that Volume IX should address. The guidance, both finalized and draft, that exists, is not yet consistent, with differences arising between the legislation and the guidelines and between guidelines (e.g. in 75/319/EEC 'serious adverse drug reaction' is defined as "an adverse reaction which is fatal, life threatening, disabling, incapacitating or which results in a prolonged hospitalisation". In 5375/93 the definition is "any untoward medical occurrence that at any dose results in death, is life threatening, requires in patient hospitalisation or prolongation of existing hospitalisation, results in persistent or significant disability, incapacity or is

Table 2 Guidance texts on pharmacovigilance (CPMP: Committee for Proprietary Medicinal Products; ICH: International Conference on Harmonization)

Description	Comment
Chapter V, Draft Notice to Applicants Vol. IIA 5944/94	Chapter V under review. Vol IX of the Notice to Applicants in draft May 1998; under discussion
Causality classification in pharmacovigilance in the EC 111/3445	Adopted 1991
Pharmacovigilance in the framework of the CPMP 111/8234/89	Adopted October 1990
Note for guidance on the procedure for competent authorities on the undertaking of pharmacovigilance 175/95	Adopted by CPMP 8.6.95 Supersedes draft 111/3963/92
Guideline on adverse reaction reporting by MA holders 111/3174/93	Draft
Guideline for marketing authorisation holders on periodic drug safety update reports 111/3173/93	Draft
Guideline for marketing authorization holders on post-marketing safety studies111/3176/93	Draft
Guideline for MA holders on ongoing pharmacovigilance evaluation during the post-marketing period 111/3177/93	Draft
Clinical safety data management: definitions and standards for expedited reporting (ICH) 337/97	Operative 1.6.95, supersedes 111/3375/93
Data elements for transmission of individual ADR reports (ICH) 287/95	Supersedes 144/95
Clinical safety data management: period safety update reports for marketed drugs (ICH) 288/95	To be incorporated in revised Chapter V of 5944/94 Operative 18.6.97 (111/3175/93 superseded)
Conduct of pharmacovigilance for centrally authorized products 183/97	Adopted April 1997

a congenital anomaly or birth defect)". As a matter of law, the position is that it is the legislation which binds and is enforceable and so must be followed. This fact is acknowledged in the recently adopted ICH guideline 288/95: "Guidelines are not legally binding. Some portions of this guideline may not be reflected in existing regulations. To that extent, until the regulations are amended, MAHs must comply with existing regulations".

EC directives (not 'regulations', which have immediate, direct application and effect upon the date earmarked following adoption by the Community) need to be implemented by member states before they can be applied and enforced by those authorities. The treatment of guidelines in this process may also differ, with some member states actually incorporating the guidance into their implementing measures. A good example of this arose in relation to the CPMP's good clinical practice (GCP) guidelines of 1990, to which specific reference was made in local legislation in Italy and the Netherlands. It is inevitable that some differences in interpretation and therefore, in the results of implementation, will arise during this process. However, member states can be brought to book by the Commission in the European Court of Justice (ECJ) for improper implementation of, or failure to implement, EC legislation.

In the UK, concern with regard to achieving complete implementation has led to a change in the approach to drafting legislation. By tradition, English law is drafted precisely with careful use of language and, until recently, efforts were made to transpose or 'translate' European requirements and to fit them into and around whatever UK legislation existed. However, particularly in the field of medicines law, following the discovery of some legislative shortcomings, the practice has developed so that the draftsmen now tend to 'lift' large sections of the text from European legislation and place it in local legislation, without any attempt to mould or interpret it or to alter the language to fit that previously used in English texts. Such 'importation' can be problematic where the text used has been drafted in accordance with a different legal culture and is comparatively ambiguous or vague. An alternative approach has merely been to cross refer to the 'relevant Community provisions' incorporating them, as they stand in full, again, bringing with them any inherent problems or issues of interpretation that are part and parcel of the European text (see SI 3144 of 1994, Article 7(1) "Every holder of an UK marketing authorisation... shall comply with all obligations which relate to him by virtue of the *relevant* Community provisions including in particular obligations relating to providing or updating information... to pharmacovigilance..."). Such problems may be less of an issue in other systems. In German legislative practice, laws are produced together with statements of reasons for both general and more specific provisions allowing regulated individuals, the national authority and the court to make use of these explanatory statements in interpreting the provisions.

In any event, it is also a requirement of EC law that local laws must be interpreted in the light of, and consistently with, the relevant EC provisions and objectives. In the context of pharmacovigilance, both the general and specific aims (above) of medicines legislation must be borne in mind.

- "The primary purpose of any rules concerning the production and distribution of medicinal products must be to safeguard public health". (Directive 65/65/EEC)
- The competent authority "shall suspend or revoke an authorisation... where that product proves to be harmful in normal conditions of use...". (Directive 65/65/EEC)
- The establishment of the CPMP was stated to be "in order to facilitate the adoption of *common* decisions by member states on the authorisation of medicinal products on the basis of scientific criteria". (Directive 75/319/EEC)

The EC provisions are set out in Chapter 12, but there are deficiencies in the law in its present form. Apart from familiar issues of definition, for example none for 'healthcare professional' (Directive 75/319/EEC, Regulation 2309/93) or 'innovative product' (Regulation 540/95), the scope of 'serious adverse drug reaction' and whether regulators wish to include congenital abnormality in its meaning (as appears in several guidelines), some of the main technical issues are summarized in Table 3.

Table 3 Unresolved issues in European Community law

Queries/Deficiencies	Comment
Scope of the requirements	The legislation (both the regulations and the directives) in imposing both recording and reporting requirements confines itself to 'information about suspected adverse drug reactions' defined in a way that is apparently equivalent to a reference to spontaneous individual ADR reports. In practice, relevant 'drug safety information' is broader than this and the authorities are evidently interested in the recording and reporting of much broader categories of data. For example, the oral contraceptives' review in the mid-1990s raised the question of MAHs' reporting obligations in respect of interim epidemiological study data—a source mentioned in draft guidance, but not covered by the direct recording and reporting requirements in the legislation. In contrast, requirements in the USA for post-marketing reporting of adverse drug experiences addresses the review of data from sources specifically including scientific literature and epidemiological studies.
	The legislation (Directive 75/319/EEC) imposes an obligation upon member states to establish a drug monitoring system and describes their function as the collection of information 'useful in the surveillance of medicinal products'. Consistency in what member states might collect/expect from MAHs and what MAHs should provide would be helpful.
	The law says that member states' systems should allow them to collate information on 'frequently observed misuse' and 'serious abuse', neither of which are defined in the legislation. (Note: In the USA the definition of 'adverse drug experience' expressly includes overdose and events due to abuse, withdrawal, or failure of expected pharmacological action). The EC legislation applies no direct equivalent reporting obligations upon MAHs. Neither occurrence is classified as an ADR, but it seems that attempts are being made through draft guidance to bridge the gap, a function that guidance cannot, in any event fulfil. If an obligation is to be imposed upon MA holders, the law will need amendment.
	Although the argument might be advanced that given the aims of the legislation, all information relevant to drug safety should be made available to regulators within a time frame and in a manner consistent with its degree of seriousness, even if this were correct, it would be preferable and would only be workable if the legislation dealt expressly with these obligations. It is not ideal, and legally doubtful, for regulators to be placed in a position where they seek to rely on provisions such as Article 21(c) in Regulation 2309/93 (see Article 29C of Directive 75/319/EEC for mutual recognition and nationally authorised products) as though it imposed a positive unilateral reporting requirement when it is not worded in such terms: "any *request* from the competent authorities for the provision of additional information necessary for the evaluation of the benefits and risks of a medicinal products is answered fully..." (emphasis added)
Source of reports	The obligations for serious ADR reporting are framed with reference to reports received by MAHs from 'healthcare professionals'. The meaning of 'healthcare professional' is addressed only in draft guideline (Guideline 111/3174/93: Adverse reaction reporting by MA holders), but in any event, leaves doubt as to how to handle reports from other sources or, in the case of some professionals, without the corroboration of the patient's doctor. (Note, however, the World Health Organization (WHO) programme on drug monitoring—36 participating countries accept reports from pharmacists (Edwards, *BMJ*, Vol 315, 30 August 1997)).

Table 3 (*Cont.*)

	Clarification of whether the provision is limited to healthcare professionals, and of what this term means (there is a possible definition, arising out of consideration of the Advertising Directive 92/28/EEC) would improve the position and arguably bring it in line with regulators' expectations. Again, this is not an issue in USA provisions where serious unexpected 15-day alert reports are reportable to the authorities, "regardless of source".
Timing	Reporting of serious ADRs is required "immediately" and within 15 days of receipt of the information. The obligation attaches to the person responsible for placing the product on the market (generally interpreted as the MAH) and so it is reasonable to interpret the relevant receipt being that of the MAH upon whom the duty rests. However, in times of commercial licensing, of co-marketing and various forms of distribution, the addition of the words "by that person" would remove doubt and obviate the possibility of an approach, which would see time running from the time of receipt by another individual even though the MAH had no actual knowledge. In USA practice, companies tend to assume that reporting time runs from receipt of data by a licensee of a product and will seek to set up their reporting systems accordingly. In fact, this is more a matter of industry practice, rather than of any express obligation in law.
Data lock points (DLPs) for periodic reporting	As written, the legislation requires 'periodic safety update reports' (PSURs) at periods calculated from the grant of the authorization of the product in the Community. As contemplated by the ICH guidelines 288/95, this leads to a multiplicity of differing reports for the same product where it is marketed globally, all with slightly differing DLPs. The ICH has acknowledged the lack of practicality or need for this, but the legislation will need amendment if it is to reflect the international consensus that the first date of marketing anywhere in the world can operate as the DLP for a unified PSUR. The legal obligation with regard to the development of EU guidance (not law), is only to "take account of international harmonization work". But politically, the ICH is subscribed to by EC legislators and, to be of value, must have strong influence upon their work in drafting or amending EC legislation.

As indicated, a particular level of complication arises in licensing situations where, as is common in the industry, companies license out products to others for commercial reasons. (For fuller discussion see Monitoring Drug Safety in Commercial Licensing Situations in Europe; *Int. J. Pharmac. Med.*, 1998, 12:55–70.) In these circumstances, doubts or complexity in legislation and guidance are magnified. There is no reference to these practicalities in the EU legislation, although guidance emerging from the ICH does acknowledge the point. However, difficulties arising in relation to the running of a pharmacovigilance unit are magnified in licensing situations where several parties may be involved. Uncertainties of interpretation such as the point of onset of the 15-day reporting period for spontaneous serious ADRs (above) could become particularly significant. A consensus view taken from major companies with EC operations during 1997 appeared to be that the period for making reports should run from the date of knowledge of the MAH fixed with the reporting obligation and not that of the licensee/licensor passing on that information to the

MAH. It would seem that during the first part of 1998 regulators working on Volume IX of the Notice to Applicants were minded to take a different view.

It will be evident that there yet remains some scope for refining the new EC legislation, not least so that it accurately reflects both the information that the regulators reasonably require in practice and that which the regulated are in a position to provide. It was always planned that there would be a review of the pharmacovigilance provisions after six years (i.e., from January 1995) of the operation of the new requirements. The Community is three years into that period without, as yet, having seen completion of its component parts in terms of guidance and the operation of the procedures. Teething troubles are to be expected from the EC legislation in such involved circumstances.

European Procedures and Powers in the event of a Product Safety Issue

The interplay between local and EC authorities on pharmacovigilance matters also raises legal issues. If the product concerned is authorized through the national route in only one member state, dealing with pharmacovigilance signals indicating product safety concerns is a matter for the national authority, following its national procedures, pursuant to national legislation. These will take account of EC provisions, in particular Article 21 of Directive 65/65/EEC, which defines the circumstances in which revocation or suspension may occur as "where the product proves harmful in the normal conditions of use or where its therapeutic efficacy is lacking or where its qualitative and quantitative composition is not as declared . . . where the particulars supporting the application as provided for in Articles 4 and 4a are incorrect or have not been amended in accordance with Article 9a or when the controls referred to in Article 8 of this Directive or Article 23 of Directive 75/319/EEC . . . have not been carried out".

In 1993 the ECJ determined in the case of Pierrel Spa v. Ministero della Sanita (C183/92) that a national authority could revoke or suspend an authorization only on the grounds provided by 65/65/EEC (or other EC legislation) and could not add other bases to their national provisions which extend beyond the scope of EC provisions. The case did not (as Article 21 does not), however, address the matter of the compulsory variation of national authorizations. This remains at local discretion for purely nationally authorized products.

Where the product is also authorized by national route elsewhere in the EC, or where it has been authorized by the mutual recognition route in several member states, there is either the potential (national) or the requirement (mutual recognition) for a safety question to be examined and determined by the CPMP. Where products are centrally authorized, the responsibility for arranging and co-ordinating consideration of the issue, is done at European level, through the European Medicines Evaluation Agency (EMEA) upon the advice of the CPMP, albeit that the alert/concern may originate from one or more member states.

EC provisions make clear arrangements for dissemination of alerts and information between member states and between member states and the EMEA (see Directive 75/319/EEC and Regulation 2309/93). Article 30 of Directive 75/319/EEC states: "Member States shall take all appropriate measures to ensure that the competent authorities concerned communicate to each other such information as is appropriate to guarantee that the requirements for the... marketing authorisations are fulfilled".

The speed and means of transmission of the information depends upon the level of seriousness assigned to the concerns arising from the information received. The system is such that an MAH cannot expect a safety issue to remain ring-fenced in a particular member state when the product is marketed in other parts of the EU.

Where a product is authorized in more than one member state, the reference provisions in Article 12 of Directive 75/319/EEC allow a member state (or the MAH, or the Commission) to refer a safety matter (amongst other issues) to the CPMP, which is obliged, under Article 8.2, to examine it. (When reference has been made by a member state, it must be notified, not only to the CPMP, but also to the MAH. Both the member state and the MAH are thereafter obliged to supply to the CPMP all available information relating to the matter in question which is in their possession. In this way, the issue and the solution for it are thrown into the European arena for a 'European solution' to be adopted.)

The nature of this CPMP obligation was, during 1996, subject to some debate, in particular, in the context of the review of oral contraceptives relating to the degree of risk of serious thromboembolic events in third generation pills. It was unclear whether the UK had made a formal reference under Article 12 of Directive 75/319/ EEC to the CPMP. In the event, the CPMP dealt with the matter on a less formalized basis. An examination of the legal obligations of the CPMP, as drafted, shows that they do not suggest any discretion as to whether to accept a reference. However, there must be a "reference" and the legislation does not spell out the method by which one is to be made or recognized. In theory, therefore, a reference under Article 12 can be made simply by a clear, identifiable request addressed to the CPMP to examine an issue adequately described where "the interests of the Community are involved". It would not require any great formality to make the request, but the question of whether the "interests of the Community" are involved leaves considerable scope for discussion and, presumably, the exercise of some discretion by the CPMP.

The Commission and CPMP view is, evidently, that it is in the general interest for there to be a less formalized process available for the CPMP's scientific experts to evaluate a product safety query without the Committee being drawn immediately into formal and time-limited procedures requiring them to reach a formal opinion that is binding in the EU (once adopted by the Commission). The referral of matters to the CPMP's Pharmacovigilance Working Party is not uncommon with the Working Party reporting its views informally to the CPMP, a practice that is not covered by legislation.

Although Article 12 makes provision for cases to be referred to the CPMP, 'before' a member state reaches a decision with regard to any application, suspension, withdrawal or variation, "which appears necessary, in particular, to take account of the information collected in accordance with Chapter V(a)" (i.e. the pharmacovigilance provisions), the reference is not compulsory ("may refer"). However, Article 15(a) of Directive 75/319/EEC provides a means by which a member state, "in respect of a mutual recognition or a concertation (Directive 87/22/EEC) product, must" refer to the CPMP in circumstances where it considers a variation of the authorization, or its suspension, or withdrawal, is "necessary in the interests of public health".

The relevant procedure for references is set out in Articles 13 and 14 of Directive 75/319/EEC. This requires a reasoned opinion to be provided by the CPMP within 90 days of the reference (with a possible extension of 90 days). However, a shorter deadline might be set where the matter is considered to be urgent. The provisions for hearings under Article 12, state only that the MAH "may" be asked to explain itself, orally or in writing, before the CPMP reaches an opinion. This appears to contrast, to the detriment of the MAH, with the provisions relating to references under Article 11, where the provision is that the MAH has a 'right' to make oral or written explanations. However, bearing in mind the principles of natural justice, it is strongly argued that the difference in drafting style should not be treated as legally significant, with the MAH in either situation, in fact being entitled to and afforded the same rights to appear before the CPMP in order to defend its product.

In the context of a product safety concern, the outcome of the CPMP's consideration may be that the MA, summary of product characteristics (or its equivalent) and labelling be varied or alternatively, that the MA should be suspended or revoked, with immediate, or phased product withdrawal. Delay can arise with regard to the procedural stages which occur 'after' the CPMP has delivered its opinion. Although there are time limits applicable to the decision making progress as to when the EMEA must forward the CPMP opinion to the Commission and when the Commission must draft the resulting licensing decision (both 30 days), time limits are absent from the point at which the standard Community decision-making procedure comes into effect. Procedure involving the Standing Committee and the process occurring between Standing Committee consideration and the Commission's finalization of the decision, is not time limited and can be lengthy. This is simply the result of application of a standard procedure applicable to all decision-making by the Commission, which in the pharmaceutical licensing context, is not ideal. Having said this, in the field of pharmacovigilance, where the decision may concern a serious matter, the sense of urgency may well be such that the formal decision, pursuant to the CPMP's opinion would be made with all due haste. Member states have 30 days to comply with the decision and also to confirm with the CPMP and the Commission that they have done so. Again, although not discussed in the legislation, member states, with due regard to their responsibility/liability to local populations, are likely to take action locally at an early stage following a CPMP opinion in an urgent case. In any event, Directive 75/319/EEC allows the suspension of marketing and use, at local level, in urgent cases in order to protect public health in advance of a "definitive decision being adopted", subject to notice within one day to the CPMP and other member states.

The extent to which member states may deal with what they perceive to be product safety issues without reference to the CPMP is questionable. In the case of an MR product, this is unlikely to be an option. In most cases where compulsory action is contemplated by the member state, it is likely to be considered "necessary for the protection of public health", the basis upon which the obligation to refer arises (Article 15a Directive 75/319/EEC). (Even reasons for revocation provided by Article 11, 65/65/EEC that are concerned with changes in licence particulars and the provision of dossier updates, may raise public safety concerns.) With purely nationally authorized products, there is no requirement in the legislation for a reference, but it should be noted that Article 11 of Directive 75/319/EEC makes provision for references to the CPMP to be made where member states have adopted divergent decisions in relation to MAs for essentially the same product. The Commission has indicated its interest in minimizing the extension and persistence of differences in

MAs granted in different member states for the same basic products. It could certainly invoke an Article 11 procedure where a member state pursued a course of regulatory action at national level on a serious matter without reference to CPMP. A member state's ability to deal on a purely local basis with a safety concern may also depend upon the content of national provisions. In the UK, parts of SI 1994 No 3144 are written in a way that rules out the national procedures applicable to taking compulsory regulatory action, together with the associated appeals rights, where the product in question is "authorised elsewhere in the Community". Perhaps the original intention was to reflect Article 15a, Directive 75/319/EEC and to deal with MR products, but that limitation was not properly applied in the local law, which would require amendment to achieve this clear result and remove the uncertainty now pertaining to local procedures in such circumstances.

In practice, where product crises have arisen since the introduction of the New Systems, as discussed above, the CPMP has not been reluctant to take a less formalized approach to assessing the position. Hence, on a number of occasions, the CPMP has preferred to adopt a position statement, to issue press releases and let matters be thrashed out in the Pharmacovigilance Working Party without being subject to formal process. There are clear advantages in such a stance, but there are, inevitably, also difficulties. 'Informal' consideration of these issues does not result in a binding opinion/decision. Member states are free to apply the outcome of the discussion 'if' and 'as', they see fit. With the non-formal approach, the MAH has no established process or rights (e.g. to make representations to adequate time) upon which to rely. The MAH can still, however, be required to supply information requested to the authorities on statutory grounds. In such circumstances, it would clearly be arguable that it would be against natural justice, even in informal circumstances, for a body charged with responsibilities of review by the Community to fail to allow such representations to be made or to take them into account. However, the lack of set time limits, procedures and requirements does mean that these rights are undetermined and thus, afforded and exercised on an ad hoc basis. Informal procedures are run according to time frames, which are determined by the CPMP and/or the Working Party and the process of evaluation may last for some considerable time, amidst a blaze of publicity. Even after a CPMP consideration that does 'not' result in any form of opinion or recommendation to limit product use or availability, a product may nevertheless be killed off in the marketplace owing to the public speculation regarding its safety.

The Consequence of Failures to Meet Adverse Drug Reaction Reporting Requirements

Common shortcomings that may lead to compliance failures, some more serious than others, include those discussed below.

Misunderstanding the requirements

The more complex the requirements become, the greater the multiplicity of requirements imposed by different authorities, the easier it is to make errors.

Poor or incomplete SOPs

SOPs must be written to cover all aspects of the procedures. Drafting fatigue can set in with the result that the procedures only cover one aspect of one half of the process required.

Insufficient staff and resources

The failure of companies to devote adequate resources to pharmacovigilance is probably becoming a thing of the past. The profile of regulatory functions within pharmaceutical companies has grown tremendously over the last 10 to 15 years with the realization that unless their regulatory affairs are in order and without regulatory input into policy and strategy making, the core of the business of pharmaceutical companies (i.e. in selling products), could be seriously undermined.

Poor inter-company communication

This may lead to unnecessary delays in relevant information being reported by the MAH. Increasingly, over recent years, regulatory authorities have shown that they are inclined to try to look through the separate legal personality of different companies within a corporate group and to expect rapid exchange of information within those corporate groups, particularly in relation to pharmacovigilance. As a matter of law, there are established principles for respecting the individuality and separate personality of companies, which although part of a global group of companies, may well be totally separate in terms of their jurisdiction, operations and internal organization. Nonetheless, from a product liability aspect, it is in the interests of the companies' and corporate headquarters to ensure efficient exchange of relevant product and market information and regulatory data between group members who have products in common.

Delay

This is usually consequential upon one of the other shortcomings above.

Low priority being given to European requirements

Again, since the advent of 'New Systems' and the legal requirement for there to be an appointed 'person responsible' for pharmacovigilance for each MAH, the previously common occurrence of corporate groups setting up their pharmacovigilance functions with the rules and regulations of another jurisdiction as the governing factor is changing. The legislation forces companies to focus upon access and accountability within the EU (e.g. see Article 7, 65/65/EEC).

Failure to train representatives

As part of the company structure, representatives in the field are often the first point of contact between the company and health care professionals. EC law makes it plain that company representatives have a clear role in pharmacovigilance (see Article 21, Regulation 2309/93 and Article 29c, Directive 75/319/EEC). Failure to train representatives, and failure to establish procedures that require and enable them to pass on within adequate time, information collected in the field from health care professionals, may well lead to companies overreaching the 15-day reporting period for spontaneous, serious reactions.

Failure to provide for regular review

Before the requirements were introduced for PSURs, it was not unusual for MAHs not to have in place adequate procedures for regular review of the totality of ADRs and safety data received within a given period to compare it against the previous product record. In this way, for example, increased incidence might be missed. The requirements under the legislation for PSURs should make such omission impossible.

Poor follow up

It is a common criticism of regulators that reports are not adequately followed up by MAHs. However, it can arise that the MAH's ability to undertake follow-up is severely curtailed by the attitude and lack of cooperation from original sources or lack of knowledge, such as when corroboration is sought from a doctor where the source is the patient or the pharmacist. This will highlight the absence of legal compulsion upon health care professionals to make reports in the first instance. The European rules 'allow' member states to make reporting by health care professionals a legal requirement. In the majority of member states, the professionals have not had this obligation imposed upon them, (but see, for example, Italy where new rules affecting doctors and pharmacists have been introduced).

Failure to tie in licensees, distributors, joint venture and other partners

It is still common for contracts between commercial partners to give low priority to the arrangements for liaison in relation to pharmacovigilance. It is also still common for these arrangements to be addressed only after a contract has been entered into and for there to be little, and in some cases, no provision, for exchange or supply of information. Although imposing obligations does not guarantee adherence by a contractual partner, total failure to set them out clearly in the first instance is a major oversight. Addressing the issue only after a contract has been completed may give rise to delay and difficulties when the parties cannot agree the arrangements in subsequent discussion, and may have more far reaching consequences when the structure and finance provisions are, or would have been affected, by the arrangements necessary for pharmacovigilance (e.g. in a large contract where the cost of IT systems is an issue).

Types of consequences of failure to meet requirements

The consequences of failures to meet requirements can be roughly divided into:

- Regulatory.
- Civil.
- Criminal.

The consequences may apply to the MAH, to the individual who is appointed as 'person responsible' for pharmacovigilance and also to other officers of the MAH. While it may be thought that the appointment of a 'person responsible' would insulate all other senior company officers from any responsibility in relation to a failure of compliance, this is not necessarily so. As a matter of law, and depending upon the provisions applicable in the member state dealing with the breach, it is possible for other officers of the company of sufficient level of authority and having some degree of responsibility, involvement and/or knowledge, to be made subject to enforcement proceedings.

Regulatory Consequences

Regulatory consequences will affect the MAH and the MA itself. A loss of credibility with regulatory authorities can be a serious commercial concern. A failure in reporting compliance may ultimately result in product safety being reviewed (see above), although it is actually more common for failures in reporting to come to light 'after' a product safety issue has already been identified within the member state.

It is a moot point, however, whether breach of pharmacovigilance requirements would justify revocation of an MA, 'in the absence' of a clear and immediate safety concern of a serious nature (i.e. whether the technical breach alone would be significant justification). As discussed above, Directive 65/65/EEC provides for suspension or revocation of authorizations 'only' where the product proves harmful in normal conditions of use, therapeutic efficacy is lacking or where qualitative and quantitative composition is not as originally declared (see Article 11 and Article 21, see also Regulation 2309/93 for equivalent provisions for centralized products). Directive 75/319/EEC refers to suspension or withdrawal taking place where it is necessary for the protection of public health—Article 15(a). As mentioned, in the case of Pierrel SPA *v.* Minstero dela Sanita (C83/92 7 December 1993), the ECJ found that the only ground upon which revocation would be justifiable by the Italian authorities were those mentioned in Directive 65/65/EEC. It is not open to competent authorities (central or national) to add to those provisions. It therefore seems that any failure in pharmacovigilance compliance must raise a question of safety, quality or efficacy for a revocation of the authorization to be justifiable, consistent with Article 11, 65/65/EEC. In contrast, US provisions for post-marketing reporting of adverse drug experiences state, "If an applicant fails to establish and maintain records and make reports as required under this section, FDA may withdraw approval of the application and thus prohibit continued marketing..." (Para 71, 423 S314.81).

There is also an issue as to whether a breach of a pharmacovigilance obligation might provoke/justify competent authority inspection. Where products are nationally authorized, local law will be applicable in respect of operations taking place within the jurisdiction and in some cases, European member states assign wide powers to competent authority inspectorates (e.g. UK Medicines Act 1968, Section 111 *et seque*). Directive 75/319/EEC envisages "repeated inspections to ensure compliance with legal requirements" (see Article 26). Although this provision was originally placed in the legislation in the context of the regulation of manufacturing operations, again coupled with whatever local provisions apply, this is now extended by expansion of the directive to provide a basis for inspections to be undertaken by certain competent authorities, in broader circumstances.

Where a product is centrally authorized, the responsibility for following up pharmacovigilance matters rests with the EMEA (CPMP). However, the EMEA has no manpower for the conduct of inspections and EC legislation generally envisages co-operation between the Community and member states. The mechanism for an inspection in those circumstances, could be a request from the EMEA or CPMP addressed to the member state in which the MAH conducts relevant operations where the pharmacovigilance function takes place. Regulation 2309/93 envisages the Commission, in such circumstances, co-ordinating the "supervisory responsibilities" of member states. Article 17 states that the "supervisory authorities shall have responsibility for exercising supervision over MAHs" in accordance with Chapter V of Directive 75/319/EEC (i.e. pharmacovigilance activities). The Regulation defines supervisory authorities as those who have granted the manufacturing authorization, or where batch control and release of third country imports takes place. This may not, however, be the same country as that in which the company bases its pharmacovigilance activities. However, 'supervision' and enforcement are not necessarily synonymous and this does not rule out action by another member state with legal jurisdiction, perhaps at the supervisory authority's request. This remains speculation in the absence of any actual examples.

Article 17.2 provides further for "serious disagreements" between member states as to MAH compliance with manufacturing or pharmacovigilance requirements to be settled by the Commission requesting an inspector from the supervisory authority to undertake a further inspection accompanied, if required, by an impartial member state, and/or a rapporteur or expert nominated by the CPMP. Member states are also obliged to refer to the CPMP (and Commission), concerns arising and proposals for action to be taken where they consider one of the measures covered in Chapter V or VI, Directive 75/319/EEC (pharmacovigilance sections) should be applied. It is up to the Commission then to refer the matter to the CPMP and it would seem that the Commission may, in these circumstances, determine the time limit for delivery of the CPMP opinion according to urgency.

Civil Consequences—product Liability

Although in the context of personal injury claims, the MAH and other parties (e.g. doctors, licensing authorities) may all be the target of proceedings, it is usually the MAH pharmaceutical company, perceived as having 'deep pockets', that is the prime target for claimants. Claims for negligence based upon a failure to act with reasonable care (e.g. to obtain or act upon pharmacovigilance data) and/or the supply of a product that is "defective" in legal terms (e.g. because its labelling was not amended, pursuant to the receipt and review of pharmacovigilance data so as to give adequate warnings and precautions) are always possible.

Tables 4 and 5 set out in very simple terms the necessary 'ingredients' for establishing product liability, either in negligence or under statute: so-called, strict liability.

All of the elements of each of these legal wrongs must be present in a given situation for liability to be established. In negligence therefore, where the claim is

Table 4 Criteria for negligence—D + L + F + C = N	
D: Duty of care	Owed to the claimant; easy to establish in the case of the supplier/ manufacturer *vis à vis* the patient who uses the product
L: Lack of reasonable care	Evidenced by a failure to conduct operations according to accepted standards applicable at the time—that is, a breach of regulatory requirements, or possibly failure to take account of or apply (industry) guidelines
F: Foreseeable injury	Of the type likely to occur following failure (e.g. side effect of the drug)
C: Causation	The lack of reasonable care must have caused/contributed to the injury; if a label would not have been read by the patient in any event, an omission from it might not have caused injury

Table 5 Criteria for Strict Liability—D + D + C = SL	
D: Defect	Widely defined—product design defect, manufacturing error, (so that the product is less safe than persons generally would be entitled to expect) deficiency in 'presentation'
D: Damage	To person or property flowing from the defect
C: Causation	see Table 4

made against the person alleged to owe the duty of care (in the context of this chapter, this will be the MAH putting the product on the market) proof of causation, without a lack of reasonable care having occurred, will not afford the claimant a remedy. However, the chief distinction between negligent liability and so-called strict liability is that in the case of the latter, fault is not required to be shown. To establish strict liability (Directive 85/374/EEC) the claimant must establish against the "producer" (manufacturer/importer into the EU), that the product was "defective" (for the purpose of the law, this could refer to shortcomings in its presentation, design or manufacture) and that it caused the injury suffered.

It would not be at all unusual for claimants in personal injury actions to look for a regulatory compliance failure on the part of a company defendant. The demonstration of a regulatory breach will significantly assist the plaintiff in establishing lack of reasonable care (i.e. conduct falling below acceptable standards). In fact, whether the failure is alleged to be directly relevant to the injury or not, it can be used to demonstrate a general lack of care in the operation of corporate systems with prejudicial effect. Failure to warn is a common element of many pharmaceutical product liability cases, where the pleadings (of negligence and strict liability) might be expected to assert that had the labelling accurately dealt with contraindications, precautions and/or warnings, the patient would have avoided the injury allegedly suffered, either because the product would not have been used/administered at all, or the patient would have been monitored, advised (by the treating doctor), or managed differently so as to avert injury.

In a case where pharmacovigilance omissions are identified that can be said to lead to no/or an insufficient response being adopted by the MAH (especially where the

---

Table 6 Scenario

Product X MA granted in 1993

Patient A prescribed product in July 1994

Company receives reports of serious unexpected possible ADRs early May 1994

Follow-up poor and protracted

Reports not filed for 12 weeks; company takes no further action thereafter

Mr A suffers serious reaction (same as those reported) end July 1994

Following receipt of reports, regulatory authority reviews product and (a) takes it off market, or (b) strictly limits its use and amends warnings and contraindications (identifying an ascertainable group of patients in whom use is discouraged) in September 1994

Mr A Sues claiming he would not and should not have been exposed to the drug at all; he falls within the contraindicated group

---

regulatory authorities have taken some form of action or simply criticized a company), the plaintiff is a significant way towards establishing a case for lack of reasonable care in negligence, or that the product was defective in strict liability terms, because it was not presented accurately and was therefore, less safe than persons were entitled to expect, given the content of the labelling.

Table 6 sets out a brief scenario that crudely illustrates the issues.

In this situation, the company has received reports of serious unexpected possible ADRs. The product has not long been on the market and is probably under intensive monitoring. Where those professionals reporting the events clearly suspect them to be ADRs, the company should have notified the authorities with basic information immediately, supplying follow-up data as obtained and affording the authorities the opportunity to pursue their own line of enquiry. To report only after follow-up and then not to consider (aside from compulsory activity by the authorities) what would be an appropriate response, would not amount to reasonable, responsible conduct, especially when the authorities subsequently take action to withdraw/amend the MA.

In such circumstances, Mr A can make a good case for saying that swifter action by the company would have resulted in earlier product withdrawal/MA amendment such that he would not have been exposed to the risk of hazard.

There are factors that might alter the legal assessment of such cases. For example, had the information received been garbled and difficult to draw any conclusions upon, or insufficient to constitute an ADR report, the delay in following up until the 'minimum' information necessary was available might not be unreasonable where action could not be taken until intelligible, assessable data were obtained. If follow-up were unsuccessful, the ability to demonstrate that all reasonable steps had been taken by the company would be crucial. (Note: in the USA, regulatory requirements require a report of "steps taken to seek additional information and the reasons why it could not be obtained" with regard to 15-day alert reports).

It may be that even had a label change been implemented earlier, Mr A's doctor would still have prescribed X, judging the potential risks to be outweighed by the potential benefit and that Mr A would have agreed to take it, so that the omission/ defect did not actually lead to the injury and the label change would not have changed the course of events. This line of argument is problematic where the compulsory regulatory action taken is MA suspension followed by revocation.

The company's failure to amend labelling or withdraw the product might still be acceptable if the company can show that it did promptly, fully and properly consider the data, but reasonably (i.e. for good, identifiable, recorded reasons) decided in all the circumstances to leave the product on the market in its current presentation. Subsequent compulsory action by the authorities, defended by the company, would not render a well-considered decision unreasonable retrospectively, although that fact is likely to test strenuously the rationale of the company's earlier decision making. In general, in any event, although certainly influential, the decision of an authority will not be determinative of whether there has been negligence or whether a product is defective.

Criminal Consequences

The possibility of criminal sanctions for breach of pharmacovigilance requirements arises in a number of member states, including the UK. They may be applied to MAH companies and to individual employees, including the 'responsible persons', with the resulting prosecution, in the worst cases, leading to a fine and/or imprisonment, loss of reputation, and in the case of individuals, loss of employment. These are clearly, for individuals, potentially very serious consequences and highlight the level of responsibility imposed upon those taking on the role of 'person responsible' for pharmacovigilance. Having said this, within Europe, individual prosecutions are relatively rare in relation to regulatory breaches generally. There has been no publicity within the EU of any prosecution of a private individual in cases of non-compliance with MAH obligations since the requirements were introduced.

Where nationally authorized products are concerned, the relevant local provisions may be applied by the member state in respect of the MAH and possibly company officers including 'person responsible' whose identity is notified to the authorities. With regard to mutual recognition products, these are still locally granted authorizations and breaches could be expected to be dealt with on a local level with liaison between authorities. However, the relevance of local sanctions to breaches occurring in relation to centrally authorized products where the competent authority is the EMEA/Commission, must be examined further.

The Commission has no powers of prosecution, no criminal competence in this context and the regulations and legislation do not contain any specific reference to types of sanction. However, the EC does expect member states to take proportionate measures to enforce EC law. It is expected that member states will enforce the law with the same effectiveness and thoroughness as national law (see Council Resolution 95/C 118/01). As with regulatory supervision, the mechanism therefore, is for authorities at EC level to request a member state or member states, to take action according to their local provisions in respect of MAHs/persons responsible etc. operating within their jurisdiction. Article 69 of Regulation 2309/93 specifically provides that member states must determine the penalties for infringement of the regulations. These penalties must be "sufficient to promote compliance". If a breach occurs in certain jurisdictions, this might constitute an offence, but the MAH could, it would seem, be subject to different enforcement action in other member states where the locally provided penalties are less strict. Table 7 shows the differences between some member states in their provisions for sanctions for breaches of pharmacovigilance regulations. For example, in the UK, the *Medicines Act* 1968 provides for

Table 7   Pharmacovigilance—member states (survey Mckenna & Co, Autumn 1996 and Spring 1997)

Country	Legislation	Offence	Sanction
Belgium	Law on Medicinal Products 25.3.1964 (as amended) Royal Decrees 3.7.69 (as amended), 7.4.95	Breach may be punished by criminal sanction or administrative fine: depends upon seriousness	• Imprisonment (eight days to one month) and/or fine (BEF 100–1000 × 200) • Administrative fine (BEF 100–500 × 200)
Germany	German Drug Law 1976 (as amended) Regulation (Pharm BetrV) Federal Health Office (BGA) 1991 (due to be replaced by announcement of Federal Institute (BfArM)	Administrative offence	Fine up to DM 50 000 (criminal liability for bodily injury or involuntary manslaughter)
Italy	Presidential Decree No. 93 25.1.91 Decree of Ministry of Health 20.4.91 Circular of Ministry of Health 29.4.93 Law 24.1.96 Legislative Decree No. 44.F18-2-97.	Administrative sanctions for breach of rules with regard to institution of pharmacovigilance services: fines from Itl 30 m to Itl 180 m (MAH and person responsible)	Penalty Itl 1 m – Itl 10 m and imprisonment up to six months in cases of violation of duty to record and notify serious ADRs to the competent authorities or to file a report upon request or period reports
Spain	Law 25/1990 Royal Decree 767/93	Administrative infringement (serious)	Fine 500 000–2 500 000 Ptas (or × 5 value of product)
UK	Medicines Act 1968 Regulation 3144 of 1994	Criminal offence	Fine and/or imprisonment. Fine £5000 (summary) unlimited (indictment) and/or imprisonment (two years on indictment)

criminal sanctions for several offences and, under Section 124, for the individual 'personal' criminal responsibility of corporate officers. Under Regulation 3144 of 1994, which implements all recent EC pharmaceutical directives, enforcement powers are expressly reserved in respect of 'EC obligations', which include those relating to pharmacovigilance (see Schedules 3, 10 and 14). The legislation makes no distinction whatsoever between action taken where centrally authorized products are concerned and where products have national authorizations. However, it would be unlikely that a member state would act in respect of breaches concerning a centralized product without first reporting/referring to or receiving a request from the competent authority—EMEA/Commission/CPMP.

It is clear from EC legislation (see above) that the member states' competent authorities are expected to monitor compliance and to keep the European authorities well informed. Under UK law, criminal prosecutions against individuals are still relatively rare and indeed prosecutions generally are undertaken only in clearcut cases, since the competent authority must make a significant commitment of its limited resources. However, EC policy in addressing regulatory obligations and allocating regulatory responsibility is increasingly to nominate individuals within MAHs for key responsibilities at the regulatory level with the intention, no doubt, of focusing activity and attention, and improving compliance. For this to be achieved, there must evidently be potential for sanctions to be imposed where standards are not achieved, particularly where there are marked consequences for patient health.

Chapter 15

Ethics, Honesty and the Pharmaceutical Industry

M. D. B. Stephens

"All research involving direct contact with patients or healthy people is to be submitted for independent ethical review and for the individual subject's prior consent" (Diamond *et al.*, 1994). The duties and composition of Independent Ethics Committees (IECs) are laid down in the 'Guideline for good clinical practice, 1996', (ICH E6 CPMP/ICH/135/95 Para. 3). Their main function is to safeguard the rights, safety and wellbeing of all trial subjects.

The IEC should consist of a reasonable number of members, who collectively have the qualifications and experience to review and evaluate the science, medical aspects and ethics of the proposed trial. It is recommended that there are at least five members, of whom there is one member whose primary area of interest is in a non-scientific area and one member who is independent of the institution/trial site. For multinational studies there is a European Ethical Review Committee (EERC) (Bennett, 1995). In the USA, France and Scandinavia the ethical committees are an integrated part of drug trial regulation (Hvidberg, 1994). Those working in pharmacovigilance with clinical trials need to be familiar with the associated ethical problems and their implications.

Ethics

Individual Ethics

What is best for the present patient? This is the approach of the practising clinician and is represented by the Bayesian methodology. It must always prevail when dealing with serious type B suspected adverse drug reactions (ADRs).

Collective Ethics

What is best for the population of patients or society? This is the approach of most statisticians and epidemiologists and is represented by standard statistical methods. This is at its strongest when applied to common mild reversible type A ADRs.

It has been suggested that individual ethics should dominate the early clinical trials (i.e. phase I and II while collective ethics should dominate phase III and IV) (Palmer, 1993).

The most important document regarding ethics in clinical trials is the Declaration of Helsinki, which should be attached to all trial protocols. The first two paragraphs of the introduction are "It is the mission of the physician to safeguard the health of the people. His or her knowledge and conscience are dedicated to the fulfilment of this mission" (collective approach).

The *Declaration of Geneva of the World Medical Association* binds the physician with the words "The health of my patient will be my first consideration" (Hurwitz and Richardson, 1997) and the International Code of Medical Ethics declares that "A physician shall act only in the patient's interest when providing medical care which may have the effect of weakening the physical and mental condition of the patient" (individual approach).

Paragraph 5 of section I entitled 'Basic principles' states "Every biomedical research project involving human subjects should be preceded by careful assessment of predictable risks in comparison with foreseeable benefits to the subject or to others. Concern for the interest of the subject must always prevail over the interest of science and society" (i.e. individual ethic must always be put before the collective ethic).

Paragraph 7 of the same section states "Physicians should abstain from engaging in research projects involving human subjects unless they are satisfied that the hazards involved are believed to be predictable. Physicians should cease any investigations if the hazards are found to outweigh the potential benefits". The problem lies here in the word "predictable" since type B ADRs are defined as being unpredictable as opposed to type A, which are predictable.

Paragraph 3 of the section entitled 'Medical research combined with professional care' (clinical research) reads "In any medical study, every patient—including those of a control group, if any—should be assured of the best proven diagnostic and therapeutic methods".

Placebo-controlled Trials

Does the last paragraph mean that a placebo control group is not ethical unless there is no proven treatment for a disease? One clinical pharmacologist has said "the blanket Helsinki recommendations which undermine the use of placebos generally, need revision" (Collier, 1995) and he goes on to say "Incidentally, it seems to preclude study of 'active' experimental drugs since proof of their efficacy cannot come until the trial is completed". Dr L. Lasagna adds weight to this argument by stressing the scientific advantages of placebo studies (Lasagna, 1995).

This has been countered "But if blind assessment can be achieved in a comparative trial of two active treatments is there any point to using a placebo group?" And later "If we adhere to these ethical guidelines, placebo controlled trials should become infrequent as medical knowledge accumulates. Then the scientific method of comparing active treatments against one another will be essential to understand" (Rothman, 1996).

In reply to Rothman three letters in the *British Medical Journal* stress the scientific need for placebo studies (Double, 1996; Georgiou, 1996; McQuay and Moore, 1996).

In an article entitled 'Comparing treatments' there is a subtitle 'Comparison should be against active treatments rather than placebos'. The authors give the reasons for the early use of placebos as "In the United States the Food and Drug Administration, historically, has required evidence from two placebo controlled trials before licensing a new compound, although some recent approvals have been based on a single trial" (Henry and Hill, 1995). The use of placebo in a fluticasone study of allergic rhinitis was said to be of little relevance to clinicians compared with the use of an active control (Galant, 1995; Weinberger, 1995). The use of a placebo group in studies in postoperative vomiting has been said to be unethical (Adams, 1996).

The ethics of using a placebo in controlled trials with odansetron have been questioned and the American Medical Association's Council on Ethics and Judicial Affairs quoted "It is fundamental social policy that the advancement of scientific knowledge must always be secondary to primary concern for the individual" (Citron, 1993).

For a placebo-controlled trial four questions must be answered:

- Was there any therapeutic intervention available that could be reasonably assumed to be less harmful than the placebo control?
- Did the placebo control pose more than a minimal risk to those patients?
- Was the study designed in every way possible to minimize potential harm to the patients receiving placebo?
- Were the patients fully and accurately informed of the additional risk of being in the placebo group? (Citron, 1993).

It must be assumed that the *Declaration of Helsinki* will not be changed within the near future, even if that is desirable. What are the objections to accepting an active control group instead of a placebo group? If the new drug seems indistinguishable from the active control "You don't really know what you've got" according to Dr Robert Temple of the FDA. "The control may be a poor drug, or the trial may have been incapable of detecting true differences between the drugs. Regulators may therefore license an inferior product" (Henry and Hill, 1995).

Early trials using a surrogate endpoint such as blood pressure may only need a few patients when comparing a new drug with placebo to show that it works; but if equivalence with another active drug is required then the trial numbers escalate as will the cost. In order to establish superiority over another active drug the number of patients required will depend upon the difference demanded. Is it possible to defend the use of placebo as a control for the second drug of a new class or performing a second study after a placebo-controlled study has shown that the first drug of a new class is efficacious? Glaxo staff have done so in regard to peptic ulcer disease in the past. Their conclusion was that although placebo-controlled trials in appropriate patient populations place additional ethical concerns on investigators, institutional review boards and sponsors, the benefits derived from the conduct of scientifically sound clinical trials that result in the approval of new drug therapies far outweigh the risks of a placebo control group (Ciociola *et al.*, 1996). This view is at odds with the *Declaration of Helsinki*, paragraph 5, section I above.

For a placebo-controlled clinical trial to be morally justified the following conditions should appertain:

- There must be an uncertainty as to whether the drug is any more likely to be better than a placebo.
- In most cases there must be no agreed alternative treatment better than placebo. Exceptions to this could arise if the statistical advantage of using a 'coarse' comparator like placebo enable a much smaller trial to be conducted as a result, though such trials give a poor picture of the rival merits of the active drugs themselves and as such may be of doubtful value.
- There must be a significant need for the knowledge to be obtained by the placebo-controlled trial (it must be important to know whether the proposed treatment is better than placebo).
- There must be a reasonable possibility that the new drug can indeed turn out to be better than placebo.
- The illness under treatment must not be so serious that any delay in receiving an active drug would be clinically harmful or dangerous.

Placebo-controlled studies should be the exception and not the norm and it should take exceptional circumstances to justify them (Evans and Evans, 1996). These conditions have been taken from a book by the authors, which is well worth reading since it has been written for members of ethical committees.

The exception mentioned in the second condition above needs amplification, since all placebo-controlled studies require fewer patients than those with an active control. In the Glaxo paper, to show a 40% difference between placebo (presumed to heal 35% of ulcers) and the new drug 28 patients are needed in each group, or if the allocation is 2:1 then 21 patients are needed in the placebo group to 42 in the active group. To show equivalence between two active drugs would require 408 patients under the same circumstances.

Although it is possible to reduce the risk run by those in the placebo group by excluding those with predisposing factors, it is extremely unlikely to make the risks equal to those taking an active control. Can one equate the increased risk of 28 patients taking placebo with the lesser risk of the 408 taking an active control? The Glaxo authors also put the point that the placebo control has fewer patients at risk from the ADRs of the new study drug. The chances of discovering ADRs with a new drug increase with the number of patients treated, so this is only relevant if the drug is scrapped and no further studies are undertaken with it. This rarely occurs. Would the FDA accept a new drug application (NDA) with only 28 patients in each group of a placebo-controlled study? If so then there was considerable overkill in the placebo studies in new drugs for peptic ulcer disease. The problem is debated further in a discussion paper (Collins, 1995). In a leading article in the *Lancet* on the defence of the FDA "the acceptance of placebo-controlled evidence in preference to comparator drug trial data is a serious flaw in the regulator process" (*Lancet leader*, 1995).

Ethics committees have been criticized for endorsing proposals for new placebo-controlled research when existing evidence shows that an active form of treatment is better than placebo (Savulescu *et al.*, 1996). In phase I studies the sponsor should consider 'Would I volunteer to take part in this study?' Ten out of 12 companies had special ethics committees for phase I studies (Baber, 1994, 1995). Unfortunately, there have been circumstances where scientists have submitted themselves as volunteers to risks that no ethics committees would ever sanction, so this question does not solve the problem. Suggested further reading is 'Clinical trials: specific problems associated with the use of a placebo control group' by T. J. M. Cleophas, J. v. d. Meulen and R. B. Kalmansohn in the *British Journal of Clinical Pharmacology* (1997) **43**, 219–221.

Many clinical trials organized by the industry have placebo run-in periods and the reasons given are:

- To weed out non-compliers (Hulley and Cummings, 1988, Spilker, 1991).
- To eliminate placebo responders (Spilker, 1991).
- To ensure the patients are stable (Pocock, 1983).
- To wash out previous treatment.
- To provide a period for baseline measurement.

This has been said to be incompatible with informed consent (Senn, 1997). However it would be justified if:

- The use of placebo has negligible risk and acceptable discomfort.
- It enhances the science or interpretation of the study.
- The 'deception' is covered adequately in the information provided to patients.
- There is agreement by an independent ethics committee that those conditions hold (Ramsay, 1997).

Stopping Studies

There are cases where ethically approved studies have become unethical either because one drug has established superiority before all the patients have been recruited or because the adverse effects of one drug have outweighed any benefit and it therefore needs to be stopped. The time when a difference becomes statistically significant may not coincide with the time when the study becomes unethical (e.g. a study comparing extracorporeal membrane oxygenation with standard therapy in newborns with persistent pulmonary hypertension was halted when there were four deaths of the ten babies on standard therapy but none of the nine babies in the oxygenation group had died ($p = 0.54$). This trial was stopped by the investigators on ethical grounds, but later it was felt that the evidence for the superiority of oxygenation was not strong and gave little scope for making reliable judgements for future use.

The basic ethical conflict in monitoring trial results is to balance the interests of patients within the trial—that is, the individual ethics of randomizing the next patient and the longer term interest of obtaining reliable conclusions on sufficient data—or the collective ethics of making appropriate treatment policies for future patients (Pocock, 1992). Professor Pocock also says as far as the example is concerned "Thus collective ethics may have been compromised by such early stopping". If one asks oneself the analogous question to the one above "Would I want my baby to be randomized and take the risk of conventional treatment?" However the *Declaration of Helsinki* says "Concern for the interest of the subject must always prevail over the interest of science and society". Professor Pocock's conclusions were "The ethical dilemma faced by data monitoring committees has no easy solution but it is important to note that premature stopping based on limited evidence can have severe consequences either by introducing exaggerated claims so that inadequate treatments enter clinical practice or by failing to collect sufficient evidence on effective treatments in order to convince rightly sceptical clinicians of their true merits".

Ethical Committees

The ethical committee has a responsibility to monitor a study and to intervene where necessary. This can be done either by a mid-term interim report or by receiving an interim report every six months (Evans and Evans, 1996). The equivalent of the ethical committee in the USA is the Institutional Review Board (IRB) (Levine, 1997). It has been suggested that the independent ethical committee (IEC)/IRB should be informed of adverse events as they occur (Sniderman, 1996). The 'Guideline for good clinical practice, 1996' (ICH E6 CPMP/ICH/135/95) states that the investigator must report to the IRB/IEC promptly all ADRs that are both serious and unexpected and new information that may affect adversely the safety of the subjects or the conduct of the trial. Also changes increasing the risk to subjects and/or affecting significantly the conduct of the trial and deviations from, or changes of, the protocol to eliminate immediate hazards to the trial subjects must be reported—paragraphs 3.3.8; 3.3.9; 5.17 (ADR reporting). An independent data monitoring committee (IDMC) may be established by the sponsor to assess, at intervals, the progress of a clinical trial, the safety data and the critical efficacy endpoints, and to recommend to the sponsor whether to continue, modify or stop a trial (ICH 'Guideline on good clinical practice, 1996' section 5.5.2).

In some large phase III studies there may be an IDMC and an IRB/IEC, both monitoring and possibly stopping a study. The company pharmacovigilance staff will need to make sure that any serious unexpected adverse event is notified to the regulatory authority, the IDMC and the IRB/IEC.

Due to problems in seeking ethical committee approval with large multicentre studies special committees, multi-centre research ethical committees (MRECs) have been set up to deal with them (National Health Service guidance note HFG(97)23, April 1997).

The need to have approval from numerous local ethical committees has been a nightmare for the industry and the recent *Ethics Committees review of multicentre research: establishment of multicentre research ethics committees, 1997* seems to have done little to relieve the situation (Evans, 1997). There is also a European Ethical Review Committee, which specifically reviews multinational trials (EERC) (Bennett, 1995, 1997; Cordier, 1997; Foster, 1997).

The 'Guidelines on the practice of ethics committees' says, referring to the situation where society rather than the individual may benefit "In such situations, however large the benefit, to expose a participant to anything more the minimal risk needs very careful consideration and would rarely be ethical". Minimal risk in everyday life could include travelling on public transport or private car, but not by pedal or motor cycle. In medicine they would be no more likely and not greater than the risk attached to routine medical or psychological examination (CIOMS and WHO, 1993; RCP of London Committee on Ethical Issues in Medicine 1996).

Suggested further reading:

- *Manual for Research Ethics Committees*, 4th edition. Ed. C. Foster, King's College London, 1996.
- *Introduction to Research Ethical Committees, ABPI, 1997.*
- *International Journal of Pharmaceutical Medicine* **11**, (3), 121–176 June 1997.
- Guidelines and recommendations for European ethics committees (1997). Int. J. Pharm. Med., **11** (3), 129–135.
- *Ethics Committees Review of Multicentre Research: Establishment of Multicentre Research Ethics Committees*. Department of Health, 1997.

Pharmaceutical Promotion

It has been argued that 'promotion of medicines by the pharmaceutical industry is, by its very nature, unethical', in that actions done out of respect of one group's interests rather than the interests of humanity at large are unethical (Collier, 1995). This was rebutted in the same issue of 'pharmaceutical medicine'; "pharmaceutical promotion is a valid and important part of the process of the discovery and development of new medicines for individual patients and the overall benefit of the health of society" (Read and Stonier, 1995). However, it is clear from comparing promotional material and the scientific literature for drugs of the same class that a balanced account of the advantages and disadvantages of a drug are rarely projected to the prescriber, but rather that the prescriber is pounded with a biased view of the drug that appeals to parts of the brain other than the intellect. This makes it difficult for the prescriber to judge what is in the best interest for a particular patient.

Conclusion

There is a conflict between the *Declaration of Helsinki* and good science. Bad science is, in itself, unethical. The prime allegiance must be to the individual patient or subject and the science must be as good as circumstances will allow.

Honesty

Several industries whose products adversely affect the health of the world have been criticized for putting profits before the wellbeing of people (e.g. tobacco, salt, sugar, breast milk substitutes and processed foods: Anand, 1996; Godlee, 1996; Wise, 1996; Taylor, 1998). Some of these industries target developing countries. It is therefore important to examine the pharmaceutical industry and its behaviour.

In the past many have criticized the honesty of the pharmaceutical industry. In recent years regulations and guidelines have restricted the possibility of dishonesty and another generation has entered the industry. Comments will, therefore, be made only on publications since 1990.

Promotional Honesty

There is an instinctive feeling that 'they' may be affected by advertisements, but that 'I' make my decisions rationally and based on scientific facts.

The drug industry spent an estimated £5000 per general practitioner (GP) promoting its products in the UK in 1985 (Smith, 1986). The large budgets of pharmaceutical companies for drug promotion and marketing, estimated at 20–30% of sales turnover, or about 2–3 times the average expenditure on research and development (*Lancet* leader, 1993) suggest that current drug promotional activities are effective in changing physicians behaviour. The estimated cost of free drug samples given to a GP over one year was £1485.22 (O'Mahony, 1993).

"Companies tend to emphasise the positive aspects of products, focussing on attributes that will give them a marketing edge, and not to provide all the objective data (including adverse effects and contraindications) required for comparative analysis" (*Lancet*, 1993). "The problem of misleading drug advertisements is real" (Kessler, 1992).

In 1994 an FDA team gave details of three techniques used by the industry which were of particular concern to the FDA.

Seeding Studies

"Some company-sponsored trials of approved drugs appear to serve little or no scientific purpose. Because they are, in fact, thinly veiled attempts to entice doctors to prescribe a new drug being marketed by the company, they are often referred to as 'seeding trials' ".

Unsubstantiated Claims of Superiority Over Competing Products

"The sponsor misrepresented the risk of drug interactions associated with its product relative to the risk with the competing products by making selective use of negative clinical reports and omitting certain important drug interactions associated with its own product".

Switch Campaigns

"Pharmaceutical companies . . . . . . are increasingly trying to cause patients to be switched from their originally prescribed medications to 'me too' drugs marketed by the companies. The manufacturer asked retail pharmacists who received prescriptions for the older form of the drug to contact the prescribing physicians and request that they change their prescriptions to the newer form . . . . . . The pharmacists would receive a payment for each prescription thus switched" (Kessler *et al.*, 1994).

Advertisements

"I found that the majority of promotional claims referred to me citing clinical studies violated the advertising regulations of the Food and Drug Administration" (Hoberman, 1995).

Tretinoin is only approved for acne, but in 1988 a study reported that it improved the appearance of 'photoaged' skin, for which it was not licenced. Subsequently there were many articles and promotional efforts supporting this use (Stern, 1994, 1995). "To promote such uses (of certain medications for unapproved indications) drug companies employ additional techniques....to disseminate material directly to physicians that discuss unapproved uses.... Another technique is the publication of sponsored symposia....In an analysis of 11 journals, 51% of those focussing on a single drug discussed products that had not received FDA approval. Furthermore, the lower the therapeutic value of the drug discussed, the more likely it was that the symposium promoted unapproved indications" (Stryer and Bero, 1995).

In answer to Dr Stern's comment "The approval process is extremely expensive, and many drugs are never approved for appropriate indications.... This problem is particularly relevant to less common diseases". (Kalish, 1995). In the case of the use of topical tretinoin for 'photoaging' (Stern, 1994) some experts viewed the initial findings as a half-full cup, whereas others argued that the cup was half empty. The company's promotional use of these findings made tretinoin appear to be a fountain of youth. Unfortunately we are unlikely ever to know the full story of the promotion of topical tretinoin by Johnson and Johnson. Because it destroyed the records, Johnson and Johnson recently pleaded guilty to charges of conspiracy to obstruct justice in government investigations of this promotional effort and the company paid a $5 million fine (Stern, 1995).

In the USA, the FDA found that Kabi illegally promoted olsalazine as being indicated for the treatment of mild, moderate and severe active ulcerative colitis; for use in children; as being superior to sulphasalazine; and as a 'first choice' therapy in the treatment of ulcerative colitis (Ahmed, 1993).

A survey of 100 Irish physicians found that when they assessed ten advertisements chosen at random, 80% were not comfortable with the fact that information relating to side effects, contraindications or precautions had been excluded. One hundred consecutive advertisements in Irish medical journals were divided into 33 full advertisements and 67 'reminder' advertisements and of the 100 only 33 had details of adverse effects, contraindications and precautions (Hemeryck *et al.*, 1995).

A survey in the USA of 109 advertisements peer-reviewed by specialist physicians concluded that in the opinion of the reviewers many advertisements contained deficiencies in areas in which the FDA has established standards of quality. Reviewers considered that side effects and contraindications in special populations were not appropriately highlighted in 47% of the 49 advertisements in which such information was considered relevant. Only 30% of 95 advertisements were considered to present information on side effects and contraindications with a prominence and readability that was reasonably comparable to the presentation of information on the drug's effectiveness, whereas 57% of advertisements were judged negatively in this respect. The reviewers recommended minor revisions of 27%, major revisions of 48% and rejection of 76% for lack of information on side effects and contraindications (Dillner, 1992; Wilkes *et al.*, 1992).

"Some of the worst examples of quackery can be found in advertisements by ethical multinational pharmaceutical companies, taking advantage of the fact that drugs can be easily bought from pharmacists and that local drug-control legislation is weak or ineffective" (Birley, 1989). Advertisements and data sheets provided for developing countries have been criticized by the Medical Lobby for Appropriate Marketing (MALAM) (Ragg, 1993).

Pharmaceutical adverts, labelling and package inserts in developing countries often show the twin problems of exaggerated indications and minimized adverse effects (Menkes, 1997).

Drug advertisements in the Indian editions of the British Medical Journal were found to be misleading and to make unsubstantiated claims when compared with the UK edition (Gitanjali *et al.*, 1997)

Comparing the *Monthly Index of Medical Specialties* (MIMS) for the UK and India it was found that side effects were omitted in 86% of advertisements in the Indian edition and 57% in the UK edition. Cost was never given in the Indian version and was missing in 57% of the UK advertisements (Dikshit and Dikshit, 1994). Despite clear statements by the World Health Organization (WHO) that antimicrobial drugs have no place in the routine treatment of acute diarrhoea, one out of two antidiarrhoeal preparations marketed in 1988–1989 contained an antimicrobial drug. In Pakistan, 25 pharmaceutical companies, including some of the largest multinationals, market antidiarrhoeal drugs worth more than $10 million, but only four companies make oral rehydration solution (Costello and Bhutta, 1992).

According to the FDA Pfizer has been making unsubstantiated claims about its antidepressant sertraline to American physicians (Barnett, 1996a).

Concealing Information

A task force appointed by the FDA has concluded that Upjohn may have obscured information regarding the safety of Halcion (triazolam), and has recommended that the department of justice investigate (Barnett, 1996a).

Nippon Shoji began marketing sorivudine, a shingles treatment sold as Usevir, in September 1996, but had to withdraw it within weeks when it was found to be fatal when combined with cancer drugs. Evidence of the dangers began emerging in 1986, but Nippon Shoji concealed information from the government about two of the deaths during clinical trials (Daily Telegraph, 1994; Hirokawa, 1996).

Pfizer received a letter from the FDA in 1996 warning that it has failed to report adverse drug experiences (ADEs) on eight drugs. In reviewing Pfizer's reporting since 1983, the FDA found "that the same or similar problems continue to recur, even though you have made promises to correct them" (Barnett, 1996b).

There have been circumstances where a company has reported AEs with another company's products, but when challenged have failed to validate them or where they appear to have encouraged a physician to report AEs to another company's drugs. This type of behaviour is rarely proven, but pharmacovigilance staff should be aware of the possibility when investigating cases, since rigorous enquiry may discourage further episodes.

Clinical Trials

In 1987 Professors Hampton and Julian stated that "companies have tried to prevent publication of unfavourable results by pressure on investigators or on journals" (Hampton and Julian, 1987).

Three physicians who had taken part in the Multicenter Isradipine Diuretic Atherosclerosis Study dropped out of the investigative group because they believed that the sponsor of the study was attempting to wield undue influence on the nature of the final paper (Applegate *et al.*, 1997).

A drug company suppressed research showing that generic thyroid drugs were as effective as its own branded product for almost seven years (Rennie, 1997; Wise, 1997; Nahata and Welty, 1998).

Bristol-Myers Squibb exerted pressure on ethical grounds to end an independent trial of one of its drugs (*Lancet* leader, 1997). Merk Sharpe and Dohme lost its battle in the Norwegian courts to stop the publication of an article that criticized one of the company's products (Goldbeck-Wood, 1997).

There may be several different ways that a figure can be calculated and again several different ways that it can be displayed graphically. Sometimes one presentation is more appealing to the company while another way may be thought to be more appropriate by independent statisticians. The decline in the incidence of a disease over the years looks quite different when displayed arithmetically rather than logarithmically (e.g. deaths due to tuberculosis when shown arithmetically show a straight line decline from 1838 with a minimal blip around 1950 when chemotherapy was introduced (Fletcher *et al.*, 1996), but when shown logarithmically there is a very sharp increase in the decline starting in 1950 (Teeling Smith, 1986). A numerator may be much smaller when a specific definition is used compared with a term written by the clinician—for example, the Council for International Organization of Medical Science (CIOMS) definition of pancytopenia (anaemia : Hb level < 100 g/l; neutropenia: polymorphonuclear count $< 1.5 \times 10^9$/l; thrombocytopenia: platelets $< 100 \times 10^9$/l) (Bénichou and Solal-Celigny, 1991) compared with the clinician's term 'pancytopenia'.

A denominator derived from the meta-analysis of publications of all the clinical trials with a drug may underestimate it due to the exclusion of unpublished studies or overestimate it by duplication of publications (Tramèr *et al.*, 1997).

It is important that when calculating incidence rates of ADRs any provisos are made clear. Frequently there will be a genuine difference of opinion about the most appropriate way to calculate or illustrate data, but when in doubt an independent point of view should be sought.

Attitude Towards Adverse Drug Reactions

Fitzgerald (1992) writing on crisis management and ADRs said "The initial response of those working within an organisation, particularly product champions, both technical and commercial, is that of denial. Until this moment, the whole culture within the company has been positively and energetically to promote the advantage of the drug. Thus before accepting that the drug is associated with a potentially serious disadvantage, drug champions tend to demand, firstly, proof of causality; secondly, to seek out alternative explanations for the clinical syndrome; and thirdly, to try to implicate other agents in the same drug class, in order to diminish the impact on the specific product".

Replies published by companies, concerning published ADRs are not too dissimilar to this pattern, giving a very one-sided viewpoint and certainly not giving the reader a balanced opinion of the problem. These letters usually contain some of the following:

- No admission of a causal relationship.
- No acknowledgement of the validity of any of the comments in the original publication.
- A list of all possible alternatives; however, tenuous.
- No mention of the number of cases that the company have received.
- References, some of which when obtained seem to have little to do with the original problem.
- Implications that it is a class effect.
- The letter may be from a clinician who has been involved with the company as a trialist or adviser without any acknowledgement of an association with the pharmaceutical company.

That is not to say that there are not some misleading ADR reports published. A Brussels physician wrote to the Lancet certain results of an enquiry among general practitioners to detect possible serious AEs of...... The company brought an action against the doctor for 'negative publicity'. The court rejected the claim but it is due to go to appeal (Law Notes, 1997).

In an editorial in *Risk and Safety in Medicine* Dr M. N. G. Dukes says...... "even with western industry one still in the nineties runs into serious instances where risk data have been concealed in the interests of commerce" (Dukes, 1996).

Investigators

Numerous incidences of investigator fraud have been proven. In the field of AEs the investigator's attitude can vary from bewildered ignorance to deliberate dishonesty:

- Some fail to document and report what they should clearly recognize as an AE.
- Some are so 'invested' in the study drug and believe so strongly in its safety that their enthusiasm overshadows sound scientific and regulatory standards.
- Some choose not to report AEs either because it requires too much effort or they are deliberately attempting to defraud.
- Some are confused over what constitutes an AE (Mackintosh and Zepp, 1996).

Sales Representatives

Fewer than 75% of representatives spontaneously volunteered information to clinicians on side effects (Bignall, 1994). In a USA survey of hospital physicians 37% of them said that their prescribing was influenced by pharmaceutical representatives and it was found that 11% of the representatives' statements were inaccurate when compared with their own literature or the data sheet—all the inaccurate statements were favourable to their own drug. However, 43% thought the representatives provided more reliable information than printed advertisements (Ziegler *et al.*, 1995).

A confidential retail card used by sales representatives said that at meetings with retail pharmacists an objective is "to persuade pharmacists to identify those patients who obtain scripts for other nasal sprays and refer them back to their GP for consideration of an alternative therapy" (Collier, 1993).

The Pharmaceutical Industry and Parliament

Clause 118 of the *UK Medicines Act, 1968*, makes it a criminal offence for the officials involved in licensing or withdrawing a licence from a drug to disclose information about their decisions. The *Medicines Information Bill* would have allowed summaries of reasons for licensing decisions to be made public (*Lancet*, **341**, 885, 1993). The bill failed to complete the report stage on April 30th 1993 "Because of 77 amendments that had been tabled, mostly by Conservative MPs representing the pharmaceutical industry" (Houghton, 1993). All the information that the Bill proposed should be disclosed is already accessible in the USA under the *Freedom of Information Act* (Scrip, 1993). The information available under this USA law has been used as a basis for scathing comments both on the industry and the regulators in a paperback published in 1996 called *Science, Politics and the Pharmaceutical Industry* (Abraham, 1996). The drugs chosen—all non-steroidal anti-inflammatory drugs (NSAIDs)—were naproxen, benoxaprofen, piroxicam, zomepirac and suprofen and are all old drugs marketed before 1983, so the book's conclusions are of historic value rather than having relevance to current processes. In regard to the European Public Assessment Report for drugs in the centralized procedure for biotechnical drugs and highly innovative drug products Abraham says 'The current regulatory situation in the UK and the EU is, therefore, one in which the commercial interest of the industry in secrecy are given priority over the interests of patients and health professionals in obtaining adequate access to information about medicine safety assessments' (Abraham, 1997).

Data Sheets or Summaries of Product Characteristics

The data sheet or summary of product characteristics (SPC) is an important channel whereby the pharmaceutical company influences the prescription of its drugs. "Headache is listed in the UK *Data Sheet Compendium* as an occasional side-effect of bromocriptine, but there was no indication of danger to the patient. In the *Physician's Desk Reference*, the US equivalent of the *Data Sheet Compendium*, there is well-documented evidence of strokes in women receiving bromocriptine for post-partum breast-milk suppression, preceded by severe unilateral headache without hypertension" (Bell, 1993). Bromocriptine was approved in 1980 but by 1983 a number of serious AE were reported, e.g. severe hypertension, seizures and strokes and the FDA requested the company to alter their labelling but the company disagreed and did so again in 1985. It was 1987 before the company agree to the change. In 1994 the FDA were sued by a consumer organization because of the 'unreasonable administrative delay in banning bromocriptine'. The company withdrew the drug from the market (Ahmed and Wolfe, 1995).

The present data sheets are unsatisfactory in that they do not contain sufficient information to enable the prescriber to make a risk–benefit judgement. Since the wording is chosen by the manufacturer they should be regarded as an advertisements rather than scientific documents. Sometimes the wording is chosen to hide rather than to reveal and this may be done by using higher level ADR terms or terms that are too vague to be of any help, (e.g. visual disturbance, motor disorder or liver function test abnormalities). Does 'usually transient' mean that sometimes they are irreversible? Since in the UK only the 'main' side effects need be included, the data sheets may not include all the known ADRs.

The medical requirements are frequently in conflict with the commercial demands in the area of information for the prescriber. A survey of pharmaceutical companies showed that eight of 22 had marketing staff on the committee that made decisions on changes in data sheets (Stephens, 1997). It is difficult to justify their presence.

Conclusions

Deception concerning ADRs may occur by telling some of the truth but not the whole truth "The truth that is told with bad intent beats all the lies you can invent" (William Blake). The exquisite use of words by pharmaceutical companies is the main tool for deceiving the regulators and prescribers. The pharmaceutical industry is another industry where on occasions profits are put before honesty.

Further Reading

Suggested further reading includes:

- *A Decent Proposal: Ethical Review of Clinical Research*, Donald Evans and Martyn Evans, John Wiley and Sons, 230 pp, £24.95, 1996.
- *Guidelines on the Practice of Ethics Committees in Medical Research involving Human Subjects, 3rd edition, The Royal College of Physicians of London, August 1996.*
- *CIOMS and WHO (1993) International Ethical Guidelines for Biomedical Research involving Human Subjects, WHO, Geneva.*
- Independent ethical review of studies involving personal medical records. *J. Roy. Coll. Physic. (London)*, **28**, 1994.

Useful Abbreviations

AAB	Antibiotic Associated Bleeding
AAG	Alpha-1-acid glycoprotein
AAH	Meditel. Amalgamated Anthracite Holding
AAP	American Academy of Paediatrics
ABOF	All Body Organs and Functions Questionnaire
ABPI	Association of the British Pharmaceutical Industry
ACE	Angiotensin Converting Enzyme or Adverse Clinical Event, USA
ACRPI	Association for Clinical Research in the Pharmaceutical Industry, UK
ACTH	Adrenocorticotrophic Hormone
ADE	Adverse Drug Experience, USA
ADH	AntiDiuretic Hormone
ADME	Administration, Distribution, Metabolism and Excretion
ADP	Approved Drug Product List
ADR	Adverse Drug Reaction
ADRAC	Australian Drug Reactions Advisory Committee
ADRIAN	ADR Interactive Advice Network, ICI, UK
ADROIT	Adverse Drug Reactions On-line Information Tracking, UK
ADRSS	ADR Reporting System of the American Academy of Dermatology
AE	Adverse event
AEGIS	Active Electrically Generated Information Service
AERS	Adverse Event Reporting System
AGIM	Association Général de l'Industrie du Médicament (Belgian Pharmaceutical Industry Association)
AICRC	Association of Independent Clinical Research Contractors
AIDS	Acquired Immunodeficiency Syndrome
AIMS	Arthritis Impact Measurement Scale or Abnormal Involuntary Movement Scale
AIOPI	Association of Information Officers in the Pharmaceutical Industry, UK
AK	AerzigKammer (Drug Commission of German Physicians)
ALT	(SGPT) Alanine Aminotransferase
AMA	American Medical Association
AMDP	Association for Methodology and Documentation in Psychiatry Germany
AMG	ArzneiMittelGesetz, Germany
AMIFE	Asociación de Medicos de la Industrira Farmacutica Espanola
AMIP	Association des Médecins de l'Industrie Pharmaceutique (French Association of Pharmaceutical Physicians)
AMK	ArzneiMittelKommission der Deutschen Ärzteschaft, Germany
AMM	Authorisation de Mise sur le Marché (France)
AMUP	ArzeneiMittel Überwachung in der Psychiatrie
ANCOVA	ANalysis of COVAriance

ANF	Anti-Nuclear Factor
ANOVA	Analysis of Variance
AP	Alkaline Phosphatase
APACHE	Acute Physiology and Chronic Health Evaluation
APMA	Australian Pharmaceutical Manufacturers' Association
APTT	Activated Partial Thromboplastin Time
APWI	Active Permanent Workshop of Imputology
APhA	American Pharmaceutical Association
ARGOS	Adverse Reaction Group Of SEAR, UK
ARME-P	Association pour la Recherche Méthologique En Pharmacovigilance
ARVI	Adverse Reaction to Vaccines and Immunizations
ASPP	Anonymized Single Patient Print, UK
AST	(SGOT) Aspartate Aminotransferase
ATC	Anatomical-Therapeutic-Chemical Classification, WHO
AUC	Area Under Plasma Concentration–Time Curve
BARDI	Bayesian Adverse Reaction Diagnostic Instrument
BCDSP	Boston Collaborative Drug Surveillance Program, USA
BCG	Bacillus Calmette-Guérin Vaccine
BDT	Basophil Degranulation Test
BFU-E	Burst Forming Units-Human Erthrocyte Colony
BGA	BundesGesundheitsAmt (Now BFARM) (Germany)
BIAM	Banque d'Information Automatisée sur le Médicament
BIRA	British Institute of Regulatory Affairs
BLIPS	Biometric Laboratory Information Processing System
BMA	British Medical Association
BMRC	British Medical Research Council
BNF	British National Formulary
BP	British Pharmacopoeia
BPI	Bundesverbund der Pharmazeutischen Industrie (Germany)
BPRS	Brief Psychiatric Rating Scale
BrAPP	British Association of Pharmaceutical Physicians, UK
BSA	Body Surface Area
BSP	Bromosuphalein Excretion Test
BUN	Blood Urea Nitrogen
BZT	Biometric Centre for Therapeutic Studies (Munich)
BZD	Benzodiazepines
CAGE	Cut, Annoyed, Guilty, Eye-opener
CAIRS	Computer Assisted Information Retrieval System
CANDA	Computer Assisted New Drug Application, USA
CAPLA	Computer Assisted PLA
CARS	Computer Assisted Review of Safety
CAT	Computerized Axial Tomography
CBC	Complete Blood Count
CBER	Center for Biologics Evaluation and Research (FDA)
CCASS	Canadian Congenital Anomalies Surveillance System
CCSI	Company Core Safety Information
CCDS	Company Core Data Sheet

CDC	Center for Disease Control, USA
CDER	Center for Drug Evaluation and Research (FDA)
CDM	Clinical Data Monitor
CDS	Core Data Sheet
CDT	Canadian Disease and Therapeutic Index
CFR	Code of Federal Regulations, USA
CG	Chorionic Gonadotrophin
CHD	Congenital Heart Disease
CHDMB	Comprehensive Hospital Drug Monitoring, Berne
CIOMS	Council for International Organization of Medical Sciences
CMR	Centre for Medicines Research, UK
CMV	CytoMegaloVirus
CNS	Central Nervous System
COP	Code of Practice
COMPASS	Computerized On-line Medicaid Pharmaceutic Analysis and Surveillance System, USA
COPD	Chronic Obstructive Pulmonary Disease
COSTART	Coding Symbols for a Thesaurus of Adverse Reaction Terms, USA
CPK	Creatine PhosphoKinase
CPMP	Committee for Proprietary Medicinal Products, Europe
CPR	Cardio-Pulmonary Resuscitation
CRA	Clinical Research Associate
CRF	Clinical Record Form, Case Record Form
CRM	Committee for Review of Medicines, UK
CRO	Clinical Research Organization or Contract Research Organization
CRPV	Centre Regional de Pharmacovigilance
CSD	Committee on Safety of Drugs
CSI	Core Safety Information
CSM	Committee on Safety of Medicines, UK
CSPV	Centre Suisse de PharmacoVigilance
CSSC	Clinical Safety Surveillance Committee (PhRMA)
CTC	Clinical Trial Certificate
CTX	Clinical Trial Exemption Certificate
CV	Coefficient of Variation
CXR	Chest Radiograph
DAP	Data Analysis Print (MCA)
DARRP	Drug Adverse Reaction Reporting Programme, Canada
DARTS	Diabetes Audit And Research Tayside
DAWN	Drug Abuse Warning Network, USA
DCF	Data Collection Form
DDD	Defined Daily Dose
DEA	Drug Enforcement Administration, USA
DELTA	Drug Effects on Laboratory Tests Awareness
DEMP	Data Exchange of Medical Products
DES	Division of Epidemiology and Surveillance, USA
DEU	Drug Epidemiology Unit, USA
DHSS	Department of Health and Social Security, UK

DIA	Drug Information Association, USA
DIC	Disseminated Intravascular Coagulation
DLP	Data Lock Point
DMARD	Disease Modifying Anti-Rheumatic Drugs
DNA	DeoxyriboNucleic Acid
DOH	Department of Health
DOI	Drugs of Interest, USA
DOTES	Dosage Record and Treatment Emergent Symptom Scale
DPHM	Direction de la Pharmacie et du Médicament, France
DRA	Drug Regulatory Authority
DRL	Drug-Related Lupus
DS	Discharge Summary
DSI	Division of Scientific Investigations (FDA)
DSMIII	Diagnostic and Statistical Manual (American Psychiatrists, 3rd edition)
DSMC	Data Safety Monitoring Committee
DSRU	Drug Surveillance Research Unit, UK
DTP	Diphtheria, Tetanus, Pertussis
DURG	Drug Utilization Research Group
DVP	Revised Side Effect (Czechoslovakia)
EBV	Epstein-Barr Virus (Mononucleosis)
EC	European Community
ECARS	European Computer Assisted Regulatory Submission
ECDEU	Early Clinical Drug Evaluation Program, USA
ECJ	European Court of Justice
ECOG	Eastern Cooperative Oncology Group, USA
EDI	Electronic Data Interchange
EDTA	EthyleneDiamine TetraAcetic acid
EEG	ElectroEncephaloGram
EERC	European Ethical Review Committee
EFPIA	European Federation of Pharmaceutical Industries Associations
ELISA	Enzyme Linked Immunosorbent Assay
EM	Erythema Multiforme
EMEA	European Medicines Evaluation Agency
EOF	Greek National Drug Organization
EORTC	European Organization for Research and Treatment of Cancer
EPI	Epidemiology in the Pharmaceutical Industry or European Product Index
EPRG	European Pharmacovigilance Research Group
EPTIS	Electronic Prescribing and Therapeutic Information System, UK
ERG	ElectroRetinoGram
ESR	Erythrocyte Sedimentation Rate or End of Study Report
EWG	Expert Working Group
EWL	EigenschaftWörte Liste
FAPI	Fachgesellschaft der Ärzte in der Pharmazeutischen Industrie (Association of German Doctors in the Pharmaceutical Industry)
FAPh	Italian National Pharmacovigilance Association
FASS	Farmaceutiska Specialiteter i Sverige

FAST	Fluorescent AllergoSorbent Test
FDA	Food and Drug Administration, USA
FDE	Fixed Drug Eruption
FEV_1	Forced Expiratory Flow in One Second
FFA	Free Fatty Acid
FGRP	Florida Geriatric Research Program
FHSA	Family Health Service Authority
FMH	Swiss Medical Federation
FOI	Freedom of Information, USA
FROST	FROSTig Developmental Test of Visual Perception
FSH	Follicle Stimulating Hormone
FTI	Free Thyroxine Index
FVC	Forced Vital Capacity
G6PD	Glucose-6–Phosphate Dehydrogenase
GBS	Guillain-Barré Syndrome
GC	Gas Chromatography
GCP	Good Clinical Practice
GFR	Glomerular Filtration Rate
GGT	Gamma Glutamyl Transpeptidase
GH	Growth Hormone
GHC	Group Health Cooperative, USA
GHR	General Health Rating Scale
GLP	Good Laboratory Practice
GM-CFC	Granulocyte/ Macrophage Colony Forming Cells
GM-CSF	Granulocyte/Macrophage Colony Stimulating Factor
GMP	Good Manufacturing Practice
GP	General Practitioner
GPASS	General Practice Administration System for Scotland
GPMSP	Good Post-Marketing Surveillance Practice
GPRD	General Practice Research Database (previously VAMP)
GVHD	Graft Versus Host Disease
GWB	General Well-being Index
HARTS	Hoechst Adverse Reaction Terminology
HAV	Hepatitis A Virus
HBD	HydroxyButyrate Dehydrogenase
HBV	Hepatitis B Virus
HDL	High-Density Lipoprotein
HGPRT	Hypoxanthine-Guanine PhosphoRibosyl Transferase
HIV	Human Immunodeficiency Virus
HLA	Human Leucocyte Antigen
HMA	Holder of the Marketing Authorization
HMO	Health Maintenance Organization
HPLC	High-Performance Liquid Chromatography
IAAAS	International Agranulocytosis and Aplastic Anaemia Study
IADR	Idiosyncratic ADR
IB	Investigator's Brochure
ICBD	International Clearing House for Birth Defects Monitoring

ICD	International Classification of Disease
ICD9CM	International Classification of Diseases, 9th Revision Clinical Modification
ICG	Indo-Cyanine Green excretion test
ICH	International Conference on Harmonization
ICHPPC	International Classification of Health Problems in Primary Care
ICU	Intensive Care Unit
ID	Incidence Density
IDMC	Independent Data Monitoring Committee
IDR	Incidence Density Ratio or Idiosyncratic Drug Reaction
IEC	Independent Ethics Committee
IF-EPI	International Forum in the Pharmaceutical Industry (Epidemiology)
IFCC	International Federation of Clinical Chemistry
IFPMA	International Federation of Pharmaceutical Manufacturers Association
IHS	International Health Services
IKS	Interkantonale KontrollStelle, Union of Swiss Cantons Drug Regulatory Authority
IMMP	Intensive Medicines Monitoring Programme, New Zealand
IMS	Intercontinental Medical Statistics
INCLEN	INternational Clinical Epidemiology Network
IND	Investigational New Drug, USA
INR	International Normalized Ratio
INN	International Non-Propietary Name
INSERM	Institut National de la Santé et de la Recherche Médicale
INTDIS	International Drug Information System, WHO
IQOLA	International Quality of Life Assessment
IRB	Institutional Review Board (USA)
IRD	International Registration Document
IRFMN	Istituto di Richerche Farmacogiche Mario Negri
ISPE	International Society for PharmacoEpidemiology
ISS	Integrated Safety Summary
ITEM	Institute for Technical Evaluation of Medicines
IUCD	IntraUterine Contraceptive Device
JAMA	Journal of the American Medical Asssociation
JPMA	Japanese Pharmaceutical Manufacturers Association
LAREB	LAndelijke Registratie Evaluatie Bijwerkingen (Netherlands Pharmacovigilance Foundation)
LDH	Lactate Dehydrogenase
LDL	Low-Density Lipoprotein
LFT	Liver Function Tests
LH	Luteinizing Hormone
LLN	Lower Limit of Normal
LTT	Lymphocyte Transformation Test
MA	Marketing Authorization
MAH	Marketing Authorization Holder
MAIL	Medicines Act Information Leaflet
MAL	Medicines Act Leaflet

MALAM	Medical Lobby for Appropriate Marketing
MANCOVA	Multivariate Analysis of Covariance
MANOVA	Multivariate Analysis of Variance
MAOI	Monoamine Oxidase Inhibitor
MAR	Monitored Adverse Reactions, USA
MARC	Medicines Adverse Reaction Centre, New Zealand
MCA	Medicines Control Agency, UK
MCH	Mean Corpuscular Haemoglobin
MCHC	Mean Corpuscular Haemoglobin Concentration
MCV	Mean Corpuscular Volume
MDI	Medical Data Index or Metered Dose Inhaler
MedDRA	Medical Dictionary for Drug Regulatory Affairs
MEDLARS	Medical Literature Analysis and Retrieval System
MEMO	Medication Events Monitoring Organization
MHW	Ministry of Health and Welfare, Japan
MIF	Migration Inhibition Factor
MIMS	Monthly Index of Medical Specialties
MIP	Medicines in the Public Interest, USA
MMA	Manufacturers Marketing Authorisation
MMIF	Macrophage Migration Inhibition Factor
MMR	Mumps, Measles, Rubella
MR	Mutually Recognized (Authorized Medicinal Product)
MRC	Medical Research Council
MREC	Multicentre Research Ethics Committee
MRI	Magnetic Resonance Imaging
MSEP	Minor Symptoms Evaluation Profile
MeSH	Medical Subject Heading
MSLT	Multiple Sleep Latency Test
MTD	Maximum Tolerated Dose
NAARAS	National Anaesthetic Adverse Reaction Advisory Service, UK
NAD	Nothing Abnormal Diagnosed
NARD	Netherlands Centre for Monitoring ADRs
NARI	NorAdrenaline Reuptake Inhibitor
NCE	New Chemical Entity
NCHS	National Center for Health Statistics, USA
NCI	National Cancer Institute, USA
NCPIE	National Council on Patient Information and Education
NDA	New Drug Application, USA
NDAB	National Drug Advisory Board, Ireland
NDE	New Drug Evaluation, USA
NDTI	National Disease and Therapeutic Index, USA
NEFA	Non-Esterified Fatty Acid
NEMC	New England Medical Center
NHANES	National Health Examination Surveys, USA
NHP	Nottingham Health Profile, UK
NHS	National Health Service
NIDA	National Institute of Drug Abuse, USA

NIH	National Institutes of Health, USA
NLN	Nordic Council on Medicines
NNHO	Number Needed to Have One (Adverse Event)
NOAEL	No Observed Adverse Effect Level
NPA	National Prescription Audit
NPIS	National Poisons Information Service
NSAID	Non-Steroidal Anti-Inflammatory Drug
NTDL	Non Toxic Dose Level
NTIS	National Technical Information Service, USA
NVFG	Nederlandse Vereniging voor Farmaceutische Geneeskundigen
OA	OsteoArthritis
OBRR	Office of Biologic Research and Review, USA
OC	Oral Contraceptive
OCHP	Oxford Community Health Project, UK
ODE	Office of Drug Evaluation, USA
OLGA	On-Line Guide to Quality of Life Assessment
ONS	Office for National Statistics, UK (previously OPCS)
OPCS	Office of Population, Censuses and Surveys, UK (now ONS)
OTC	Over-The-Counter
OXMIS	OXford Medication Information System, UK
ODRR	Office of Drug Research and Review, USA
PACT	Philadelphia Association for Clinical Trials or Prescribing Analysis and Costs
PAH	Para-amino Hippuric Acid Clearance
PAR	Pseudoallergic Reaction
PAS	Para-aminosalicylic Acid
PC	*Post-Cibum* (After Meals)
PCC	Poisons Control Center, USA
PCV	Packed Cell Volume
PDR	Physician's Desk Reference, USA
PE	Pharmacoepidemiology
PEFR	Peak Expiratory Flow Rate
PEM	Prescription Event Monitoring
PEN	Pharmaco-Epidemiological Newsletter
PERI	Education and Research Institute
PhRMA	Pharmaceutical Research and Manufacturers of America
PhVWP	Permanent CPMP Working Group on Pharmcovigilance
PID	Prescription Information Document
PIL	Patient Information Leaflet
PLA	Product Licensing Authority/Application
PMA	Pharmaceutical Manufacturers' Association
PMN	PolyMorphoNuclear Leucocytes
PMS	Post-marketing Surveillance
POM	Prescription Only Medicine
POMS	Profile of Mood States
PPA	Prescription Pricing Authority, UK
PPI	Patient Package Insert, USA

PQVS	Profil de la Qualité de la Vie Subjective
PRIST	Paper RIST
PRN	*Pro Re Nata* (When Required)
PRR	Proportional Reporting Ratio
PSA	Prescription Sequence Analysis, Netherlands
PSUR	Periodic Safety Update Report
PT	Prothrombin Time
PV	PharmacoVigilance
QALY	Quality Adjusted Life Year
QoL	Quality of Life
QWB	Quality of Well-Being Index
RA	Rheumatoid Arthritis
RADAR	Risk benefit Assessment Detection And Response
RADS	Retrospective Assessment of Drug Safety
RAST	Radio-AllergoSorbent Test
RBC	Red Blood Count, Red Blood Cells
RCGP	Royal College of General Practice, UK
RCT	Randomized Clinical Trial
RIA	RadioImmunoAssay
RIDURS	Rhode Island Drug Use Reporting System
RIST	RadioImmunoSorbent Test
ROC	Receiving Operating Characteristic
RR	Relative Risk
SADRAC	Swedish ADR Advisory Committee
SADRRS	Spontaneous Adverse Drug Reaction Reporting System
SAE	Serious Adverse Event
SAFTEE	Systematic Assessment For Treatment Emergent Events
SAMM	Safety Assessment of Marketed Medicines
SANZ	Schweizerische Arzneimittel Nebenwirkungs-Zentrale (Swiss Pharmacovigilance System)
SAS	Statistical Analysis Software Institute, USA
SD	Standard Deviation
SDI	Selective Dissemination of Information Profile
SDMC	Safety Data Monitoring Committee
SEAR	Safety, Efficacy and Adverse Reaction Subcommittee
SEER	Surveillance, Epidemiology and End Results (Cancer), USA
SER	Standardized Event Rate, USA
SGOT	(AST) Serum Glutamic Oxaloacetic Transaminase
SGPT	(ALT) Serum Glutamic Pyruviate Transaminase
SI	Statutory Instrument
SI	Système Internationale
SIGAR	Special Interest Group on Adverse Reactions
SIP	Sickness Impact Profile
SLE	Systemic Lupus Erythematosus
SMAC	Sequential Multiple Analyser Channel
SMART	Stuart Medical Adverse Reaction Thesaurus, USA
SMON	Subacute Myelo-Optic Neuropathy

SNIP	Syndicat National de l'Industrie Pharmaceutique, France
SNOMED	Systematized NOmenclature of MEDicines
SNRI	Selective Serotonin Noradrenaline Reuptake Inhibitor
SOC	System Organ Class
SPC	Summary of Product Characteristics
SPDP	Saskatchewan Prescription Drug Plan
SRS	Spontaneous Reporting System
SSAP	Subjective Symptoms Assessment Profile
SSRI	Selective Serotonin Reuptake Inhibitor
STD	Sexually Transmitted Disease
STESS	Subject's Treatment Emergent Symptom Scale
SUD	Sudden Unexpected Death
TAIWAN	Triage Application for Imputologists Without An Interesting Name
TBG	Thyroxine Binding Globulin
TCA	Tricyclic Antidepressants
TDM	Therapeutic Drug Monitoring
TEN	Toxic Epidermal Necrolysis
TESS	Treatment Emergent Symptom Scale/Treatment Emergent Symptom and Signs
TIBC	Total Iron Binding Capacity
TOP	Termination of Pregnancy
TPMT	ThioPurine MethylTransferase
TPN	Total Parenteral Nutrition
TRH	Thyroid Releasing Hormone
TSH	Thyroid Stimulating Hormone
TT	Thrombin Time
T_3	Tri-iodothyronine
T_4	Thyroxine
TREO	Therapeutic Research and Education Organization
TTO	Time to Onset
U and E	Urea and electrolytes
UKEQA	UK External Quality Assessment Scheme (Laboratory Data)
ULN	Upper Limit of Normal
URTI	Upper Respiratory Tract Infection
UTI	Urinary Tract Infection
VAERS	Vaccines Adverse Event Reporting System
VAMP	Value Added Medical Products
VAS	Visual Analogue Scale
VLDL	Very Low Density Lipoprotein
VMA	VanillylMandelic Acid
WBC	White Blood Cell/white blood count
WHO	World Health Organization
WHOART	WHO Adverse Reaction Terminology
WUG	WHO User's Group

Useful Web Sites

ABPI
http://www.abpi.org.uk/

Adverse Drug Reactions Bulletin
http://www.thomsonscience.co

Association of Clinical Biochemists
http://www.leeds.ac.uk/acb/
Items of general medical interest and an assay finder to help researchers find methods or labs to measure a wide variety of hormones, metals, enzymes and drugs in body fluids (Pallen, 1997).

Australian Therapeutic Goods Administration (TGA)
http://www.health.gov.au/tga

BioMedNet
http://www.cursci.co.uk/BioMedNet/biomed.html/ OR
http://BioMedNet.com
The world wide web club for the biological and medical community (free membership).

Canadian Health Protection Board (HPB)
http://www.hwc.ca/hpb

CBER What's New
http://www.fda.gov/cber/whatsnew.htm
FDA Center for Biologics Evaluation and Research

CDER What's New
http://www.fda.gov/cder/whatsnew.htm
FDA Center for Drug Evaluation and Research

Centre for Medicines Research
http://www.cmr.org/

Clinical Pharmacology Drug Monograph Service
http://www.cponline.gsm.com

Clinician's Computer-Assisted Guide to the Choice of Instruments for Quality of Life Assessment in Medicine
http://www.glamm.com/ql/guide.htm

This contains hypertext with references to QoL measurements divided into (a) general diseases, (b) specific diseases and therapies, (c) health organisations, (d) bibliography.

ClinWeb
http://www.ohsu.edu/clinweb (Kiley, 1997)
Oregon Health Sciences University.

CNN interactive (health)
http://www.cnn.com/HEALTH/index.html
Up-to-date information on health issues including drug safety concerns and withdrawals.

Code of Federal Register
http://www.access.gpo.gov/nara/cfr/index.html OR
http://www.access.gpo.gov/su_docs/aces/aces140.html
For proposed rules and guidelines.

Committee on Safety of Medicines (CSM)
http://www.open.gov.uk/mca/csmhome.htm

Current Problems in Pharmacovigilance
http://www.open.gov.uk/mca/mcahome.htm

Cutaneous Drug Reactions
http://triz.dermatology.uiowa.edu/home.html

DIA home page
http://www.diahome.org
Home page of the Drug Information Association

Doctor's Guide to the Internet
http://www.psigroup.com (Johnson and Wordell, 1998)

Documents for Clinical Research
http://www.ams.med.unigoettingen.de/~rhilger/Document.html
Declaration of Helsinki, other documents and collection of related sites.

Druginfonet
http://www.druginfonet.com (Johnson and Wordell, 1998)

EC DGXIII Telecommunications
http://www.ispo.cec.be/
Information

EMBASE
http://www.healthgate.com/healthGate/price/embase.html
(Kiley, 1997).

EMEA
http://www.eudra.org/emea.html
http://www.eudra.org/home.html

Eudra Net: Network Services for the European Union Pharmaceutical Regulatory Sector
http://www.eudra.org
Includes information on the European Agency for the Evaluation of Medicinal Products.

Europa
http://www.cec.lu
Official web site of the European Union.

European Pharmacovigilance Research Group
http://www.ncl.ac.uk/~neprg/

Food and Drug Administration
http://www.fda.gov/

FDA Adverse Events database
http://www.fda.gov/cder/adr

Health on the Net
http://www.hon.ch

Health Information on the Internet
http://www.wellcome.ac.uk/healthinfo/
New bimonthly newsletter from the Wellcome Trust and the RSM.

Hyppos Project
http://www.ifinet.it/hypposnet
Information in Italian and English about the Hyppos project, which has led to the development of a QoL tool for the measurement of hypertensive patients in Italy. It contains a description of the project, the tool, publications about the development of the tool and its application, plus general references to QoL and hypertension.

International Classification of Disease (ICD)-10
http://www.cihi.ca.newinit/scope.htm

International Conference of Harmonization (ICH) 3 Home Page
http://cc.umin.u-tokyo.ac.jp/ich/ich3.html
Official ICH web site with documents; (needs a password).
Applied Clinical Trials, June 1996, page 54.
or http://www.ifpma.org/ichl.html

ICH documents

http://www.ifpma.org/ich1.html
or via the FDA home page (http://www.fda.gov/cder/guidance/index.htm)
or ICH home page (http://www.pharmweb.net/pwmirror/pw9/ifpma/ich1.html)

International Society of Pharmacoepidemiology

http://www.pharmacoepi.org/

InterPharma

http://www.interpharma.co.uk
The latter are vast sites with links to other databases for pharmaceutical support
sites—http://www.MedsiteNavigator.com

JAMA

http://www.ama-assn.org/jama
This gives many other useful USA sites (Sikorski and Peters, 1997).

Market and Exploitation of Research

http://www.cordis.lu

Medicines Control Agency (MCA)

http://www.opengov.uk/mcahome.htm

Medical Matrix

http://www.medmatrix.org

Medical Research Council

http://www.nimr.mrc.ac.uk/MRC/

MEDLINE (free)

http://www.ncbi.nlm.nih.gov/PubMed
or http://www.medmatrix.org/SPages/medline.asp
List of free sites (Kiley, 1997a)

MEDLINE

http://www.medmatrix.org/SPages/medline.asp (Kiley, 1997)
or http://www.medsitenavigator.com/medline/medline.html
A metasite with full and changing MEDLINE search engines (Sikorski and Peters, 1997)
List of freesites

Medscape

http://www.medscape.com

Multilingual glossary of medical terms

http://allserv.rug.ac.be/~rvdstich/eugloss/welcome.html (Pallen, 1997)

National Institute of Health (USA)

http://www.nih.gov

Organised Medical Networked Information
http://www.omni.ac.uk (Kiley, 1997b)

PharminfoNet
http://pharminfo.com/or http://pharminfo.com/phrmlink.html
Independent assessment of therapeutics and advances in new drug development
(Kiley, 1997c)

Pharmweb
http://www.pharmweb.net
Information resource for pharmaceutical and health-related information

Quality of Life
http://www.glamm.com/ql/guide.htm
The choice of instrument.
http://www.glamm.com/q1/ursl.htm
Quality of Life Assessment in Medicine
This contains hypertext with references to QoL measurements divided into (a) assessment tools, (b) reference organizations and groups, (c) diseases, symptoms and specific populations, (d) the top ten journals that publish articles of interest to QoL assessment in medicine, (e) methodology, (f) bibliographical research.

Reuters Health Information Services
http://www.reutershealth.com

SCRIP: World Pharmaceutical News
http://www.pjbpubs.co.uk/scrip

Swedish Medical Products Agency
http://www.mpa.Se

World Health Organization (WHO) Collaborating Centre for International Drug Monitoring
http://www.who.ch/ or http://www.who.pharmasoft.se

SNOMED
http://snomed.org/
Systematised Nomenclature of Human and Veterinary Medicine

Further reading:
The Internet, adverse events and safety. B. L. Colbert and J. Silvey. *Int. J. Pharma. Med.* 1998, **12**, 83–86
Physicians' guide to the Internet. L. Hancock, Lipincott-Raven, 1996
A selective guide to Pharmacovigilance resources on the Internet. M. Maistrello, M. Morgutti, A. Rossignoli and M. Posca. *Pharmacoepidemiology and Drug Safety*, May–June 1998, **7(3)**, 183–189.

Bibliography

Some books published before 1990 have been retained in the bibliography because of their unique value; although they may not still be in print they may be available in libraries. It has not been possible to exclude the possibility of later editions for some publications.

Drug-induced Diseases

A Guide to Drug Eruptions. The European File of Side-effects in Dermatology. 6th edition. W. Bruinsma. Free University of Amsterdam. P.O. Box. 21, 1474 HJ, Oosthuizen. The Netherlands, 1996.
Brief but invaluable. Contains lists of drugs causing each type of skin reaction. Useful general text. Annual supplements between frequent editions.

ADR to Drug Formulation Agents—A Handbook of Excipients. Eds: N. Weiner and I. L. Bernstein, Marcel Dekker, 1989.
The first part of the book is an excellent account of allergic mechanisms. Every possible excipient is discussed including materials in devices, propellants in aerosols, flavours and colouring agents. Excellent reference book.

Adverse Drug Reactions and the Skin. S. M. Breathnach and H. Hintner, Blackwell Scientific Publications, 1992.

Adverse Drug Reactions in Dentistry, 2nd edition. R. Seymour, J. Meecham and J. Walton, Oxford University Press, 1996.
£55.00.

Adverse Drug Reactions, A Practical Guide to Diagnosis and Management. Ed: C. Bénichou. John Wiley & Sons, 1994.
Improved and extended English version of the above French title. Superb. $49.95. Absolutely essential if dealing with clinical trials.

Adverse Effects of Herbal Drugs. Eds: P. De Smet, K. Keller, R. Hansel and R. F. Chandler. 220 pp, Vol. 3. Springer Verlag, Heidelberg, 1996.
£46, DM 98, FF 370, Lit 108. 240.

Adverse Effects of Psychotropic Drugs. Eds: J. M. Kane and J. A. Lieberman. Guildford Press, New York, 1992.

Adverse Events Associated with Childhood Vaccines. Evidence bearing on Causality. Ed: R. K. Stratton, C. J. Howe and R. B. Johnston, Division of Health Promotion and Disease Prevention. Institute of Medicine, National Academy of Sciences, 2101 Constitution Ave, N. W. Washington, DC 20418, 1994.

Allergic Reactions to Anaesthetics. Monographs in Allergy. Vol. 30. Ed: E. SK. Assem. Karger, 1992.
£128.30, $256.50.

Allergic Reactions to Drugs. Eds: A. L. de Weck and H. Bundgaard. *Handbook of Experimental Pharmacology.* Vol. 63. Springer-Verlag, 1983.
Excellent.

Blood Disorders Due to Drugs and Other Agents, Eds: R. H. Girdwood. Excerpta Medica, Amsterdam, 1973.

Cutaneous Drug Reactions: An Integral Synopsis of Today's Systemic Drugs, 2nd edition. Eds: K. Zurcher and A. Krebs, Karger, Basel, 1992.
570 pages, $397.00, DM 594.

Cutaneous Side-effects of Drugs. K. Bork, W. B. Saunders Company, 1988.
422 pages with many coloured photographs. Out of print.

Drug Eruption Reference Manual, 5th edition. J. Z. Litt and W. A. Pawlak. Cleveland Ohio, Wal-Zac Enterprises, 1997.
452 pages, also DERM-On-Disk.

Drug Induced Injury to the Digestive System. Ed: M. Guslandi and P. C. Braga, Springer-Verlag, 1993.
£58.50.

Drug Reactions and the Liver. Eds: M. Davis, J. M. Tredger and R. Williams, Pitman Medical, 1981.
All the authors originate from the Liver Unit at King's College Hospital. This is an important book with background discussion on mechanisms of ADRs and the liver.

Drug-induced Disorders, Vol. 2. *Drug-induced Diseases in the Elderly.* F. I. Caird and P. J. W. Scott, Elsevier Science, 1986.
Out of print.

Drug-induced Disorders, Vol. 3. Series ed. M. N. Dukes.

Drug-induced Disorders, Vol. 5. Series ed. M. N. Dukes.

Drug-induced Disorders, Vol. 4. *Drug-induced Immune Diseases*, Ed: J. Descotes, Elsevier Science, 1990.
Out of print.

Drug-induced Heart Disease, Vol. 5. Ed: M. R. Bristow, Elsevier, North Holland, Biomedical Press, Amsterdam, 1980.
Most of the many contributors are from the USA. A lot of physiopathological details. Well produced. Out of print.

Drug-induced Hepatic Injury, 2nd edition. B. H. Ch. Stricker, Elsevier Science, 1992.
Details of individual drug reactions as well as general information.

Drug-Induced Hepatotoxicity, Vol. 121. Ed: R. Cameron, G. Feuer and F. de la Iglesia Springer Verlag, 1996.
681 pages, DM 530, £247.50, FF 1997, Lit 585. 389.

Drug-induced Infertility and Sexual Dysfunction. Eds: R. Foreman, S. Gilmour-White and N. Foreman. Cambridge University Press, New York, 1996.
55 pages.

Drug-induced Liver Disease. Ed: G. C. Farrell, Churchill Livingstone, 1994.
£120.

Drug-induced Neurological Disorders. K. K. Jain, Hografe and Huber Publishers, 1996.
400 pages.

Drug-induced Nutritional Deficiencies, 2nd edition. D. A. Roe, AVI Publications Co. Inc., Westport, Connecticut, 1985.

Drug-induced Ocular Side-effects, 4th edition. Ed: F. T. Fraunfelder and J. A. Grove, William and Wilton, 1996.
650 pages. A well-structured textbook on individual drugs. Based on experience of the *American National Registry of Drug-induced Ocular Side Effects.* Yearly supplements.

Drug-Induced Pathology. Ed: E. Grundmann, Springer Bln, 1980.

Drug-induced Pulmonary Disease. Clinics in Chest Medicine, Vol. 11, No. 1. Ed: J. A. D. Cooper. W. B. Saunders Company, March 1990.
Out of print.

Drug-related Damage to the Respiratory Tract, Ed: P. Grosdanoff, W. König, D. Müller, H. Otto, G. K. Reznik, T. Wolfgang, unter Mitarb. V. Günther, Karin, MMV, 1986.

Drugs and Sexual Function, A Pharmacological Approach. M. A. Davies and A. D'Mello. Ridge Publications.
66-page paperback.

Formulation Factors in Adverse Reactions. Eds: A. T. Florence and E. G. Salole, Wright (Butterworth & Co.), 1990.
Out of print.

Guide Pratique de Pharmacovigilance. Ed: C. Bénichou, Editions Pradel, 1992.
Superb.

Guidelines for Detection of Hepatotoxicity Due to Drugs and Chemicals. Eds: C. S. Davidson, C. M. Leevy and E. C. Chamberlayne. US Department of Health Education and Welfare, NIH Publication No. 79-313.
An American book with all the world experts participating. This is a unique book.

Handbook of Pharmaceutical Excipients, 2nd edition. Eds: A. Wade and P. J. Weller. The American Pharmaceutical Association and The Pharmaceutical Society of Great Britain, 1994.
672 pages, £150 in UK, £160 in rest of world.

Iatrogenic Diseases, 3rd edition. Eds: P. F. D'Arcy and J. P. Griffin. Oxford University Press, 1986.

Will tend to be compared with the Textbook of Adverse Drug Reactions. This edition is a considerable improvement on the second edition with many more contributors, the first hundred pages being given to general topics.

Neuroleptic Induced Movement Disorders. Ed: K. Yassa, N. P. V. Nair and D. V. Jeste, Cambridge University Press, 1997.
484 pages.

Neurotoxic Side-effects of Prescription Drugs. Ed: C. M. Brust. Butterworth-Heineman, 1996.
435 pages, $40.

PAR Pseudo-allergic Reactions, Vol. 1, *Genetic Aspects and Anaphylactoid Reactions.* Karger, 1980.
Each of the series contains 6-11 chapters which are essays on various subjects.

PAR Pseudo-allergic Reactions, Vol. 2, *Cytotoxic and Complement Mediated Reactions.* Karger, 1980.

PAR Pseudo-allergic Reactions, Vol. 3, *Cell Mediated Reactions Miscellaneous Topics.* Karger, 1982.

PAR Pseudo-allergic Reactions, Vol. 4, *Involvement of Drugs and Chemicals. Idiopathic and Food- or Drug-induced Pseudo-allergic Reactions.* Eds: P. Dukor, P. Kallos, M. D. Schlumberger and G. B. West. Karger, 1985.

Pathology of Drug-induced and Toxic Diseases. Ed: R. H. Ridell, Churchill Livingstone, 1982.
The majority of contributors are American with a sprinkling from the UK. Excellent, authoritative basic textbook. Out of print.

Textbook of Adverse Drug Reactions, 4th edition. Ed: D. M. Davies. Oxford University Press, 1991.
A new edition will be out during 1998. Superb textbook dealing with all aspects; includes individual drugs (well referenced) as well as a few general chapters. £112.50.

Toxicology of the Eye, 3rd edition. Ed: W. Morton Grant. Thomas, Springfield, Illinois, 1986.
Exhaustive tome. Covers disorders of function as well.

Treatment-induced Respiratory Disorders. Eds: G. M. Akoun and J. P. White. Elsevier. 1989.
Out of print.

Teratogenesis, Pregnancy and Lactation

Chemically Induced Birth Defects, 2nd edition. J. L. Schardein, Marcel Dekker, 1993.

Congenital Malformation Syndromes. Ed: D. Donnai and R. Winter, Chapman and Hall. 640pp, £115.00.

Congenital Malformations Worldwide. A report from the International Clearing House for Birth Defects Monitoring System. Elsevier, 1991.
£85.50.

Drug Safety in Pregnancy. Eds: P. I. Folb and M. N. G. Dukes. Elsevier, 1990.
$242.75.

Drugs and Human Lactation, 2nd edition. Eds: P. N. Bennett *et al.* Elsevier, 1996.
722 pages.

Drugs and Pregnancy. Ed: L. C. Gilstrap and B. B. Little, Chapman and Hall, 1992.
£69.00.

Drugs and Pregnancy. Human Teratogenesis and Related Problems, 2nd edition. Ed: D. F. Hawkins, Churchill Livingstone, 1987.
350 pages. In two sections: the first background information and the second the effect of different drugs in pregnancy and lactation. Out of print.

Drugs in Pregnancy and Lactation: A Reference Guide to Fetal and Neonatal Use of Drugs in Pregnancy and Lactation, 4th edition. G. G. Briggs, R. K. Freeman and S. J. Yaffe. Williams and Wilkins, Baltimore/London, 1994.

Maternal – Fetal Toxicology. A Clinician's Guide, 2nd edition. Ed: G. Koren, Marcel Dekker, 1994.
848 pages, $175.00.

Reproductive Toxicity. Ed: Sullivan, Watkins and Venne, European Community, 1993.

REPRORISK includes TERIS teratogen information system, Shepard's catalogue of teratogen agents, REPROPTEXT reproductive hazard reference and REPROTOX, which includes over 3000 chemicals, OTC, prescription, recreational and nutritional agents (see Europharm for address).

Teratogenic Effects of Drugs: A Resource for Clinicians (Teris). Ed: J. Friedman and J. Polifka, John Hopkins University Press.
680 pages, £86.00.

The Effects of Drugs on the Fetus and Nursing Infant. J. M. Friedman and J. E. Polifka, John Hopkins University Press.
648 pages, £34.

Drug Interactions

A Manual of Adverse Drug Interactions, 5th edition. Eds: J. P. Griffin and P. F. D'Arcy. Elsevier Press, 1997.
664 pages, $227.00. NLG395.00.

A good introduction to interaction mechanisms. Interactions presented in tabulated form in pharmacological groups. The only one with medical authors.

Clinical Pharmacology of Drug Interactions. Ed: R. Rondanelle Piccin, 1988.
Elegant, by four pharmacologists from the Policlinic S. Matteo, Pavia.

Diet and Drug Interactions. Ed: Roe, D. A. Chapman and Hall, 1995. 350 pages, £39.95.

Drug Interaction Facts. Ed: D. S. Tatro, A. W. Kluwer, 1998. $54.95.

Drug Interaction Index, 2nd edition. Eds: R. T. Weibert and W. A. Norcross. Medical Economic Books, 1988.

Drug Interactions and Side Effects Diskette. Physician's Desk Reference. 1991.

Drug Interactions in Psychiatry, 2nd edition. Eds: D. A. Ciraule, R. I. Shader, D. J. Greenblatt and W. L. Creelman. Williams and Wilkinson. £34.

Drug Interactions Newsletter. A Clinical Perspective and Analysis of Current Developments. Eds: P. D. Hansten and J. R. Horn. Applied Therapeutics Inc.

Drug Interactions, 6th edition. Eds: P. D. Hansten and J. R. Horn. Philadelphia, 1989.
Half the book deals with drug effects on clinical laboratory results; 264 pages on interactions.

Drug Interactions, 4th edition. Ivan Stockley, The Pharmaceutical Press, 1996.
Succinct data on a large number of interactions, each dealt with individually. Easy to read. 1008 pages on interactions. I found this book easiest to read. This edition is hardbacked. £58.00 in UK, £62 in rest of world.

Drug Interferences and Drug Effects in Clinical Chemistry, Apoeksbolaget, 4th edition. N. Tryding and K.-A. Roos. Swedish Society for Clinical Chemistry, 1986.
Two ways: A. *in vitro* (i.e. analytical interference), B (i.e. biological effects). Analysed component, effect + or –.

DRUG-REAX interactive drug interactions consisting of five modules on CD-ROM (see Europharm for address).

Drug Test Interactions Handbook. Ed: J. G. Salway. Chapman and Hall Medical, 1989. 1104 pages, £295.

INTERLEX. Ed: L. Beeley.
A PC-based information system that can be obtained from Exeter Data Base Systems Ltd. Updated every six months.

Manual of Drug Interactions for Anaesthesiology, 2nd edition. Eds: R. A. Mueller and D. B. A. Lundberg. Churchill Livingstone, 1992.

Mechanisms of Drug Interactions, Vol. 122. Eds: P. F. D'Arcy, J. C. McElnay and P. G. Welling. Springer Verlag, Berlin, 1996.
363 pages, £208.50, DM 446, FF 1680, Lit 492. 600.

Clinical Trials

Clinical Drug Trials and Tribulations. Ed: A. Cato. Marcel Dekker, 1988.
Covers many of the problems met in clinical trials. It has a very good chapter on laboratory data.

Clinical Measurement in Drug Evaluation. Ed: W. S. Nimmo and G. T. Tucker. John Wiley and Sons, 1995.
344 pages; £49.95.

Databases for Pharmacovigilance. What can we do? Ed: S. R. Walker. Medical Benefit Risk Foundation, April 1996.
Copies from Centre for Medicines Research, Woodmanstone Road, Carshalton, Surrey, SM5 4DS, UK.

Drug Safety Assessment in Clinical Trials, Vol. 138, *Statistics, Textbooks and Monographs.* Ed: G. S. Gilbert. Marcel Dekker, 1993.
American book mostly devoted to statistical treatment of safety data and is therefore unique.

Guide to Clinical Interpretation of Data. B. Spilker. Raven Press, New York, 1986.
A large number of tables. Very useful.

Guide to Clinical Studies and Developing Protocols. B. Spilker. Raven Press, New York, 1984.
A vast number of tables. A valuable reference book.

Guide to Clinical Trials. B. Spilker. Raven Press, New York, 1991.
On CD ROM, Lippincott-Raven, 1996.

Guidelines for Pre-clinical and Clinical Testing of New Medicinal Products, Part 2: Investigations in Man. ABPI, 1977.

Handbook of Clinical Research, ACRPI, 2nd edition. Eds: J. Lloyd and A. Raven. Churchill Livingstone, 1994.

Handbook of Phase I/II Clinical Drug Trials. Eds: J. O'Grady and P. Joubert, CRC Press.
1997

Measuring Health: A Guide to Rating Scales and Questionnaires, 2nd edition, Eds: I. McDowell and C. Newell. Oxford University Press, 1996.

Measuring Health: a Guide to Rating Scales and Questionnaires. I. McDowell and C. Newell. University of Ottawa, Oxford University Press, Oxford and Walton, OX2 6DP, 1987.

Presentation of Clinical Data. B. Spilker and J. Schoenfelder. Raven Press, 1990.
There are chapters on laboratory data, ADR and quality of life. Almost every page has an example for 540 pages. Exhaustive. It states clearly that data analysis and statistical presentations are not described.

Randomised Controlled Clinical Trials. C. J. Bulpitt, Martinus Nijhoff, 1983.

One of the very few books that deals adequately with both sides of the cost/benefit ratio. Forms, questionnaires and the quality of life are dealt with very fully; but the latter are now dated.

Requirements for the Assessment of Clinical Safety. Proceedings of the First International Conference on Harmonization, Brussels, 1991. Eds: Prof. P. F. D'Arcy and D. W. G. Hamon. The Queen's University of Belfast, 1993.

Safety Requirements for the First Use of New Drugs and Diagnostic Agents in Man. The Council for International Organisation of Medical Sciences (CIOMS), 1983.
Subtitled: A review of safety issues in early clinical trials of drugs. Essential reading for those involved in phase I and 2 studies. 61 pages.

Safety Testing of New Drugs, Laboratory Predictions and Clinical Performance. Eds: D. R. Laurence, A. E. M. McLean and M. Weatherall. Academic Press, 1984.

Quality of Life Tools

The Quality of Life. L. Fallowfield. Souvenir Press, London, 1990.

Quality of Life and Pharmacoeconomics in Clinical Trials. Ed: B. Spilker, Lippincott-Raven Publishers, 1995.
1259 pages, £114.50.

Quality of Life Assessment. Key Issues in the 1990s. Eds: S. R. Walker and R. M. Rosser. Kluwer Academic Publishers, Dordrecht, 1993.

Quality of Life Assessment in Clinical Trials. Ed: B. Spilker, Raven Press Ltd, New York, 1990. Awaiting the second edition.

The Quality of Life of Cancer Patients. Eds: N. K. Aaronson and J. Beckmann. Monograph series of the European Organisation for Research on Treatment of Cancer (EORTC) Volume 17. Raven Press, 1987.

Measuring Functioning and Well-being. The Medical Outcomes Study Approach. Eds: A. L. Stewart and J. E. Ware, Jr. Duke University Press Durham and London, 1992.

Qualita Della Vita in Oncologia, a Cura di Cortesi. E. Roila, F. Tamburini and M. Citta di Castello. 43–55, 1995.

Introduzione alla Farmaceconomia. Bootman, J. L., Townsend, R. J. and McGhan, R. F. Versione Italiana a Cura di Recchia, G. and Carli, G.F. Milano, OEMF, 1993.

Jaeschke, R., Singer, J. and Guyatt, G. H. (1989). Measurement of health status. Ascertaining the minimal clinically important difference. *Contr. Clin. Trials*, **10**, 407–415.

The WHO QoL Group (1995). The World Health Organisation quality of life assessment (WHOQOL), position paper from the World Health Organisation. *Soc Sci Med.*, **10**, 1403–1409.

Testa, M. A. and Simonson, D.C. (1996). Assessment of Quality of Life outcomes. *New Engl. J. Med.*, **334** (13), 835–840.

Scientific Advisory Board of the Medical Outcomes Trust. (1995). Instrument Review Criteria. *Med. Outcomes Trust Bull.*, I–IV.

SF36 Physical and Mental Component Summary Measures, A User's Manual. Ware, J. E., Kosinski, M. and Keller, S. D. The Health Institute, New England Medical Center, 1994.

Fletcher, A. (1995). Quality of life measurements in the evaluation of treatment, proposed guidelines. *Br. J. Clin. Pharmacol.* **39**, 217–222.

Gill, T.M. and Feinstein, A.R. (1994). A critical appraisal of the quality of life measurements. *JAMA*, **272**, 619–626.

Guyatt, G. H., Naylor, C. D., Juniper, E., Heyland, D. K., Jaeschke, R. and Cook, D. J. for the Evidence-based Medicine Working Group. (1997). Users' guide to the medical literature. XII How to use articles about health-related quality of life. *JAMA*, **277**, 1232–1237.

Lepiege, A. and Hunt, S. (1997). The problem of quality of life in medicine. *JAMA*, **278**, 47–50.

CD-ROM for Windows Quality of Life Assessment in Medicine, Glamm Interactive srl, Issue 1, December 1996. Periodically updated, containing 9000 bibliographical references and 100 QoL tools developed over the past 20 years.

Quality of Life Newsletter. Published by the Mapi Research Institute.

British Journal of Medical Economics.

Toxicology

Casarett and Doull's Toxicology, 5th edition. The Basic Science of Poisons. Ed: C. D. Klaasen, McGraw Hill, 1996.

General and Applied Toxicology, Vols 1 and 2. Eds: B. Ballantyne, T. Marrs and P. Turner, Macmillan Publishers Ltd, Basingstoke, 1993.

Principles and Methods of Toxicology, 3rd edition. Hayes, A. W. (1994), Raven Press, New York.

Pharmaceutical Medicine. Eds: D. M. Burley and T. B. Binns, Edward Arnold, USA, 1985.

Reference Books

A Dictionary of Pharmacology and Clinical Drug Evaluation. Eds: D. R. Laurence and J. R. Carpenter, UCL Press Ltd, London. 1994.

Abbreviations in Medicine, 3rd edition. Karger, Albrecht Scherkl.

ABPI Compendium of Patient Information Leaflets. Datapharm Publications Ltd. 12 Whitehall, London, SW1A 2DY.

ABPI Data Sheet Compendium. Datapharm Publications Ltd.
1500 pages on UK drug products. Annual.

Avery's Drug Treatment, 4th edition. Eds: T. M. Speight and N. H. G. Holford, Adis International Ltd, 1997.
1820 pages, $155, £120, Sfr 165.

British National Formulary. British Medical Association and Royal Pharmaceutical Society of Great Britain. The Pharmaceutical Press, FREEPOST WC 1124, London, SE1 1BR.
Cloth backed bi-annual. £13.50. Now on CD-ROM or floppy disc.

Common Abbreviations in Clinical Medicine. Kai Haber. Raven Press, 1988.

Compendium of Quality of Life Instruments. Ed: S. Salek, J. Wiley, 1997.
Biannual update, electronic version and newsletter.

Dictionary of Pharmaceutical Medicine. Ed: G. Nahler, Springer Verlag, 1994.
177 pages, DM 39, £18, FF 147, Lit 43.070.

Dictionnaire Vidal. OVP, 11 rue Quentin-Bauchart, 75384, Paris.
Details of all the French drug products. Annual (see Europharm).

Drug Epidemiology. Ed: A. Bertelsman, Springer Verlag, 1993.
English–German Dictionary with German–English subject index and critical appraisal forms for literature review. 183 Pages. DM 78, £36.50, FF 294, Lit 86.150.

Europharm. (OVP).
On CD-ROM. Total annual subscription £2350. This includes:

Compendium Suisse des Médicaments.
£275.
L'Informatore Farmaceutico. Farmadisco.
£385.
Martindale. The Extra Pharmacopoeia.
£265.00.
PDR Physician's Desk Reference.
£480.
Rote Liste.
£ 130.
Simposium Terapeutica.
The Portuguese database.
£220.
The Spanish database.
£265.
Vademecum Internacional.
Vidal and Vidal Interactions.
£330.

Available from Microinfo Ltd. CD-ROM Division, PO Box 3, Omega Park, Alton, Hampshire, GU34 2PG, England. Tel: 01420 86848.

Global Adverse Drug Reaction Reporting Requirements. Scrip Report. B. Arnold. PJB Publications Ltd, August 1997.
Ref. BS, 879 pages 240+, £450, $945, ¥108,000.

International Drug Directory 1994/95. Swiss Pharmaceutical Society, 1995.
Synonyms, formulas and therapeutic classes of over 7000 drugs and over 28 000 proprietary preparations from 27 countries, 1300 pages. 1995.

International Monitoring of Adverse Reactions to Drugs. Adverse Reaction Terminology. WHO Collaborating Centre for International Drug Monitoring, Uppsala, Sweden, 1996.

Japan Pharmaceutical Reference (JPR), 4th edition. Japan Medical Products International Trade Association, 7-1 Nihonbashi Honcho 4-chome, Chuo-ku, Tokio 103, Japan.
1367 pages, $200.

Japanese Adverse Drug Reaction Terminology. Safety Division, Pharmaceutical Affairs Bureau, MHW. Ijken, Tokyo, 1996.

L'informatore Farmaceutico, Organisazione. Editorali, Medico-Farmaceutica SRL, Via Edolo 42, 20125, Milano.
Two-volume annual giving details of all Italian drug products (see Europharm).

Martindale. The Extra Pharmacopoeia.
£265.00.

Martindale. The Extra Pharmacopoeia, 31st edition. Ed: J. E. F. Reynolds. The Pharmaceutical Press, I996.
2800 pages, best source of brand names in other countries £176.00, also available on CD-ROM and online via Tel: +44 (0) 171 930 5503.

MEDIS Diseases Code, 3rd edition. Medical Information System Development Center, Tokyo, 1993.

Meyler's Side Effects of Drugs, 13th edition, 1996 and *The Side Effects of Drugs Annual*, Nos. 4-19, 1996, Excerpta Medica.
Absolutely essential. The most exhaustive available text on ADRs of individual drugs. Also available as CD-ROM, SEDBASE, from Elsevier Science B. V. Contact: Silver-Platter Information Ltd, 10, Barley Mow Passage, Chiswick, London, W4 4PH, UK or embase-europe@elsevier. nl.

National Pharmacovigilance Systems. Ed: Sten Olsen, The Uppsala Monitoring Centre (WHO), 1997.
63 pages, loose-leaf.

PDR Physician's Desk Reference.
£480.

Pharmacogenetics. Ed: W. W. Weber. Oxford Monograph on Medical Genetics No. 32, Oxford University Press, 1997.
£45.

Pharmacology: Drug Actions and Reactions. Ed: R. R. Levine, Parthenon Publishers, Carnforth, UK. 1996.
569 pages, $44.95.

Physician's Desk Reference Guide to Drug Interactions, Side-Effects, Indications, 50th edition. BSP Medical Economic.
1552 pages, £37.50.

Physician's Desk Reference, 50th edition. Medical Economics Comp. Inc., USA. 1996.
3060 pages of USA drug products; annual (see Europharm); also in disk format, electronic Library; £455.00.

Quick Guide to Japanese Ethical Products. JMRC Co., Medical Department, Metatex Co. Ltd, 3-12-4I. Komaba Meguro Ku Tokyo 153.
Check price before ordering!.

Rote Liste. Bundesverband der Pharmazeutischen Industrie, V. Karlstr. 21, 6000 Frankfurt am Main.
Details of all the German drug products; annual (see Europharm).

The Davis Book of Medical Abbreviations. F. A. Davis. S. L. Mitchell-Hatton Publishers, 1991.
A deciphering guide.

The Relevance of Ethnic Factors in the Clinical Evaluation of Medicines. Ed: S. Walker. CMR Workshop Series, Kluwer Academic, 1994.
$85.

Laboratory Data

Clinical Chemistry in Diagnosis and Treatment, 5th edition. J. F. Zilva, P. R. Pannell and P. D. Mayne. Edward Arnold, 1988.
Excellent.

Clinical Diagnosis, Management by Laboratory Methods, 19th edition. Ed: J. B. Henry, W. B. Saunders, Philadelphia, 1997.
£28.95.

Clinical Haematology, 7th edition. Ed: R. D. Eastham and R. Slade. Butterworth-Heinemann, 1992.

Drug Effects in Clinical Chemistry, 2nd edition. Eds: N. Tryding and C. - G. Lindblad, Apoteksbolaget, Stockholm, 1981.

Effects of Drugs on Clinical Laboratory Tests, 3rd edition. AACC Press, 1990.

Introduction to Biochemical Toxicity, 2nd edition. Eds: E. Hodgeson and P. Levi, Appleton Lange Con, 1994.

Multivariate Interpretation of Clinical Laboratory Data. Statistics: Textbooks and Monographs, Vol. 75. Eds: A. Albert and E. K. Marion. Marcel Dekker Inc, 1987.

The Drug Etiology of Agranulocytosis and Aplastic Anemia, Monographs in Epidemiology and Biostatistics, Vol. 18. D. W. Kaufman, J. P. Kelly, M. Levy and S. Shapiro. Oxford University Press, 1991.
Results of a very large case–control study.

General

A Decent Proposal—Ethical Review of Clinical Research. Evans & Evans, Wiley & Sons, 1994.
230 Pages, $35.00.

Adverse Reactions—A Changing Challenge. Eds: L. Lasagna and M. M. Reidenberg. Proceedings of the 2nd World Congress on Clinical Pharmacology and Therapeutics, 1983.

Analyse D'incidence en Pharmacovigilance, Application à la Notification Spontanée. ARME-Pharmacovigilance Editions, Bordeaux, 1992.
191 pages in French. (2nd edition).

Arzneimittelneben- und -wechselwirkungen. Ein Handbuch für Ärzte und Apotheker. Eds: P. Herman, C. J. Estler, O. Hockwin, E. Kallenberger, K. A. Kovar, H. Kurz, U. Müller-Breitenkamp, E. Noack, H. J. Ruoff, E. J. Verspohl, V.-G. Wissenschaftliche, 1991.

Assessing Causes of Adverse Drug Reactions. Ed: J. Venulet. Academic Press, 1982.
Based on a workshop held at Morges, Switzerland, in June 1981. Almost half the participants were Ciba-Geigy staff, but with contributors from most of the world authorities. Dominated by standardized methods with few voices in opposition.

Clinical Epidemiology. A Basic Science for Clinical Medicine. Eds: D. L. Sackett, R. B. Haynes and P. Tugwell. Little, Brown and Co., Bosoton/Toronto, 1985.
Well written—comprehensive.

Communication in Pharmaceutical Medicine. A Challenge for 1992. Eds: J. R. Ferran, J. Lahuerta Dal Rè and R. Lardinois. Prous Scientific Publ., 1991.
Publication of the papers presented at the 7th International Conference on Pharmaceutical Medicine. Quite a few papers on ADRs.

Detection and Prevention of Adverse Drug Reactions. 1984. Eds: H. Boström and N. Ljungstedt, Skandia International Symposia 1983. Almqvist Wiksell International, 1984.
Excellent discussions between world experts.

Drug Epidemiology and Post-marketing Surveillance. Eds: B. L. Strom and G. Velo. NATO ASI Series, Series A: Life Sciences Vol. 224, Planum Press Ltd, 1992.

This is the proceedings of a NATO Advanced Study Institute meeting held in Sicily between 27th September and 8th October 1990. 172 pages. Excellent. Still very relevant.

Drug Safety, A Shared Responsibility. Churchill Livingstone, 1991.
Written by the staff of the International Drug Safety Department of Glaxo Group Research.
126 pages.

Drug-induced Sufferings. Medical, Pharmaceutical and legal Aspects. Ed: T. Soda. Excerpta Medica, 1980.
Proceedings of the Kyoto (Japan) International Conference against drug-induced sufferings held in 1979. Contributors worldwide, but the majority Japanese. Not as emotional as the title implies. Contains reports on most of the world ADR problems.

Drug-safety Progress and Controversies, Eds: M. Auriche, J. Burke and J. Duchier. Pergamon Press, 1982.
The proceedings of the IVth International Congress of Pharmaceutical Physicians, April 1981. Largely given to adverse drug reactions and post-marketing surveillance, especially within the industry.

Epidemiologia da Medicamento, Principiis gerahs. Eds: J. R. Leopard, G. Tognoni and S. Rezenfeld. Hucitec-Abrasco, Sao Paulo-Rio de Janeiro, 1989.

Erfassung und Bewertung unerwünschter Wirkungen von Arzneimitteln. Ed: H. P. Ferber, P. Grosdanoff, O. Kraupp, T. Lehnert, W. Schütz. De Gruyter, 1990.

European Medicines Research, Perspective in Pharmacotoxicology and Pharmacovigilance. Ed: G. N. Fracchia. IOS Press, 1994.
Out of the 420 pages there are 148 dealing with pharmacovigilance.

Farmaco Sorveglianza. Eds: G. Casadea and A. Silve. Presentazione di Radoffo Paoletti, Massoni, Milano, 1989.

Farmacoepideiología. Ed: Alfonso Carvajal. Univ. De Valladolid, Spain, Secretaiade de Pullicacione, 1993.
162 pages.

Idiosyncratic ADR: Impact on Drug Development and Clinical Use after Marketing, Eds: C. A. Naranjo and J. K. Jones. International Congress Series 878, Excerpt Medica, 1990. Out of print.
Proceedings of the Satellite Symposium to the IV World Conference on Clinical Pharmacology and Therapeutics, Mannheim-Heidelberg, 29-30 July 1989. Covers idiosyncratic ADR very well.

Imaging Drug Reactions and Toxic Hazards, 3rd edition. Ed: G. Ansell. Chapman & Hall.
Paperback £24.50, hardback £90.

Immunotoxicology and Immunopharmacology, 2nd edition. J. Dean, M. Luster, A. Munson and I. Kimber. Raven Press.
770 pages.

Immunotoxicology. Eds: G. G. Gibson, R. Hubbard and D. V. Parke. Academic Press, 1983.

Comprehensive. The proceedings of the first international symposium on immunotoxicology in 1982. About half of its 500 pages are on drug-related topics. It is well produced and well referenced and has a very good chapter on drug allergy.

Improving Drug Safety—A Joint responsibility. Eds: R. Dinkel, B. Horisberger and K. W. Tolo. Springer Verlag, 1991.

A publication of a RAD-AR meeting in Wolfsberg in 1990. Interesting reading, but too many communications in too little space.

Living with Risk, The BMA. Guide. John Wiley and Sons, 1987.

Medicines and Risk/Benefit Decisions. Eds: S. R. Walker and A. W. Asscher, MTP Press, 1987.

This is the proceedings of a Centre for Medicines Workshop held in October 1985. An excellent coverage of the situation.

Medicines Regulation, Research and Risk. Ed: J. P. Griffin. The Queen's University, Belfast. 1989.

Monitoring Drug Safety. Ed: R. D. T. Farmer and J. W. van der Velden.

On CD-ROM. Contact: Interactive Educational Systems. Tel: 0181 3989217; fax: 0181 3982939; E-mail: 74214. 16@ compuserve. com.

Monitoring for Adverse Drug Reactions. Ed: S. R. Walker. Kluwer Academic Publisher, 1985.

£73.25.

Monitoring for Drug Safety, 2nd edition. Ed: W. H. Inman, MTP Press Ltd, 1986.

An interesting book on postmarketing surveillance with a wide ranging list of international contributors. Now needs updating.

Pharmacoepidemiology, 2nd edition. Ed: B. L. Strom. Churchill Livingstone Inc., New York, 1994.

741 pages. All there is to know about the subject: details of all the main databases and therefore mostly USA oriented. $135.00.

Pharmacoepidemiology. S. A. Edlavitch. Lewis Pub., 1990.

Papers at 3rd International Conference on Pharmacoepidemiology, Sept 9–11, 1987. Out of print, Jan, 1992.

Pharmacoepidemiology: An Introduction, 3rd edition. Eds: A. G. Hartzema, M. S. Porta and H. H. Tilson. Harvey Whitney Books. P. O. Box 42696/ Cincinnati, OH 45242 USA, 1998.

Post-marketing Drug Safety Management: a Pharmaceutical Industry Perspective. Willem K. Amery, IOS Press (Van Diemenstraat 94, 1013 CN Amsterdam, Fax: 31–20/620 34 19), 1998.

$120.

Risk and Consent to Risk in Medicine. Ed: R. D. Mann. Parthenon Publishing Group, 1989.

Proceedings of a Management Forum conference in 1988.

Risk Factors for ADR—Epidemiological Approaches. Eds: E. Weber, D. H. Lawson and R. Hoigné. Birkhäuser Verlag, 1990.

Publication of the 4th World Conference on Clinical Pharmacology and Therapeutics in Heidelberg, 1989.

Side Effects of Drugs Essays. Ed: M. N. G. Dukes. Elsevier. 1990.

These are 14 essays, each taken from a *Side-effects of Drugs Annual.*

The Perception and Management of Drug Safety Risks. Eds: B. Horis Berger and R. Dinkel. Springer Verlag, 1989.

Paperbacks

A Regional Spontaneous Surveillance Program for Adverse Drug Reactions as a Tool to Improve Pharmacotherapy. G. H. P. de Koning, CIP-Gegevens Koninklijke Bibliotheek, Den Haag, Netherlands, 1993.

190 pages. A translated Dutch PhD thesis on the Netherlands Pharmacovigilance Foundation (LAREB).

Adverse Event Monitoring and its Implementation in Clinical Trials. M. A. Wallander. Uppsala University, Almqvist & Wiksell International Stockholm, 1991.

An excellent doctoral thesis. 147 pages.

Analyse d'Incidence en Pharmacovigilance: Application à La Notification Spontanée, 2nd edition. ARME-Pharmacovigilance, Bordeaux. 1992.

Cadre Juridique des Études de Cohortes en Pharmacovigilance, 2nd edition. ARME-Pharmacovigilance Editions, Bordeaux, 1995.

Databases for Pharmacovigilance: What Can We Do? Ed: S. R. Walker. Medical Benefit-Risk Foundation. April 1996.

Copies from Centre for Medicines Research, Woodmanstone Road, Carshalton, Surrey, SM5 4DS, UK.

Diccionario de Farmacoepidemiologia. Eds: B. Bégaud and L. H. Martin-Arias. Masson, Barcelona, 1997.

151 pages.

Dictionnaire de Pharmaco-épidémiologie, 2nd edition, Ed: B. Bégaud, ARME-Pharmacovigilance Editions, Hôpital Pellegrin, 33076 Bordeaux Cédex, 1995.

92 pages.

Données Françaises de Morbidité Utiles en Pharmacovigilance, 2nd edition, ARME-Pharmacovigilance Editions, Bordeaux, 1997.

Drug Surveillance: International Cooperation Past, Present and Future. Proceedings of the XXVth CIOMS Conference, Geneva, 14–15 September, 1993. Eds: Z. Bankowski and J. F. Dunne, 1994.
198 pages.

Etudes de Cohortes en Pharmacovigilance, 2nd edition. ARME-Pharmacovigilance Editions, 1995.
100 pages in French.

Farmaco Sorveglianza. Eds: G. Casadea and A. Salve. Presentazione di Radoffo Paoletti, Massoni, Milano, 1989.
In Italian.

Farmacoepidemiología. A. Carvajal, Secreterade de Pullicaciones University of Valladolid, 1993.
162 pages. In Spanish. Details available from: Centro Regional de Farmacovigilancia de Castilla y León, Avenida Ramón y Cajal, 7, 47005 Valladolid, Spain.

Guideline for Preparing Case Clinical Safety Information on Drugs. Report of CIOMS working group III, 1995.
69 pages.

Importance de la Pharmaco-épidémiologie pour l' Industriel du Médicament. Eds: B. Bégaud and A. Fourrier, Cahiers Techniques du SNIP No. 16: L'epidémiologie dans l'entreprise: pour quoi faire? Syndicat National de l'Industrie Pharmaceutique, Paris, 1997.
151 pages.

Improving Drug Safety: The Assessment, Management and Communication of the Therapeutic Benefits and Risks of Pharmaceutical Products. Eds: N. Shimizu, Y. Tanaka, J. Jones and D. Taylor. PharMa International Inc. 1990.
The Official proceedings of the RAD-AR symposium 1989 held in Japan. 346 pages.

Interethnic Differences in Clinical Responsiveness. Eds: J. A. M. McAuslane, K. Thomas, C. E. Lumley and S. R. Walker. CMR 95-4R, March 1995.

International Reporting of Adverse Drug Reactions. CIOMS Working Group I, Final Report, 1990.
66 pages.

International Reporting of Periodic Drug Safety Update Summaries. Final report of CIOMS working group II, 1992.
21 pages.

List of References (On causality assessment). Third International APWI meeting, ARME-Pharmacovigilance Editions, 1992.
58 pages in English.

Methodological Approaches in Pharmacoepidemiology: Application to Spontaneous Reporting. ARME-P, Elsevier Science Publishers. 1993.
174 pages. Actually a hardback but it is better here with the other ARME-P publications. An excellent French statistical guide to the subject.

Monitoring and Assessment of Adverse Drug Effects. Council for International Organisation of Medical Sciences (CIOMS), 1986.
The advantages and disadvantages of various methods covered in 30 pages.

Nombre de Sujets Nécessaires pour Démontrer l'Equivalence entre deux Risques. Eds: P. Tubert-Bitter, R. Manfredi and B. Bégaud. ARME-Pharmacovigilance Editions, 1996.
41 pages.

Reporting Adverse Drug Reaction: A BMA policy document. Board of Science and Education. BMA Professional Division Pub., 1996.
£5.95.

Second European Pharmacovigilance Symposium, Abstracts. Editions du Vidal, Paris, 1992.
In French or English. 109 pages.

The Extent of Population Exposure Required to Assess Clinical Safety. Eds: J. A. M. McAuslane and K. Thomas. CMR 94-IOR, September 1994.
Check the price before ordering for all CMR publications. Address above.

The Relevance of Ethnic Factors in the Clinical Evaluation of Medicines. Ed: S. R. Walker, Kluwer Academic, Boston, 1994.
262 pages, $85.

Tollerabilità di un Farmaco: Valutazione Clinica. Ed: C. Borghi and D. Canti, Organizzazione Editorale Medico Farmaceutica, Via Edolo, 42-20125, Milano, 1986.
210 pages, In Italian.

Books critical of the industry and/or regulators

Warning, these books can affect your peace of mind!

A Healthy business? World Health and the Pharmaceutical Industry. A. Cheatley, Zed Books, London, 1990.

Adverse Reactions. T. Maeder, William Morrow and Co., 1994.
480 pages. The story of chloramphenicol.

Bad Medicine: the Prescription Drug Industry in the Third World. M. Silverman, M. Lydecker and P. R. Lee. Stanford University Press, Stanford, 1992.

Cured to Death. A. Melville and C. Johnson, New English Library, 1983.

Deadly Medicine. T. J. Moore, Simon and Schuster, 1995.
349 pages. The stories of flecanide, moricizine and encainide.

Deception by Design: Pharmaceutical Promotion in the Third World. J. Lexchin. Consumers International Regional Office for Asia and the Pacific, 1996.
91 pages.

Merck V Glaxo, The Million Dollar Battle. M. Lynn. Heineman, London, 1991.

Power And Dependence—Social Audit on the Safety of Medicines. C. Medawar. Eds:
L. Ramsay and B Guthrie, Social Audit Ltd., 1992.
Box 111, London NW1 8XG, £11.

Prescription for Death: The Drugging of the Third World. M. Silverman, University of
California Press; Berkeley, CA, 1982.

Problem Drugs. A. Chetley, ZED books, 7 Cynthia St, London N1 9JF, 1995.

Roche versus Adams. S. Adams, Fontana/Collins, 1985.

*Science, Politics and the Pharmaceutical Industry; Controversy and Bias in Drug
Regulation.* J. Abraham, University College London Press, 1995.

Strong Medicine. A. Hailey, Pan Books, 1984.
476 pages.

Thalidomide and the Power of the Drug Companies. S. Sjöstrom and R. Nilsson,
Penguin Books, 1972.

The Health Conspiracy. J. Collier. Century Hutchinson Ltd, 1989.

There's Gold in Them Thar Pills. A. Klass. Penguin Books, 1975.

Journals

Adverse Drug Reaction Bulletin. Ed: R. E. Ferner.
Bi-monthly. In English, Italian, French and Spanish editions. Each issue deals with
one particular ADR problem area.

Adverse Drug Reactions and Acute Poisoning Reviews. Ed: J. P. Griffin, Oxford
University Press. Quarterly journal.
Excellent monographs on specific areas.

Clin-Alert.
An American semi-monthly giving the latest ADRs. Published by Clin-Alert Inc.,
143 Old Marlton Pike, Medford, NJ 08055, USA.

Current Problems.
Published by the CSM 3–4 times a year or when necessary.

Drug Information Journal.
Quarterly journal of the Drug Information Association. Excellent source of information on methodology and data management. Absolutely essential.

Drug Safety. Adis Press Ltd.
Bimonthly. Used to be called Medical Toxicology and Adverse Drug Experiences.
Excellent.

Drugs and Therapeutics Bulletin.
Fortnightly bulletin published by the Consumers' Association, 2 Marylebone Road,
London, NW1 4DX, UK. Independent and objective.

International Journal of Pharmaceutical Medicine.
Journal of the Society of Pharmaceutical Medicine. Eds: B. Dickson and M. Young, Blackwell Scientific Publications.
The official Quarterly. Started 1997.

Journal of Clinical Epidemiology, including Pharmacoepidemiological Reports.

Journal of Clinical Research and Pharmacoepidemiology. Elsevier.
Official publication of the Association of Clinical Pharmacologists. Quarterly.

Journal of Pharmacoepidemiology. Eds: J. E. Fincham. The Howarth Press, USA.
A quarterly.

Pharmacoepidemiology and Drug Safety. Ed: R. Mann. Wiley.
Bimonthly. Journal of the International Society of Pharmacoepidemiology.

Quality of Life Research. Rapid Science Publishers.
Official journal of the International Society of Quality of Life Research.

Reactions Weekly. Adis Press, New Zealand.
Quarterly and cumulative annual index. Current adverse drug reaction problems. Fills in the time lag before ADRs are published in Meyler's.

Scrip. Ed: P. Brown. PJB Publications Ltd.
Published at frequent but irregular intervals. Essential reading to find out what is happening in your own company and to your own drugs, as well as the changes in the regulations and practices around the world.

The International Journal of Risk and Safety in Medicine. Ed: M. N. Dukes. Elsevier.
A quarterly that started in May 1990.

British Journal of Medical Economics.

Quality of Life Research.

Quality of Life Newsletter.
Published by the Mapi Research Institute.

Appendices

Appendix 1: Products withdrawn from sale due to safety reasons in UK and/or USA 1961–1995 (Fr, France; Ger, Germany; pers. comm., personal communication)

INN	Trade name	Therapeutic class	Reason(s) for withdrawal/ suspension of product licence	Launch date	Countries	PL Suspension (S) / Withdrawal (W)	Countries	Years on market	Reference
Acetylsalicyclic acid (paediatric)	Aspirin	Analgesic	Reye's syndrome	1899	UK	1986	UK		Spriet-Pourra (1994)
Alclofenac	Prinalgin	Non-steroidal anti-inflammatory drug (NSAID)	Skin and renal reactions Mutagenic metabolite	1972	UK	1979	UK	8	Bakke (1984)
Alphoxalone	Althesin	Anaesthetic	Allergic-type reaction due to Cremophor EL	1972 1973 1977	UK Fr. Ger.	1984 1984 1984	UK Fr. Ger.	12 11 7	CSM (pers. comm. 1995)
Aminoglutethimide	Elipten	Anticonvulsant	Endocrinological Reintroduced—Cushing's Syndrome	1960 1978	USA USA	1966	USA	6	Bakke (1984)
Aminopyrine		Analgesic	Haematological	1900 1900	USA UK	1970 1975	USA UK	70 75	Spriet-Pourra (1994)
Azaribine	Triazure	Antipsoriatic	Neuropsychiatric Coagulation disorders	1975	USA	1976	USA	1	Bakke (1984)
Benoxaprofen	Opren	NSAID	Cholestatic jaundice Photosensitivity	1980 1982 1982	UK USA Ger	1982 1982 1982	UK USA Ger	2 < 1 < 1	CSM (pers. comm. 1995)
Benziodarone	Amplivix	Uricosuric Coronary dilator	Hepatic	1962 1962	UK Fr	1964 1987	UK Fr	2 25	Bakke (1984)
Bismuth		Gastrointestinal drug	Neuropysychiatric		Fr	1978	Fr		Spriet-Pourra (1994)
Bithionol	Actamer	Anthelminthic	Dermatological	?	USA	1967	USA	?	Spriet-Pourra (1994)
Buformin		Antidiabethc	Metabolic	1978	Ger	1978		?	Spriet-Pourra (1994)

Drug	Trade name	Type	Reason	Year intro	Country	Year withdrawn	Country	No.	Reference
Chloramphenicol		Antibiotic	Aplastic anaemia	1950	Fr	1978	Fr	28	Spriet-Pourra (1994)
Chlormadinone	Normenon	Hormone	Animal carcinogenicity	1965	USA	1970	USA	5	Bakke (1984)
				1966	UK	1970	UK	4	
Clioquinol	Enterovioform	Antidiarrhoeal	Neuropsychiatric	1930	UK	1981	UK	51	Bakke (1984)
				1930	USA	1973	USA	43	
				1930	Fr	1985	Fr	55	
				1930	Ger	1985	Ger	55	
Centoxin	HA-1A	Hu-anti-lipid A IgM monoclonal	Gram-negative septicaemia	?	UK	1992	UK	?	CSM (pers. Comm., 1995)
Danthron	Dorbanex	Laxative	Animal carcinogenicity Reintroduced with restrictions	1959	USA	1987	USA	28	Spriet-Pourra (1994)
				1964	UK	1987	UK	23	
				1964	Fr	1987	Fr	23	
				1989					
Desensitizing vaccines		Vaccine	Allergic-type reactions	?	UK	1989	UK		Spriet-Pourra (1994)
Diamthazole	Asterol	Antifungal	Neuropsychiatric	?	USA	1977	USA	17	Spriet-Pourra (1994)
				1955	Fr	1972	Fr		
Dihydrost-reptomycin		Antibiotic	Neuropsychiatric	?	USA	1970	USA	?	Spriet-Pourra (1994)
Dinoprostone	Propess	Hormone	Uterine hypertonus and fetal distress	1989	UK	1990	UK	< 1	CSM (pers. comm., 1995)
Dipyrone		Analgesic	Haematological	1930	UK	1977	UK	47	Bakke (1984)
				1930	USA	1977	USA	47	
Dithiazanine		Anthelminthic	Metabolic Cardiovascular	?	USA	1964	USA		Spriet-Pourra (1994)
					Fr	1964	Fr		
Domperidone (injection)	Motilium	Antiemetic	Cardiovascular Risk of overdose	?	UK	1986	UK	?	Spriet-Pourra (1994)
				1983	Fr	1986	Fr	3	
					Ger	1986	Ger	?	
Doxylamine Dicyclomine	Bendectin Debendox	Antihistamine	?: Teratogenicity— dysmorphogenicity?	1956	USA	1983	USA	27	Hays (1983)
				1957	UK	1983	UK	26	

Appendix 1 (*Contd.*)

INN	Trade name	Therapeutic class	Reason(s) for withdrawal/suspension of product licence	Launch date	Countries	PL Suspension (S) / Withdrawal (W)	Countries	Years on market	Reference
Encainide	Enkaid	Antiarrhythmic	Cardiovascular Excess mortality risk	1987	USA	1991	USA	4	Spriet-Pourra (1994)
Factor VIII	Factorate	Coagulation factor	Manufacture problem Risk of AIDS transmission	1972	UK	1986	UK	14	Spriet-Pourra (1994)
Factor XIII	Fibogammin	Coagulation factor	Manufacture problem Progressive scleroderma	1976 1979 ?	UK Fr Ger	NW 1992 1992	UK Fr Ger	? 13	Spriet-Pourra (1994)
Fenclofenac	Flenac	NSAID	Multiple—especially skin reactions	1978	UK	1984	UK	6	CSM (pers. comm., 1995)
Feprazone	Methrazone	NSAID	Multiple	1976	UK	1984 1984	UK Ger	8	CSM (pers. Comm., 1995)
Flosequinan	Manoplax	Heart failure	Increased mortality Lack of long-term efficacy	1992	UK	1993 1993	UK USA	9 months	CSM (pers. comm., 1995)
Growth hormone (natural)	Crescormon	Hormone	Manufacture problem Creutzfeldt-Jakob disease transmission	1970 1970 1970 1970	UK USA Fr Ger	1985 1985 1985 1985	UK USA Fr Ger	15	Spriet-Pourra (1994)
Guanethidine	Ganda (high dose)	Anti-glaucoma eye drops	Ophthalmological	1977 1973	UK Fr	1986 NW	UK	9	Spriet-Pourra (1994)
Ibufenac	Dytransin	NSAID	Hepatic	1966	UK	1968	UK	2	Bakke (1984)
Indomethacin-R	Osmosin form	NSAID	Multiple gastrointestinal—36 fatal small intestine perforations	1982	UK	1983 1983	UK Ger	9 months	CSM (pers. comm., 1995)
Indoprofen	Flosint	NSAID	Gastrointestinal carcinogenicity	1982	UK	1983 1984	UK Ger	1 ?2	Spriet-Pourra (1994)

Drug	Trade name	Class	Indication	Year	Country	Year	Country	Number	Reference
Iodinated casein strophantin	Coratose	Anorexiant	Metabolic	?	?	1964	USA	?	Spriet-Pourra (1994)
Mebanazine	Actomol	Antidepressant	Hepatic Drug interactions	1963	UK	1975	UK	12	Bakke (1984)
Megestrol acetate	Volidan 21	Hormone	Carcinogenicity	1963	UK	1970 1969 1975	UK Fr Ger	7	Bakke (1984)
Methandrostenolone	Dianabol	Hormone	Endocrinological	1960 1960 1962 1963	USA Fr UK Ger	1982 1982 1982 1982	USA Fr UK Ger	12 12 10 9	Script report
Methapyrilene		H1 antihistamine	Carcinogenicity	1947 1950	USA UK	1979 1979	USA UK	31 29	Bakke (1984)
Metipranolol	Glauline	Antiglaucoma eye drops	Ophthalmological — uveitis (high dose) Low-dose preparation	?	UK	1990 1991	UK	?	CSM (pers. comm., 1995)
Metofoline	Versidyne	Analgesic	Experimental toxicity	?	?	1965	USA	?	Spriet-Pourra (1994)
Mumps vaccine Urabe AM9 strain	Pariorix	Vaccine	Neuropsychiatric Meningitis	1988 1986	UK Fr	1992 NW 1992	UK Fr USA	4	Anon (1992)
Neomycin (injection)		Antibiotic	Misuse Irrigation of open wounds	?	USA	1989	USA	?	Spriet-Pourra (1994)
Nialamide	Niamid	Antidepressant (MAOI)	Hepatic Drug interactions	1959 1959 1960	UK USA Fr	1978 1974 NW	UK USA Fr	19 15	Bakke (1984)
Normifensin	Merital	Antidepressant	Haemolytic anaemia Hepatotoxicity-fatal hepatitis	1977 1976 1978 1985	UK Ger Fr USA	1986 1986 1986 1986	UK Ger Fr USA	9 9 8 1	Stonier (1992)
Oxphenbutazone	Tanderil	NSAID	Haematological Multiple	1960 1961 1962 1962	USA Fr UK Ger	1985 1985 1984 1985	USA Fr UK Ger	25 24 22 23	Spriet-Pourra (1994)
Oxyphenisatin	Veripaque	Laxative	Hepatic	1955 1957	UK USA	1978 1972 1976 1981	UK USA Ger Fr	23 15	Bakke (1984)

Appendix 1 (*Contd.*)

INN	Trade name	Therapeutic class	Reason(s) for withdrawal/ suspension of product licence	Launch date	Countries	PL Suspension (S) / Withdrawal (W)	Countries	Years on market	Reference
Penicillins (topical use)		Antibiotic	Allergic-type reactions	?		1972	USA	?	Spriet-Pourra (1994)
Perhexiline maleate	Pexid		Hepatic damage Peripheral neuropathy	1975	UK	1985	UK	10	CSM (pers. comm., 1995)
Phenacetin		Analgesic	Renal Carcinogenicity	<1900 1900	UK USA	1980 1983 1986 NW	UK USA Ger Fr	80 83	Bakke (1984)
Phenformin	Insoral Dibotin	Antidiabetic	Metabolic	1959 1959 1964	UK USA Fr	1982 1977 1977	UK USA Fr	23 18 13	Bakke (1984)
Phenoxypropazine	Drazine	Antidepressant (MAOI)	Hepatic Drug interactions	1961	UK	1966	UK	5	Bakke (1984)
Phenylbutazone	Butazolidine	NSAID	Haematological Multiple	1952	Ger	1985 Restriction	Ger USA Fr	33	Spriet-Pourra (1994)
Pituitary chorionic hormone		Hormone	Hypersensitivity	?	UK	1972	UK	?	Spriet-Pourra (1995)
Polidexide	Secholex	Antihyper-lipidaemic	Experimental toxicity Toxic impurities	1974	UK	1975	UK	1	CSM (pers. comm., 1995)
Practolol	Eraldin	Beta blocker	Oculomuco-cutaneous syndrome Deafness Sclerosing peritonitis	1970 1973 ?	UK Fr Ger	1975 1975 1975	UK Fr Ger	5 2	CSM (pers. comm., 1995)
Prenylamine	Segontin Synadrin	Antianginal	Cardiovascular	1973 1965 1965	UK Ger Fr	1989 1989 1989	UK Ger Fr	16 24 24	Spriet-Pourra (1994)
Pronethalol	Alderlin	Beta blocker	Animal carcinogenicity	1963	UK	1965	UK	2	Bakke (1984)

Drug	Trade name(s)	Class	Adverse reaction	Year	Country	Year withdrawn	Country	No.	Reference
Propanadid	Epontol	Anaesthetic	Allergic-type reactions	1967	Fr	NW 1983	Fr UK	?	Spriet-Pourra (1994)
Remoxipride	Roxiam	Antipsychotic	Haematological—aplastic anaemia	1991	UK	1994	UK	3	CSM (pers. comm., 1995)
Somatropin	Crescormone	Natural growth hormone	Creutzfeldt-Jakob diesease	1973	UK	1985	UK	12	Bakke (1995)
Sulfamethoxy-pyridazine	Lederkyn	Antinfective	Haematological Dermatological	?	UK	1986	UK	?	Spriet-Pourra (1994)
Suprofen	Suprol	NSAID	Renal	1986	USA	1987 1987	USA UK	1	CSM (pers. comm., 1995)
Temafloxacin	Omniflox Teflox	Antinfective	Hepatic dysfunction Haemolytic anaemia Nephrological Anaphylaxis Metabolic	1991 1992 1992	UK USA Ger	1992 1992 1992	UK USA Ger	?4 months	Davey (1993)
Terolidine	Micturin	Urinary incontinence	Cardiac arrhythmia	1986 1990	UK Ger	1991 1991	UK Ger	5 1	Wild (1992)
Tetracycline (paediatric form)	Achromycin V	Antibiotic	Teeth discolouration	1952	USA	1979	USA	27	Spriet-Pourra (1994)
Thalidomide	Contergan Distaval	Sedative Orphan Drug Inds	Teratogenicity Phocomelia	1956 1956	UK Ger	1961 1961	UK Ger	5 5	Spriet-Pourra (1994)
Thenalidine		H1 antihistamine	Haematological	1961	UK	1961	UK	?	Spriet-Pourra (1994)
Ticrynafen	Selacryn Diflurex	Diuretic	Hepatic	1979 1976	USA Fr	1980 1991	USA Fr Ger	1 15 ?	Bakke (1984)
Tranylcypromine	Parnate Parstelin	Antidepressant (MAOI)	Cardiovascular Drug interactions	1963	Fr	1987 1964	Fr USA	24	Spriet-Pourra (1994)
Triazolam	Halcion	Hypnotic	Neuropsychiatric—memory loss, depression	1979 1980 1983 ?	UK Fr USA Ger	1991 1992 NW NW	UK Fr USA Ger	12 12	CSM (pers. comm., 1995)

Appendix 1 (*Contd*)

INN	Trade name	Therapeutic class	Reason(s) for withdrawal/ suspension of product licence	Launch date	Countries	PL Suspension (S) / Withdrawal (W)	Countries	Years on market	Reference
Triparanol	MER-29	Antihyper-lipidaemic	Ophthalmological	1959	USA	1962 1962	USA Fr	3	Spriet-Pourra (1994)
Tryptophan	Pacitron Optimax	Low protein diet Re-introduced -r OPTICs monitor.	Eosinophilic myalgia syndrome	1974	USA	1989 1990 1990 1990	USA UK Ger Fr	15	Wood (1992)
Urethane	Various	Solvent	Carcinogenicity	1933	Fr	1985 1977	Fr USA	52 ?	Spriet-Pourra (1994)
Vitamin E	E-Ferol	Vitamin	Haematological Hepatic Renal	1983	USA	1984	USA	1	Spriet-Pourra (1994)
Zomepirac	Zomax	NSAID	Allergic-type reactions—fatal anaphylaxis	1980 1981	USA UK	1983 1983	USA UK	3 2	CSM (pers. comm., 1995)
Zimeldine	Zelmid	Antidepressant	Hepatotoxicity Neurological—peripheral neuropathy, Guillain-Barré syndrome	1982 1982	UK Ger	1983 1983	UK Ger	1 1	CSM (pers. comm., 1995)

Tolerstat, an aldose-reductase inhibitor developed for treatment of serious diabetes complications was withdrawn by one of the manufacturers in October 1996 because of cases of deaths due to hepatic necrosis (Foppiano and Lombardo, 1997)
Dexfenfluramine and fenfluramine were withdrawn worldwide by the manufacturers because of heart valve defects in the US in September 1997 (In Brief, 1997)
Mibefradil, the first selective T-channel blocker, was withdrawn by the manufacturers in June 1998 because of potential interactions with 25 other drugs (In Brief, 1998)
NW Not withdrawn.

Appendix 2: The Van Arsdel Classification of Allergic Reactions

1. Mast cell-mediated
2. T cell-mediated
3. Photodermatitis (systemic)
4. Other cutaneous reactions (mechanism unknown)
5. Drug fever
6. Systemic lupus erythematosus (SLE) and other autoimmune reactions
7. Grouped into organ classes

1.   Mast Cell-mediated

These are Gell and Coombs' class one reactions. There are two types:

(a) Anaphylactoid reactions, which are type 'A' reactions where the drug causes immediate release of histamine, leukotrienes and chemotactic factors. There is a dose–response relationship. Intravenous injections can cause a massive release of cardiac histamine and cause cardiac arrest. No latent period for sensitization is necessary, but the same mediators are released as in the anaphylactic-type reactions. These are sometimes called pseudoallergic reactions (PARS). Drugs causing these are typically iodinated radiographic contrast media and TTO is immediate or usually within one hour. (Hoigné *et al.*, 1993).

(b) True type 'B' hypersensitivity reactions requiring several days of treatment before the reaction occurs or occuring immediately in a person previously sensitized to the drug (e.g. anaphylaxis, urticaria, angioneurotic oedema) TTO is immediate or usually within one hour when sensitized. Most are within 30–60 minutes, but in a small percentage of cases they may be delayed for an hour or more (Yunginger, 1992). The latent period before the onset of a hypersensitivity reaction is 10–20 days (Patterson and Anderson, 1982; Anderson and Adkinson, 1987). However, neutralizing antibodies to streptokinase are elevated from four days after its administration (Jennings, 1996).

Serum Sickness

TTO is 6–12 days (Rocklin, 1978). In 11 of 12 patients it was 8–13 days (Lawley *et al.*, 1984) and 8–14 days (Roujeau and Stern, 1994).

Angioedema

Of cases of angioedema with angiotensin-converting enzyme ACE inhibitors, 83% occur within the first week, one occurred after five hours (Slater *et al.*, 1988), 47% within the first week, 77% within three weeks and with one exception all resolved within one week (Hedner *et al.*, 1992). Less than four weeks (Roujeau and Stern, 1994). Angioedema with ACE inhibitors. In one study 35 of 36 patients were clear within one week (Hedner *et al.*, 1992) whereas with erythromycin, recovery begins within 24 hours (Huang, 1989). Typically after 7–21 days (Rieder, 1994), but can be as late as 13 months (Venable, 1992). Angioedema with penicillins, cephalosporins, contrast media, TTO is a few minutes to a few hours. Angioedema with non-steroidal anti-inflammatory drugs (NSAIDs) TTO is 1–7 days (Roujeau and Stern, 1994).

Urticaria

This may start hours or days after initiation of treatment. After haemophilus B–diphtheria toxoid conjugate vaccine urticaria developed within 48 hours (Scheifele, 1989).

Anticoagulant Necrosis

TTO with heparin is 5–10 days and warfarin, 3–5 days (Roujeau and Stern, 1994).

2. T-cell Mediated

Eczematous Contact Dermatitis

In sensitized patients the reaction is evident 6–48 hours after contact (Kaplan, 1984).

3. Photodermatitis (Systemic)

Photosensitivity TTO is minimum of five days (Roujeau and Stern, 1994). Photoallergy after 5–10 days (Van Arsdel, 1982). Phototoxicity within 24 hours (Emmett, 1978).

4. Other Cutaneous Reactions (Mechanism Uncertain)

Erythematous (Maculopapular) Rashes

TTO is 5–10 days. Can occur up to two weeks after administration (Breathnach, 1993). Incidence of erythematous eruptions peaks at about nine days, but can be as late as three weeks, but if already sensitized it is within 2–3 days (Stewart and Beeley, 1988). With phenytoin approximately it is 10 days or 1–3 days on re-exposure. (Shear, 1990).

Toxic Epidermal Necrolysis

TTO is typically 1–3 weeks. After a single dose of sulfadoxone TTO is an average 22 days, range 3–46 days.

Stevens–Johnson Syndrome

TTO is typically 1–3 weeks (Roujeau and Stern, 1994). May appear as late as six days after dechallenge. In Stevens-Johnson syndrome and toxic epidermal necrolysis, after dechallenge, the regrowth of epidermis may begin within days, but usually takes about three weeks (Roujeau and Stern, 1994). Erythema multiforme due to sulfonamides TTO is approximately 10 days (Shear, 1990).

Fixed Drug Eruptions

TTO is a few hours to 72 hours.

Alopecia

For alopecia with cytotoxic drugs (a type A reaction) TTO is 3–6 weeks. Anticoagulant alopecia occurs after 2–3 months (Levantine and Almeyda, 1973).

Vasculitis

TTO is 1–3 weeks (Roujeau and Stern, 1994). With clindamycin a case occurred after five days (Lambert *et al.*, 1982). For urticarial vasculitis TTO is 4–12 days (Shear, 1990).

Hypersensitivity Syndrome

With anticonvulsants, sulphonamides and allopurinol, TTO has been found to be 7–10 days (Rieder, 1994) and 2–6 weeks (Roujeau and Stern, 1994).

5. Drug Fever

TTO is usually 7–10 days (Rieder, 1994). After mumps, measles and rubella (MMR) vaccine TTO is usually 7–10 days with a peak on days 9 and 10 (Roberts *et al.*, 1995).

6. SLE and Other Autoimmune Reactions

TTO is at least two weeks and usually more the one month (Uetrecht, 1992), being less than six months in 35 of 69 patients (*Current Problems*, 32). Malaise, pyrexia and a rash may occur from 5–15 days after immunization with MMR (Calman and Moore, 1994).

7. Other Systems—grouped into Organ Classes

Haematologic

Agranulocytosis Most commonly occurs 1–3 months after starting the drug (Uetrecht, 1992). May occur up to a few days after dechallenge (Heimpel, 1988) as follows:

- Mianserin—TTO has a mean 17 weeks, with a range of 3–164 months. Mean time is almost 14 weeks (Uetrecht, 1992). Mean 13.7 weeks, range 3–164 weeks, but if the two extreme high values are excluded the mean exposure time to diagnosis was 6.3 weeks (Coulter and Edwards, 1990).
- Tricyclic antidepressants—TTO is 4–8 weeks (Albertini and Penders, 1978).
- Nitrogen mustards—TTO is within a few days and lasts for 10–21 days (Uetrecht, 1992).
- Phenylbutazone—TTO is less the one month to seven years.
- Captopril—TTO is typically 1–2 months.
- Clozapine—among those who died average TTO was 58 days, with a range of 16–107 days; median 8 weeks, range 0.5–24 weeks. (*Current Problems*, 32).
- Methimazole—TTO averages 37 days.
- Propylthiouracil—TTO averages 18 days.
- Chlorpromazine—TTO averages 61 days, with a range of 13–318 days. On dechallenge an increase in lymphocytes is seen on the fourth or fifth days and this will recur each time on rechallenge after 20 days or more rather than the usual response with other drugs, which is immediate. (Pisciotta, 1978).
- Phenothiazines—20–40 days usually required (Young and Vincent, 1980).

- Dapsone—TTO is from three weeks to three months.
- Sulfonamides—TTO has a median period of 13 days.
- Procainamide—TTO is usually 1–3 months, but in one case 459 days (Uetrecht, 1992).

After agranulocytosis on dechallenge the granulocytes have been found to increase within a few days (IAAAS, 1991) and in—International Agranulocytosis and Aplastic Anaemia Study 7–14 days (Young and Vincent, 1980). They were normal within two weeks in one study and 50% were normal within 30 days in another study (IAAAS, 1991). Neutropenia recovered in 16 of 16 patients within 14 days and in 14 patients within one week (Weitzman and Stossei, 1978).

Haemolytic Anaemia   With nomifensine TTO is one week to five months (Stonier, 1992).

With autoimmune haemolytic anaemia TTO is at least four months, while for immune complex haemolytic anaemia TTO is days; drug adsorption. TTO is days to a few weeks (Driscoll and Knodel, 1986).

For acute immunoallergic haemolytic anaemia TTO is over 15 days except where an antibody can be shown to be present before 15 days (Habibi *et al.*, 1988).

Thrombocytopenia   In immunological thrombocytopenias it takes at least 5–10 days for the antibodies to any antigen to develop (McVie, 1973) and on dechallenge it often recovers within 1–3 days (Hoigné *et al.*, 1993) and usually within 7–10 days, but can persist for 3–4 weeks (McMillan, 1983). Thrombocytopenia with heparin has been found to occur after 7–11 days (*Current Problems*, 29) and 3–14 days, but usually after one week (Hackett *et al.*, 1982). A survey of 309 cases showed the median time to occurrence was 21 days with a wide range of one day to 11 years; 32% occurred within two weeks and 16% occurred after one year (Pedersen-Bjergaard *et al.*, 1997).

Aplastic Anaemia   With cytotoxic drugs (type A reaction) the TTO is usually 14–212 days (Vincent, 1986). Immunological aplastic anaemia may occur at any time during or after treatment. The induction period is thought not to exceed six months. The average time from the onset of symptoms to diagnosis of the disease is 6.5 weeks (the same is true when it is due to chloramphenicol) (Gordon-Smith, 1979). The interval between the last course of chloramphenicol and the recognition of anaemia was five months or less in seven patients, 8–9 months in two and two years in one patient (Wallerstein *et al.*, 1969).

Hepatic

Cholestatic Injury   This may occur during or after dechallenge. Three weeks after the last drug dose is the longest acceptable interval for a reaction attributed to a drug (Perez *et al.*, 1972). However, cholestatic hepatitis with co-amoxicillin may occur up to six weeks after stopping the drug (*Current Problems*, 32).

General Hypersensitivity   This usually develops within four weeks (Sherlock, 1986) and hypersensitivity within 1–5 weeks.

Metabolic Aberration   This is difficult to prove and is very variable in onset from one week to 12 months or more (Zimmerman, 1990).

Individual drugs are difficult to characterize as to whether they are part of a general hypersensitivity or a metabolic aberration:

- Labetalol—median TTO is 60 days, range 21–189 days (Clark *et al.*, 1990).
- Halothane hepatocellular injury occurs between the second and fifth postoperative days (Rieder, 1994). It is usually a week, but it may be as late as three weeks. (Ranek, 1978).
- Amiodarone—TTO is usually more than one year but can be within one month (Tharakan *et al.*, 1993).
- Paracetamol jaundice (type A reaction) occurs 3–4 days after overdose (Sherlock, 1979).

Pulmonary

Pneumonitis   With nitrofurantoin, TTO is generally within one month (Israel-Biet *et al.*, 1991). For chronic nitrofurantoin lung disease, the duration of therapy is six months to seven years (White and Ward, 1985).

For pneumonitis with amiodarone, the duration of therapy is one month to nine years (White and Ward, 1985). Pulmonary toxicity occurs within the first 30 months, occasionally as early as 2–3 weeks (Banarjee and Honeybourne, 1996).

Pneumonitis due to bleomycin usually occurs within 1–3 months, but can occur after dechallenge (White and Ward, 1985).

Eosinophilic Pneumonitis   This normally starts within one month (White and Ward, 1985) as follows

- Gold—TTO varies from 1–26 months (Israel-Biet *et al.*, 1991) and the duration of therapy 5–16 weeks.
- Sulfasalazine—TTO is several months to even years.
- Methotrexate—may be acute or delayed a few weeks after discontinuation (Israel-Biet *et al.*, 1991), but may occur as early as 12 days or as late as five years.

Asthma   Asthma with ethylenediamine normally occurs within 24–48 hours, but may occur sooner (White and Ward, 1985).

Pulmonary Oedema   With hydrochlorothiazide, TTO is 15–60 minutes after ingestion (White and Ward, 1985).

ACE Cough   TTO is after one day to 12 months (O'Hollaren and Porter, 1990), 59% after one month, average 14.5 months (Olsen, 1995). After dechallenge 50% improvement in less than three days and resolved by ten days (Yecsil *et al.*, 1994). Three days to 12 months (Bowman *et al.*, 1995). Median TTO is 19 days, range 17–20 days; median TT off is 26 days, range 24–36 days (Ramsay and Yeo, 1995). This is probably the most accurate estimate from a controlled trial, but the patients were only included if they developed the cough within six weeks and lost it on dechallenge within four weeks.

Renal

Interstitial Nephritis This usually occurs within 15 days, range 2–44 days (Hoitsma *et al.*, 1991). The time from exposure to onset of symptoms ranged from 4–30 days in nine cases. It may vary from a few days to several months (Pusey *et al.*, 1983) and 5–21 days (Galpin, 1975).

With penicillins and cephalosporins, TTO is at least 7–10 days (Cooper and Bennett, 1987). With NSAIDs, mean TTO is 6.8 months, range two weeks to 19 months (D'Angio, 1987). With Chinese herbs, only after a lag time of about one year (Ronco and Flahault, 1994).

Acute Renal Necrosis With aminoglycosides, renal failure develops 7–10 days after the start of treatment, while with amphotericin B, there is a reduction of glamerular filtration rate (GFR) within two weeks. With radiocontrast media, there is a rise in serum creatinine in the first few days.

Nephrotic Syndrome This occurs as follows:

- Penicillamine—TTO is several months.
- Captopril—proteinuria can occur as early as the first month.
- NSAIDs—TTO is from two weeks to two years.
- Lithium—TTO is several months (Hoitsma *et al.*, 1994).
- Aminoglycosides—TTO is 7–10 days (Cooper and Bennett, 1987).

Benoxaprofen Hepatorenal Syndrome Mean TTO in fatal cases is 8.5 months, SD 1.2 months, range 1–24 months. Mean TTO in non-fatal cases is 6.9 months, SD 1.9 months, range 0.5–15 months (Griffin, 1983).

Cardiac

Arrhythmias With terodiline, TTO is one week to three years, average 13 months (*Current Problems*, 32) (Wild, 1992).

Hypersensitivity Myocarditis TTO is very variable, from days to months (Fenoglio *et al.*, 1980), or from hours to many months (Taliercio *et al.*, 1985).

Gastrointestinal

Pseudomembranous Colitis This may start up to three weeks post dechallenge.

Mucositis
TTO is 7–14 days.

Paralytic Ileus
With cytotoxic drugs, TTO is 3–7 days.

Pancreatitis TTO can occur from a few hours to three months. It resolves after dechallenge from within a few days to three weeks. (*Prescribe*, 1994).

Neurological

Peripheral Neuropathy   With sulfonamides, TTO is usually 1–3 weeks after completion of treatment (Mastaglia and Argov, 1981). With nitrofurantoin, TTO is within 45 days.

Phenothiazine Retinopathy   TTO is usually within days or weeks rather than months (Dickey and Morrow, 1990).

Neuroleptic Malignant Syndrome   TTO usually starts shortly after start of treatment, one case occurred after five hours (Dickey and Morrow, 1990), but can be from hours to months after the start (Caroff, 1980), soon after the first dose or after prolonged treatment (Smego and Durack, 1982). The TTO for neuroleptics is not related to the duration of exposure, but typically develops over a period of 24–72 hours (Guzé and Baxter, 1985).

Optic Neuropathy   With chloramphenicol, TTO is 3–8 months, while with thioridazine, TTO is 1–2 months (Davidson and Rennie, 1986).

Extrapyramidal Reactions   TTO of dystonic reactions is within a few hours to one week, at least 75% within 72 hours.

After depot intramuscular injection they usually start on the second day (Lader, 1970). With paroxetine most cases start within three days (*Current Problems*, 1993).

Of dyskinesias 90% occur within 4.5 days. TTO of Dystonic–dyskinetic reactions with metoclopramide is often within 24 hours, 94% occuring within 72 hours, and all but 1% occuring within 14 days (Bateman *et al.*, 1985).

TTO of akathisia is after one week, but may be delayed (Lader, 1970). Acute akathisia can occur within one hour with droperidol and metoclopramide (*Lancet* leader, 1986). Of cases of akathisia, 90% have been found to occur within 73 days (Ayd, 1961). Resolution on dechallenge is uncertain, most resolving in days or weeks, but some persisting (Ball, 1985).

TTO of parkinsonism is within 72 days in 90% of cases (Ayd, 1961), resolving permanently in 65% of cases in a mean time of seven weeks range 1–36 weeks (Stephen and Williamson, 1984).

TTO of tardive dyskinesia is after 3–4 months, and up to nine years (Crane, 1968). It may occur two months to two years after dechallenge. During long-term treatment (for at least one month in someone aged over 60 years and for at least three months in others) or within a few weeks of withdrawal of a dopamine antagonist (four weeks for oral formulations and eight weeks for depot formulations) (Launer, 1996).

Convulsions   Those following diphtheria, tetanus, pertussis (DTP) vaccine can occur up to 14 days after vaccination. Tricyclic antidepressant-induced seizures usually appear within a few days after starting the drug or changing to a higher dose (Zaccara *et al.*, 1990).

Guillain-Barré Syndrome   When this occurs after swine influenza vaccine it can occur up to at least six weeks and possibly eight weeks later but not longer

(Langmuir *et al.*, 1984). The onset is about 2–3 weeks, with a median of 12 days (Haber *et al.*, 1994).

Ear

Aminoglycoside ototoxicity may occur within the first 3–5 days and is reversible in approximately 50% of cases. Tinnitus may continue for several days to two weeks after dechallenge (Seligman *et al.*, 1996).

TTO of streptomycin ototoxicity is a few weeks to as long as six months. It usually occurs 4–8 days after starting the drug (range 12 hours to 32 days). Resolution usually begins within 24 hours to three days after dechallenge and may be completed in two weeks (range 2–30 days) (Seligman *et al.*, 1996).

TTO of neomycin ototoxicity is after 4–6 weeks (Ballantyne, 1970).

Ototoxicity with diuretics is usually reversible, while that with antineoplastic drugs and aminoglycosides is usually irreversible.

Tinnitus and deafness with NSAIDs clears within 48–72 hours (Huang and Schacht, 1989).

Minocycline vestibulotoxic symptoms (dizziness, vertigo, ataxia and lightheadedness) usually occur within 1–3 days, reversibility occuring within 48–72 hours after dechallenge. Tolerance to tricyclic antidepressant tinnitus is likely to develop within 2–4 weeks (Seligman *et al.*, 1996).

Other

Gynaecomastia has been reported with finasteride after 3 to 13 months (end of monitoring). This may include a delay before reporting (Wilton *et al.*, 1996).

Appendix 3: TAIWAN (Triage Application for Imputologists Without an Interesting Name)

This is a method for triage that has been developed from that used by Dr Jain (see method number 24). It has been improved and computerized by Dr D. Lewis and the staff at SmithKlineBeecham. The answers to each question are given a numerical score. When the answers are confirmed by the operator the total score is divided by the number of questions answered. Each report is assessed according to the following algorithm:

Probable ('A') = 2.
Possible ('B') = 1–1.99.
Unclassified ('O') = 0.99.

Questions

1. Is there a biological explanation for the adverse event (AE) (pathomechanism known)?
   Yes = 2.5, No, but hypothesis = 1.5, No = 1.
2. Is there a temporal relation between the product and the AE?
   Yes, strong = 2.5, Yes, plausible = 1, Weak= 0, No = −2.

3.   Did the AE disappear on dose reduction or dechallenge?
     Resolved = 3, Partially recovered or not specified = 2, Yes, with treatment = 1, No, organic lesion found = −2, No = −1.
4.   Is rechallenge positive?
     Yes = 3, No, but AE treated = 2, Yes (same class) = 2, Yes (same therapeutic area) = 1.5, No = −1.
5.   Is the event previously known and documented?
     Yes, published/labelled = 2.5, Yes, one/two publications = 1.5, Only spontaneous cases = 1, No = −1.
6.   Is the AE known to occur with intercurrent disease?
     Yes = 0, Rarely = 1.5, No = 2.
7.   Is the AE known with concomitant drug with temporal relation?
     Yes = 0, Rarely (< 1 drug) = 1, Rarely (one drug) = 1, No = 2, Interaction, published/labelled = 2.5, Interaction, hypothetical = 1.5.
8.   Does the patient have any relevant medical history?
     Yes, significant = 0, Yes (rarely causes AE) = 1, No = 2.

Contact person: Dr D. Lewis, International Product Safety and Pharmacovigilance, Glaxo Wellcome Research and Development, Greenford Rd, Greenford, Middlesex, UB6 0HE. Tel: 0181 4223434.

Appendix 4: UK Databases for Pharmacoepidemiology

Medicines Monitoring Unit (MEMO) (Dr T. MacDonald, Ms J. M. M. Evans)

MEMO is based within Ninewells Hospital and medical school at the University of Dundee. It is a record linkage system developed for the post-marketing surveillance of drugs in the population of Tayside, Scotland (approximately 400 000 people).

Patients in Tayside are allocated a unique ten-digit patient identifier (the community Health Index Number CHNo.) when they register with a general practitioner (GP). Dispensed prescriptions are obtained by MEMO from the Pharmacy Practice Division and MEMO allocates the CHNo. on the basis of name and address details on the prescription. Information from the prescription is then entered onto the database. MEMO also has access to CHNo.-specific records of hospital admissions with diagnosis and procedure codes, which can be linked to the CHNo.-specific dispensed prescribing database. Many other outcome databases are also available. The original patient records can be accessed to check computerized diagnosis when necessary.

The system has been used to conduct many case–control and cohort studies on drug safety.

Collaborative record linkage studies in the entire population of Scotland (approximately five million) are also being piloted by MEMO.

Suggested further reading is:

MacDonald, T. M. and McDevitt, D. G. (1994). The Tayside Medicines Monitoring Unit (MEMO). In: B. L. Strom (ed). *Pharmacoepidemiology*. 2nd edition. 245–255 (John Wiley & Sons Ltd, Chichester).

Evans J. M. M., McDevitt, D. G. and MacDonald, T. M. (1995). The Tayside Medicines Monitoring Unit (MEMO): A record linkage system for pharmacovigilance. *Pharmaceut. Med.* **9**, 177–184.

Contact person is Dr T. MacDonald, MEMO, Ninewells Hospital and Medical School, Dundee, Scotland, DD1 9SY. Tel: 01382 632575, Fax: 01382 644972, E-mail: Postbox @MEMO.dundee.ac.uk

Prescription Event Monitoring (PEM) (Dr M. D. B. Stephens, Dr R. Mann, Drug Safety Research Unit)

Some of the principles of PEM were first put forward by Dr Inman in 1977 as 'Recorded release' (Inman, 1977) when he was responsible for the management of the National yellow card spontaneous reporting scheme. Later the Committee for the Safety of Medicines (CSM) proposed 'Retrospective Assessment of Drug Safety' (RADS) (CSM, 1977). Sadly the government of the time turned the scheme down because of the cost. Dr Inman then left the CSM in 1980 to set up the Drug Surveillance Research Unit (DSRU) (Inman, 1981; DSRU, 1983, 1984, 1985, 1987). The DSRU is managed by a charitable trust known as the Drug Safety Research Trust.

Method

Prescriptions written by doctors within the National Health Service (NHS) are sent by the pharmacist to the Prescription Pricing Authority (PPA), which is responsible for arranging the payment of pharmacists. At the same time the PPA send prescriptions of all new drugs being monitored by PEM to the DSRU. At a subsequent time (now usually six months) a simple green form questionnaire is sent to the GP who originally wrote the prescription. The questionnaire is in two parts. The top half defines an adverse event (AE) and is detached by the GP to preserve patient anonymity. The bottom half of the questionnaire has space for the following details:

1. Indication for the drug.
2. Patient's date of birth and sex.
3. Date the drug was started.
4. Whether the drug has been stopped and, if so, the date of stopping and the name of any drug substituted.
5. Any events subsequent to the first prescription and their outcome.
6. Any events after stopping the drug, with dates.

The form is returned to the DSRU after detachment of the top half by the GP. The results for one drug can be compared with results from other similar drugs that have been through the system.

Dr Inman gave ten main objectives:

1. To enable estimation of the incidence of AEs.
2. To record all events and not merely those thought to have been drug-induced.
3. To include all users of a drug for at least as long as required to assemble a population capable of revealing comparatively uncommon drug events (e.g. in the range 0.1–1%).
4. To permit long-term follow-up.

5. To have no influence on prescribing (i.e. no inducements).
6. To cause no increase in medicolegal risk.
7. To permit fast communication between researchers, prescribers, regulatory authorities and manufacturers.
8. To be standardized so that groups of patients treated with one drug can be compared with other groups.
9. To be 'doctor-friendly'.
10. To be inexpensive (Inman, 1991).

Several factors prevent a 100% return of forms (apart from the occasional unco-operative doctor) and include patients changing doctor (see page 216) and doctors moving, retiring or dying.

PEM can now monitor all new chemical entities marketed for use in general practice on a national scale, but does not monitor new formulations, new doses, or new routes of administration. All prescriptions are collected from the date of marketing and they are usually followed up six months later or after a pre-determined interval; further follow-up is always possible (Mackay *et al.*, 1997a). All deaths are followed up routinely by inspecting the records of each patient and by examining the death certificate; all pregnancies are followed-up. When necessary hospital records of any patient living or dead in whom an adverse reaction has been suspected are followed up with an 85% success rate.

Advantages

These are:

1. PEM provides independent reports on large cohorts, median size 11 215 patients (e.g salmeterol and finasteride) (Mann *et al.*, 1996; Wilton *et al.*, 1996; Freemantle *et al.*, 1997).
2. PEM allows meaningful comparisons between drugs in the same therapeutic group (e.g. comparison of five antibiotics) (Wilton *et al.*, 1996) and comparison of five selective serotonin reuptake inhibitors (SSRIs) (Mackay *et al.*, 1997b).
3. PEM is the only database that can give incidence densities for AEs from the first 10 000 patients treated (Freemantle *et al.*, 1997).

Disadvantages

These are:

1. Like all 'unrandomized' studies comparison of different drugs of the same class by PEM is biased by the different reasons for their prescription. This phenomenon is known as 'channelling' (Petri and Urquhart, 1991). It can be minimized by adding additional questions to the green form to try to differentiate channelling from other possible biases.
2. PEM may fail to pick up very rare adverse drug reactions since the cohorts are limited to about 20 000.
3. It is difficult to establish events and drug use in the elderly when they have moved into old people's homes and terminal care hospitals.
4. There is a time lag in detecting ADRs to new drugs.

5. There is a presumption that unreturned forms do not differ substantially from those returned. This should not influence comparisons between drugs of the same class, but might do so for the first of an entirely new class of drugs.
6. It depends upon funding by the industry despite recommendations that it should be funded from central government (BMA Scientific Affairs Department, 1996).

The *Drugs and Therapeutic Bulletin* (Herxheimer, 1988) added three more disadvantages:

1. Incompleteness of doctors' records (probably true of all databases relying on GP notes).
2. The lack of control data (drugs of the same class can be used as controls, but the attendant biases must be recognized).
3. Exclusion of prescriptions dispensed in hospitals (Herxheimer, 1988).

Dr Waller has said that it is difficult to adapt PEM to study drugs that have been available for some time (Waller, 1991a).

PEM is best at generating new hypotheses and strengthening hypotheses from other sources. Its unique quality is that it monitors the first 10 000 patients taking a new drug and that it covers all of England.

Suggested further reading is:

- Mann, R.D., Wilton, L.V., Pearce, G.L., MacKay, F.J. and Dunn, N.R. (1997). Prescription Event Monitoring (PEM) in 1996—A method of non-interventional observational cohort pharmacovigilance. *Pharmacoepidemiol Drug Safety*, **6**, Suppl. S5–11.

Contact person is Dr R. Mann, Drug Safety Research Unit, Bursledon Hall, Southampton, SO31 1AA. Tel: (01703) 406122/3; fax: (01703) 406551.

Mediplus

This commercial database covers 567 GPs and 1.8 million patients from 139 practices. Previously it was called the Amalgamated Anthracite Holding (AAH) Meditel Group. The data are collected directly from the GPs computers. The Read code system is used. It is early in its history as a pharmacovigilance database, but hopes to expand soon. It was one of the many databases used to challenge the hypothesis that third generation oral contraceptives (OCs) doubled the rate of thromboembolism in women compared with second generation OCs (Farmer *et al.*, 1997).

Contact person is Dr P. Harrison, Mediplus Information, IMS House, 107, Marsh Road, Pinner, Middlesex, HA5 5HQ. Tel: 0181 723 3400; fax: 0181 969 1272.

General Practice Administration System for Scotland (GPASS)

GPASS covers 1 900 000 patients. It is difficult to find out more about this database.

Contact person is J. Hamlon, GPASS, Seaforth House, Seaforth Road, Hillington, Glasgow. Tel: 0141 882 9996.

General Practice Research Database (GPRD) (Dr F. J. Mackay, Clinical Research fellow, Drug Safety Research Unit and Ms J. Hollowell, Office of National Statistics)

The GPRD was originally set up by the Value Added Medical Products (VAMP) software company in May 1987 (Office for National Statistics, 1996). Practices were offered advantageous terms for purchasing computer equipment in exchange for following an agreed protocol for the recording of clinical data and for transferring anonymized patient-based clinical records on a regular basis to the VAMP research database. The research database was officially transferred to the Department of Health in September 1994 to be managed by the Office for National Statistics (ONS) on their behalf. As of mid 1997 the number of GPRD practices is 450. Around 90 of these have now moved to a new version of VAMP software, VAMP Vision. Data are continuing to be collected from all GPRD practices, but recent data from Vision practices will not be available until next year.

The GPRD covers a total population of around 3.5 million, with more than 30 million patient years of observation and covers over 5% of the population of England and Wales.

Participating practices are encouraged to record all events resulting in the prescription or withdrawal of a drug or other treatment, including the indication for acute treatments, the original indication of every repeated treatment, and the indication for any change in or addition to medication. Similarly, all adverse drug reactions and details of every prescription issued by the practice should be entered. Over 50 studies have been published using data from GPRD including pharmacoepidemiological studies, drug safety studies and analysis of prescribing habits (Office for National Statistics, 1997).

Suggested further reading is *A Major Resource for Drug Safety Studies*, Herschel Jick. Centre for Medicines Research, 1995.

Contact persons are:

Jen Hollowell, Office for National Statistics, GPRD, Room B6/04, 1 Drummond Gate, London, SW1V 2QQ. Tel: 0171 533 5217; fax: 0171 533 5252; gprd@ons.gov.uk for general/other customer enquiries.
Patrick Irwin at the Department of Health (for licence enquiries). Tel: 0171 972 6186.
Dr Alan Dean (for studies in all disciplines including pharmacoeconomics). Tel: 0171 542 5533.

The Doctors' Independent Network Database (Dr R. M. Martin, Clinical Research fellow, Drug Safety Research Unit and N. Richards, Director, CompuFile Ltd, 1 Tannery House, Tannery Lane, Woking, Surrey, GU23 7EF)

The Doctors' Independent Network is a database of 226 computerized general practices who provide anonymized routinely collected data to a central database (Martin, 1995). A panel of 142 general practices (617 doctors) have been identified as providing particularly high quality data. There are a total of over 3.07 million records in the database and 2.03 million patients are currently alive and registered with the panel of selected practices. Most practices (98.6%) have provided data for at least five years.

The GPs who provide data use the AAH Meditel System 5 general practice computer system. They record registration, demographic, prescribing, morbidity and mortality data on their computer system using the Read code clinical coding system. Read codes have been adopted as the standard coding system for the NHS and have a number of advantages which have been detailed elsewhere (Buckland, 1993).

Anonymized and encrypted data are extracted on a daily basis from the practices via a modem and transmitted electronically to the central database in Surrey, UK. Each patient is assigned a number, which forms part of the extracted data. Therefore individual patients can be followed up with the GP's consent. The confidentiality procedures conform to guidelines specified by the Royal College of General Practitioners and the British Medical Association Joint Computing Group (1987).

The panel includes doctors from England, Scotland and Wales. There are fewer single-handed GPs (4%) and slightly more fundholding (64%) and dispensing doctors (20%) when compared with national figures (10%, 53%, and 13%, respectively). The age-sex distribution of the patients is broadly similar to national statistics.

An important advantage of the Meditel computer system is that a specific number links prescription to a diagnosis. Therefore when designing research studies there is no need to create artificially definitions to determine likely drug–diagnosis linkages—a problem reported with other automated databases (Mackay *et al.*, 1997c).

The database has recently realised its potential for scientific research and a number of papers have been published in peer-reviewed journals. These include observational analyses of antidepressant prescribing in general practice (Donoghue and Tylee, 1996; Donoghue *et al.*, 1996), a review of asthma treatment in children (Warner, 1995), and changes in prescribing of the OCs after the UK 'pill-scare' in October 1995 (Martin *et al.*, 1997).

Continued development of the database for the purposes of academic research is being facilitated in a joint venture between the Doctors' Independent Network and the Division of General Practice and Primary Care at St. George's Hospital Medical School, London.

Suggested further reading is Walker, S. R. (ed.) *Databases for Pharmacovigilance* (1996). (Medicines Benefit Risk Foundation), which is available from the Centre for Medicines Research.

Appendix 5: Forms

Medicines Control Agency (MCA) report form for investigational durgs

IN CONFIDENCE

MEDICINES ACTS 1968 AND 1971
REPORT ON SERIOUS UNEXPECTED ADVERSE REACTIONS

1. Report only serious unexpected adverse reactions.
2. Record all other drugs, including self-medication, taken in the previous 3 months. With congenital abnormalities, record all drugs taken during pregnancy.
3. Please do not be deterred from reporting because some details are not known.
4. Has this patient's reaction been reported to us previously [YES/NO].
5. To show the clinical trial approval under which the drug reaction occurred please tick the relevant box and provide identifying number and protocol number.
6. 'Country' refers to the country where the reaction occurred.

APPROVAL	CTX	CTC	CTMP	PROTOCOL NUMBER		COMPANY'S REACTION REPORT NO	COUNTRY
IDENTIFYING NUMBER (CTX, CTX, CTMP, MA, PMS etc)						DATE RECEIVED:	

NAME AND ADDRESS OF COMPANY DOCTOR
or other representatives of marketing authorisation holder.

NAME OF PATIENT'S OWN DOCTOR
(and address if known)

Signed: _____ Date: _____

NAME OF PATIENT (to allow for linkage with other reports for same patient. Please give record number for hospital patients).

NAME OR INITIALS	SEX	AGE or DATE OF BIRTH	WEIGHT (kg)	HEIGHT (cms)

DRUGS, VACCINES (Inc Batch No) DEVICES, MATERIALS etc. (Please give Brand Name if known)	ROUTE	DAILY DOSE	DATE		INDICATION
			STARTED	ENDED	
SUSPECTED DRUG (inc dosage form and strength)					
OTHER DRUGS (Inc non-prescription/OTC medicinal produts; please state if no other drug given).					
SUSPECTED REACTIONS			STARTED	ENDED	OUTCOME (eg. fatal, recovered)
ADDITIONAL NOTES					

Date:

MCA yellow form (for marketed products)

IN CONFIDENCE - REPORT ON SUSPECTED ADVERSE REACTIONS

1. Report reactions and effects as instructed by MAIL 49
2. Record all other drugs, including self-medication taken in the previous 3 months. With congenital abnormalities, record all drugs taken during pregnancy.
3. Please do not be deterred from reporting because some details are not known.
4. Has this patient's reaction been reported to us presiouvly: Previous Adverse Reaction Registration No:
5. Please state the licensing status under which the drug reaction occurred (ring status box and give identifying number):

LICENSING STATUS	CTX	CTC	CTMP	LICENSED/ SPONTANEOUS REPORT	LICENSED/ PMS	COMPANY'S REACTION REPORT NO.
IDENTIFYING NUMBER (CTX, CTC, CTMP, PL, PMS, ETC.)						

NAME AND ADDRESS OF COMPANY DOCTOR or other representative of product license holder.	NAME OF PATIENT'S OWN DOCTOR (and address if known)
Signed: _____ Date: _____	

NAME OF PATIENT (To allow for listings with other reports for same patient. Please give record number for hospital patients).

FAMILY NAME	SEX	AGE or DATE OF BIRTH	WEIGHT (kg)
FORENAMES			

DRUGS, VACCINES (Inc. Batch No.), DEVICES, MATERIALS etc. (Please give Brand Name if known)	ROUTE	DAILY DOSE	DATE STARTED	ENDED	INDICATION
SUSPECTED DRUGS, etc					
Other drugs, etc. (Please state if no other drug given.) NONE					

SUSPECTED REACTIONS	STARTED	ENDED	OUTCOME (eg. fatal, recovered)

ADDITIONAL NOTES

Food and Drug Administration (FDA) 3500A

MED WATCH
THE FDA MEDICAL PRODUCTS REPORTING PROGRAM

Approved by FDA on 3/27

Mfr report #

UF/Dist report #

FDA Use Only

A. Patient information

1. Patient identifier

in confidence

2. Age at time of event:

or_____

Date of birth:

3. Sex

☐ female
or
☐ male

4. Weight

_____ lbs
or
_____ kgs

B. Adverse event or product problem

1. ☐ **Adverse event** and/or ☐ **Product problem** (e.g., defects/malfunctions)

2. Outcomes attributed to adverse event
(check all that apply)

☐ death _____
(mo/day/yr)

☐ life-threatening

☐ hospitalization - initial or prolonged

☐ disability

☐ congenital anomaly

☐ required intervention to prevent permanent impairment/damage

☐ other: _____

3. Date of event
(mo/day/yr)

4. Date of this report
(mo/day/yr)

5. Describe event or problem

6. Relevant tests/laboratory data, including dates

7. Other relevant history, including preexisting medical conditions (e.g., allergies, race, pregnancy, smoking and alcohol use, hepatic/renal dysfunction, etc.)

C. Suspect medications(s)

1. Name (give labeled strength & mfr/labeler, if known)
#1

#2

2. Dose, frequency & route used
#1

#2

3. Therapy date (if unknown, give duration) from/to (or best estimate)
#1

#2

4. Diagnosis for use (indication)
#1

#2

5. Event abated after use stopped or dose reduced
#1 ☐ yes ☐ no ☐ doesn't apply

#2 ☐ yes ☐ no ☐ doesn't apply

6. Lot # (if known)
#1

#2

7. Ex. date (if known)
#1

#2

8. Event reappeared after reintroduction
#1 ☐ yes ☐ no ☐ doesn't apply

#2 ☐ yes ☐ no ☐ doesn't apply

9. NDC # - for product problems only (if known)
#1   #2

10. Concomitant medical products and therapy dates (exclude treatment of event)
NI

G. All manufacturers

1. Contact office - name/address (& mfring site for devices)

2. Phone number

3. Report source
(check all that apply)
☐ foreign
☐ study
☐ literature
☐ consumer
☐ health professional
☐ user facility
☐ company representative
☐ distributor
☐ other:

4. Date received by manufacturer (mo/day/yr)

5.
(A)NDA #_____
IND #_____
PLA #_____

pre-1938 ☐ yes
OTC
product ☐ yes

6. If IND, protocol #

7. Type of report (check all that apply)
☐ 5-day ☐ 15-day
☐ 10-day ☐ periodic
☐ Inital ☐ follow-up #

9. Mfr. report number

8. Adverse event terms(s)

E. Initial reporter

1. Name, address & phone #

2. Health professional?
☐ yes ☐ no

3. Occupation

4. Initial reporter also sent report to FDA
☐ yes ☐ no ☐ unk

FDA

Domain Facsimile of FDA
Form 3500A

Submission of a report does not constitute an admission that medical personnel, user facility, distributor, manufacturer or product caused or contributed to the event

Appendix 6: Guidelines for Company-sponsored Safety Assessment of Marketed Medicines (SAMM)

Introduction

It is well-recognised that there is a continuous need to monitor the safety of medicines as they are used in clinical practice. Spontaneous reporting schemes (e.g. the UK yellow card system) provide important early warning signals of potential drug hazards and also provide a means of continuous surveillance. Formal studies to evaluate safety may also be necessary, particularly in the confirmation and characterisation of possible hazards identified at an earlier stage of drug development. Such studies may also be useful in identifying previously unsuspected reactions.

Scope of Guidelines

These guidelines apply to the conduct of all company-sponsored studies which evaluate the safety of marketed products. They take the place of previous guidelines on post-marketing surveillance which were published in 1988 (BMJ, 296: 399–400). Studies performed under those guidelines were found to have some notable limitations (BMJ, 1992, 304: 1470–1472) and these new guidelines have been prepared in response to the problems identified. The major changes may be summarised as follows:

1. The scope of the guidelines has been expanded to include all company-sponsored studies which are carried out to evaluate safety of marketed medicines. It should be emphasised that this includes both studies conducted in general practice and in the hospital setting. The name of the guidelines has been changed to reflect the emphasis on safety assessment rather than merely surveillance.

2. The guidelines have been developed to provide a framework on which a variety of data collection methods can be used to improve the evaluation of the safety of marketed medicines. Whilst it is recognised that the design used needs to be tailored to particular drugs and hazards, the guidelines define the essential principles which may be applied in a variety of situations. The study methods in this field continue to develop and therefore there will be a need to review regularly these guidelines to ensure that they reflect advances made in the assessment of drug safety.

The guidelines have been formulated and agreed by a Working Party which includes representation from the Medicines Control Agency (MCA), Committee on Safety of Medicines (CSM), Association of the British Pharmaceutical Industry (ABPI), British Medical Association (BMA) and the Royal College of General Practitioners (RCGP). Other guidelines exist for the conduct of 'Phase IV clinical trials' where the medication is provided by the sponsoring company (see section 2(b) below). Some of these studies will also meet the definition of a SAMM study (see below) and should therefore also comply with the present guidelines.

1. Definition of Safety Assessment of Marketed Medicines

(a) Safety assessment of marketed medicines (SAMM) is defined as 'a formal invest-igation conducted for the purpose of assessing the clinical safety of marketed medicine(s) in clinical practice'.

(b) Any study of a marketed drug which has the evaluation of clinical safety as a specific objective should be included. Safety evaluation will be a specific objective in postmarketing studies either when there is a known safety issue under investigation and/or when the numbers of patients to be included will add significantly to the existing safety data for the product(s). Smaller studies conducted primarily for other purposes should not be considered as SAMM studies. However, if a study which is not conducted for the purpose of evaluating safety unexpectedly identifies a hazard, the manufacturer would be expected to inform the MCA immediately and the section of these guidelines covering liaison with regulatory authorities would thereafter apply.

In cases of doubt as to whether or not a study comes under the scope of the guidelines the sponsor should discuss the intended study plan with the MCA.

2. Scope and Objectives of SAMM

(a) SAMM may be conducted for the purpose of identifying previously unrecog-nised safety issues (hypothesis-generation) or to investigate possible hazards (hypothesis-testing).

(b) A variety of designs may be appropriate including observational cohort studies, case-surveillance or case-control studies. Clinical trials may also be used to evaluate the safety of marketed products, involving systematic allocation of treatment (for example randomisation). Such studies must also adhere to the current guidelines for Phase IV clinical trials.

(c) The design to be used will depend on the objectives of the study, which must be clearly defined in the study plan. Any specific safety concerns to be investigated should be identified in the study plan and explicitly addressed by the proposed methods.

3. Design of Studies

Observational Cohort Studies

(a) The population studied should be as representative as possible of the general population of users, and be unselected unless specifically targeted by the objectives of the study (for example a study of the elderly). Exclusion criteria should be limited to the contraindications stated in the data sheet or summary of product characteristics (SPC). The prescriber should be provided with a data sheet or SPC for all products to be used. Where the product is prescribed outside the indications on the data sheet, such patients should be included in the analysis of the study findings.

(b) Observational cohort studies should normally include appropriate comparator group(s). The comparator group(s) will usually include patients with the disease/indication(s) relevant to the primary study drug and such patients will usually be treated with alternative therapies.

(c) The product(s) should be prescribed in the usual manner, for example on an FP10 form written by the general practitioner or through the usual hospital procedures.

(d) Patients must not be prescribed particular medicines in order to include them in observational cohort studies since this is unethical (see section 15 of the 'Guidelines on the Practices of Ethics Committees in Medical Research involving Human Subjects', Royal College of Physicians, 1990).

(e) The prescribing of a drug and the inclusion of the patient in a study are two issues which must be clearly separated. Drugs must be prescribed solely as a result of a normal clinical evaluation, and since such indications may vary from doctor to doctor a justification for the prescription should be recorded in the study documents. In contrast, the inclusion of the patient in the study must be solely dependent upon the criteria for recruitment which have been specifically identified in the study procedures. Any deviation from the study criteria for recruitment could lead to selection bias.

(f) The study plan should stipulate the maximum number of patients to be entered by a single doctor. No patient should be prospectively entered into more than one study simultaneously.

(g) Case-control studies are usually conducted retrospectively. In case-control studies comparison is made between the history of drug exposure of cases with the disease of interest and appropriate controls without the disease. The study design should attempt to account for known sources of bias and confounding.

Case-surveillance

(h) The purpose of case-surveillance is to study patients with diseases which are likely to be drug-related and to ascertain drug exposure. Companies who sponsor such studies should liaise particularly closely with the MCA in order to determine the most appropriate arrangements for the reporting of cases.

Clinical Trials

(i) Large clinical trials are sometimes useful in the investigation of post-marketing safety issues and these may involve random allocation to treatment. In other respects, an attempt should be made to study patients under as normal conditions as possible. Exclusion criteria should be limited to the contraindications in the data sheet or SPC unless they are closely related to the particular objectives of the study. Clinical trials must also adhere to the current guidelines for Phase IV clinical trials (see 2(b) above). Studies which fulfil the definition of SAMM but are performed under a clinical trial exemption (CTX) or under the clinical trial on a marketed product (CTMP) scheme are within the scope of these guidelines.

4. Conduct of Studies

(a) Responsibility for the conduct and quality of company-sponsored studies shall be vested in the company's medical department under the supervision of a named medical practitioner registered in the United Kingdom, and whose name shall be recorded in the study documents.

(b) Where a study is performed for a company by an agent, a named medical practitioner registered in the United Kingdom shall be identified by the agent to supervise the study and liaise with the company's medical department.

(c) Consideration should be given to the appointment of an independent advisory group(s) to monitor the safety information and oversee the study.

5. Liaison with Regulatory Authorities

(a) Companies proposing to perform a SAMM study are encouraged to discuss the draft study plan with the Medicines Control Agency (MCA) at an early state. Particular consideration should be given to specific safety issues which may require investigation.

(b) Before the study commences a study plan should be finalised which explains the aims and objectives of the study, the methods to be used (including statistical analysis) and the record keeping which is to be maintained. The company shall submit the study plan plus any proposed initial communications to doctors to the MCA at least one month before the planned start of the study. The MCA will review the proposed study and may comment. The responsibility for the conduct of the study will, however, rest with the sponsoring pharmaceutical company.

(c) The company should inform the MCA when the study has commenced and will normally provide a brief report on its progress at least every six months, or more frequently if required by MCA.

(d) The regulatory requirements for reporting of suspected adverse reactions must be fulfilled. Companies should endeavour to ensure that they are notified of serious suspected adverse reactions and should report these to the MCA within 15 days of receipt. Events which are not suspected by the investigator to be adverse reactions should not be reported individually as they occur. These and minor adverse reactions should be included in the final report.

(e) A final report on the study should be sent to the MCA within 3 months of follow-up being completed. Ideally this should be a full report but a brief report within 3 months followed by a full report within 6 months of completion of the study would normally be acceptable. The findings of the study should be submitted for publication.

(f) Companies are encouraged to follow MCA guidelines on the content of progress reports and final reports.

6. Promotion of Medicines

(a) SAMM studies should not be conducted for the purposes of promotion.

(b) Company representatives should not be involved in SAMM studies in such a way that it could be seen as a promotional exercise.

7.   Doctor Participation

(a)   Subject to the doctor's terms of service, payment may be offered to the doctor in recompense for his time and any expenses incurred according to the suggested scale of fees published by the BMA.

(b)   No inducement for a doctor to participate in a SAMM study should be offered, requested or given.

8.   Ethical Issues

(a)   The highest possible standards of professional conduct and confidentiality must always be maintained. The patient's right to confidentiality is paramount. The patient's identity in the study documents should be codified and only his or her doctor should be capable of decoding it.

(b)   Responsibility for the retrieval of information from personal medical records lies with the consultant or general practitioner responsible for the patient's care. Such information should be directed to the medical practitioner nominated by the company or agent, who is thereafter responsible for the handling of such information.

(c)   Reference to a Research Ethics Committee is required if patients are to be approached for information, additional investigations are to be performed or if it is proposed to allocate patients systematically to treatments.

9.   Procedure for Complaints

A study which gives cause for concern on scientific, ethical or promotional grounds should be referred to the MCA, ABPI and the company concerned. Concerns regarding possible scientific fraud should be referred to the ABPI. They will be investigated and, if appropriate, referred to the General Medical Council.

10.   Review of Guidelines

The Working Party will review these guidelines as necessary.

Association of the British Pharmaceutical Industry (ABPI)
British Medical Association (BMA)
Committee on Safety of Medicines (CSM)
Medicines Control Agency (MCA)
Royal College of General Practitioners (RCGP)

References

Abadie, E. and Souetre, E. (1993). Aspects économiques de la pharmacovigilance dans l'industrie pharmaceutique. *Thérapie*, **48**, 125–127.

ABPI (1977). Guidelines for preclinical and clinical testing of new medicinal products. Part 2: Investigations in man. *Ass. Br. Pharm. Ind.*, 13.

Abraham, J. (1996). In *Science, Politics and the Pharmaceutical Industry. A controversy and bias in drug regulation.* UCL Press, London.

Abraham, J. W. (1997). Secrecy and drug regulation in Europe: who is being protected? *Int J. Risk Safety Med.*, **10**, 143–146.

Abstract 1063 (1988). *J. Clin. Epidemiol.*, **41**, 35–45.

Abt, K. (1987). Descriptive data analysis: A concept between confirmatory and exploratory data analysis. *Methods Inf. Med.*, **26**, 77–88.

Abt, K. (1990). Statistical aspects of neurophysiologic topography. *J. Clin. Neurophysiol.*, **7**, 519–534.

Abt, K. and Krupp, P. (1986). Pooling of laboratory safety data in multicenter studies. *Drug Inf. J.*, **20**, 311–313.

Abt, K., Cockburn, I. T. R., Guelich, A. and Krupp, P. (1989). Evaluation of adverse drug reactions by means of the life table method. *Drug Inf. J.*, **23**, 143–149.

Adams, A. K. (1996). Use of placebo in studies of postoperative vomiting is unethical. *Br. Med. J.*, **313**, 233.

Adie, E. and Souetre, E. (1993). Aspects économiques de la pharmacovigilance dans l'industrie pharmaceutique. *Thérapie*, **48**, 125–127.

Ahmed, S. R. (1993). FDA and olsalazine. *Lancet*, **342**, 487.

Ahmed, S. R. and Wolfe, S. M. (1995). Lesson from a drug indication withdrawal. *Pharmacoepidemiol. Drug Safety*, **4**, S78.

Aitken, R. C. B. (1969). Measurement of feelings using analogue scales. *Proc. R. Soc. Med.*, **62**, 989–993.

Akesson, A., Berglund, K. and Karlsson, M. (1980). Liver function in some common rheumatic disorders. *Scand. J. Rheumatol.*, **9**, 81–88.

Albengres, E., Gauthier, F. and Tillement, J. P. (1990). Current French system of post-marketing drug surveillance. *Int. J. Clin. Pharmacol. Therap. Toxicol.*, **27**(7), 312–314.

Albertini, R. S. and Penders, T. M. (1978). Agranulocytosis associated with tricyclics. *J. Clin. Psych.*, **39**, 483–485.

Albin, H., Bégaud, B., Boisseau, A. and Dangoumau, J. (1980). Validation des publications d'effets indésirables par une methode d'imputatilité. *Thérapie*, **35**(5), 571–576.

Alexander, W. J. (1991). Adverse events: A classification system for use in clinical trials. *Drug Inf. J.*, **25**, 457–459.

Allport, S. (1994). Resource planning – where do we go from here? Presented at the 5th Drug Information Association European Workshop in statistical methodology in clinical research and development. Edinburgh.

Alvarez-Requejo, A., Carvaajal, A., Vega, T. L. and Bégaud, B. (1994). Under-reporting of adverse drug reactions in a Spanish regional centre of pharmacovigilance. *Drug Safety*. Abstr. 249, Suppl. 1, S104.

An experiment in early PMS of new drugs: Prepared for the FDA, 24 Oct 1978. 214–231 (IMS America Ltd, Ambler, PA.).

Anand, R. K. (1996). Health workers and the baby food industry. *Br. Med. J.*, **312**, 1556–1557.

Anderson, M. D. (1990). Comprehensive criteria (MDA), National Cancer Institute common toxicity criteria (CTC). *Proc. Ann. Meet. Am. Clin. Oncol.*, **9**, A340.

Andersson, O. (1979). Registration of side-effects by means of a questionnaire. *Acta. Med. Scand. Suppl.*, **628**, 29–32.

Andrew, M., Beerman, B., Klauka, T., Mørkøre, H., Nissen, A., Peura, S., Sakshaug, S. and Sigfússon, E. (1996). ADR warning has decreased the use of third-generation oral contraceptives in the Nordic countries. Abstr 305. 12th International Conference on Pharmacoepidemiology 1996.

Andrews, G. R., Caird, F. I. and Leask, R. G. S. (1975). *Age and Ageing*, **2**, 14.

Anello, C. (1983). The use, design and limitations of selected Phase IV studies in the USA. *Droit et Pharmacie Essais Cliniques Postmarketing*. Editions de Santé.

Anello, C. (1986). *Scrip*, **1146**, 16.

Anello, C. (1988). PMS legislation. Structure and results. *Pharm. Med.*, **879**(2), 11–22.

Anello, C. (1991a). FDA's revised extramural research program. *Clinical Kinetics in Focus. Drug Information Association Meeting June 18th*.

Anello, C. (1991b). ADR monitoring across Europe. Management Forum meeting.

Anon. (1975). Rauwolfia and breast cancer. *Lancet*, **2**, 312.

Anon. (1976). Thalidomide's long shadow. *Br. Med. J.*, **2**, 1155.

Anon. (1981a). Hunting rare adverse drug reactions. *Br. Med. J.*, **282**(6261), 342.

Anon. (1981b). Pertussis vaccine. *Br. Med. J.*, **282**, 1563.

Anon. (1982a). Lessons from the benoxaprofen affair. *Lancet*, 529.

Anon. (1982b). Crying wolf on drug safety. *Br. Med. J.*, **284**, 219.

Anon. (1983a). How the yellow card system might be improved? *Pharm. J.*, **231**, 160.

Anon. (1983b). Manufacturer sponsored symposia. *Drug Ther. Bull.*, **21**(6), 24.

Anon. (1992). PL/CHO (92), Department of Health, London.

Anon. (1995). Good practices in pharmacovigilance. Drugs for human use. *Thérapie*, **50**(6), 547–555.

Ansell, P., Bull, D. and Roman, E. (1996). Childhood leukaemia and intramuscular vitamin K: findings from a case–control study. *Br. Med. J.*, **313**, 204–205.

Applegate, W. B., Furberg, C. D. and Grimm, R. (1997). The multicenter Isradipine diuretic atherosclerosis study (MIDAS). *JAMA*, **277**, 297.

Appolone, G. *et al.* (1997) Il progetto IQOLA. In: *Questionario Sullo Stato Di Salute SF 36, Manuale D'uso e Guida Alla Interpretazione Dei Risultati*. (Ed. Guerrini and Associati, Milano, Italy). p. 142.

Appolone, G. and Mosconi, P. The Italian SF 36 Health Survey: translation, validation and norming. *J. Clin. Epidemiol*. (in press).

Arneborn, P. and Palmbled, J. (1982). Drug-induced neutropenia a survey for Stockholm 1973–1978. *Acta. Med. Scand.*, **212**, 289–292.

Arnold, B. (1997), Global ADR reporting requirements. *Scrip*, PJB Publications Report August.

Aronson, J. K. and White, N. J. (1996). Principles of clinical pharmacology and drug therapy. In: *Oxford Textbook of Medicine*, 3rd edition. On compact disc. (Oxford University Press, Oxford).

Ashton, C. H. (1981). Disorders of the foetus and infant. In: Davies, D. M. (ed.) *Textbook of Adverse Drug Reactions*. 71–117 (Oxford Medical, Oxford University Press, Oxford).

Ashton, C. H. (1984). Benzodiazepine withdrawal an unfinished story. *Br. Med. J.*, **288**, 1135–1140.

Ashton, H. (1991). Adverse effects of nicotine. *ADR Bulletin*, **149**,.

Assenzo, J. R. and Sho, V. S. (1982). Use of statistics in the analysis of side-effect data from clinical trials of psychoactive agents *Prog. Neuropsychopharmacol. Biol. Psychiat.*, **6**, 543–550.

Association of Anaesthetists of Great Britain and Ireland and the British Society of Allergy and Clinical Immunology. (1995). *Suspected Anaphylactic Reactions Associated with Anaesthesia*. Revised edition 2.

Atkin, P. A. and Shenfield, G. M. (1995). Medication related adverse reactions and the elderly: a literature review. *Adv. Drug React. Toxicol. Rev.*, **14**(3), 175–191.

Atkins, M. J. (1995). Who discovered inhalation anaesthesia? *Pharmaceutical Medicine*, **9**, 33–43.

Auriche, M. (1985). Approche bayésienne de l'imputabilitées phénomènes indésirables aux médicaments. *Thérapie*, **40**, 301–306.

Austrian, M. L. (1996). Informed consent and women of childbearing age in investigational studies: a lawyer's perspective. *Drug Inf. J.*, **30**, 365–370.

Avery, C. W., Bertram, P. L., Allison, B. and Mandell, N. (1967). Systematic errors in the evaluation of side effects. *Am. J. Psychiat.*, **123**, 875–878.

Avorn, J. (1997). Including elderly patients in clinical trials. *Br. Med. J.*, **315**, 1033–1034.

Avorn, J., Everitt, D. E., Bright, R. A., Gurnitz, J. and Chown, H. (1989). AIDS related diagnoses and drug use among AZT users in New Jersey Medicare. *J. Clin. Res. Drug Dev.*, (Abstract) **3**, 201–229.

Ayd, F. J. (1961). A survey of drug-induced extrapyramidal reactions. *JAMA*, 1054–1061. Vol. 175.

Azarnoff, D. L. (1972). Physiologic factors in selecting human volunteers for drug studies. *Clin. Pharmacol. Ther.*, **13**(5) Pt 2, 796–802.

Azarnoff, D. L., Abrams, W. B., Cuttner, J., Hewitt, W. L. and Hallman, H. (1975). Phase III investigations. *Clin. Pharmacol. Ther.*, **18**(5) Pt 2, 650–652.

Baber, N. S. (1994). Volunteer studies: are current regulations adequate? The ethical dilemma. *Pharm. Med.*, **8**, 153–159.

Bader, J.-P. (1981). *Scrip, no.* 639, 1.

Bakke, O. M., Manocchia, M., Abajo, F. de, Kaitin, K. I. and Lasagna, L. (1995). Drug safety discontinuations in the United States and Spain from 1974 through 1993: a regulatory perspective. *Clin. Pharmacol. Ther.*, **58**, 108–117.

Bakke, O. M., Wardell, W. M. and Lasagna, L. (1984). Drug discontinuations in the United Kingdom and the United States, 1986 to 1983: issues of safety. *Clin. Pharmacol. Ther.*, **35**(3), 559–567.

Ball, C. J., McLaren, P. M. and Morrison, P. J. (1993). The personality structure of 'normal' volunteers. *Br. J. Clin. Pharmacol.*, **36**, 369–371.

Ball, R. (1985). Drug induced akathisia; a review. *J. Roy. Soc. Med.*, **78**, 748–752.

Ballantyne, J. (1970). Iatrogenic deafness. *J. Laryngol. Otol.*, 967–1000.

Banerjee, D. J. and Honeybourne, D. (1996). Drug-induced pulmonary alveolar disease. *Adverse Drug React. Bull.*, **181**, 687–690.

Bardham, K. D. (1987). Unfavourable results and drug company trials. *Lancet.*

Barnett, A. A. (1996a). Upjohn and FDA criticised over Halcion. *Lancet*, **347**, 1616.

Barnett, A. A. (1996b). FDA warns Pfizer on sertraline marketing. *Lancet*, **348**, 469.

Barrington, P., Bowden, M. W. and Dewland, P. M. (1990). Arrhythmias in the normal heart. *7th International Conference on Pharmaceutical Medicine.* Abstract 24–5 108.

Bartlett, A., Costa, A., Estruch, J., Sánchez, J. and PUIG, A. (1990). Basis for the recruitment of healthy volunteers in phase 1 studies. *7th International Conference on Pharmaceutical Medicine.* Abstract 12–14.

Barton, B. (1989). D. I. A. conference. *Scrip*, **1472**, 20.

Barton, F., Moore, R., Terrin, M., Charache, S. and Koshy, M. *et al.* (1996). Treatment guesses by patients and investigators in a double-blind clinical trial. *Control. Clin. Trials.*, Abstract A05, 17, 25th April.

Bashaw, E. D. (1992). Application of clinical pharmacological tools to facilitate clinical drug development. *DIA Conference, Methods and Examples for Assessing Benefit/Risk and Safety for New Drug Application*, July 20–21.

Bass, R. (1987). Risk-benefit decisions in product licence applications. In: Walker, S. R. and Asscher, A. W. (eds), *Medicines and Risk/benefit Decisions.* 127–135. (MTP Press Ltd).

Batchelor, J. R., Welsh, K. L., Mansilla, Tonoco, R., Dollery, C. T., Hughes, G. R. V., Bernstein, D., Ryan, P., Naish, P. F., Aber, G. M., Bing, R. F. and Russell, G. I. (1980). Hydralazine induced S. L. E. and influence of H. L. A.-D. R. and sex on susceptibility. *Lancet*, **1**, 1107–1108.

Bateman, D. N. and Elhatton, P. (1997). National system for monitoring all drug use in pregnancy already exists. *BMJ*, **314**, 1414-1415.

Bateman, D. N., Lee, A., Rawlins, M. D. and Smith, J. M. (1991). Geographical differences in adverse drug reaction reporting rates in the northern region. *Br. J. Clin. Pharmacol.*, 188–189.

Bateman, D. N., Rawlins, M. D. and Simpson, J. M. (1985). Extrapyramidal reactions with metoclopramide. *Br. Med. J.*, **291**, 930–932.

Bates, D. W. (1996). Medication errors. *Drug Safety*, **15**(5), 303–310.

Bates, D. W., Cullen, D. J., Laird, N., Petersen, L. A., Small, S. D., Servi, D., Laffel, G., Sweitzer, B. J., Shea, B. F., Hallisey, R., Vander Vliet, M., Nemeskal, R. and Leape, L. L. (1995). Incidence of adverse drug events and potential adverse drug events. *JAMA*, **274**, 29–34.

Bates, D. W., Spell, N., Cullen, D. J., Burdick, E., Laird, N., Peterson, L. A., Small, S. D., Sweitzer, B. J. and Leape, L. L. (1997). The cost of adverse drug events in hospitalised patients. *JAMA*, **277**, 307–311.

Baum, C., Faich, G. A. and Anello, C. (1987). Differences in manufacturers reporting of ADR to the FDA in 1984. *Drug Inf. J.*, **21**, 257.

Baum, C., Anello, C., Faich, G. A., Dreis, M. and Tomita, D. (1988). National ADR surveillance. *Arch. Intern. Med.*, **148**, 785.

Beard, K. (1991). Special considerations in the assessment of adverse drug reactions in the elderly. *Pharm. Med.*, **5**, 37–48.

Beardon, P. H. G., McGilchrist, M. M., McKendrick, A. D., McDevitt, D. G. and MacDonald, T. M. (1993). Primary non-compliance with prescribed medication in primary care. *Br. Med. J.*, **307**, 846–848.

Bechtel, P. R. (1995). Relevance and limits of pharmacogenetics to detect patients at risk of adverse drug reactions. *Pharmacoepidemiol. Drug Safety*, **4**, 31–36.

Beck, A.T., Ward, C.H., Mendelson, M., Mock, J. and Erbaugh, J. (1961). An inventory for measuring depression. *Arch. Gen. Psychiat.*, **4**, 561–571.

Beecher, N. H. (1955). The powerful placebo. *JAMA*, **159**, 1602–1606.

Beeley, L., Elliott, D. and Griffiths, K. (1986). Patterns in spontaneous reports sent to a regional ADR reporting centre. Abstract 423. *Acta. Pharm. Toxicol.*, Suppl. V. 159.

Bégaud, B. (1984). Standardized assessment of adverse drug reactions: The method used in France Special Workshop–Clinical. *Drug Inf. J.*, **18**, 275–281.

Bégaud, B. (1993). Pharmacovigilance. In '*Methodological approaches in pharmaco-epidemiology*'. Ed. ARME-P, Bordeaux, Pub. Elsevier.

Bégaud, B., Péré, J.-C. and Dangoumau, J. (1981). Mise en oeuvre d'un critère, la bibliographie. *Thérapie*, **36**, 233–236.

Bégaud, B., Chaslerie, A. and Haramburu, F. (1994). [Organization and results of drug vigilance in France]. *Rev. Epidemiol. Santé Publique*, **42**(5), 416–423.

Bégaud, B., Doermann, F., Fourrier, A. and Haramburu, F. (1996). Is age a risk factor for adverse drug reactions? *Pharmacoepidemiol. Drug Safety*, **5**, S84.

Bégaud, B., Haramburu, F., Moride, Y., Tubert-Bitter, P., Alvarez-Requejo, A., Carvajal, A., Vega, T. and Chaslerie, A. (1994). Assessment of reporting and under reporting in pharmacovigilance. In: Fracchia, G. N. (ed.) *European Medicines Research. Perspectives in Pharmacotoxicology and Pharmacovigilance*. 276–283. IOS Press.

Bégaud, B., Tubert-Bitter, P., Chaslerie, A. and Haramburu, F. (1995). Signal generation in pharmacoepidemiology: a new rule of three. Abstract 148. *Pharmacoepidemiol. Drug Safety*, **4**, S67.

Begg, N and Miller, E. (1990). Role of epidemiology in vaccine policy. *Vaccine*, **8**, 180–189.

Bell, T. (1993). Bromocriptine and drug information. *Lancet*, **342**, 1118.

Belton, K. and the European pharmacovigilance research group. (1997). Attitude survey of adverse drug-reaction reporting by health care professionals across the European union. *Eur. J. Clin. Pharmacol.*, **52**, 423–427.

Bénichou, C. (1990). Criteria of drug-induced liver disorders. Report of an international consensus meeting. *J. Hepatol.*, **11**(2), 272–276.

Bénichou, C. (ed.) (1994) *Adverse Drug Reactions, A Practical Guide to Diagnosis and Management.* (John Wiley and Sons).

Bénichou, C. and Danan, G. (1989). Lack of definitions of adverse drug reaction. *Drug Inf. J.*, **23**, 71–74.

Bénichou, C. and Danan, G. (1991). Guidelines for the management of adverse events occurring during clinical trials. *Drug Inf. J.*, **25**, 565–571.

Bénichou, C., Danan, G. and Solal-Celigny, P. (1991). Standardisation of International databases: definitions of drug-induced blood cytopenias. *Int. J. Clin. Pharmacol. Toxicol.*, **29**, 75–81.

Bénichou, C. and Solal-Celigny, P. (1991). Standardization of definitions and criteria of causality assessment of adverse drug reactions. Drug-induced cytopenia. *Int. J. Clin. Pharmacol. Ther. Toxicol.*, **29**(2), 75–81.

Bénichou, C. and Solal-Celigny, P. (1991). Standardisation of definitions and criteria for causality assessment of adverse drug reactions. Drug-induced blood cytopenias: report of an international consensus meeting. *Nouv. Rev. Hematol.*, **33**, 257–262.

Bénichou, C., Danan, G and Flahault, A. (1993). Causality assessment of adverse reactions to drugs—II. An original model for validation of drug causality assessment methods: Case reports with positive rechallenge. *J. Clin. Epidemiol.*, **46**(11), 1331–1336.

Bénichou, C., Danan, G. and Vigeral, Ph. (1988). Conduites à tenir devant l'apparition d'anomalies cliniques ou biologiques au course d'un essai thérapeutique. *Thérapie.*, **43**, 465–468.

Bénichou, C., Eliaszewicz, M. and Flahault, A. (1994). Adverse drug reactions in HIV positive patients. *Pharmacoepidemiol. Drug Safety*, **3**, 31–40.

Bénichou, C., Eliaszewicz, M. and Flahaut, A. (1995). Adverse drug reactions in HIV-seropositive patients. In: *A Practical Guide to Diagnosis and Management*. Ed. C. Benichou, Chichester, Wiley.

Benjafield, J. and Adams-Webber, J. (1976). The golden section hypothesis. *Br. J. Psychol.*, **67**, 11–17.

Bennett, B. S. and Lipman, A. G. (1977). Comparative study of prospective surveillance and voluntary reporting in determining the incidence of adverse drug reactions. *Am. J. Hosp. Pharm.*, **34**, 931–936.

Bennett, P. (1995). Ethical review of multi-location clinical trials and the work of the European Ethical Review Committee. *Pharm. Med.*, **9**, 123–127.

Bennett, P. (1997). Transnational ethical review and education. *Int. J. Pharmaceut. Med.*, **11**, 213–216.

Beral, V. (1977). Mortality among oral contraceptive users. Royal College of General Practitioners' Oral Contraception Study. *Lancet*, **2**, 727–731.

Bernheim, J. L. (1994). The clinical activity biases on the estimation of attributable drug side-effects. In: Fracchia, G. N. (ed.) *European Medicines Research, Perspectives in Pharmacotoxicology and Pharmacovigilance*. 310–321. IOS Press.

Berto, D., Milleri, S., Squassante, L. and Baroldi, P. A. (1996). Evaluation of personality as a component of the healthy condition of volunteers participating in Phase I studies. *Eur. J. Clin. Pharmacol.*, **51**, 209–213.

Bethge, H., Czechanowski, B., Gundert-remy, U., Hasford, J., Kleinsorge, H., Kreutz, G., Letzel, H., Müller, A. A., Selbmann, H. K. and Weber, E. (1991). Recommendations for the detection, recording, collection and evaluation of adverse events in the clinical investigations of drugs. *Drugs in Germany*, **34**, 10–15.

Bhowmick, B. K. (1991). Hazards of abrupt drug withdrawal. *Geriatr. Med.*, **21**, 6–9.

Bianchi-Bosisio, A., D'agrosa, F., Gaborardi, F., Gianazza, E. and Righetti, P. G. (1991). Sodium dodecyl sulphate electrophoresis of urinary proteins. *J. Chromatogr., Biomed. Appl.*, **569**, 243–260.

Bignall, J. (1994). *Lancet*, **344**, 536.

Biour, M., Wagniart, F., Jablonka, J., Hamel, J. D., Weissenburger, J. and Cheymel, G. (1986). Interêts de la micro-informatique dans la recherche des doublons. *Thérapie*, **41**, 383–384.

Bird, H. A., Legalley, P. and Hill, J. (1985). In: *Combined Care of the Rheumatic Patient*. (Springer-Verlag, Berlin).

Biriell, C. (1988). The WHO project for intensified signal review. In: *ADR—A Global Perspective on Signal Generation and Analysis. Proceedings of WHO Anniversary Symposium*, 57–58.

Birley, J. L. T. (1989). Drug advertisements in developing countries. *Lancet*, 220.

Bixler, E. O., Kales, A., Manfredi, R. L., Vgontzas, A. N., Tyson, K. L. and Kales, J. D. (1991). Next-day memory impairment with triazolam use. *Lancet*, **337**, 827–831.

Blanc, S., Leuenberger, P., Berger, J. P., Brooke, E. M. and Schelling, J. L. (1979). Judgements of trained observers on adverse drug reactions. *Clin. Pharmacol. Ther.*, **25**(5), 493–498.

BMA Scientific Affairs Department (1996). *Reporting Adverse Drug Reactions.* (British Medical Association, London).

BMJ Leader. (1880). pp. 2984.

Boisseau, A., Bégaud, B., Albin, H. and Dangoumau, J. (1980). Evaluation d'un diagnostic d'effets indesirables des médicaments avec un recul de six mois. *Thérapie*, **35**, 577–580.

Bolton, D. P. G. and Cross, K. W. (1974). Further observations on cost of preventing retrolental fibroplasia. *Lancet*, **1**, 445–458.

Boman, G. (1986). The nordic countries. In: W. H. W. Inman (ed.) *Monitoring for Drug Safety.* MTP Press.

Boman, G. Lundgren, P. and Stjernström, G. (1975). Mechanism of the inhibiting effect of P. A. S. granules on the absortion of rifampacin by an excipient, bentonite, *Eur. J. Clin. Pharmacol.*, **8**, 293–299.

Bond, A. and Lader, M. (1974). The use of analogue scales in rating subjective feelings. *Br. J. Med. Psychol.*, **47**, 211–218.

Borden, E. K., Gardner, J. S., Westland, M. and Gardner, S. D. (1984) Post-marketing surveillance. *JAMA*, **251**(6), 729.

Borghi, C. and Canti, D. (1986). Il concetto storico di farmaco e di terapia. In: *Tollerabilita di un Farmaco, Valutazione Clinica.* 3–23 (Organizzazione Editoriale Medico Farmaceutica S.r.l., Milan).

Borghi, C., Pallavivi, G., Comi, D., Lombardo, M., Mantero, O., Minetti, L., Selvini, A. and Suppa, G. (1984). Comparison of three different methods of monitoring unwanted effects during antihypertensive therapy. *Int. J. Clin. Pharmacol. Ther. Tox.*, **22**(6), 324–328.

Bortnichak, E. A. (1990). Pharmacoepidemiological training opportunities. In: *Improving Drug Safety. The Assessment, Management and Communication of the Therapeutic Benefits and Risks of Pharmaceutical Products, October 1989.* (Pharma. International).

Bottiger, L. E. and Westerholm, B. (1973). Drug-induced blood dyscrasias in Sweden. *Br. Med. J.*, **3**, 339–343.

Bottiger, M., Romanus, V., Deverdier, C. and Boman, G., (1982). Osteitis and other complications caused by generalised BCGitis. Experiences in Sweden. *Acta. Paediatr. Scand.*, **71**, 471–478.

Bowman, L., Carlstedt, B. C., Miller, M. E. and Mcdonald, C. J. (1995). Evaluation of ACE-inhibitor (ACE-1) associated cough using modified prescription sequence analysis (PSA). *Pharmacoepidemiol. Drug Safety*, **4**, 17–22.

Bowman, L., Carlstedt, B. C., Hancock, E. F. and Black, C. D. (1996). Adverse drug reactions (ADR) occurrence and evaluation in elderly inpatients. *Pharmacoepidemiol. Drug Safety*, **5**, 9–18.

Br. Med. J., (1958) H. P. 'Stalinon': a therapeutic disaster. *Br. Med. J.*, **1**, 515.

Bracchi, R. (1996). Drug companies should report side effects in terms of frequency. *Br. Med. J.*, **312**, 442.

Bradford Hill, A. (1965). The environment and disease: association or causation. *Proc. Roy. Soc. Med.*, **58**, 295–300.

Bradley, C. P. (1992). Factors which influence the decision whether or not to prescribe: the dilemma facing general practitioners. *Br. J. Gen. Pract.*, **42**, 454–458.

Brass, E. P. and Thompson, W. L. (1982). Drug-induced electrolyte abnormalities. *Drugs*, **24**, 207–220.

Breathnach, S. M. (1993). Drug eruptions. *Hospital Update*, June, 344–351.

Breathnach, S. M. (1995). Management of drug eruptions: Part II. Diagnosis and treatment. *Australas. J. Dermatol.*, **36**, 187–91.

Brenner, N., Frank, O. S. and Knight, E. (1993). Chronic nutmeg psychosis. *J. Roy. Soc. Med.*, **86**, 179–180.

British Medical Journal Leader. (1985). *Br. Med. J.*, **290**, 1369–1370.

British Medical Journal Leader. Benoxaprofen. *Br. Med. J.*, **285**(6340), 459–450.

British Medical Journal Leader. (1996). Secrets about drugs are not healthy. *Br. Med. J.*, **348**, 765.

Brooks, R. (1983). Health indicators in arthritis. In: Teeling-Smith G. (ed.) *Measuring the Social Benefits of Medicine* 84–91 (Office of Health Economics, London).

Brown, J. S., Kaitin, K. I., McAuslane, N., Thomas, K. E. and Walker, S. R. (1996). Population exposure required to assess clinical safety: report to the international conference on harmonization working group. *Drug Inf. J.*, **30**, 17–27.

Brown, K. R., Getson, A. J., Gould, A. L., Martin, C. M. and Ricci, F. M. (1979). Safety of cefoxitin: An approach to the analysis of laboratory data. *Rev. Infect. Dis.*, **1**, 228–231.

Brown, W. J., Buist, N. R., Gipson, H. T., Huston, R. K. and Kennaway, N. G. (1982). Fatal benzyl alchol poisoning in a neonatal intensive care unit. Lancet, **1**, 1250.

Bruinsma, W. (1996). *A Guide to Drug Eruptions*, 6th edition. (De Zwaluw, P. O. Box 21, Oosthuisen, The Netherlands).

Buckland, R.(1993). The language of health. *Br. Med. J.*, **306**, 287–288.

Buist, A. S., Burney, P. G. J. and Feinstein, A. R. (1989). Fenoterol and fatal asthma. *Lancet*, **1**, 1071.

Bulpitt, C. J. (1983). *Randomised Controlled Clinical Trials*. (Martinus Nijhoff, The Hague).

Bulpitt, C. J. and Fletcher, A. E. (1990). The measurement of quality of life in hypertensive patients, a practical approach. *Br. J. Clin. Pharmacol.*, **30**, 353–364.

Bulpitt, C. J., Dollery, C. T., and Carne, S. (1974). A symptom questionnaire for hypertensive patients. *J. Chron. Dis.*, **27**, 309–323.

Bulpitt, C. J., Dollery, C. T. and Carne, S. (1976) Change in symptoms of hypertensive patients after referral to hospital clinics. *Br. Hosp. J.*, **38**, 121–128.

Burley, D. M. (1988). The rise and fall of thalidiomide. *Pharm. Med.*, **3**, 231–237.

Burley, D. M. and Binns, T. B. (1976). Erroneous adverse reaction reports. *Lancet*, 1193.

Burns-Cox, C. J. (1970). Negative Coombs in Chinese on methyl-dopa. *Lancet, 2, 673.*

Busto, U., Sellers, E. M., Naranjo, C. A., Cappell, H., Sanchez-Craig, M. and Sykora, K. (1986). Withdrawal reaction after long-term therapeutic use of benzodiazepines. *N. Engl. J. Med.,* **315,** 854–859.

Bystritsky, A. and Waikar, S. V. (1994). Inert placebo versus active medication. *J. Nerv. Ment. Dis.,* **182**(9), 485–487.

Byyny, R. L. (1976). Withdrawal from glucocorticoid therapy. *N. Engl. J. Med.,* **295,** 30–32.

Cahal, D. A. (1965). Adverse reactions to nalidixic acid. *Lancet,* **i,** 441.

Caird, F. I. (1973). Problems of interpretation of laboratory findings in the old *Br. Med. J.,* **4,** 348–351.

Calman, K. (1996a). On the state of public health. *Health Trends,* **28,** 3, 79–88.

Calman, K. (1996b). UK medical chief calls for risk debate. *Scrip,* **5,** 2169.

Calman, K. (1996c). Risks of new drugs and procedures should be rated. *Reactions,* **625,** 3.

Calman, K. C. and Moores, Y. (1994). Measles and rubella immunisation campaign. PL.CMO (94) 12, PL.CMO (94) 15. Department of Health Store, Health Publication Unit P5.

Calman, K. C. and Royston, G. H. D. (1997). Risk language and dialects. *Br. Med. J.,* **315,** 939–942.

Cambell, C. M. A. (1997). Baby milk companies accused of breaching code. *Br. Med. J.,* **314,** 830.

Cameron, H. M. and McGregor, E. (1981). Prospective study of 1152 hospital autopsies, 1: Inaccuracies in death certification. *J. Pathol.,* **133,** 273–283.

Cancer Research Campaign Working Party. (1980). Trials and tribulations: thoughts on the organisation of multicentre clinical studies. *Br. Med. J.,* **281,** 918–920.

Cardon, P. V., Dommel, F. W. and Trumble, R. R. (1976). Injuries to research subjects a survey of investigators. *N. Engl. J. Med.,* **295,** 650–654.

Carlsson, A. M. (1983). Assessment of chronic pain: 1. Aspects of the reliability and validity of the visual analogue scale, *Pain,* **16,** 87–101.

Carlsson, C. (1990). Herbs and hepatitis, *Lancet,* **2,**1068.

Carmen Del Rio, M. and Alvarez, F. J. (1996). Medication use by the driving population. *Pharmacoepidemiol. Drug Safety,* **5,** 255–261.

Carmignoto, F. (1991). L'interpretazione degli esami di laboratorio nella sperimentazione clinica dei farmaci. *Progr. Med. Lab.,* **6,** 587–592.

Caroff, S. N. (1980). The neuroleptic malignant syndrome. *J. Clin. Psychiat.,* **41,** 79–83.

Carson, J. L. (1984). COMPASS data base. An epidemiologist's viewpoint. *Proceedings of the 20th annual meeting of Drug Information Association,* 97–100.

Carson, J. L. and Strom, B. L., (1986). Technique of postmarketing surveillance. An overview. *Med. Toxicol.,* **1,** 237–246.

Carson, J. L. Strom, B. L. and Morse, M. L. (1989) Medicaid. In: Strom, B. L. (ed.) *Pharmacoepidemiology* 14.

Castle, W. M. (1989). The ICI approach: possible adverse reaction information system. *Drug Inf. J.,* **23,** 183–188.

Castle, W. (1991). Adverse drug reactions: scope and limitations of causality assessment and the use of algorithms. *Int. J. Risk Safety Med.,* **2,** 185–192.

Castle, W., Fuller, N., Hall, J. and Palmer, J. (1993). Serevent nationwide surveillance study: comparison of salmeterol with salbutamol in asthmatic patients who require regular bronchodilator treatment. *Br. Med. J.*, **306**, 1034–1037.

Castle, W., Williams, P. M., Grob, P. R., Ellis, R., Robinson, N. D. P. and Battersby, L. A. (1987). ADRIAN: Adverse Drug Reaction Interactive Advice Network. Abstracts 6th International Meeting of Pharmaceutical Physicians, UK.

Cato, A. E., Cook, L., Starbuck, R. and Heatherington, D. (1983). Methodologic approach to adverse events applied to Bupropion clinical trials. *J. Clin. Psychiat.*, **44**(5) (Sec. 2), 187–190.

Caulfield, M. and Cafferkey, M. (1998). Gene therapy: the possibilities and the problems. *Int. J. Pharm. Med*, **12**, 5–7.

Chalmers, D. (1985). A PMS study of captopril utilising viewdata technology. Abstract. International Symposium: Evaluation of the Risk Benefit Profile in the PMS of the Drug, Bergamo, Italy.

Chalmers, D., Dombey, S. L. and Lawson, D. H. (1987). Post marketing surveillance of captopril for hypertension—a preliminary report. *Br. J. Clin. Pharmacol.*, **24**, 343–349.

Chalmers, D. M., Rinsler, M. G., MacDermott, S., Spicer, C. C. and Levi, A. J. (1981) Biochemical and haematological indicators of excessive alcohol consumption. *Gut*, **22**, 992–996.

Chan, T. Y. K. and Critchley, J. A. J. H. (1994). Drug-related problems as a cause of medical admissions in Hong Kong. Abstract 103. *Pharmacoepidemiol. Drug Safety*, **3**, Suppl. 1, S41.

Chan, T. K. and Critchley, J. A. J. H. (1995). Drug-related problems as a cause of hospital admissions in Hong Kong. *Pharmacoepidemiol. Drug Safety*, **4**, 165–170.

Chang, R. W. and Fineberg, H. V. (1983). Risk-benefit consideration in the management of polymyalgia rheumatic. *Med. Decis. Making*, **3**, 459–475.

Chaslerie, A., Dartiques, J. F. and Bégaud, B. (1995). Under-reporting of adverse drug reactions in the elderly. *Pharmacoepidemiol. Drug Safety*, **4**(6), 379–381.

Chen, R. T. (1996). Special methodological issues in pharmacoepidemiology studies of vaccine safety. In: *Pharmacoepidemiology*. Ed. Strom, B. L., Wiley, Chichester. 581–595.

Chen, R. T. and Haber, P. (1995). Safety profiles and similarity index: New tools for assessing vaccine safety. Abstract 095. *Pharmacoepidemiol. Drug Safety*, **4**, Suppl. 1, S43.

Chen, R. T. and DeStephano, F. (1998). Vaccine adverse events 'causal or coincidental?' *Lancet*, **351**, 611–612.

Cherng, N. C., Ali, M. W., Trost, D. C. and Li, M. Y. (1996). Some approaches to the evaluation and display of laboratory safety data. Presented at the 1996 Joint Statistical Meetings in Chicago IL.

Chick, J., Kreitman, N. and Plant, M. (1981). Mean cell volume and gamma glutamyl-transpeptidase as markers of drinking in working class men. *Lancet*, **1**, 1249–1251.

Choonara, I., Gill, A. and Nunn, A. (1996). Drug toxicity and surveillance in children. *Br. J. Clin. Pharmacol.*, **42**, 407–410.

Chouinard, G., Ross-Chouinard, A., Annable, L. and Jones, B. D. (1980). Extrapyramidal symptom rating scale. *Can. J. Neurol. Sci.*, **7**(3), 233.

Chuang-Stein, C. (1992). Safety analysis: Too much? not enough? and how? (with discussion) *Biopharm. Rep.*, **1**, 3, 1–11.

Chuang-Stein, C. (1992). Summarizing laboratory data with different reference ranges in multicenter clinical trials. *Drug Inf. J.*, **26**, 77–84.

Chuang-Stein, C. (1993). The regression fallacy. *Drug Inf. J.*, **27**, 1213–1220.

Chuang-Stein, C. (1994). A new proposal for benefit-less-risk analysis in clinical trials. *Control Clin. Trials.*, **15**, 30–43.

Chuang-Stein, C. (1995). Points for consideration in the collection and analysis of safety data. *Drug Inf. J.*, **29**, 37–44.

Chuang-Stein, C. and Tong, D. M. (1997). The impact and implication of regression to the mean on the design and analysis of medical investigations. *Stat. Method Med. Res*, **6**, 115–128.

Chuang-Stein, C., Mohberg, N. R. and Sinkula, M. S. (1991). Three measures for simultaneously evaluating benefits and risk using categorical data from clinical trials. *Stat. Med.*, **10**, 1349–1359.

Chuang-Stein, C., Mohberg, N. R. and Musselman, D. M. (1992). Organization and analysis of safety data using a multivariate approach. *Stat. Med.*, **11**, 1075–1089.

Chuang-Stein, C. (1998). Laboratory data in clinical trials: a statistician's perspective. *Control Clin Trials*, **19** (2), 167–178.

Ciccolunghi, S. N. and Chaudri, H. A. (1975). A methodological study of some factors influencing the reporting of symptoms. *J. Clin Pharmacol.*, **10**, 496–505.

Ciccolunghi, S. N., Fowler, P. D. and Chaudry, M. J. (1979). Interpretation of haematological and biochemical laboratory data in large-scale, multicenter clinical trials. *J. Clin. Pharmacol.*, **19**, 302–312.

Cimons, M. (1993). The deadly risks of research. *Los Angeles Times*. 25th August. A15–17.

Ciociola, A. A., Webb, D. D. and McSorley, D. J. (1996). The continued use of placebo-controlled clinical trials in the study of peptic ulcer disease: a sponsor perspective. *Drug Inf. J.*, **30**, 433–439.

CIOMS (1983). *Safety Requirements for the First Use of New drugs and Diagnostic Agents in Man.* (Council for International Organisation of Medical Sciences, Geneva).

CIOMS Working Group. (1990). *International Reporting of Adverse Drug Reactions. Final Report of the CIOMS Working Group.*

CIOMS Working Group II. (1992). *International Reporting of Periodic Drug Safety Update Summaries. Final Report of the CIOMS Working Group II.*

CIOMS Working Group III. (1995). Guidelines for Preparing Core Clinical Safety Information on Drugs. CIOMS Geneva. 17.

CIOMS and WHO (1993). *International Ethical Guidelines for Biomedical Research Involving Human Subjects.* (WHO, Geneva).

Citron, M. L. (1993). Placebos and principles: A trial of Ondansetron. *Ann. Int. Med.*, **118**, 470–471.

Clark, A. and Fallowfield, L. J. (1986). Quality of life measurements in patients with malignant disease: a review. *J. Roy. Soc. Med.*, **79**, 165–168.

Clark, J. A. Zimmerman, H. J. and Tanner, L. A. (1990). Labetalol hepatotoxicity. *Ann. Intern. Med.*, **113**, 210–213.

Clark, P. M. S., Holder, R., Mullet, M. and Whitehead, T. P. (1983). Sensitivity and specificity of laboratory tests for alcohol abuse. *Alcohol*, **18**(3), 261–269.

Classen, D. C., Pestotnick, S. L., Evans, R. S. and Burke, J. P. (1991). Computerized surveillance of adverse drug events in hospital patients. *JAMA*, **266**, 2847–2851.

Classen, D. C., Pestotnik, S. L., Scott Evans, R., Lloyd, J. F. and Burke, J. P. (1997). Adverse drug events in hospitalized patients. *JAMA*, **277**, 301–306.

Clinical Trials Unit, Department of Pharmacology and Therapeutics, London Hospital Medical College. (1977). Aide-memoire for preparing clinical trial protocols. *Br. Med. J.*, 1323–1324.

Cocchetto, D. M. and Nardi, R. V. (1986). Benefit–risk assessment of investigational drug, current methodology, limitations and alternative approaches. *Pharmacotherapy*, **6**(6), 286–303.

Cohen, M. R. (1974). A compilation of abstracts and an index of articles published by the BCDSP. *Hosp. Pharm.*, **9**, 437–448.

Cohen, S. N. (1995). Drug promotion. *N. Engl. J. Med.*, **332**, 1032.

Cohen, J. A. and Kaplan, M. M. (1975). The S.G.O.T./S.G.P.T. ratio in liver disease. *Gastroenterology*, **69**, 813,.

Colburn, W. (1989). Controversy IV: Population pharmacokinetics, NONMEM and the pharmacokinetic screen. Academic, industry and regulatory perspectives. *Pharmacokinetics*, **29**, 1–6.

Collier, J. (1993). Drug company representatives and sales priorities. *Lancet*, **341**, 1031–1032.

Collier, J. (1995). Can the promotion of medicines by the pharmaceutical industry be ethical? *Pharm. Med.*, **9**, 45–47.

Collier, J. (1995). Confusion over use of placebos in clinical trials. *Br. Med. J.*, **311**, 821–822.

Collier, J. and Herxheimer, A. (1987). Roussel convicted of misleading promotion. *Lancet*, **1**, 113–114.

Collins, J. and Johnston, A. (1995). Motivation of volunteers to participate in clinical research. *Br. J. Clin. Pharmacol.*, **41**, 437P-475P.

Collins, M. (1995). Placebo-controlled trials and alternatives. *Drug. Inf. J.*, **29**, 493–496.

Committee for Proprietary Medicinal Products *Working Party on Efficacy of Medicinal Products. Good Clinical Practice (G. C. P.) for Trials on Medicinal Products in the European Community.* Guidelines. 111/3976/88–EN.

Committee for Safety of Medicines (1983). Osmosin (controlled release indomethacin). *Curr. Prob.*, **11**.

Committee for Safety of Medicines. Suggestions for monitoring adverse drug reactions, *Pharm. J.*, **219**, 30–31.

Committee of Principal Investigators. (1978). A co-operative trial in the primary prevention of ischaemic heart disease using clofibrate. *Br. Heart J.*, **40**, 1069–1118.

Committee of Principal Investigators. (1980). WHO co-operative trial on primary prevention of ischaemic heart disease using clofibrate to lower serum cholesterol: mortality follow-up. *Lancet*, **2**, 279–385.

Conforti, A., Leone, R., Moretti, L., Guglielomo, L. and Velo, G. P. (1995). Spontaneous reporting of adverse drug reactions in an Italian region: six years of analysis and observations. *Pharmacoepidemiol. Drug. Safety*, **4**, 129–135.

Conover, W. J. and Salsburg, D. S. (1988). Locally most powerful tests for detecting treatment effects when only a subset of patients can be expected to "respond" to treatment. *Biometrics*, **44**, 189–196.

Conrad, K. A. (1995). Clinical pharmacology and drug safety: lessons from hirudin. *Clin. Pharmac. Therap.*, **58**(2), 123–126.

Constant, K. W., Worlledge, S., Dollery, C. T. and Breckenridge. A. (1966). Methyl dopa and haemolytic anaemia. *Lancet*, **i**, 201.

Cook, M. and Ferner, R. E. (1993). Adverse drug reactions: who is to know? *Br. Med. J.*, **307**, 480–481.

Coombs, R. R. A. and Gell, P. G. H. (1968). Classification of allergic reactions responsible for clinical hypersensitivity and disease. Ed. Coombs, R. R. A. and Gell, P. G. H. (eds) In: *Clinical Aspects of Immunology*, 2nd edition. 575–596.

Cooper, K. and Bennett, W. M. (1987). Nephrotoxicity of common drugs used in clinical practice. *Arch. Intern. Med.*, **147**, 1213–1218.

Cordier, L. (1997). Is there a European ethical framework for clinical research? *Int. J. Pharm. Med.*, **11**, 137–140.

Cornelia, I. R. L., Kipferler, P. and Hasford, J. (1997). Drug use assessment and risk evaluation in pregnancy—The PEGASUS-project. *Pharmacoepidemiol. Drug. Safety*, **6**, Suppl. 3, S37–S42.

Cornelli, U. (1984). The phase IV monitoring studies. Example of naproxen Na multi-centre Italian trial. In: *Postmarketing clinical trials-the phase IV studies*. Ed. C. Crescioni and J. M. James. Editions de Santé, 89–105.

Corre, K. A. and Spielberg, T. E. (1988). Adverse drug reaction processing in the United States and its dependance on physician reporting: zomepirac (Zomax) as a case in point. *Ann. Emerg. Med.*, **17**, 145–149.

Correspondent. (1990). Switzerland: monitored release not what it seems. *Lancet*, **2**, 496.

Corso, D. M., Pucino, F., Deleo, J. M., Calis, K. A. and Gallelli, F. (1992). Development of a questionnaire for detecting potential adverse drug reactions. *Ann. Pharmacother.*, **26**, 890–896.

Costello, A. M de L. and Bhutta, T. (1992). Antidiarrhoeal drugs for acute diarrhoea in children. *Br. Med. J.*, **304**, 1–2.

Costongs, G. M. P. J., Janson, P. C. W., Bas, B. M., Hermans, J., Van Wersch, J. W. J. and Brombacher, P. J. (1985). Short-term and long-term intra-individual variations and critical differences of clinical chemical laboratory parameters. *J. Clin. Chem. Clin. Biochem.*, **23**, 7–16.

Coulter, D. M. (1988). Eye pain with nifedipine and disturbance of taste with captopril: a mutually controlled study showing a method of PMS. *Br. Med. J.*, **296**, 1086–1088.

Coulter, D. M. and Edwards, I. R. (1990). Mianserin and agranulocytosis in New Zealand. *Lancet*, **336**, 785–787.

Craig, J. J. and Morrow, J. I. (1997). Register of women who take drugs during pregnancy has been set up. *Br. Med. J.*, **314**, 603.

Crane, G. E. (1968). Tardive dyskinesia in patients treated with major neuroleptics: a review of the literature. *Am. J. Psychiat.*, **124**(8), 40–49.

Crane, J., Flatt, A., Jackson, R., Ball, M., Pearce, N., Burgess, C., Kwong, T. and Beasley, R. (1989). Prescribed fenoterol and death from asthma in New Zealand, 1981–83: case–control study. *Lancet*, **1**, 917–922.

Croog, S. H., Levine, S., Testa, M. A., Brown, B., and Bulpitt, C. J. (1986). The effects of anti-hypertensive therapy on the quality of life. *N. Engl. J. Med.*, **314**, 1657–1664.

Crooks, J. (1977). The detection of adverse drug reactions. *J. Roy. Coll. Physic. Lond.*, **11**(3), 239–244.

Cross. K. W. (1973). Cost of preventing retrolental fibroplasia. *Lancet*, **2**, 954–956.

Curran, C. F. and Bawa, O. (1990). Implementation of a worldwide drug safety surveillance system. *Drug. Inf. J.*, **240**, 605–614.

Curran, C. F. and Engle, C. (1997). An index of United States federal regulations and guidelines which cover safety surveillance of drugs. *Drug. Inf. J.*, **31**, 833–841.

Curran, C. F. and Sills, J. M. (1997). An index of United States federal regulations and guidelines which cover clinical safety surveillance of biological products. *Drug. Inf. J.*, **31**, 843–847.

Current Problems. (1990). **29**.

Current Problems. (1990). **30**.

Current Problems. (1991). **32**.

Current Problems. (1993). **19**(2).

Czerwinski, A. W. (1974). The Phase 1 drug study. In: McMahon F. G. (ed.) *Drug-induced Clinical Toxicity* 374. Futura.

Dahlstrom, W. G., Welsh, G. S. and Dahlstrom, L. E. (1996). An MMPI handbook, Vol. 1, Clinical Interpretation. University of Minnesota Press, Mineapolis.

Daily Telegraph. (1981). 3 June-25 June.

Daily Telegraph. (1996). Abortions rise after pill scare. *Daily Telegraph*, 22nd November.

Danan, G. and Bénichou, C. (1990). Standardisation in International databases: Definitions of drug induced liver disorders. *J. Hepatol.*, **11**, 272–276.

Danan, G. and Bénichou, C. (1993). Causality assessment of adverse reactions to drugs—1. A novel method on the conclusions of international consensus meetings: Application to drug-induced liver injuries. *J. Clin. Epidemiol.*, **46**(11), 1323–1330.

Danan, G., Lagier, G., Bégaud, B. and Couzigou, P. (1985). Guide d'imputation des hépatites médicamenteuses. *Thérapie*, **40**, 247–251.

D'Angio, R. G. (1987). Nonsteroidal antiinflammatory drug-induced renal dysfunction related to inhibition of renal prostaglandins. *Drug. Intell. Clin. Pharm.*, **21**, 954–960.

Dangoumau, J., Bégaud, B., Boisseau, A. and Albin H. (1980). Les effets indésirables des médicaments, Diagnostics comparés de cliniciens et pharmacologues cliniciens. *Nouv. Presse Méd.*, **9**(9), 1607–1609.

Dangoumau, J., Bégaud, B., Péré, J. C. and Albin, H. (1981). De l'imputabilité origenelle a l'imputabilité terminale. *Thérapie.*, **361**, 219–227.

Dangoumau, J., Evreux, J. C. and Jouglard, J. (1978). Méthode d'imputabilité des effets indésirables des médicaments. *Thérapie*, **33**, 373–381.

D'Arcy, P. F. and Griffin, J. P. (1994). Thalidomide revisited. *Adv. Drug. React. Toxicol. Rev.*, **13**(2), 65–76.

Darragh, A., Lambe, R., Kenny, M. and Brick, I. (1985). Sudden death of a volunteer. *Lancet*, **1**, 93–95.

Davey, P. and McDonald, T. (1993). Postmarketing of Quinolones 1990–1992. *Drugs.*, **45, S3**, 46–53.

Davidson, C. S., Leevy, C. M. and Chamberlyne, E. E. (1979). *Guidelines for Detection of Hepatotoxicity due to Drugs and Chemicals.* Fogarty conference, USA Department of Health, Education and Welfare, NIH publication no. 79–113.

Davidson, S. I. and Rennie, I. G. (1986). Ocular toxicity from systemic drug therapy, an overview of clinically important adverse reactions. *Med. Toxicol.*, **1**, 217–274.

Davies, D. M. (1984). Special report. *Adv. Drug. React. Ac. Pois. Rev.*, **3**(4), 249–250.

Davis, J. M. (1994). Current reporting methods for laboratory data at Zeneca Pharmaceuticals. *Drug Inf. J.*, **25**, 403–406.

Davis, M. (1989) Drugs and abnormal liver function tests. *Adv. Drug. Reac. Bull.*, **139**.

Davis, T. G., Pickett, D. L. and Schlosser, J. M. (1980). Evaluation of a worldwide spontaneous reporting system with cimetidine. *JAMA*, **243**(19), 1912–1914.

Dawnay, A. (1990). Measurement of renal side effects. In: O'Grady, J. and Lind, O. (eds) *Early Phase Drug Evaluation in Man.* Macmillan.

Day, T. K. (1983). Intestinal perforation associated with slow release indomethacin capsules. *Br. Med. J.*, **287**, 1671–1672.

De Caester, M. P. and Ballarde, F. W. (1990). Unexplained haematuria, *Br. Med. J.*, **301**, 1171–1172.

De Gier, J. (1997). Annual meeting of the Society of Pharmaceutical Medicine. *Pharm. Med.*, **11**, 353.

De Smet, P. A. G. M. (1995a). Should herbal medicine-like products be licensed as medicines? *Br. Med. J.*, **310**, 1023–1024.

De Smet, P. A. G. M. (1995b) Health risks of herbal remedies. *Drug Safety*, **13**(2), 81–93.

De Smet, P. A. G. M., Van Den Eertwegh, A. J. M. and Stricker, B. H. (1996). Hepatotoxicity associated with herbal tablets. *BMJ*, **313**, 92.

De Vries, B. M., Hughes, G. S. and Huysen, L. S. (1991). Screening for illicit drug use in drug development studies. *Drug. Inf. J.*, **25**, 49–53.

Dean, M. (1993). A new prescription for drug industry. *Lancet*, **341**, 883–884.

Decoster, G., Rich, W. and Brown, S. L. (1994). Safety profile of Filigrastim. In *Filigrastim in Clinical Practice.* Ed. Mostyn, G. and Dexter, T. H., Marcel Dekker, New York.

Delamothe, T. (1992). Reporting adverse drug reactions. *Br. Med. J.*, **304**, 465.

Delap, R. J. Fourcroy, J. L. and Fleming, G. A. (1996). Fetal harm due to paternal drug exposure: a potential issue in drug development. *Drug. Inf. J.*, **30**, 359–364.

DeMets, D., Friedman, L. M. and Furberg, C. (1980). Counting in clinical trials. *N. Engl. J. Med.*, **302**(16), 924–925.

Denkers, J., Ahlfors, U. G., Bech, P., Elgin, K. and Lingjaerde, O. (1976). Classification of side effects in psychopharmacology. *Pharmacopsychiat.*, **19**, 40–42.

Department of Health and Human Services, Food and Drug. Administration. (1993). Guideline for the study and evaluation of gender differences in clinical evaluation of drugs. *Federal Register Notice*, **58**(139), 39406–39416.

Deshazo, R. D. and Kemp, S. F. (1997). Allergic reactions to drugs and biologic agents. *JAMA*, **278**, 1895–1906.

Di Masi, J. A., Hansen, R. W., Grabowski, H-G. and Lasagna, L. (1991). Cost of inovation in the pharmaceutical industry. *J. Health Economics.*, **10**, 107–142.

Diamond, A., Hall, S., Jay, M., Laurence, D., Mayon-White, R., Peckham, C., Rawlins, M., Turner-Warwick, M. and Wald, N. (1994). Independent ethical review of studies involving personal medical records. *J. Roy. Coll. Physicians Lond.*, **28**, 5, 439–443.

Dickey, W. and Morrow, J. I. (1990). Drug-induced neurological disorders. *Prog Neurobiol.*, **34**, 331–342.

Dijkman, J. H. M. and Querton, J. (1994). Feasibility of Europe-wide specimen shipments. *Drug. Inf. J.*, **28**, 385–391.

Dikshit, R. K. and Dikshit, N. (1994). Commercial source of drug information: comparison between the United Kingdom and India. *Br. Med. J.*, **309**, 990–991.

Dillner, L. (1992) Drug advertisements misleading. *Br. Med. J.*, **304**, 1526.

Dimenäs, E., Dahlof, C., Olofsson, B. and Wiklund, I. (1989). CNS related subjective symptoms during treatment with β adrenoceptor antagonists (atenolol and metropolol) two double-blind controlled studies. *Br. J. Clin. Pharmacol.*, **28**, 527–534.

Dimenäs, E., Dahlof, C., Olofsson, B. and Wiklund, I. (1990). An instrument for quantifying subjective symptoms among untreated and treated hypertensives: Development and documentation. *J. Clin. Res. Pharmacoepidemiol.*, **4**, 205–217.

Dimenäs, E., Wallander, M-A., Svärdsudd, K. and Wiklund, I. (1991). Aspects of quality of life with felodipine, *Eur. J. Clin. Pharmacol.*, **40**, 141–147.

Dinman, B. D. (1980a). Occupational health and the reality of risk—an eternal dilemma of tragic choice. *J. Occup. Med.*, **22**(3), 153–157.

Dinman, B. D. (1980b). The reality and acceptance of risk. *JAMA*, **244**(11), 1226–1228.

Distillers Company (Biochemicals Ltd). (1961). Distival. *Lancet*, **2**, 1262.

Division of Drug Experience, Food and Drug Administration. (1980). *Procedural Manual for Handling Drug Experience Reports. Glossary, Paper Flow and Algorithms.*

Dixon, J. S. and Bird, H. A. (1981). Reproducibility along a 10 cm, vertical visual analogue scale. *Ann. Rheum. Dis.*, **40**, 87–89.

Dobbs, J. H. (1988). Exchange of Worldwide Safety Surveillance Data via an International Computer Database. *Drug. Inf. J.*, **22**, 71–74.

Dollery, C. T. (1977). Clinical trials of new drugs. *J. Roy. Coll. Phys. Lond.*, **11**(3), 226–233.

Dollery, C. T. and Rawlins, M. D. (1977). Monitoring adverse reactions to drugs. *Br. Med. J.*, **1**, 96–97.

Domecq, C., Naranjo, C. A., Ruiz, I. and Busto, U. (1980). Sex-related variations in the frequency and characteristics of adverse drug reactions. *Int. J. Clin. Pharmacol. Ther. Toxic*, **18**, 362–366.

Dong, M. H., Ariello, C., Juergens, J. P., Turner, W. M., Gelberg, A. and Armstrong, G. D. (1988). A microcomputer based data entry system for reporting adverse drug reactions in the United States. *Drug. Inf. J.*, **22**, 61–70.

Donoghue, J. and Tylee, A. (1996). The treatment of depression: prescribing pattern of antidepressants in primary care in the UK. *Br. J. Psychiat.*, **168**, 164–168.

Donoghue, J., Tylee, A. and Widgust, H. (1996). Cross-sectional database analysis of antidepressant prescribing in general practice in the UK, 1993–5. *Br. Med. J.*, **313**, 861–862.

Donovan, S., Mills, J., Goulder, M. A., Dumelow, N. W., Amos, R. and Carlisle, L. (1996). Electronic patient diaries: a pilot study. *Applied Clinical Trials*, **5**, 40–49.

Double, D. B. (1996). Placebo controlled trials are needed to provide data on effectiveness of active treatment. *Br. Med. J.*, **313**, 1008–1009.

Dowell, A. C. and Britton, J. F. (1990) Microhaematuria in general practice: is using urine microscopy misleading? *Br. J. Gen. Pract.*, **40**, 67–68.

Downey, W., Baker, M., Melston, D., McNutt, M., Quinn, T., Strand, L. M. and West, R. (1990). Pharmacoepidemiology in Saskatchewan. *J. Clin. Res. Pharmacoepidemiol.*, **4**, 113–145.

Downing, R. W., Rickels, K. and Meyers, F. (1970). Side reactions in neurotics, 1: A comparison of two methods of assessment. *J. Clin. Pharmacol.*, **10**, 289–297.

Drici, M-D., Raybaud, F., De Lunardo, C., Iacono, P. and Gustovic, P. (1995). Influence of the behaviour pattern on the nocebo response of healthy volunteers. *Br. J. Clin. Pharmacol.*, **39**, 204–206.

Driscoll, M. S. and Knodel, L. C. (1986). Induction of haemolytic anaemia by non-steroidal anti-inflammatory drugs. *Drug Intelligence and Clinical Pharmacy.*, **29**, 925–34.

Druce, H. (1990). Impairment of function by antihistamines. *Ann. Allergy*, **64**, 403–405.

Drug Information C. P. E. Study 67 (1983) Patient receipt of prescription drug information USA, F and D.A.

Drug Surveillance Research Unit: *PEM News*, vol. 1 1983; *PEM News*, vol. 2 1984; *PEM News*, vol. 3 1985; *PEM News*, vol. 4 1987; Hamble Valley Press, Southampton.

Drug induced acute pancreatitis. (1994). *Prescrire Int.*, **3**(12), 111–112.

Dukes, M. N. G. (1996). Drug safety—can more be done? *Risk and Drug Safety Med.*, **9**(2), 71–73.

Dukes, M. N. G. and Lunde, I. (1979). Common sense and communities. *Pharm. Weekblad.*, **144**, 1283–1284.

Dunnett, C. and Goldsmith, C. (1981). When and how to do multiple comparisons. In Buncher, C. R. and Tsay, J. V. (eds.), Statistics in the Pharmaceutical Industry, 1981, pp. 397–432.

Dupont, R. L. (1996). Books, journals, new media—tobacco. *JAMA*, **275**, 1285.

Dusheiko, G, Dibisceglie, A., Bowyer, S., Sachs, E., Ritchie, M., Schoub, B. and Kew, M. (1985). Recombinant leukocyte interferon treatment of chronic hepatitis B. *Hepatology*, **5**(4), 556–560.

Edwards, I. R. (1993). Drug safety monitoring: an international perspective. *Ann. Acad. Med. Singapore*, **22**(1), 107–110.

Edwards, I. R. (1997). Editorial. *Br. Med. J.*, **315**, 500.

Edwards, I. R., Lindquist, M., Wiholm, B-E. and Napke, E. (1990). Quality criteria for early signals of possible adverse drug reactions. *Lancet*, **336**, 156–158.

Edwards, I. R., Wiholm, B-E. and Martinez, C. (1996). Concepts in risk–benefit assessment. A simple merit analysis of a medicine. *Drug Safety*, **15**, 1–7.

Ehrmeyer, S. S. and Laessig, R. H. (1994). Monitoring clinical trials in multiple testing sites: can good laboratory practice and proficiency testing assure uniform testing? *Drug. Inf. J.*, **28**, 1212–1223.

Einarson, A., Koren, G. and Bergman, U. (1996). Treatment of nausea and vomiting in pregnancy. *Abstract.* 1st Congress of the European Drug Utilization Research Group. Rational Drug Use in Europe. Challenges for the 21st century. June 27–30th.

Elashoff, J. D. (1981) Down with multiple 't' tests. *Gastroenterology*, **80**, 615–620.

Ellenberg, S. S. (1994). New adverse experience reporting requirements for licensed biological products. *DIA Conference, The Management of Adverse Drug Reactions—Diagnoses and Issues, 3–6th December.*

Ellenberg, S. S. (1996). The use of data monitoring committees in clinical trials. *Drug Inf. J.*, **30**, 553–559.

Elwood, P. C. and Hughes, D. (1970). Clinical trial of iron therapy of psychomotor function in anaemic women. *Br. Med. J.*, **3**, 254–255.

Emanueli, A. and Sacchetti, G. (1978). An algorithm for the classification of untoward events in large scale clinical trials. *Agents Actions*, **7**, 318–322.

Emanueli, A. and Sacchetti, G. (1982). Post-marketing surveillance methodology as applied in a pharmaceutical medical department. In: Auriche, M., Burke, J. and Duchier, Y. (eds.) *Drug safety Progress and Controversies*. 265–273, (Pergamon Press, France).

Emmett, E. A. (1978). Drug photoallergy. *Int. J. Dermatol.*, **17**, 370–379.

Enas, G. G. (1991). Making decisions about safety in clinical trials—The case for inferential statistics. *Drug Inf. J.*, **25**, 439–446.

Enas, G. G., Dornseif, B. E., Sampson, C. B., Rockhold, F. W. and Wuu, J. (1989). Monitoring versus interim analysis of clinical trials: A perspective from the pharmaceutical industry. *Contr. Clin. Trials*, **10**, 57–70.

Enstellung von Monographie-Entwürfen Pharm. Ind. (1986). **48**(IIa), 1293.

Erickson, P. and Patrick, D. L. (1988). Guidelines for selecting quality of life assessment: methodological and practical considerations. *J. Drug Ther. Research*, **13**, 5.

Erickson, P., Taeuber, R. C. and Scott, J. (1995). Operational aspects of quality of life assessment. Choosing the right instrument. *Pharmacoeconomics*, **7**(1), 39–48.

Ernst, E. and Resch, K. L. (1995). Concept of true and perceived placebo effects. *Br. Med. J.*, **311**, 551–553.

Ernst, E. and Resch, K. L. (1996). Risk–benefit ratio or risk–benefit nonsense. *J. Clin. Epidemiol.*, **49**(10), 1203–1204.

European Forum for Good Clinical Practice. (1997). Guidelines and recommendations for European ethics committees. *Int. J. Pharmaceut. Med.*, **11**, 129–135.

Evans, D. (1997). The reform of multicentre ethical review: MRECS for better or worse. *Int. J. Pharmaceut. Med.*, **11**, 217–220.

Evans D. and Evans, M. (1996). *A Decent Proposal: Ethical Review of Clinical Research*. (John Wiley and Sons).

Evans, G. O. (1996). Factors affecting the choice of laboratories for clinical trials. *Drug Inf. J.*, **30**, 815–820.

Evans, R. S., Pestotnick, S. L., Classen, D. C., Horn, S. D., Bass, S. B. and Burke, J. P. (1994). Preventing adverse drug reactions in hospitalised patients. *Ann. Pharmacother.*, **28**, 523–527.

Evens, R. P., Flynn, J. F. and Mapes, D. M. (1996). Preventing the pitfalls in planning phase IV clinical trials: a biotechnical experience. *Drug Inf. J.*, **30**, 583–591.

Faich, G. A., (1986a). *Postmarketing Surveillance of Prescription Drugs*. (Current status, Clinical Real Life Studies Program, Clinical Medicine Research Institute, 800 Second Ave, New York).

Faich, G. A. (1986b). Special report ADR monitoring. *N. Engl. J. Med.*, **314**(24), 1589–1592.

Faich, G. A., Castle, W., Bankowski, Z. and The C.I.O.M.S. ADR working group. International ADR reporting. The C.I.O.M.S. project. *Drug Inf. J.*, **34**, 419–425.

Faich, G. A., Guess, H. A. and Kuritsky, J. M. (1988). Post-marketing surveillance for drug safety. In: Cato, A. E. (ed.) *Clinical Trials and Tribulations*. (Marcel Dekker, New York).

Fairweather, W. R. (1996). Integrated safety analysis statistical issues in the assessment of safety in clinical trials. *Drug Inf. J.*, **30**, 875–879.

Farina, J. L., Krupp, P. and Tobler, H. J. (1978). Computer tools in spontaneous reporting of adverse drug reactions. A multinational company approach. In: *Computer Aid to Drug Therapy and to Drug Monitoring*. Ed. Ducrot *et al.*, IFIF North Holland Publishing Company.

Farmer, R. D. T., Lawrenson, R. A., Thompson, C. R., Kennedy, J. G and Hambleton, I. R. (1997). Population-based study of risk of venous thromboembolism associated with various oral contraceptives. *Lancet*, **349**, 83–88.

Farmer, R. D. T., Todd, J-C., MacRae, K. D., Williams, T. J. and Lewis, M. A. (1988). Oral contraceptives were not associated with venous thromboembolic disease in recent study. *BMJ*, **316**, 109–1091.

Farrington, C. P., Nash, J. and Miller, E. (1996). Case series analysis of adverse reactions to vaccines: a comparative evaluation. *Am. J. Epidemiol.*, **143**(11), 1165–73.

Farrington, P., Pugh, S., Colville, A., Flower, A., Nash, J., Morgan-Capner, P., Rush, M. and Miller, E. (1995). A new method for active surveillance of adverse events from diphtheria/tetanus/pertussis and measles/mumps/rubella vaccines. *Lancet*, **345**, 567–569.

Fauchald, P., Helgeland, A. and Storm-Mathison. (1978). Treatment of hypertension with prazosin. An open study in general practice. *Proceedings of the European Prazosin Symposium*. Excerpta Medica.

Fayers, P. M. and Jones, S. D. R., (1983). Measuring and analysing the quality of life in cancer clinical trials. A review. *Stat. Med.*, **2**, 429–446.

FDA Guideline (1993). Guidelines for the study and evaluation of gender differences in the clinical trials of new drugs.

FDA Task Force (1993). Fialuridine: Hepatic and pancreatic toxicity. November 12th 1993.

Federal Register. (1994). Adverse experience reporting requirements for human drug and licensed biological products. *Federal Register*, Docket no. 93N-0181.

Federal Register. (1997). *Rules and Regulations FDA 21 CFR parts 312.32*. Volume 62, no. 194, 52250.

Federspiel, C. F., Ray W. A. and Schaffner, W. (1976). Medicaid records as a valid data source: The Tennessee experience. *Med. Care*, **14**, 166–172.

Feger, H. (1996). Pill scare led to abortion misery for thousands. *Daily Express*, 23rd November, 17.

Fennerty, A., Campbell, I. A. and Routledge, P. A. (1988). Anticoagulants in venous thrombo-embolism. Guidelines for optimum treatment. *Br. Med. J.*, **197**, 1285–1288.

Fenoglio, J. J., McAllister, H. A. and Mullick, F. G. (1981). Drug related myocarditis. I. Hypersensitivity myocarditis. *Hum. Pathol.*, **12**, 900–907.

Fields, H. L. and Levine, J. D. (1981). Biology of placebo analgesia. *Am. J. Med.*, **70**(4), 745–746.

Fieldstad, L. M., Kurjatkin, O. and Cobert, B. L. (1996). A template for adverse event reporting in licensing agreements. *Drug Inf. J.*, **30**, 965–971.

Figueiras, A., Tato, F., Takkouche, B. and Gestal-Otero, J. J. (1997). An algorithm for the design of epidemiologic studies applied to drug surveillance. *Eur. J. Clin. Pharmacol.* **51**, 445–448.

Finkle, W. D. (1985). Studies of drug effects within the Kaiser Foundation Health Plan, Southern California region. *Drug Inf. J.*, **19**, 243–247.

Finn, R. (1992). Food allergy—fact or fiction: a review. *J. Roy. Soc. Med.*, **85**, 560–564.

Finney, D. J. (1965). The design and logic of a monitor of drug use. *J. Chron. Dis.*, **18**, 77–98.

Finney, D. J. (1996). Statistical aspects of pharmacoepidemiology. *Drug Inf. J.*, **30**, 987–990.

Fisher, S., Bryant, S. G. and Kluge, P. M. (1987). Detecting adverse drug reactions in post-marketing surveillance: interview validity. *Drug Inf. J.*, **21**, 173–183.

Fisher, S., Bryant, S.G. and Kluge, P.M. (1986). Measuring ADRs in a PMS system. *Psychopharm. Bull.*, **22**, 272–277.

Fitzgerald, J. D. (1992). Crisis management: The medical director's response. *Pharmacoepidemiol. Drug Safety*, **1**, 155–161.

Fitzsimmons, S. C., Burkhart, G. A., Borowitz, D., Grand, R. J., Hammerstrom, T., Durie, P. R., Lloyd-Still, J. D. and Owenfels, A. B. (1997). High-dose pancreatic-enzyme supplements and fibrosing colonopathy in children with cystic fibrosis. *N. Engl. J. Med.*, **336**, 1283–1289.

Fleming, D. M., Knox, J. D. E. and Crombie, D. L. (1981). Debendox in early pregnancy and foetal malformation. *Br. Med. J.*, **283**, 99–101.

Fleming, J. J. (1984). Comparison of tubular proteinuria, using sodium dodecyl sulphate polyacrylamide gel electrophoresis, in patients during methotrexate or aminoglycoside treatment or with cadmium or balkan nephropathy. *Clin. Chim, Acta.*, **140**, 267–277.

Fletcher, A. E. and Bulpitt, C. J. (1986). Assessment of Q of L in C.V.S. therapy. *Br. J. Clin. Pharmacol.*, 1986, **21**, 173S–181S.

Fletcher, A. P. and Griffin, J. P. (1991). International monitoring for adverse drug reactions of long latency. *Adv. Drug React. Toxicol. Rev.*, **10**(4), 209–230.

Fletcher, P. (1991). Paper-based PMS in Europe. *Management Forum*, March 1991.

Fletcher, R. H., Fletcher, S. W. and Wagner, E. H. (1996). In: *Clinical Epidemiology: The Essentials*, 3rd edition, 233, Williams and Wilkinson.

Flicker, M. R. (1995). *Ethnic Factors Influences on Safety and Efficacy: a Perspective. DIA Conference, New Orleans, December 4th.*

Fogarty Conference. (1979). Davidson, C. S., Leevy, C. M. and Chamberlayne, E. C. (eds.) *Guidelines for Detection of Hepatotoxicity due to Drugs and Chemicals.* (USA Department of Health Education and Welfare. NIH Publication number 79–313).

Follath, F., Burkart, F. and Schweizer, W. (1971). Drug-induced pulmonary hypertension. *Br. Med. J.*, **1**, 265.

Fonseca, M., Freitas, A., Pfafffenbach, G. and Mendes, G. B. B. (1997). Drug use in pregnancy: a pharmacoepidemiological study. Late breaker abstract. *13th International Conference on Pharmacoepidemiology.* Aug. 24–27th, Florida, USA.

Food and Drug Administration. (1986). FDA criteria for identifying laboratory values as 'clinically significantly abnormal' Appendix 5. In: Supplementary suggestions for preparing an original N. D. A. submission and for organising information in periodic safety updates. From *Draft Guidelines for the Format and Content of the Clinical Data Section of an Application*. FDA.

Foppiano, M. and Lombardo, G. (1997). Worldwide pharmacovigilance systems and tolrestat withdrawal. *Lancet*, **349**, 399–400.

Forbat, A., Lond, M. B., Lehmann, H. and Silk, E. (1953). Prolonged apnoea following injection of succinylcholine. *Lancet*, **2**, 1067–1068.

Foster, C. (1997). The current status of ethical review procedures in the United Kingdom. *Int. J. Pharmaceut. Med.*, **11**, 155–159.

Fox, A. W. (1995). Women in clinical trials. *Appl. Clin. Trials*, Oct. 12.

Franklin, H. R., Van Der Putten, E, P., Simonetti, G. P., Dubbelmann, A. C., Ten Bokkel Huinnick, W. W., Taal, B. G., Hilton, A. M. and Aaronson, N. K. (1989). Toxicity grading systems for oncological trials. *Contr. Clin. Trials*, **10**(3), 351.

Fraser, C. G. (1986). In: *Interpretation of Clinical Chemistry Laboratory Data*, 42 (Blackwell Scientific Publications, Oxford).

Fraser, C. G. and Fogarty, Y. (1989). Interpreting laboratory results. *Br. Med. J.*, **298**, 1659–1660.

Fraser, H. S. (1996). Reserpine: a tragic victim of myth, marketing and fashionable prescribing. *Clin. Pharmacol. Ther.*, **60**(4), 368–373.

Fraumeni, J. F. (1967). Bone marrow depression induced by chloramphenicol and phenylbutazone. *JAMA*, **20**(1), 828.

Freed, G. L., Katz, S. L. and Clark, S. J. (1996). Safety of vaccines. *JAMA*, **276**(23), 1869–1872.

Freedman, L. S., Simon, R., Foulkes, M. A., Friedman, L., Geller, N. L., Gordon, D. J. and Mowery, R. (1995). Inclusion of women and minorities in clinical trials and the NIH revitalization act of 1993—The perspective of NIH clinical trialists *Contr. Clin. Trials*, **16**, 277–285.

Freemantle, S., Pearce, G. L., Wilton, L. V., Mackay, F. J. and Mann, R. D. (1997). The incidence of the most commonly reported events with 40 newly marketed drugs—a study by prescription-event monitoring. *Pharmacoepidemiol. Drug Safety*, **6**, Suppl. 1, 1–8.

Friedman, G. D.,(1972). Screening criteria for drug monitoring. The Kaiser-Permanente drug reaction monitoring system. *J. Chron. Dis.*, **25**, 11–20.

Friedman, G. D., Collen, M. F., Harris, L. E., Van Brunt, E. E. and Davis, L. S. (1971). Experience in monitoring drug reactions in outpatients. The Kaiser-Permanente drug monitoring system. *JAMA*, **217**(5), 567–572.

Friedman, L. M., Furberg, C. and Demets, D. L. (1985). *Fundamentals of Clinical Trials*. 2nd edition. 270 (PSG Publishing Company).

Fries, J. F. (1985). The ARAMIS (American Rheumatism Association Medical Information System) PMS program. *Drug Inf. J.*, **19**, 257–262.

Fukuhara, S., Tanabe, N., Sato, K., Ohashi, Y. and Kurokawa, K. (1997). Good clinical practice in Japan before and after ICH: Problems and potential impacts on clinical trials and medical practice. *Int. J. Pharmaceut. Med.*, **11**, 147–153.

Fulgraff, G. (1977). General discussion. In: Gross, F. H., Inman, W. H. W. (eds), *Drug Monitoring* 156. Academic Press.

Galant, S. P. (1995). Placebo-controlled versus comparative studies of drug effects. *J. Paediat.*, **126**, 681.

Galpin, J. E., Shinaberger, J. H., Stanley, T. H., Blumenkrantz, M. G., Baver, A. S. *et al* (1978). Acute interstitial nephritis due to methicillin. *Am. J. Med.*, **65**, 756–765.

Gambert, S. R., Csuka, M. E., Duthie, E. H. and Tiegs, R. (1982). Interpretation of laboratory results in the elderly. *Postgrad. Med.*, **72**(3), 147–152.

Gans, K. R., Clark, P., Burka, M. and Smith, C. (1996). Preparing modular labeling for pharmaceuticals and radiopharmaceuticals. *Drug Inf. J.*, **30**, 769–783.

Garvey, T. Q. (1991). Can there really be an integrated safety summary? *Drug Inf. J.*, **25**, 501–511.

Gau, D. W. and Diehl, A. K. (1982). Disagreement among general practitioners regarding cause of death. *Br. Med. J.*, **284**, 239–242.

Gauci, L. (1991). Meeting summary report: biotechnology and drug development. *Drug Inf. J.*, **25**, 551–563.

Geiling, E. M. K. and Cannon, P. R. (1938). Pathological effects of elixir of sulphanil-amide (diethylene glycol) poisoning. *JAMA*, **111**, 919–926.

Gelberg, A. and Armstrong, G. D. (1990). A study of the utilization of the FDA's adverse drug reaction database. *Drug Inf. J.*, **24**, 785–793.

General Considerations for the Clinical Evaluation of Drugs, USA Department of Health, Education and Welfare, Public Health Service Food and Drug Administration, Sept. 1977, 10.

Georgiou, A. (1996). High quality placebos should be used. *Br. Med. J.*, **313**, 1009.

Gershanik, J., Boecler, B., Ensley, H., McCloskey, S. and George, W. (1982). The gasping syndrome and benzyl alcohol poisoning. *N. Engl. J. Med.*, **307**, 1384–1388.

Gerstman, B. B., Lundin, F. E., Stadel, B. V. and Faich, G. A. (1990). A method of pharmacoepidemiologic analysis that uses computerised Medicaid. *J. Clin. Epidemiol.*, **43**(12), 1387–1393.

Ghajar, B. M., Lanctôt, K. L., Shear, N. H. and Naranjo, C. A. (1989). Bayesian differential diagnosis of a cutaneous reaction associated with the administration of sulfonamides. *Semin. Dermatol.*, **8**, 213–218.

Gilbert, G. S., Ting, N, and Zubkoff, L. (1991). A statistical comparison of drug safety in controlled clinical trials: The Genie score as an objective measure of lab abnormalities. *Drug Inf. J.*, **25**, 81–96.

Gill, G. V., Bayliss, P. H., Flear, C. T. G., Skillen, A. W. and Diggle, P. H. (1983). Acute biochemical responses to moderate beer drinking. *Br. Med. J.*, **285**, 1770–1773.

Gill, L. S. and Baber, N. S. (1995). Ethical and scientific review procedures in the pharmaceutical industry: a survey of 12 British-based companies. *Pharm. Med.*, **9**, 11–20.

Gillum, T. (1990). Adverse reaction design for clinical data management. *Drug Inf. J.*, **24**, 769–774.

Girard, M. (1987). Conclusiveness of rechallenge in the interpretation of adverse reactions. *Br. J. Clin. Pharmacol.*, **23**, 73–79.

Girdwood, R. H. (1974). Deaths after taking medicaments. *Br. Med. J.*, **1**, 501–504.

Gitanjali, B., Shashindran, C. H., Tripathi, K. D. and Sethuraman, K. R. (1997). Are drug advertisements in Indian edition of *BMJ* unethical? *BMJ*, **315**, 459.

Gittins, J. (1996). Quantitative methods in planning of pharmaceutical research. *Drug Inf. J.*, **30**, 479–487.

Glynn, J. R. (1993). A question of attribution. *Lancet*, **342**, 530–532.

Godlee, F. (1996). The food industry fights for salt. *Br. Med. J.*, **312**, 1239–1240.

Goettler, M., Schneeweiss, S. and Hasford, J. (1997). Adverse drug reaction monitoring—cost and benefit considerations Part II: cost and preventability of adverse drug reactions leading to hospital admission. *Pharmacoepidemiol. Drug Safety*, **6**, Suppl. 3, S79–S90.

Goldbeck-Wood, S. (1997). Drug company loses battle to stop article. *BMJ*, **315**, 1563.

Goldberg, L. I., Besselaar, G. H., Arnold, J. D., Lamberger, L., Mitchell, J. R. and Whitsett, T. L. (1975). Phase I investigations. *Clin. Pharmacol. Ther.*, **18**(5), 643–646.

Golding, J., Greenwood, R. Birmingham, K. and Mott, M. (1992). Childhood cancer i.m. vitamin k and pethidine given during labour. *Br. Med. J.*, **305**, 341–346.

Golding, J., Paterson, M. and Kinlen L. J. (1990). Factors associated with childhood cancer in a national cohort study. *Br. J. Cancer*, **62**, 304–308.

Goldsmith, D. I., Yen, C. C. and Greenberg, B. P. (1986). A comprehensive system for international pharmaceutical company monitoring of ADR. *Drug Inf. J.*, **20**, 305–310.

Goldstein, D. J., Corbin, L. A. and Sandell, K. L. (1997). Effects of first-trimester fluoxetine exposure on the newborn. *Obstet. Gynecol.*, **89**, 713–718.

Golightly, L. K., Smolinske, S. S., Bennett, M. L., Sutherland, E. W. and Rumack, B. H. (1988). Adverse effects associated with inactive ingredients in drug products. *Med. Toxicol.*, **3**, 128–165, 209–240.

Good practices in pharmacovigilance. Drugs for human use. (1995). *Thérapie*, **50**(6), 547–555.

Gordon, A. J. (1985). Numerators, denominators, and other holy grails: Management and interpretation of worldwide drug safety data. *Drug Inf. J.*, **19**, 319–328.

Gordon-Smith, E. C. (1979). Clinical features in aplastic anaemia. In: *Aplastic Anaemia-Pathophysiology and Approaches to Therapy*. Ed. H. Heimpel, W. Heit and B. Kubanck. Springer, Heidelberg. 9–13.

Gracely, R. H., Dubner, R, Deetez, W. R. and Wolskes, P. T. (1985). Clinicians expectations influence placebo analgesia. *Lancet*, **8419**, 43.

Graham, D. J. and Smith, C. R. (1985). Misclassification in epidemiologic studies of adverse reactions using large managerial data bases. *Progr. Pharmacoepidemiology*. 15–24.

Graham, G. K. (1993). Can safety labeling be harmonized? *Drug Inf. J.*, 27, 447–451.

Grahame-Smith, D. G. (1982). Preclinical toxicological testing and safeguards in clinical trials. *Eur. J. Clin. Pharmacol.*, **22**, 1–6.

Grahame-Smith, D. G. and Aronson, J. K. (1992). *Oxford Textbook of Clinical Pharmacology and Drug Therapy*. (Oxford University Press, Oxford).

Graille, V., Lapeyre-Mestre, M. and Montastruc, J. L. (1994). Drug vigilance: opinion survey among residents of a university hospital. *Thérapie*, **49**(5), 451–454.

Grandjean, P., Sandoe, S. H. and Kimbrough, R. D. (1991). Non-specificity of clinical signs and symptoms caused by environmental chemicals. *Hum. Exp. Toxicol.*, **10**, 167–173.

Green, D. M. (1964). Pre-existing conditions, placebo reactions and 'side effects'. *Ann. Intern. Med.*, **60**(2), 255–265.

Greenhalgh, T. (1986). Drug marketing in the Third World beneath the cosmetic reforms. *Lancet*, 1318–1320.

Greenhouse, J. and Silliman, N. P. (1996). Applications of a mixture survival model with covariates to the analysis of a depression prevention trials. *Stat. Med.*, **15**, 2077–2094.

Griffin, J. P. (1981). Postmarketing surveillance of licensed medicinal and other products. *Health Trends*, **13**, 87.

Griffin, J. P. (1984). Voluntary reporting. In: Walker, S. R. and Goldberg, A. (eds.) *Monitoring for Adverse Drug Reactions.* 21–31. MTP Press.

Griffin, J. P. (1986). Survey of the spontaneous ADR reporting schemes in 15 countries. *Br. J. Clin. Pharmacol.*, **22**, 83S-100S.

Griffin, J. P. and Weber, J. C. P. (1986). Voluntary system of adverse drug reaction reporting. Part II, *Adverse Drug react. Toxicol. Rev.*, **1**, 23–5.

Griffin, M. R., Piper, J. M., Daugherty, J. R., Snowden, M. and Ray, W. A. (1991). Nonsteroidal anti-inflammatory drug use and increased risk for peptic ulcer disease in elderly persons. *Ann. Intern. Med.*, **114**, 257–263.

Grohmann, R., Koch, R. and Schmidt, L. G. (1990). Extrapyramidal symptoms in neuroleptic recipients. In: Weber, E., Lawson, D. H. and Hoigné, R. (eds.), *Agents Actions.* Supplement. **29**.

Grohmann, R., Rütter, E., Sassim, N. and Schmidt, L. G. (1989). Adverse effects of clozapine. *Psychopharm.*, **99**, S101–S104.

Grymonpre, R. E., Mitenko, P. A., Sitar, D. S., Aoki, F. Y. and Montgomery, P. R. (1988). Drug-associated hospital admissions in older medical patients. *J. Am. Geriatr Soc.*, **36**, 1092–1098.

Güdeke, R. (1972). Unwanted effects of drugs in neonates, premature and young children. In Meyler, L. and Peck, H. M. *Drug Induced Diseases.* 585–606, (Excerpta Medica, Amsterdam).

Guess, H. A. (1996). Premarketing applications of pharmacoepidemiology. In: *Pharmacoepidemiology*, 2nd edition. 353–365. Wiley, Chichester.

Guess, H. A. (1991). Pharmacoepidemiology in pre-approval clinical trial safety monitoring. *J. Clin. Epidemiol.*, **44**(8), 851–857.

Guess, H. A., West, R., Strand, L. M., Helston, D., Lydick, E. G., Bergman, U. and Wolski, K. P. (1983). Fatal gastro-intestinal bleeding amongst users and non-users of non-steroidal anti-inflammatory drugs (NSAID) in Saskatchewan, Canada. *J. Clin. Epidemiol.*, **41**, 35–45.

Guideline for Good Clinical Practice. (ICH Harmonised Tripartite Guideline), (1996).

Guideline for the Format and Content of the Clinical and Statistical Sections of New Drug Applications. (1988). 71–74 (Center for Drug Evaluation and Research, U.S. Department of Health and Human Services, Public Health Service, Food and Drug Administration).

Guidelines for Preclinical and Clinical Testing of New Medicinal Products. (1977). Part 2: Investigations in Man. *Ass. Br. Pharm. Ind.*, **13**.

Gurdon, H. (1994). Japan drug firm shut after 15 patients die. *Daily Telegraph*, September 2nd. pp13.

Gurwitz, G. H. and Avorn, J. (1990). Old age, is it a risk for ADR?. In: Weber, E., Lawson, D. H., and Hoigné, R (eds.) *Risk factors for ADR—Epidemiological Approaches.* Agents Actions, Birkhauser, Suppl. 29, 13–25.

Guy, W. (1976) Dosage record and treatment emergent symptom scale. In: *ECDU Assessment Manual for Psychopharmacology.* (US Department of Health, Education and Welfare, intercom issues; 6–F1).

Guy, W. and Ban T.A. (1982). *The AMDP System. A Manual for Assessment and Documentation in Psychopathology.* (Springer Verlag, Heidelberg).

Guyatt, G. H. (1984). *The Questionnaire in the Assessment of Cardio-respiratory disease. The McMaster Approach.* An ICI publication of a workshop held in April 1984 on the assessment of the effect of drug therapy on the quality of life in cardiorespiratory disease.

Guyatt, G. H., Berman, L. B., Townsend, M. and Wayne Taylor, D. (1985). Should study subjects see their previous responses?. *J. Chron. Dis.*, **38**, (12), 1003–1007.

Guyatt, G. H., Thompson, P. J., Berman, L. B., Sullivan, M. J., Townsend, M., Jones, M. L. and Pugsley, S. O. (1985). How should we measure function in patients with chronic heart and lung disease? *J. Chron. Dis.*, **38**(6), 517–524.

Guyatt, G. H., Townsend, M., Berman, L. B. and Keller, J. L. (1987). A comparison of Likert and visual analogue scales for measuring change in function. *J. Chron. Dis.*, **40**, 1129–1133.

Guzé, B. H. and Baxter, L. R. (1985). Neuroleptic malignant syndrome. *N. Engl. J. Med.*, **313**(3), 163–166.

H. P. (1958). 'Stalinon': A therapeutic disaster. *Br. Med. J.*, **1**, 515.

Haber, P., Gordon, S., Elterman, D., House, S., Chen, R. T. (1994). Assessing extent of misclassification of early Guillain-Barré syndrome—vaccine adverse reporting system, US, 1990–94. *Pharmacoepidemiol Drug Safety*, **3**, Suppl. 1, S34.

Habibi, B., Solal-Céligny, P. H., Benichou, C., Castot, A., Danan, G., Lagier, G., Lavarenne, J. and Soubrie, C. (1988). Anémies hémolytiques d'origine médicamenteuse. *Thérapie*, **43**, 117–120.

Hackett, T., Kelton, J. G. and Owers, P. (1982). Drug-induced platelet destruction. *Semin. Thromb. Haem.*, **8**(2), 116–137.

Hagman, M., Jönsson, D. and Ilhelmson, L. (1977). Prevalence of angina pectoris and myocardial infarction in a general population sample of Swedish men. *Acta. Med. Scand.*, **201**, 571–577.

Hale, M. (1996). Exploring relationships between adverse events and pharmacokinetics. Presented at the *Adverse Events Workshop, Oct 1996, Washington D.C.*

Hale. W. E., May, F. E., Marks, R. G. and Tewart, R. B. (1987). Drug use in an ambulatory elderly population: A 5–year update. *Drug. Intell. Clin. Pharm.*, **21**, 530–535.

Hall, C. (1997). Rise in abortions after thrombosis scare over pill. *Daily Telegraph.* 21.2.1997.

Hallas, J., Gram, L. F., Grodum, E., Damster, N., Brosen, K. *et al.* (1992). Drug-related admissions to medical wards: a population based survey. *Br. J. Clin. Pharmacol.*, **33**, 61–68.

Hamilton, M. A. (1960). A rating scale for depression. *J. Neurol. Neurosurg. Psychiat.*, **23**, 56.

Hampton, J. R. and Julian, D. G. (1987). Role of the pharmaceutical industry in major clinical trials. *Lancet*, 1258.

Hanif, M., Mobarek, M. R., Ronan, A., Rahman, D., Donovan, J. J. and Bennish, M. L. (1995). Fatal renal failure caused by diethylene glycol in paracetamol elixir: the Bangladesh epidemic. *Br. Med. J.*, **311**, 88–91.

Hanley, J. A. and Lippman-Hand, A. (1983). If nothing goes wrong, is everything alright? Interpreting zero numerators. *JAMA*, **249**, 1743–1745.

Hansson, O. (1980). The voice of the consumer. In: Soda, T. (ed.) *Drug-induced Sufferings. Medical, Pharmaceutical and Legal Aspects.* 20. (Excerpta Medica, Amsterdam).

Hansson, O. and Herxheimer, A. (1984). Halogenated hydroxyquinolines still no end. *Lancet,* 13 Oct.

Haramburu, F. (1993). Estimation of under reporting. In: Arme, P. (ed.) *Methodolog. App. Pharmacoepidemiol.,* 39–49.

Haramburu, F., Abraham, E. and Bégaud, B.(1993). Users of a regional center of pharmacovigilance. *Thérapie,* **48**(5), 475–477.

Haramburu, F., Bégaud, B. and Moride, Y. (1997). Temporal trends in spontaneous reporting of unlabelled adverse drug reaction. *Br. J. Clin. Pharmacol.,* **44**, 299–301.

Haramburu, F., Bégaud, B., Péré, J. C., Marcel, S. and Albin, H. (1985). Role of medical journals in adverse drug reaction alerts. *Lancet,* **2**, 550–551.

Harkins, R. D. (1996). Uses of laboratory data in antiinfective drug approval processes. *Drug. Inf. J.,* **30**, 811–813.

Harlow, B. J. (1972). Monitoring of adverse reactions by a pharmaceutical company before marketing. In: Richards D. J. and Rondel R. K. (eds.) *Adverse Drug Reactions.* (Churchill Livingstone, Edinburgh).

Harris, E. K. and Yasaka, T., (1983) On the calculation of a 'reference change' for comparing two consecutive measurements. *Clin. Chem.,* **29**(1) 25–30.

Harris, T. A. J. (1994). Clinical research aspects of sampling, storage, and shipment of blood samples. *Drug Inf. J.,* **28**, 377–381.

Harrow, D. W. G., Griffiths, K. and Shanks, R. G. (1980). Debendox and congenital malformations in Northern Ireland. *Br. Med. J.,* **281**, 1274–1381.

Harry, J. D., Baber, N. and Posner, J. (1995). HIV screening in healthy volunteers. *Br. J. Clin. Pharmacol.,* **39**, 213.

Hartl, P. W. (1973). Drug-induced agranulocytosis. In: Girdwood, R. H. (ed.) *Blood Disorders due to Drugs and Other Agents.* 147–186.

Hasford, J. (1996). Drug utilization during pregnancy and its effects on fetal outcome. The Pegasus Project. Abstract. *1st Congress of the European Drug Utilization Research Group. Rational Drug Use in Europe. Challenges for the 21st century. June 27–30th.*

Hayashi, K. and Walker, A. M. (1996). Japanese and American reports of randomised trials: differences in the reporting of adverse effects. *Control. Clin. Trials,* **17**, 99–110.

Hays, D. R. (1993). Bendectin, a case of morning sickness. *Drug Intelligence in Clinical Pharmacy.,* **17**(11), 826–7.

Hecht, A. (1987). Diet, drug dangers – déjà vu. *FDA Consumer.,* 22nd Feb. 22–27.

Hedner, T., Samuelson, O., Lunde, H., Lindholm, L., Andrew, L. and Wiholm, B-E. (1992). Angioedema in relation to treatment with ACE inhibitors. *Br. Med. J.,* **304**, 941–6.

Hegarty, J. and Williams, R. (1987). Investigation of the jaundiced patient, *Practitioner,* **231**, 441–417.

Heilman, K. (1988). The perception of drug-related risk. In: Burley, D. and Inman, W. H. W. (eds.) *Therapeutic Risk: Perception, Measurement, Management.* 1–11, Wiley and Sons Ltd, Chichester.

Heimpel, H. (1988). Drug-induced agranulocytosis. *Med. Toxicol,* **3**, 449–462.

Heimpel, H. and Heit, W. (1980). Drug-induced aplastic anaemia: clinical aspects. *Clin. Haematol,* **9**, 641–662.

Helander, A., Voltaire Carlsson, A. and Borg, S. (1995). Longitudinal comparison of carbohydrate-deficient serum transferrin and gamma-glutamyl transferase: Complementary markers of excessive alcohol consumption. *Alcohol*, **30**.

Helling-Borda, M. S., Manell, P. and Madall, H. (1986). Use of computers in drug monitoring. In: Inman, W. H. W. *Monitoring for Drug Safety*, 2nd edition. 305–322 (MTP Press).

Helzberg, J. H. (1986). 'LFTs' test more than the liver. *JAMA*, **256**, 3006–3007.

Hemeryck, L., Chan, R., McCormack, P. M. E., Condren, L. and Feely, J. (1995). Pharmaceutical advertisements in Irish medical journals. *J. Pharm. Med.*, **5**, 147–151.

Hemeryck, L., McGettigan, P., Chan, P., McCormack, P., Condren, L. and Feely, J. (. . . An audit of pharmaceutical advertisements).

Hemminki, E. (1980). Study of information submitted by drug companies to licensing authorities. *Br. Med. J.*, 833–836.

Henry, D. and Hill, S. (1995). Comparing treatments. *Lancet*, **310**, 1279.

Herbst, A. L., Ulfelder, H. and Poskanzer, D. C. (1971). Association of maternal stilboestrol therapy with tumour appearance in young women. *N. Engl. J. Med.*, **284**, 878.

Herman, R. L. and Lorgus, L. Y. (1983). Computer generation of the FDA 1639 form. *Clin. Res. Pract. Drug. Reg. Affairs* **1**, 209–225.

Herson, J. (1996). Risk vs benefit in safety analysis. Presented at the *Adverse Event Workshop*. Washington D.C.

Herxheimer, A. (1987). Basic information that prescribers are not getting about drugs. *Lancet*, **1**, 31–33.

Herxheimer, A. (1988). *Drugs and Therapeut. Bull.*, **26**(23), 89–91.

Herxheimer, A. (1991). How much drug in the tablet? *Lancet*, **337**, 346–348.

Herxheimer, A. and Lionel, N. D. W. (1970). Assessing reports of therapeutic trials. *Proc. Br. Pharm. Soc.*, 204–205P.

Herxheimer, A. and Lionel, N. D. W. (1978). Minimum information needed by prescriber. *Br. Med. J.*, **2**, 1129–1132.

Herxheimer, A., Collier, J., Rawlins, M. D., Schonhofer, P., Medewar, C., Melrose, D., Bannenberg, W. and Beardshaw, V. (1985). Butazones under fire. *Lancet*, **1**, 580.

Hibberd, P. L. and Meadows, A. J. (1980). Information contained in clinical trial reports. *J. Inform. Sci.*, **2**, 165–168.

Higginbotham, F. M. and Rolan, P. E. (1997). Clinical pharmacology studies in women of child-bearing potential. *Intern J. Pharmaceut. Med.*, **11**, 7–9.

Hilden, J. (1987). Reporting clinical trials from the viewpoint of a patients choice of treatment. *Stat. Med.*, **6**, 745–752.

Hiller, J. L., Benda, G. I., Rahatzad, M., Allen, J. R., Culver, D. H *et al.* (1986). Benzyl alcohol toxicity: impact on mortality and intraventricular haemorrhage among very low birth weight infants. *Pediatrics*, **77**, 500–506.

Hilts, P. J. (1993). After deaths, FDA is proposing stiffer rules on drug experiments. *New York Times*, November 16th, A1.

Hirokawa, K. (1996). Clinical pharmacologists and drug regulations—future perspective in Japan. *Br. J. Clin. Pharmacol*, **42**, 63–71.

Hoberman, D. (1995). Drug promotion. *N. Engl. J. Med.*, **332**, 1031.

Hoek, R., Stricker, B. H. Ch., Ottervanger, J. P. and Van der Velden, K. (1995). Reporting of suspected adverse reactions to drugs in primary care. *Pharmacoepidemiol Drug Safety*, **4**, S23.

Hoekman, K., Von Blomberg-Van der Flier, B. M. E., Wagstaff, J., Drexhage, H. A. and Pinedo, H. M. (1991). Reversible thyroid dysfunction during treatment with GM-CSF. *Lancet*, **338**, 541–542.

Hoigné, R. V. (1997). Should 'Idiosyncrasy' be defined as equivalent to 'Type B' adverse drug reactions? *Pharmacoepidemiol Drug Safety*, **6**, 213.

Hoigné, R., D'Andrea Jaeger, M., Wymann, R., Egli, A., Müller, U., Hess, T., Galeazzi, R., Maibach, R. and Künze, U. P. (1990).Time pattern of allergic reactions to drugs. *Agents and Actions, Risk factors for ADR* Vol.29. Birkhauser, Basel. 39–57.

Hoigné, R., Schlumberger, H. P., Vervloet, D. and Zoppi, M. (1993). Epidemiology of allergic drug reactions. *Monogr Allergy.*, **31**, 147–170.

Hoigné, R., Sollberger, J., Zopp, M., Müller, U., Hess, T. Fritshy, D., Stocken, F. and Maibach, R. (1984). Die Bedeutung von Alter, geschelch Nierenfunktion, Atopie und Anzahl verabreichter Medikamente für das Auftreten von Nebenwirkungen, untersucht mit Methoden der multivariaten Statistik. Ergebnisse aus dem komprehensiven Spital-Drug-Monitoring Bern (C.H.D.M.B.). *Schweizer. Medizi. Wochenschr.*, **114**, 1854–1857.

Hoitsma, A. J., Wetzels, J. F. M. and Koene, R. A. P. (1991). Drug-induced nephrotoxicity, aetiology, clinical features and management. *Drug Safety*, **6**(2), 131–147.

Hollenberger, N. K., Testa, M. and Williams, G. H. (1991). Quality of life as a therapeutic end-point. An analysis of therapeutic trials in hypertension. *Drug Safety*, **6**(2), 83–93.

Hollister, L. E. (1972). Prediction of therapeutic users of psycho-therapeutic drugs from experience with normal volunteers. *Clin. Pharmacol. Ther.*, **13.5**(2), 803–808.

Hollister, L. E., Martz, B. L., Carr, E. A., Cohn, H. D., Crout, J. R. and Levine, J. (1975). Phase II investigations. *Br. J. Clin. Pharmacol*, **18**(5), 647–649.

Holmes, D., Holms, M. and Teresi, J. (1988). Routine collection of medication side effect data using computer terminals located in a senior centre. *Practice Concepts*, **28**(1), 105–107.

Homma, M., Hirayama, H., Noguchi, T. and Ichikawa, K. (1994). Studies on requirements for the assessment of clinical safety in nonsteroidal anti-inflammatory drugs. *Drug Inf. J.*, **28**, 413–418.

Horace, V. (1994). Good clinical practice in Europe. PJB publications, 4th edition. Scrip report.

Horton, R. (1994). The context of consent. *Lancet*, **344**, 211–212.

Horwitz, R. I. and Feinstein, A. R. (1980). The problem of protopathic bias in case control studies. *Am. J. Med.*, **68**, *255–258*.

Horwitz, R. I. and Feinstein, A. R. (1981). The application of therapeutic trial principles to improve the design of epidemiological research—a case control study suggesting that anticoagulants reduce mortality in patients with myocardial infarction. *J. Chron. Dis.*, **34**, 575–581.

Hoskins, R. E. and Mannino, S. (1992). Causality assessment of adverse drug reactions using decision support and information tools. *Pharmacoepidemiol. Drug Safety.*, **1**, 235–249.

Hostelley, L. (1989). Report and tracking spontaneous adverse experience, reports on a computer database. *Drug Inf. J.*, **23**, 171–177.

Houghton, R. (1993). Medicines Information Bill. *Br. Med. J.*, **341**, 1208–1209.

Hounslow, N. J., Tamarazians, S., Wisema, W. T., Mann, S. and Vandenburg M. J. (1987). Use of a visual analogue meter. *Br. J. Clin. Pharmacol.*, **23**(I), 117–118.

Howse, J. G. R. and Clark, G. A. (1970). Double blind trial of early dimethyl-chlortetracycline in minor respiratory illness in general practice. *Lancet.*, **2**, 1099–1102.

Hsu, P. W. and Stoll, R. W.(1993). Causality assessment of adverse events in clinical trials: I. How good is the investigator drug causality assessment? *Drug Inf. J.*, **27**, 377–385.

Hsu, P. W. and Stoll, R. W. (1993). Causality assessment of adverse events in clinical trials: II. An algorithm for drug causality assessment. *Drug. Inf. J.*, **27**, 387–394.

Hu, D. N., Qin, W. Q., Wu, B. T., Fang, L. Z., Zhou, F., Gu, Y. P., Zhang, Q. H., Yan, J. H., Ding, Y. Q. and Wong, H. (1991). Genetic aspects of antibiotic-induced deafness: mitochondrial inheritance. *J. Med. Genet.*, **28**, 79-83.

Huang, M. Y. and Schacht, J. (1989). Drug induced ototoxicity, pathogenesis and prevention. *Med. Toxicol. Adv. Drug Exp.*, **4**(6), 452–467.

Hughes, J. R., Higgins, S. T., Bickel, W. K., Hunt, W. K., Fenwick, J. W., Gulliver, S. B. and Mireault, G. C. (1991). Caffeine self-administration, withdrawal and adverse effects among coffee drinkers. *Arch. Gen. Psychiat.*, **48**, 611–617.

Hurn, B. A. L. and Tilson, H. H. (1988). Electronic drug safety surveillance in North America. *Pharm. Med.*, **2**, 359–369.

Hurwitz, N. (1969). Intensive hospital monitoring of adverse reactions to drugs, *Br. Med. J.*, **1**, 531–536.

Hurwitz, B. and Richardson, R. (1997). Swearing to care: the resurgence in medical oaths. *BMJ*, **315**, 1671–1674.

Huskisson, E. C. (1973). Good and bad clinical trials: a checklist. *J. Hosp. Pharm.*

Huskisson, E. C. (1974). Measurement of pain. *Lancet*, **2**, 1127–1131.

Huskisson, E.C. (1976). Assessment of clinical trials. *Clin. Rheum. Dis*, **2**(1), 37–49.

Huskisson, E. C. and Wojtulewski, J. A. (1974). Measurement of side effects of drugs. *Br. Med. J.,* **2**, 698–699.

Huster, W. J. (1991). Clinical trial adverse events: The case for descriptive techniques. *Drug. Inf. J.*, **25**, 447–456.

Hutchings, A. D. and Routledge, P. A. (1986). A simple method for determining acetylator phenotype using isoniazid. *Br. J. Clin. Pharmacol.*, **22**, 343–345.

Hutchinson, T. A. (1986). Standardised assessment methods for adverse drug reactions: a review of previous approaches and their problems. *Drug Inf. J.*, **20**, 439–444.

Hutchinson, T. A. (1992). Causality assessment of suspected adverse drug reactions. In: *Detection of New Adverse Drug Reactions.* Ed. M. D. B. Stephens, Macmillan Press, London.

Hutchinson, T. A. and Lane, D. A. (1989). Assessing methods for causality assessment of suspected adverse drug reactions. *J. Clin. Epidemiol.*, **42**, 5–16.

Hutchinson, T. A., Dawid, A. P., Spiegelhalter, D. J., Cowell, R. G. and Roden, S. (1991a). Computerized aids for probabilistic assessment of drug safety I: A spreadsheet program. *Drug. Inf. J.*, **25**, 29–39.

Hutchinson, T. A., Flegel, K. M., Kramer, M. S., Leduc, D. G. and Ho Ping Kong, H. (1986). Frequency, severity and risk factors for adverse drug reactions in adult out-patients: a prospective study. *Chron. Dis.*, **9**(7), 533–542.

Hutchinson, T. A., Leventhal, J. M., Kramer, M. S., Karch, F. E., Lipman, A. G. and Feinstein, A. R. (1979). An algorithm for the operational assessment of adverse drug reactions. II: Demonstration of reproducibility and validity. *JAMA.*, **242**, 633–8.

Hvidberg, E. F. (1994). Continuous improvement of ethics committees. *Drug. Inf. J.*, **28**, 1125–1128.

ICH E6 Guideline. (1996). Good Clinical Practice – Step 4.

ICH3 Topic EZC (1996). *Clinical safety Data Management, Periodic Safety Update Reports for Marketed Drugs.*

Idänpään-Heikkilä, J. (1983). *A Review of Safety Information Obtained From Phase I, II and III Clinical Investigation of Sixteen Selected Drugs.* (USA Department of Health and Human Services, Public Health Service Food and Drug Administration).

In brief (1997). Slimming drugs withdrawn following heart scare. *Br. Med. J.*, **315**, 698.

In brief (1998). Calcium channel blocker withdrawn. *BMJ*, **316**, 1766.

Inman, W. H. W. (1986). The United Kingdom. In: *Monitoring for Drug Safety.* MTP Press, Lancaster.

Inman, W. H. W. (1972). Monitoring by voluntary reporting at national level. In: Richards, D. J. and Rondel, R. K. (eds.) *Adverse Drug Reactions.* (Churchill Livingstone, Edinburgh).

Inman, W. H. W. (1977). Study of fatal bone marrow depression with special reference to phenylbutazone and oxyphenbutazone. *Br. Med. J.*, **1**, 1500–1505.

Inman, W. H. W. (1981a). Postmarketing surveillance of adverse drug reaction in general practice. I: Search for new methods. *Br. Med. J.*, **282**, 1131–1132.

Inman, W. H. W. (1981b). Postmarketing surveillance of adverse drug reaction in general practice. II: PEM at the University of Southampton. *Br. Med. J.*, **282**, 1216–1217.

Inman, W. H. W. and Adelstein, A. M. (1969). Rise and fall of asthma mortality in England and Wales in relation to pressurised aerosols. *Lancet*, **2**, 279.

Inman, W. H. W. and Mustrin, W. W. (1974). Jaundice after repeated exposure to halothane: an analysis of reports to the Committee on Safety of Medicines. *Br. Med. J.*, **1**(5).

Inman, W. H. W. and Rawson, N. S. B. (1983). Erythromycin estolate and jaundice. *Br. Med. J.*, **286**, 1954–1955.

Inman, W. H. W. and Vessey, M. P. (1968). Investigation of deaths from pulmonary, coronary and cerebral thrombosis and embolism in women of childbearing age. *Br. Med. J.*, **2**, 193–199.

Inman, W. H. W., Vessey, M. P., Westerholm, B. and Engelind, A. (1970). Thromboembolic disease and the steroidal content of oral contraceptives. *Br. Med. J.*, **2**, 203.

Inman, W. H. W., Wilton, L. V., Pearce, G. L. and Waller, P. C. (1990). Prescription event monitoring of Nabumetone. *Pharm. Med.*, **4**, 309–317.

International conference on Harmonisation (1993). *Clinical Safety Data Management: Definitions and Standards for Expedited Reporting. Draft Consensus Text. June 24th.*

International Conference on Harmonization. (1994) *Clinical Safety Data Management: Definitions and Standards for Expedited Reporting, a Step 4 Paper, ICH-2 EWG E2.*

Irey, N. S. (1972). Diagnostic problems in drug-induced diseases. In: *Drug-Induced Diseases*. **Vol. 4**, Ed. L. Meyler, H. M. Peck. Amsterdam, Excerpta Medica, pp1–24.

Isaacs, A. J. (1988). Driving and drug regulations. *Int. Clin. Psychopharmacol.*, **3** Suppl. 1, 141–146.

Isaacs, B., MacArthur, J. G. and Taylor, R. M. (1955). Jaundice in relation to chlorpromazine therapy. *Br. Med. J.*, **ii**, 1122.

Israel-Biet, D., Labrune, S., Huchon, G. J. (1991). Drug-induced lung disease: 1990 review. *Eur. Respir. J.*, **4**, 465–478.

Iwarson, S. (1985). Pharmaceutical companies and unexpected drug side effects. *Lancet*, 580.

Jachuck, S. J., Brierley, H., Jachuck, S. and Willcox, P. M. (1982). The effect of hypotensive drugs on the quality of life. *J. Roy. Coll. Gen. Pract.*, **32**, 103–105.

Jackson, D. (1990). The assessment of tolerance and side effects in non-patient volunteers. In: O'Grady, J. and Linit, O. I. (eds.) *Early Phase Drug Evaluation in Man.* 197 Macmillan.

Jackson, D. (1990). The assessment of tolerance and side-effects in non-patient volunteers. In: Weber, E., Lawson, D. H. and Hoigné, R. (eds.) Risk factors for ADR—Epidemiological Approach. *Agents Actions*, Suppl. 29, 199.

Jacobson, A. F., Goldstein, B. J., Dominguez, R. A. and Steinbook, R. M. (1986). Interrater agreement and interclass reliability measures of SAFTEE in psychopharmacological clinical trials. *Psychopharm. Bull.*, **22**(2), 382–388.

Jacubeit, T., Drisch, D. and Weber, U. (1990). Risk factors as reflected by an intensive drug monitoring system. In Weber, E., Lawson, D. H. and Hoigné, R. (eds.) *Risk factors for ADR-Epidemiological approaches. Agents Actions*, Supple. 29, 117–125.

Jaeschke, J., Singer, J. and Guyatt G. H. (1990). Comparison of seven-point and visual analogue scales. *Contr. Clin. Trials*, **11**, 43–51.

Jagathesan, R., Lewis, L. D. and Mant, T. G. K. (1995). A retrospective analysis of the prevalence of HIV seropositivity and its demographics in the normal healthy volunteer population of a phase I clinical drug study unit. *Br. J. Clin. Pharmacol.*, **39**, 463–464.

Jain, K. K. (1995). A short practical method for triage of adverse drug reactions. *Drug Inf. J.*, **29**, 339–342.

James, B. C. (1997). Every defect a treasure: learning from adverse events in hospitals. *Med. J. Aust.*, **166**, 484–487.

Jandl, J. H. (1987). *Blood: Textbook of Haematology.* Little Brown and Co.

Jefferys, D. B. (1995). Children in research: ethical and practical issues. *DIA Conference, Future Outlook for New Pharmaceuticals Post-1995*, April 2–5.

Jefferys, D. B. (1995). The marketing authorization application. In: Mann, R. D., Rawlins, M. D. and Auty, R. M. (eds.) *Pharmaceutical Medicine Current Practice.* 205. Parthenon Publishing Group.

Jefferys, D. B., Matthews, B. R. and Ritchie, J. C. (1991). Defects in applications – an analysis. In: Cartwright, A. C. and Matthews, B. R. (eds.) *Pharmaceutical Product Licensing; Requirements for Europe.* Ellis Horwood.

Jenkins, W. (1985). Adverse event reporting for UK product licence. Pre-marketing adverse drug experience. *Data Management Procedures Drug Information Workshop, December.*

Jenkinson, C., Peto, V., Fitzpatrick, R., Greenhall, R. and Hyman, N. (1995). Self-reported functioning and well-being in patients with Parkinson's disease: Comparison of the short-form health survey (SF-36) and the Parkinson's disease questionnaire (PDQ-39). *Age Ageing,* **24**, 505–509.

Jenner, P. N. (1990). A 12–month post-marketing surveillance study of Nabumetone. A preliminary report. *Drugs,* **40**, Suppl. 5, 80–86.

Jennings, K. (1996). Antibodies to streptokinase. *Br. Med. J.,* **312**, 393–4.

Jick, H. (1984). Boston collaborative drug surveillance program. In: Walker, S. R. and Goldberg, A. (eds.) *Monitoring for ADR.* (MTP Press, Lancester).

Jick, H., Jick, S. S. and Derby, L. E. (1991). Validation of information recorded on general practitioner based computerised data resource in the United Kingdom. *Br. Med. J.,* **302**, 766–768.

Jick, H., Madsen, S., Nudelman, P. M., Perera, D. R. and Stergachis, A. (1984). Postmarketing follow-up of Group Health co-operative of Puget Sound. *Pharmacotherapy,* **4**(2), 99–100.

Jick, H., Slone, D., Shapiro, S., Lewis, G. P., Worcester, J., Westerholm, B., Inman, W. H. W. and Vessey, M. P. (1969). *Lancet.,* **1**, 539–542.

Joelson, S., Joelson, I. B. and Wallander, M. A. (1997). Geographical variation in adverse event reporting rates in clinical trials. *Pharmacoepidemiol Drug Safety,* **6**, Suppl. 3, S31–S35.

Johnson, B. F., Fowle, A. S. E., Lader, S., Fox, J. and Munro-Faure, A. D. (1973). Biological availability of digoxin from Lanoxin produced in the U.K. *Br. Med. J.,* **4**, 323–326.

Johnson, J. M., Tanner, L. A. and Barash, D. (1993). Safety signals from adverse drug experience reports at FDA: Part II. *Drug Inf. J.,* **27**, 1167–1171.

Johnson, S. T. and Wordell, C. J. (1998). Internet utilization among medical information specialists in the pharmaceutical industry and academia. *DIJ,* **32**, 547–554.

Johnson-Pratt, L. R. and Bush, J. (1996). Activities of the pharmaceutical industry relative to the FDA gender guidelines. *Drug Inf. J.,* **30**, 709–714.

Johnston, J. D. and Hawthorne, S. W. (1997). How to minimise factitious hyperkalaemia in blood samples from general practice. *Br. Med. J.,* **314**, 1200–1201.

Joint Committee of ABPI, BMA, CSM and RCGP. (1988). Guidelines on Post-marketing surveillance. *Br. Med. J.,* **296**, 399–400.

Jones, D. R., Fayers, P. M. and Simons, J. (1987). Measuring and analysing quality of life in cancer clinical trials: a review. In: Aaronson, N. K. and Beckmann, J. (eds.) *The Quality of Life of Cancer Patients Monograph Series of the European Organisation for Research on Treatment of Cancer (EORTC),* **17**, 41–62.

Jones, J. K. (1982). Adverse drug reactions in the community health setting: Approaches to recognizing, counselling, and reporting. *Fam. Commun. Health,* **5**, 58–67.

Jones, J. K. (1982). Criteria for journal reports of suspected adverse drug reactions. *Clin. Pharm.,* **1**, 554–555.

Jones, J. K. (1992). Causality assessment of suspected adverse drug reactions: a tranatlantic view. *Pharmacoepidemiol. Drug Safety.,* **1**, 251–260.

Josefson, D. (1996). Herbal stimulant causes US deaths, *Br. Med. J.*, **312**, 1378–1379.

Joseph, M. C., Schoeffler, K., Doi, P. A., Yefko, H., Engle, C. and Nissman, E. F. (1991). An automated COSTART coding scheme. *Drug Inf. J.*, **25**, 97–108.

Joubert, P. H., Van Rijssen, F. W. J. and Venter, J. P. (1977). Drug side effects assessed in a 'naturalistic' setting. *S. Afr. Med. J.*, **52**, 34–36.

Joubert, P., Rivera-Calimlim, L. and Lasagna, L. (1975). The normal volunteer in clinical investigation. How rigid should selection criteria be? *Clin. Pharmacol. Ther.*, **17**(3), 253–256.

Joyce, C. R. B. (1982). Placebos and other comparative treatments. *Br. J. Clin. Pharmacol.*, **13**, 313–318.

Joyce, C. R. B. and Joyce, J. (1983). Pyramidal publication. *Eur. J. Clin. Pharmacol.*, 25, 1–2.

Joyce, C. R. B., Zutshi, D. W., Hrubes, V. and Mason, R. M. (1975). Comparison of fixed interval and visual analogue scales for rating chronic pain. *Eur. J. Clin. Pharmacol.*, **8**, 415–420.

Kafader, D. (1997). The internet information avalanche: How not to get buried. *Regul. Affairs Focus*, **2**, 8.

Kalish, R. S. (1995). Drug promotion. *N. Engl. J. Med.*, **332**, 1032.

Kalow, W. and Genest, K. (1957). A method for the detection of atypical forms of serum cholinesterase. Determination of dibucaine numbers. *Biochem. Cell. Biol.*, **35**, 339–346.

Kalra, L., Jackson, S. H. D. and Swift, C. G. (1993). Assessment of changes in psychomotor performance of elderly subjects. *Br. J. Clin. Pharmacol.*, **36**, 383–389.

Kando, J. C., Yonkers, K. A. and Cole, J. O. (1995). Fatal renal failure caused by diethylene glycol in paracetamol elixir: the Bangladesh epidemic. *Drugs*, **50**(1), 1–6.

Kaplan, A. P. (1984). Drug-induced skin disease. *J. Allerg. Clin. Immunol.*, **74**, 573–579.

Karch, F. E. and Lasagna, L. (1975). Adverse drug reactions. *JAMA.*, **234**, (12), 1236.

Karch, F. E. and Lasagna, L. (1977). Toward the operational identification of adverse drug reactions. *Clin. Pharmacol. Ther.*, **21** (3), 247–254.

Karch, F., Smith, C., Kerzner, B., Mazullo, J., Weintraub, M. and Lasagna, L. (1976). Adverse drug reactions a matter of opinion. *Clin. Pharmacol. Ther.*, **19**, 489–492.

Katz, J., Marmary, Y., Livneh, A. and Danon, Y. (1991). Drug allergy in Sjögren's syndrome. *Lancet*, **337**, 239.

Kearns, I. (1996). Introduction: drug development for infants and children: rescuing the therapeutic orphan. *Drug Inf. J.*, **30**, 1121–1123.

Kershner, R., Marsters, P., Ebrahimi, R., Fitzpatrick, S. and Cater, J. (1990). *Development of International Clinical Pooling and Reporting Strategy for Laboratory Abnormalities. D.I.A. Euromeeting, Amsterdam.*

Kessler, D. A. (1991). Drug promotion and scientific exchange: the role of the clinical investigator. *N. Engl. J. Med.*, **325**(3), 201–203.

Kessler, D. A. (1992). Addressing the problem of misleading advertisements. *Ann. Intern. Med.*, **116**, 950–951.

Kessler, D. A. (1993). Introducing MEDWatch; a new approach to reporting medication and device adverse effects and product problems. *JAMA*, **269**, (21), 2765–2768.

Kessler, D. A., Hass, A. E., Feiden, K. L., Lumpkin, M. and Temple, R. (1996). Approval of new drugs in the United States. *JAMA*, **276**, (22), 1826–1831.

Kessler, D. A., Rose, J. L., Temple, R. J., Schapiro, R. and Griffin, J. P. (1994). Therapeutic-class wars—drug promotion in a competitive marketplace. *N. Engl. J. Med.*, **331**, 1350– 1353.

Kessler, D. A., Rose, J. L., Temple, R. J., Schapiro, R. and Griffin, J. P. (1995). Drug promotion. *N. Engl. J. Med.*, **332**, 1033.

Kevany, J. (1996). Extreme poverty: an obligation ignored. *Br. Med. J.*, **313**, 65–66.

Kiley, R. (1997). Current awareness services on the Internet. *J. R. Soc. Med.*, **90**, 540–542.

Kiley, R. (1997). How to get medical information from the internet. *J. Roy. Soc. Med.*, **90**, 488–490.

Kiley, R. (1997). Medical databases on the Internet: Part 1. *J. Roy. Soc. Med.*, **90**, 610–611.

Kimbel, K. H. (1992). Secrecy and product information. *Lancet.*, **339**, 312.

Kimmel, S. E., Goldberg, L., Sekeres, M., Berlin, J. and Strom, B. L. (1995). Incidence and predictors of under reporting of serious adverse events following protamine administration. Abstract 080. *Pharmacoepidemiol. Drug Safety*, **4**, Suppl. 1, S35.

King, S. W., Statland, B. E. and Savery, J. (1976) The effect of a short burst of exercise on activity values of enzymes in sera of healthy young men. *Clin. Chim. Acta*, **72**, 211–218.

Kinney, E. L., Trautmann, J., Gold, J. A., Vesell, E. S. and Zeiis, R. (1981). Under-representation of women in new drug trials: ramifications and remedies. *Ann. Intern. Med.*, **95**(4), 495–499.

Kirkpatrick, M. A. F. (1991). Factors that motivate healthy adults to participate in phase I drug trials. *Drug Inf. J.*, **25**, 109–113.

Kitaguchi, T., Nojiri, T, Suzuki, S., Fukita, T. and Kawana, T. (1983). Some assessment systems for industry post-marketing adverse drug reaction (ADR) information. *Iyakuhin Kenkyu*, **14**(6), 980–992.

Kitchener, S., Malekottodjary, N. and McClelland, G. R. (1996). Adverse effects from placebo-treated healthy volunteers. *Br. J. Clin. Pharmacol.*, **41**, 473.

Kitler, M. E. (1989). The elderly in clinical trials: Regulatory concerns. *Drug Inf. J.*, **23**, 123–137.

Klebanoff, M. A., Read, J. S., Mills, J. L. and Shiono, P. H. (1993). The risk of childhood cancer after neonatal exposure to vitamin K. *N. Engl. J. Med.*, **329**, (13), 905–908.

Klotz, U. and Ammon, E. (1998). Clinical and toxicological consequences of the inductive potential of ethanol. *Eur. J. Clin. Pharmacol.*, **54**, 7–12.

Knowles, J. B. and Lucas, C. J. (1960). Experimental studies of the placebo response. *J. Ment. Sci.*, **106**, 231– 240.

Knox, E. G. (1975). Negligible risks to health. *Community Health.*, **6**, 244–251.

Koch, G., Schmid, J., Begun, J. and Maier, W. (1993). Meta-analysis of drug safety data. In: Sogliero-Gilbert, G. (ed.) *Drug Assessment in Clinical Trials.* (ed.), Marcel Dekker, New York.

Koch-Weser, J., Sellers, E. M. and Zacest, R. (1977). The ambiguity of adverse drug reactions. *Eur. J. Clin. Pharmacol.*, **11**, 75–78.

Kono, R. (1980). Trends and lessons of SMON research. In: *Drug Induced Sufferings.* ed. Soda, T. pp. 11 Princeton; Excerpta Medica.

Koren, G. (1990). In: *Maternal-Fetal Toxicology. A Clinician Guide.* 436 (Marcel Dekker, New York).

Kost, G. J. (1990). Critical limits for urgent clinician notification at US medical centres. *JAMA*, **263**, 704–707.

Kramer, M. S. (1986). Assessing causality of adverse drug reactions: Global introspection and its limitations. *Drug Inf. J.*, **20**, 433–437.

Kramer, M. S., Lane, D. A. and Hutchinson, T. A. (1987). Analgesic use, blood dyscrasias and case–control pharmacoepidemiology. A critique of the International Agranulocytosis and Aplastic Anaemia Study *J. Chron. Dis.*, **40**(12), 1073–1081.

Kramer, M. S., Leventhal, J. M., Hutchinson, T. A. and Feinstein, A. R. (1979). An algorithm for the operational assessment of adverse drug reactions 1: Background description and instructions for use. *JAMA*, **242**, 623–632.

Kristensen, M. B. (1976). Drug interactions and clinical pharmacokinetics. *Clin. Pharmacokinet.*, **1**, 351–372.

Kunin, C. M. and Halstead, S. (1990). Pharmacoepidemiology for developing countries. *Lancet*, 617–618.

Kunsman, G. W., Manno, J. E., Manno, B. R., Kunsman, C. M. and Przekop, M. A. (1992). The use of microcomputer-based psychomotor tests for the evaluation of benzodiazepine effects on human performance: a review with emphasis on temazepam. *Br. J. Clin. Pharmacol.*, **34**, 289–301.

La Puma, J. (1995). Drug promotion. *N. Engl. J. Med.*, **332**(15), 1031.

Lack, I., Record, R. G., McKeowen, T. and Edward, J. H. (1968). The incidence of malformations in Birmingham 1956–59. *Teratology.*, **1**, 263–80.

Lader, M. and Olajide, D. (1987). A comparison of buspirone and placebo in relieving benzodiazepine withdrawal symptoms. *J. Clin. Psychopharm.*, **7**, 11–15.

Lader, M. H. (1970). Drug-induced extrapyramidal syndromes. *J. Roy. Coll. Phys. Lond.*, **5**(1), 87–98.

Laganière, S. and Biron, P. (1979). Clinical trials: incomplete reporting of side effects. *Curr. Ther. Res.*, **25**(6), 743–746.

Lagier, G. and Royer, R. J. Information to the physician: Role of French regional pharmacovigilance centres. *Drug Inf. J.*, **24**, 203–206.

Lagier, G., Vincens, M. and Castot, A. (1983). Imputabilité en pharmacovigilance. *Thérapie*, **38**, 303–318.

Laird, N. and Dersimonian, R. (1986). Meta-analysis in clinical trials. *Contr. Clin. Trials*, **7**, 177–188.

Lambert, W. C., Kolber, L. R. and Proper, S. A. (1982). Leukocytoclastic angiitis induced by clindamycin. *Cutis*, **30**, 615–619.

Lamy, P. P. (1991). Physiological changes due to age: pharmacodynamic changes of drug action and implications for therapy. *Drugs Aging*, **1**, 385–404.

Lancet Leader. (1975a). *Lancet*, **1**, 592.

Lancet Leader. (1975b). Beta-blockade withdrawal. *Lancet*.

Lancet Leader. (1983). *Lancet*, **ii**, 624.

Lancet Leader. (1986). Akathisia and antipsychotic drugs. *Lancet*, 1131–1132.

Lancet Leader. (1993). Freedom for drug information. *Lancet*, 341.

Lancet Leader. (1995). In defence of the FDA. *Lancet*, **346**, 981.

Lancet Leader. (1996). Pill scares and public responsibility. *Lancet*, **347**, 1707.

Lancet Leader. (1997). Good manners for the pharmaceutical industry. *Lancet*, **349**, 1635.

Lancet Leader. (1993). Drug promotion: stealth, wealth and safety. *Lancet*, **341**, 1507–1508.

Lanctôt, K. L. and Naranjo, C. A. (1990). Using microcomputers to simplify the Bayesian causality assessment of adverse drug reactions. *Pharm. Med.*, **4**, 185–195.

Lanctôt, K. L., Turksen, L. B., Bazoon, M. and Naranjo, C. A. (1996). Evaluation of adverse drug events using fuzzy reasoning. Abstract PII-5 *Clin. Pharmacol. Ther.*, **59**, 2.

Lane, D. A. (1984). A probabilist's view of causality assessment. *Drug Inf. J.*, 18, 323–30.

Lane, D. A. and Hutchinson, T. A. (1986). *Assessing Causality Assessment Methods.* (University of Minnesota, Technical Report, no. 460).

Lane, D. A and Hutchinson, T. A. (1987). The notion of 'acceptable risk': The role of utility in drug management. *J. Chron. Dis.*, **40**(6), 621–625.

Lane, D. A, Kramer, M. S., Hutchinson, T. A., Jones, J. K. and Naranjo, C. (1987). The causality assessment of adverse drug reactions using a Bayesian approach. *Pharm. Med.*, **2**, 265–283.

Lane, R. J. M. and Routledge, P. A. (1983). Drug-induced neurological disorders. *Drugs*, **28**, 127–147.

Langman, M. J. S. (1991). Postmarketing surveillance: problems of confounded conclusions. *Drug Inf. J.*, **25**(2), 187–189.

Langmuir, A. D., Bregman, D. J., Kurland, L. T., Nathanson, N. and Victor, M. (1984). An epidemiologic and clinical evaluation of Guillain-Barré syndrome reported in association with the administration of swine influenza vaccine. *Am. J. Epidemiol.*, **119**(6), 841–879.

Lapierre, Y. D. (1975). Evaluation des effects secondaire chez les neurotics. Un essai avec les mesoridazin et le placebo. *Can. Psychiat. Ass. J.*, **26**, 60–61.

Laporte, J. R. (1900), *Lancet*, 658.

Larson, S. K., Elwin, C. E., Gabrielsson, J., Paalryow, L. and Wachtmeister, C. A. (1982). Do teratogenicity tests serve their objective? *Lancet*, **2**, 439.

Lasagna, L. (1980). The Halcion story, trial by media. *Lancet.*, **1**, 815.

Lasagna, L. (1981). Bias in the elucidation of subjective side effects. *Br. J. Clin. Pharmacol.*, **11**, 111S–113S.

Lasagna, L. (1984). Techniques for A. D. R. reporting. In: Böstrom, N. and Ljungstedt, N. (eds.) *Detection and Prevention of Adverse Drug Reactions.* 146. (Almqvist and Wiksell International, Stockholm).

Lasagna, L. (1986). On reducing waste in foreign clinical trials and post regulation experiences. *Clin. Pharm. Ther.*, **40**(4), 369–372.

Lasagna L. (1995). The Helsinki Declaration: timeless guide or irrelevant anachronism. *J. Clin. Psychopharmacol.*, **15**(2), 96–98.

Lasagna, L. and Von Felsinger, J. M. (1954). The volunteer subject. *Science*, **120**, 35–61.

Lasagna, L., Laties, V. G. and Dohan, J. L. (1958). Further studies on the 'pharmacology' of placebo administration. *J. Clin. Invest.*, **37**, 533–537.

Lasagna, L., Mosteller, F., Von Felsinger, J. M. and Beecher, H. K. (1954). A study of placebo response. *Am. J. Med.*, **16**, 770–779.

Launer, M. (1996). Selected side-effects: 17. Dopamine-receptor antagonists and movement disorders. *Prescribers J.*, **16**, 37–41.

Lauritson, K., Havelund, T., Laursen, L. S. and Rask-Madsen, J. (1987). Withholding unfavourable results in drug company sponsored clinical trials. *Lancet*, **1**, 1091.

Law Notes (1997). Publication of unfavourable drug information. *Int. J. Risk Safety Med.*, **10**, 133–135.

Lawley, T. J., Bielory, L., Gascon, P., Yancey, K. B., Young, N. S. and Frank, M. M. (1984). A prospective clinical and immunologic analysis of patients with serum sickness. *N. Engl. J. Med.*, **311**, 1497–1413.

Lazarou, J., Pomeranz, B. H. and Corey, P. (1998). Incidence of adverse drug reactions in hospitalised patients: a meta-analysis of prospective studies. *JAMA.* **279** (15), 1200–1205.

Le Vay, M. K. (1960). Placebo effect in mental nursing. *Lancet*, 1403.

Leape, L. L., Brennan, T. A., Laird, N., Lawthers, A. G., Localio, A. R., Barnes, B. A., Hebert, L., Newhouse, J. P., Weiler, P. C. and Hiatt, H. (1995). The nature of adverse events in hospitalised patients. *N. Engl. J. Med.*, **324**, 377–384.

Leck, I., Record, R. G., McKeown, T. and Edward, J. H. (1968). The incidence of malformations in Birmingham 1950–59. *Teratology*, **1**, 263–280.

Lee, P. R., Lurie, P., Silverman, M. M. and Lydecker, M. (1991). Drug promotion and labeling in developing countries: an update. *J. Clin. Epidemiol.*, **44**, Suppl. II, 49s–55s.

Lee, T. R. (1987). Risks in society. In: Walker, S. R. and Asscher, A. W. (eds.) *Medicines and Risk/Benefit Decisions.* 5–13. (MTP Press Ltd, Lancaster).

Leigh Thompson, W., Brunelle, R. L., Enas, G. G., Simpson, P. J. and Walker, R. L. (1988). Routine laboratory tests in clinical trials. In: *Clinical Drug Trials and Tribulations.* Ed. A. E. Cato. Drugs and the Pharmaceutical Sciences Vol. 34, Marcel Dekker.

Lessof, M. H. (1992). Reactions to food additives, *J. Roy. Soc. Med.*, **85**, 513–515.

Letemendia, F. J. J. and Harris, A. D. (1959). The influence of side effects on the reporting of symptoms. *Psychopharmacologia*, **1**, 39–47.

Levantine, A. and Almeyda, J. (1973). Drug-induced alopecia. *Br. J. Dermatol.*, **89**, 549–552.

Leveille, S. G., Buchner, D. M., Koepsell, T. D., McCloskey, L. W., Wolf, M. E. and Wagner, E. H. (1994). Psychoactive medications and injurious motor vehicle collisions involving older drivers. *Epidemiology*, **5**(6), 591–598.

Leventhal, J. M., Hutchinson, T. A., Kramer, M. and Feinstein, A. R. An algorithm for the operational assessment of adverse drug reactions. III: Results of tests among clinicians. *JAMA.*, **242**, 1991–4.

Levine, J. and Schooler, N. R. (1986). SAFTEE A technique for the systematic assessment of side effects in clinical trials. *Psychopharm. Bull.*, **22**(2), 343–381.

Levine, J. D., Gordon, N. C. and Fields, H. L. (1978). The mechanism of placebo analgesia. *Lancet*, **23**, 654–657.

Levine, J. G. and Szarfman, A. (1996). Standardized data structures and visualization tools: A way to accelerate the regulatory review of the integrated summary of safety of new drug applications. *Biopharmaceut. Rep.*, **4**(3), 12–17.

Levine, M. A. H. (1992). A guide for assessing pharmacoepidemiologic studies. *Pharmacotherapy*, **12**(3), 232–237.

Levine, M. A. H., Bennett, K., Grace, E. and Tugwell, P. (1990). Development of a disease specific adverse drug effects index. Abstract. *J. Clin. Res. Pharmacoepidemiol.*, **4**, 127–128.

Levine, M. A. H., Bennett, K., Grace, E. and Tugwell, P. (1991). Adverse Symptoms Index. Abstract PII–8. *Clin. Pharm. Therap.*, **49**(2), 151.

Levine, R. J. (1987). The apparent incompatibility between informed consent and placebo-controlled clinical trials. *Clin. Pharm. Ther.*, **42**, 247–249.

Levine, R. J. (1997). Institutional review boards. *Int. J. Pharmaceut. Med.*, **11**, 141–146.

Lewis, J. A. (1981). Postmarketing surveillance: How many patients? *Trends Pharmacol. Sci.*, **2**(4), 93–94.

Lewis, K. O. and Paton, A. (1981). ABC of alcohol. Tools of detection. *Br. Med. J.*, **283**, 1531–1532.

Lewis, M. A., Heinemann, L. A. J., MaCrae, K., Bruppacher, R. and Spitzer, W. O. (1997). The role of healthy users in studies on risk of venous thromboembolism and the use of third-generation progestagens. Abstract 213. *Pharmacoepidemiol. Drug Safety* 6, Suppl. 2, S102.

Lewis, R. V. (1987). Quantifying side-effects of ß-blockers: The role of visual analogue scales. *Human Toxicol.*, **6**, 195–201.

Lewis, R. V., Jackson, P. R. and Ramsay, L. E. (1985a). Side-effects of β-adrenoceptor blocking drugs assessed by visual analogue scales *Br. J. Clin. Pharmacol.*, **19**, 255–257.

Lewis, R. V., Jackson, P. R. and Ramsay, L. E. (1985b). Measuring β-adrenoceptor blocker side-effects by visual analogue scales: reproducibility of scoring. *Proceedings of the B. P. S., 10–12 April 1985*. 275. *Br. J. Clin. Pharmacol.*

Lewis, R. V., Jackson, P. R. and Ramsay L. C. (1985c). Measuring side-effects of β-adrenoceptor antagonists: a comparison of two methods. *Br. J. Clin. Pharmacol.*, **19**, 826–828.

Lewis, R. V., Jackson, P. R. and Ramsay, L. E. (1984). Quantification of side-effects of β-adrenoceptor blockers using visual analogue scales. *Br. J. Clin. Pharmacol.*, **18**, 325–330.

Li, D., Lindquist, M. and Edwards, I. R. (1992). Evaluation of early signals of drug-induced Stevens-Johnson syndrome in the WHO ADR database. *Pharmacoepidemiol. Drug Safety.*, **1**(1), 11–19.

Liang, M. H., Cullen, K. E. and Larson, M. G. (1983). Measuring function and health status in rheumatic disease clinical trials. *Clin. Rheum. Dis.*, **9**(3), 531–539.

Libeer, J.-C. (1994). Do external quality assessment programs guarantee quality?. *Drug Inf. J.*, **28**, 1201–1206.

Liddell, F. D. K. (1988). The development of cohort studies in epidemiology: a review. *J. Chron. Epidemiol.*, **41**(12), 1217–1237.

Lieberman, D. and Phillips, D. (1990). 'Isolated' Elevation of alkaline phosphatase: significance in hospital patients. *J. Clin. Gastroenterol.*, **2**(4), 415–416.

Lieberman, P. (1991). Anaphylactic reactions to radio-contrast media. *Ann. Allergy*, **67**, 91–100.

Liljestrand. (1980). In: Soda, T. (ed.) *Drug Induced Sufferings. Medical, Pharmaceutical and Legal Aspects.* 234. (*Excerpta Medica*, Amsterdam).

Lin, K. H., Nuccio, I. and Anderson, D. (1994). Studies of drug response in multi-ethnic populations. *Appl. Clin. Trials*, **3**(10), 36–41.

Linberg, S. E. (1996). Handling serious adverse events. DIA Conference, 'Assessing safety of investigational drugs'.

Lindeman, R. D. (1992). Changes in renal function with aging; Implications for treatment. *Drugs Aging*, **2**, 423–431.

Linden, C. V. and Barry, W. S. (1986). Drug experience reporting in a US based multinational corporation. Abstract 425, *Acta. Pharm. Toxicol.*, Suppl. V: *III World Conference on Clinical Pharmacology and Therapeutics 1986*, 159.

Lineberry, C. (1991). Approaches to describing common adverse events in the integrated safety summary. *Drug Inf. J.*, **25**, 493–500.

Lingjaerde, O., Ahlfors, U. G., Bech, P., Denkers, S. J. and Elgen, K. (1977). The U. K. U. side effects rating scale. *Acta. Psychiatrica Scand*, Suppl. 334, **76**.

Lipsky, B. A. and Hirschmann, J. V. (1981). Drug fever. *JAMA*, **245**(8), 851–854.

Longo, D. R., Brownson, R. C., Johnson, J. C., Hewett, J. E., Kruse, R. L., Novotny, T. E. and Logan, R. A. (1996). Hospital smoking bans and employee smoking behaviour. *JAMA*, **275**, 1252–1257.

Loupi, E., Ponchon, A. C., Ventre, J. J. and Evreux, J-Cl. Imputabilité d'un effet tératogène. *Thérapie.*, **41**, 207–10.

Lumley, C. E., Walker, S. R., Hall, G. C., Staunton, N. and Grob, P. R. (1986). The under-reporting of adverse drug reactions seen in general practice. *Pharm. Med.*, **1**, 205–212.

Lumpkin, M. (1994). New FDA iniatives in safety reporting. *DIA conference, Bethesda, Maryland.*

Lundberg, R. K. (1980). Assessment of drugs' side-effects: visual analogue scale versus checklist format. *Percept Motor Skills*, **50**, 1067–1073.

Lundström, S. (1993). Electronic patient diaries. *Appl. Clin. Trials.*, **2**(5), 35–37.

Lunsers, (1994). Self-rating scale to detect neuroleptic side effects. *Pharm. J.*, **253**, 695.

Lydick, E., Blumenthal, S. J. and Guess, H. A. (1990). Twenty years of renal adverse experience reporting. *J. Clin. Res. Pharmacoepidemiol.*, **4**, 183–189.

MacKay, F., Wilton, L. V., Pearce, G. L., Freemantle, S. N. and Mann, R. D. (1997a). Safety of long-term Lamotrigine in epilepsy. *Epilepsia*, **38**(8), 881–886.

MacKay, F., Dunn, N. R., Wilton, L. V., Pearce, G. L., Freemantle, S. N. and Mann, R. D. (1997b). A comparison of Fluvoxamine, Fluoxetine, Sertraline and Paroxetine examined by observational cohort studies. *Pharmacoepidemiol. Drug Safety*, **6**, 235–247.

MacKay, F. Pearce, G., Freemantle, S. and Mann, R. D. (1997c). The safety of risperidone, chlorpromazine and haloperidol: A comparative exercise using the General Practice Research Database. Poster presentation. *13th International Conference on Pharmacoepidemiology, August 24–27th.*

Mackintosh, D. R. and Zepp, V. J. (1996). Detection of negligence, fraud and other bad faith efforts during field auditing of clinical trial sites. *Drug Inf. J.*, **30**, 645–653.

Maclay, W. P. (1984). Chapter 2.4: Cohort or case approach to validation of ADRs. In: Walker, S. R. and Goldberg, A. (eds.) *Monitoring for ADR.* 69–72 (MTP Press Ltd).

Maclay, W. P., Crowder, D., Spiro, S. and Turner, P. (1984). PMS practical experience with ketotifen. *Br. Med. J.*, **288**, 911–914.

Maggini, M., Raschetti, R., Di Giovambattista, G. and Rossi, A. (1997). A population based study on drug use during pregnancy. *13th* International Conference on Pharmacoepidemiology. Aug. 24th–27th, Abstract 192. *Pharmacoepidemiol. Drug Safety,* **6**, Suppl. 2. Wiley, Chichester.

Magnani, H. (1994). The interpretation of laboratory data. *Drug Inf. J.,* **28**, 361–373.

Maistrello, I., Morgutti, M., Maltempi, M. and Dantes, M. (1995). Adverse drug reactions in hospitalised patients: an operational procedure to improve reporting and investigate under reporting. *Pharmacoepidemiol. Drug Safety,* **4**, 101–106.

Malone-Lee, J. and Wiseman, P. (1991). Terodiline and torsades de pointes. *Br. Med. J.,* **303**, 520.

Mann, R. D. (1988). From Mithridatium to modern medicine: the management of drug safety. *J. Roy. Soc. Med.,* **81**, 725–728.

Mann, R. D., Kubota, K., Pearce, G. L. and Wilton, L. V. (1996). Salmeterol: a study by prescription event monitoring in a UK cohort of 15,407 patients. *J. Clin. Epidemiol.,* **49**, 247–250.

Mannesse, C. K., Derkx, F. H. M., De Ridder, M. A. J., Man In't Veld, A. J. and Van Der Cammen, T. J. M. (1997). Adverse drug reactions in elderly patients as contributing factor for hospital admission: cross sectional study. *Br. Med. J.,* **315**, 1057–1058.

Manning, F. J. and Swartz, M. (1995). *Review of the Fialuridine (FIAU) Clinical Trials.* National (Academic Press, Washington, DC).

Mantel, N. and Haenszel, W. (1959). Statistical aspects of the analysis of data from retrospective studies of disease, *J. Natl. Cancer Inst.,* **22**(4), 719–748.

Marion, M. N. and Simon, P. (1984). Signification des adverbes utilisés pour indiquer la frequence des effets secondaires d'un médicament. *Thérapie,* **39**, 47–63.

Marken, P. A., Stoner, S. C. and Bunker, M. T. (1994). Anticholinergic drug abuse and misuse: epidemiology and therapeutic implications. *CNS Drugs* **5**, 190–199.

Marley, J. E. (1989). Safety and efficacy of nifedipine 20 mg tablets in hypertension using electronic data collection in general practice. *J. R. Soc. Med.,* **82**, 272–275.

Martin, R. M. (1995). The Doctor's Independent Network database: background and methodology. *Pharm. Med.,* **9**, 165–176.

Martin, R. M., Kerry, S. M. and Hilton, S. R. (1997). The impact of the October 1995 'pill-scare' on prescribing of the oral contraceptive pill: analysis of a UK automated database. *Fam. Pract.,* **14**(4), 279–284.

Martin, R. M., Kapoor, K. V., Witton, L. V. and Mann, R. D. (1998). Underreporting of suspected adverse drug reactions to newly marketed ▼ drugs in general practice: observational study. *BMJ.* **317**, 119–120.

Martinez, C. and Weidman, E. (1995). Methodological approach for the evaluation of adverse drug-attributed public health impacts. *11th International; Conference on Pharmacoepidemiology, Montreal.*

Martone, W. J., Williams, W. W., Mortenson, M. L., Gayner, R. P., White, J. W. *et al.* (1986). Illness with fatalities in premature infants associated with an intravenous vitamin E preparation, E-Ferol. *Pediatrics,* **78**, 591–600.

Martys, C. R. (1979). Adverse reactions to drugs in general practice. *Br. Med. J.,* **2**, 1194–1197.

Mashford, M. L. (1984). The Australian method of drug-event assessment. *Drug Inf. J.,* **18**, 271–3.

Maskell, L. J. E. (1989). Wellcome Group computer-based system for worldwide adverse drug reactions report management. *Drug Inf. J.*, **23**, 203–210.

Mastaglia, F. L. and Argov, Z. (1981). Drug-induced neuromuscular disorders in man. In: *Disorders of Voluntary Muscle*, 4th edition. 873–906.

Masters, P. W., Lawson, N., Marenah, C. B. and Maile, L. J. (1996). High ambient temperature: a spurious cause of hypokalaemia. *Br. Med. J.*, **312**, 1652–1653.

Matsumoto, C. (1991). Implementation and use of the COSTART dictionary at Lilley: Would we do it again? *Drug Inf. J.*, **25**, 201–203.

Matsuyama, Y., Ohashi, Y., Uchino, H., Takaku, F., Otsuka, Y and Suzuki, A. (1996). Vesnarinone-induced WBC disorders in Japan. *Pharmacoepidemiol. Drug Safety*, **5**, 87–93.

Matthew, N. T., Kurnan, R. and Percy, F. (1990). Drug-induced refractory headache. Clinical features and management. *Headache*, **30**, 634–638.

Maxwell, C. (1978). Sensitivity and accuracy of the visual analogue scale: a psyco-physical classroom experiment. *Br. J. Clin. Pharmacol.*, **6**, 15–24.

May, G. S., Demets, D. L., Friedman, L. M., Furberg, C. and Passamani, E. (1981). The randomised clinical trial: bias in analysis. *Circulation*, **64**(4), 669–673.

Mayo, E. (1949). In: *The Social Problems of an Industrial Civilization*.

McBride, W. G. (1961). Thalidomide and congenital abnormalities. *Lancet*, 1358.

McCarthy, M. (1996). DNA vaccination: a direct line to the immune system. *Lancet*, **348**, 1232.

McCormack, H. M., Horne, J. De L. and Sheather, S. (1988). *Psychol. Med.* 18, 1001–1019.

McCormick, P. A., Hughes, J. E., Burroughs, A. K. and Mcintyre, N. (1990). *Br. Med. J.*, **301**, 924.

McDevitt, D. (1990). The assessment, management and communication of the therapeutic benefits and risks of pharmaceutical products. In: Shimizo, N., Tanaka, Y., Jones, J. and Taylor, D. (eds.) *Improving Drug Safety*. (PharMa Inter. Inc.).

McDevitt, D. G., Beardon, P. H. G. and Brown, S. V. (1986). Mortality amongst cimetidine takers: results of a long term follow-up study using record linkage. Abstracts 414 and 415. *Acta. Pharm. Toxicol.*, Suppl. V.

McDevitt, D. G., Beardon, P. H. G. and Brown, S. T. (1987). Record linkage in Tayside: an assessment of present development. In: Mann, R. (ed.) *Adverse Drug Reactions*. 107–114, (Parthenon publishing).

McDonald, C. J., Mazzuca, S. A. and McCabe, G. P. J. (1983). How much of the placebo 'effect' is really statistical regression? *Stat. Med.*, **2**, 417–427.

McDonald, C. J., Mazzuca, S. A. and McCabe, G. P. J. (1989). How much of the placebo 'effect' is really statistical regression? (Authors' Reply) *Stat. Med.*, **8**, 1301–1302.

McEwen, J. and Vhrovac, C. B. (1985). Panel on management of ADR reports in selected national centres. *Drug Inf. J.*, **19**, 329–344.

McGettigan, P., Chan, R., McManus, J., O'Shea, B. and Feely, J. (1994). Sources of drug information in prescribing in general practice. *Br. J. Clin. Pharmacol.*, **37**, 521P.

McGettigan, P., Golden, J., Chan, R. and Feely, J. (1995). Sources of information used by hospital doctors when prescribing new drugs. *Br. J. Clin. Pharmacol.*, **41**, 437–475.

McGinley, L. (1994). FDA finds Lilly, others violated rules in tests of hepatitis drug that killed 5. *Wall Street J.* May 16th, B6.

McKenzie, R., Fried, M. W., Sallie, R., Conjeevaram, H., Di-Bisceglie, A. M., Park, Y., Savarese, B., Kleiner, D., Tsokos, M., Luciano, C. *et al.* (1995). Hepatic failure and lactic acidosis due to fialuridine (FIAU), an investigational nucleoside analogue for chronic hepatitis B. *N. Engl. J. Med.*, **333**, 1099–1105.

McMahon, F. G. (1983). How safe should drugs be? *JAMA*, **4**, 481–482.

McMillan, R. (1983). Immune thrombocytopenia. In: *Clin. Haematol.*, **12**(1), 69–88.

McNeil, B. J., Pauker, S. G., Sox, H. C. and Tversky, A. (1982). On the elictation of preferences for alternative therapies. *N. Engl. J. Med.*, **306**, 1259–1267.

McPherson, K. (1996). Third generation oral contraception and venous thromboembolism. *Br. Med. J.*, **312**, 68–69.

McQuay, H. and Moore, A. (1996). Placebo mania, placebos are essential when extent and variability of placebo response are unknown. *Br. Med. J.*, **313**, 1008.

McVie, J. G. (1973). Drug-induced thrombocytopenia. In: Girdwood, R. H. (ed.) *Blood Disorders Due to Drugs and Other Agents*. 187–208.

McVie, J. G. (1973). The adverse effects of drugs on the blood. *Br. J. Clin. Pract.*, **27**(8), 300–308.

Meade, T. W. (1981). Pertussis vaccine. *Br. Med. J.*, **283**, 59.

Medawar, C. (1989). On our side of the fence. In: Dukes, M. N. G. and Beeley, L. (eds.) *Side Effects of Drugs Annual 13*. Elsevier Science Publishers, Amsterdam.

Medawar, C. (1993). Drug Information. *Lancet*, **342**, 1490–1491.

Medicines Act 1968, Chapter 67, Part III, P. 97.

Medicines Act. (1968). *Guidance Notes on Applications for Clinical Trial Exemptions and Clinical Trial Certificates.* 94–99. (Medicines Control Agency, revised December 1995).

Meenan, R. F., Gertman, P. M. and Mason, J. H. (1980). Measuring health status in arthritis. The arthritis impact measurement scale. *Arthr. Rheum.*, **23**(2), 146–152.

Mehlman, P. T., Highley, J. D., Faucher, P., Lilly, A. A., Taub, D. M., Vickers, J., Suomi, Vickers, M. J., Painter, J. M. J., Heptonstall, J., Yusof, S. H. and Craske, J. (1994). Hepatitis B outbreak in a drug trial unit; investigation and recommendation. *Commun. Dis. Rep. Rev.*, **1**, R1–5.

Meinert, C. L. (1996). An open letter to the FDA regarding changes in reporting procedures for drugs and biologics proposed in the wake of the FIAU tragedy. *Control. Clin. Trials.*, **17**, 273–284.

Mellin, G. W. and Katzenstein, M. (1962). The saga of thalidomide. *N. Engl. J. Med.*, **267**, 1184–1193.

Melmon, K. L. and Nierenberg, D. W. (1981). Drug interactions and the prepared observer. *N. Engl. J. Med.*, **304**(12), 723–725.

Menkes, D. B. (1997). Hazardous drugs in developing countries. *BMJ*, **315**, 1557.

Merkatz, R. B., Temple, R., Sobel, S., Felden, K. and Kessler, D. A. (1993). Women in the clinical trials of new drugs. *N. Engl. J. Med.*, **329**(4), 292–296.

Merz, M., Seiberling, M., Höxter, G., Hölting, M. and Wortha, H. P. (1997). Elevation of liver enzymes in multiple dose trials during placebo treatment: are they predictable? *J. Clin. Pharmacol.*, **37**, 791–798.

Merz, W. A. and Ballmer, U. (1983). *J. Psychoact. Drug.*, **15**, 71–84.

Mesoglea, and Argov, Z. (1994). Drug-induced acute pancreatitis. *Prescrire International.*, **3**, 111–2.

Meyboom, R. and Stricker, B. (1988). National signal generation: detailed case analysis. *Proceeding of WHO Anniversary Symposium, Uppsala.*

Meyboom, R. H. B. and Royer, R. J.(1992). Causality classification at pharmacovigilance centres in the European Community. *Pharmacoepidemiol. Drug safety*, **1**, 87–97.

Meyboom, R. H., Egberts, A. C., Edwards, I. R., Hekster, Y. A., De Koning, F. H. and Gribnau F, W. (1997). Principles of signal detection in pharmacovigilance. *Drug Safety*, **16**(6), 355–365.

Meyer, B. H., Scholtz, H. E., Schall, R., Müller, F. G., Hundt, H. K. L. and Maree, J. S. (1995). The effect of fasting on total serum bilirubin concentrations. *Br. J. Clin. Pharmacol*, **39**, 169–171.

Meyer, F. P., Tröger, U. and Röhl, F. W. (1996). Adverse nondrug reactions: An update. *Clin. Pharmacol. Ther.*, **60**, 347–352.

Michels, K. B. and Faich, G. A. (1991). Linked databases (LDs) and epidemiology. *J. Clin. Res. Pharmacoepidemiol.*, **5**, 11–18.

Mikhail, M. (1993). The importance of the investigator's brochure. *Appl. Clin. Trials*, **2**(6), 56–58.

Miller, D. L., Ross, E. M., Alderslade, R., Bellman, M. N. and Rawson, N. S. B. (1981). Pertussis immunisation and serious acute neurological illness in children. *Br. Med. J.*, **282**(6276), 1565.

Miller, L. L. (1992). Pitfalls in the drug approval process: Dose–effect, experimental design, and risk–benefit issues. *Drug Inf. J.*, **26**, 251–260.

Miller, R. R. (1973). Comprehensive prospective drug surveillance, a report from the BCDSP. *Pharmaceut. Weekblad.*, **109**(20), 461–481.

Milstein, J. B., Faich, G. A., Hsu, J. P., Knapp, D. C., Baum, C. and Dreis, M. W. (1986). Factors affecting physician reporting of ADR. *Drug Inf. J.*, **20**, 157–164.

Mitchell, A. A. (1996). Special considerations in studies of drug-induced birth defects. In: *Pharmacoepidemiology*, 595–609, 2nd. B. L. Strem. Wiley, Chichester.

Mitchell, A. A. and Lesko, S. M. (1995). When a randomised controlled trial is needed to assess drug safety. The case of paediatric ibuprofen. *Drug Safety*, **13**(1), 15–24.

Mitchell, A. A., Lacoutrure, P. G., Sheehan, J. E., Kauffman, R. E. and Shapiro, S. (1988). Adverse drug reactions in children leading to hospital admission. *Pediatrics*, **82**, 24–29.

Mitchell, J. R., Thorgeirsson, V. P. *et al.* (1975). *Clin. Pharmacol. Exp. Ther.*, **18**, 70–79.

Mohberg, N. (1987). Some observations on the collection of medical events data. Drug Information Association Workshop. Arlington, December 1985. *Drug Inf. J.*, **21**(1), 55–63, 289.

Montastruc, J. L., Cathala, R. and Richard, J. P. *et al.* (1988). Médicaments et accidents de la circulation. *Thérapie*, **43**, 313–315.

Montgomery, C., Lydon, A. and Lloyd, K. (1997). Patients may not understand enough to give their informed consent. *Br. Med. J.*, **314**, 1482.

Moore, D., Walker, P. and Ismail, A. (1989) The alteration of serum potassium level during sample transit. *Practitioner*, **233**, 395–396.

Moore, M. R. (1980). International review of drugs in acute porphyria—1980. *Int. J. Biochem.*, **12**, 1089–1092.

Moore, N., Biour, M., Paux, G. *et al.* (1985). Adverse drug reaction monitoring: doing it the French way. *Lancet*, **2**(8463), 1056–1058.

Moore, N., Briffaut, C., Noblet, C., Normand, C. A. I. and Thuillez, C. Indirect drug-related costs. *Lancet.*, **345**, 588–589.

Moore, N., Lecointre, D., Noblet, C. and Mabille. M. (1995). Serious adverse drug reactions in a department of internal medicine: incidence and cost analysis. Abstract 160. *Pharmacoepidemiol. Drug Safety*, **4**, Suppl 1, S74.

Moore, N., Lecointre, D., Nobelt, C. and Mabille, M. (1998). Frequency and cost of serious adverse drug reactions in a department of general medicine. *Br. J. Clin. Pharmacol.*, **45**, 301–308.

Moore, N., Mammeri, M., Carrara, O., Desechalliers, J.-P. and Hoblet, C. (1995). Incidence and cost of adverse drug reactions in a department of a general hospital management system. Abstract 158. *Pharmacoepidemiol. Drug Safety*, **4**, Suppl. 1, S72.

Moore, N., Montero, D., Coulson, R. *et al.* (1994). Communication in pharmacovigilance. *Pharmacoepidemiol. Drug Safety*, **3**, 151–155.

Moride, Y., Haramburu, F. and Bégaud, B. (1994). Assessment of under reporting of adverse events in pharmacovigilance. Abstract 179. *Pharmacoepidemiol. Drug Safety*, **3**, Suppl. 1, S73.

Moride, Y., Haramburu, F., Requejo, A. A. and Bégaud, B. (1997). Under-reporting of adverse drug reactions in general practice. *Br. J. Clin. Pharmacol.*, **43**, 177–181.

Morris, L. A. and Kanouse, D. E. (1982). Informing patients about drug side effects. *J. Behav. Med.*, **5**(3), 363–373.

Morse, M. L. (1985). The COMPASS data base. *Drug Inf. J.*, **19**(3), 249–253.

Morse, M. L., Le Roy, A. A. and Strom, B. L. (1986). The Computerised On-line Medicaid Pharmaceutical Analysis and Surveillance System (COMPASS). In: W. H. Inman (ed.) *Monitoring for Drug Safety*, 2nd edition, (MTP Press).

Moscucci, M. (1990). Randomisation and baseline characteristics in clinical trials. *Lancet*, 335.

Moscucci, M., Byrne, L., Weintraub, M. and Cox, C. (1987). Blinding, unblinding and the placebo effect: an analysis of patients' guesses of treatment assignment in a double-blind clinical trial. *Clin. Pharmacol. Ther.*, **41**, 259–256.

Moss, D. W. (1981). Diagnostic enzymology: Some principles and applications. *Hospital Update*, 999–1010.

Mossinghoff, G. J. (1993). Drug labelling in developing countries. *Lancet*, **342**,.

Mossinghoff, G. J. (1995). Drug promotion. *N. Engl. J. Med.*, **332**(15), 1032.

Muehlberger, N., Schneeweiss, S. and Hasford, J. (1997). Adverse drug reaction monitoring—cost and benefit considerations. Part I: frequency of adverse drug reactions causing hospital admissions. *Pharmacoepidemiol. Drug Safety*, **6**, Suppl. 3, S71–S77.

Mullen, J. R., Chen, R. T., Hayes, S. R. and Knapp, G. (1991). The new vaccine AE reporting system. Abstract. *J. Clin. Res. Pharmacoepidemiol.*, **5**, 174.

Mulroy, R. (1973). Iatrogenic disease in general practice: Its incidence and effects. *Br. Med. J.*, **2**, 407–410.

Murray, M. (1992). P450 enzymes: inhibition mechanisms, genetic regulation and effects of liver disease. *Clin. Pharmacokinet*, **23**, 132–146.

Myers, M. G., Cairns, J. A. and Singer, J. (1987). The consent form as a possible cause of side-effects. *Clin., Pharm. Ther.*, **42**, 250–253.

Nagano, K., Onishi, Y. and Ozaki, J. (1980). Comparison of the drug affairs acts of different countries and problems of the amendment of the Japanese Drug Affairs Act in session. In: T. Soda (ed.) *Drug-induced sufferings.* Medical, Pharmaceutical and Legal Aspects. 281 (*Excerpta Medica*, Amsterdam).

Nahata, M. C. and Welty, T. E. (1998). Troubling issues with research publications. *Ann. Pharmacother.*, **32**, 126–128.

Nanra, R. S., Stuart-Taylor, J., De Leon, A. H. and White, K. H. (1978). Analgesic nephropathy: Etiology, clinical syndrome, and clinicopathologic correlations in Australia. *Kidney International*, **13**, 79–92.

Napke, E. and Stevens, D. G. H. (1984). Excipients and additives: hidden hazards in drug products and in product substitution. *Can. Med. Assoc. J.*, **131**, 1449–1452.

Naranjo, C. A. and Lanctôt, K. L. (1991a). Towards the development of international standards for the differential diagnosis of adverse drug events In: J. Ruiz-Ferran, J. Lahuerta Dal Re and R. Lardinois (eds.) *Communication in Pharmaceutical Medicine: A Challenge for 1992.* 175–181 (J. R. Prous S. A.).

Naranjo, C. A., Busto, U., Sellers, E. M., Sandor, P., Ruiz, I., Roberts, E. A., Janecek, E., Domecq, C. and Greenblatt, D. J. (1981). A method for estimating the probability of adverse drug reactions. *Clin. Pharmacol. Ther.*, 239–245.

Naranjo, C. A., Lanctôt, K. L. and Lane, D. A. (1990). The Bayesian differential diagnosis of neutropenia associated with antiarrhythmic agents. *J. Clin. Pharmacol.*, **30**, 1120–1127.

Naranjo, C. A. and Lanctôt, K. L. (1991b). Microcomputer-assisted Bayesian differential diagnosis of severe adverse reactions to new drugs: A 4-year experience. *Drug Inf. J.*, **25**, 243–250.

Naranjo , C. A. and Lanctôt, K. L. (1991c). Recent developments in computer-assisted diagnosis of putative adverse drug reactions. *Drug Safety*, **6**, 315–322.

Naranjo, C. A. and Lane, D. (1986). The value of standardised decision aids for assessing the causality of adverse drug reactions. *Proceedings of III World Conference on Clinical Pharmacology and Therapeutics.* Abstract. 716.

Naranjo , C. A., Lane, D., Ho-Asjoe, M. and Lanctôt, K. L. (1990). A Bayesian assessment of idiosyncratic adverse reactions to new drugs: Guillain-Barré syndrome and Zimeldine. *J. Clin. Pharmacol.*, **30**, 174–180.

Nelson, R. C. (1988). Drug safety, pharmacoepidemiology and regulatory decision making. *Drug Intell. Clin. Pharm.*, **22**, 336–344.

Neutel, C. L. (1995). Risk of traffic accident injury after a prescription for a benzodiazepine. *Ann. Epidemiol.*, **5**(3), 239–244.

Nevin, N. C. (1998). Gene therapy: supervision, obstacles and the future. *Int. J. Pharm. Med.*, **12**, 19–22.

New Zealand Hypertension Study Group. (1979). A multicentre open trial of labetalol in New Zealand. *Br. J. Clin. Pharmacol.*, 179S-182S.

Newman, T. B. (1995). If almost nothing goes wrong, is almost everything all right? Interpreting small numbers, *JAMA*, **274**, 1013.

Newman, T. J. (1995). From bedside to package insert: Presentation of AEs in product labeling. *Drug Inf. J.*, **29**, 1263–1267.

Nicholl, A., Elliman, D. and Ross, E. (1998). MMR vaccination and autism 1998. *BMJ*, **316**, 716–717.

Nicholls, J. J. (1977). The practolol syndrome: a retrospective analysis. In: *Post-marketing Surveillance of Adverse Reactions to New Medicines.* (Medico-Pharmaceutical Forum, Publication no. 7).

Nicholls, D. P., Husaini M. H., Bulpitt, C. J., Stephens, M. D. B. and Butler, A. G. (1980). Comparison of labetalol and propanolol in hypertension. *Br. J. Clin. Pharmacol.*, **9**, 233–237.

Nicholson, A. N. (1978). Visual analogue scales and drug effects in man. *Br. J. Clin. Pharmacol.*, **6**, 3–4.

Nicholson, A. N. (1986). Impaired performance. In: D'Arcy, P. F. and Griffin, J. P. (eds.) *Iatrogenic Diseases.* (Oxford University Press, Oxford).

Nickas, J. (1995). Adverse event data collection and reporting: a discussion of two grey areas. *Drug Inf. J.*, **29**, 1247–1251.

Nickas, J. (1997). Clinical trial safety surveillance in the new regulatory and harmonization environment: Lessons learned from the "Fialuridine crisis". *Drug Inf. J.*, **31**, 63–70.

Nickens, D. J. (1998). Using tolerance limits to evaluate laboratory data. *Drug Inf. J.*, **32**, 261–269.

Nilsson, A. (1996). Reasons for excluding healthy volunteers from participation in phase I clinical trials. Abstract book, poster 8. *Ninth International Conference on Pharmaceutical Medicine.*

Nived, O., Sturfelt, G., Eckernäs, S. and Singer, P. (1994). A comparison of 6 months compliance of patients with rheumatoid arthritis treated with tenoxicam and naproxen. Use of patient computer data to assess response to treatment. *J. Rheumatol.*, **21**, 1537–1541.

Nony, P., Boissel, J. P., Girard, P., Lion, L., Haugh, M. C., Fareh, S. F. and De Breyne, B. (1994). The role of an initial single-blind placebo period in phase I clinical trials. *Fundam. Clin. Pharmacol.*, **8**, 185–187.

Nony, P., Delair, S., Girard, P., Rachet, F. and Boissel, J. P. (1994). The role of placebo in early phase I trials. *J. Clin. Trials Meta-analysis*, **29**, 282–283.

Nordkvist Olsson, T., Backstrom, M. and Mjorndal, T. (1997). Interaction between the Drug Information Centre and the Regional Centre for Adverse Drug Reaction Monitoring in northern Sweden. *Pharm. World. Sci.*, **19**(2), 114–115.

Norrby, S. R. and Pernet, A. G. (1991). Assessment of adverse events during drug development: experience with temafloxacin. *J. Antimicrobial. Chemotherap.*, **20**, 111–119.

Northington, R. (1996). A review of issues in the collection and reporting of adverse events. *Biopharmaceut. Rep.*, **4**(2) 1–5.

Norwegian Multicenter Study Group. (1981). Timolol-induced reduction in mortality and reinfarction in patients surviving acute myocardial infarction. *N. Engl. J. Med.*, **304**(14), 801–807.

Nunn, A. (1997). Annual meeting of the Society of Pharmaceutical Medicine. *Pharm. Med.*, **11**, 352.

Oates, J. A. (1972). A scientific rationale for choosing patients rather than normal subjects for phase I studies. *Clin. Pharmacol. Ther.*, **13**(5) Pt 2, 809–811.

O'Brien, A. (1995). Licensing of drugs for the elderly. *Pharm. Med.*, **9**, 185–190.

O'Brien, K. L., Selanikio, J. D., Hecdirert, C., Placide, M. F., Louis, M., Barr, D. B., Barr, J. R., Hospedales, C. J., Lewis, M. J., Schwartz, B., Philan, R. M., St Victor, S., Espindola, J., Needham, L. L. and Denerville, K. (Acute Renal Failure Team) (1998). Evidence of Pediatric deaths from acute renal failure caused by diethyleneqlycol poisoning. *JAMA*. **279** (15), 1175–1180.

O'Brien, P. C. (1986). Comparing two samples: Extensions of the t, rank-sum, and log-rank tests. *J. Am. Stat. Assoc.*, **83**, 52–61.

O'Connor, P. C., McCabe, J. and Lawson, D. H. (1982). Report of ADR in general medical journals. *Irish. J. Med. Sci.*, **151**, 184–187.

Offerhaus, L. (1979). Guidelines for evaluation of antihypertensive drugs in man. *Eur. J. Clin. Pharmacol.*, **16**, 427–430.

Office for National Statistics. (1996). *The General Practice Research Database. Information for Researchers.* (ONS).

Office for National Statistics. (1997). *Publication Based on Data from the General Practice Research Database.* (GPRD) *Bibliography, November 1996, Update April 1997.* (ONS).

O'Hanlon, J. F. and De Gier, J. J. (1986). *Drugs and Driving*, Taylor Francis.

O'Hoolaren, M. T. and Porter, G. A. (1990). Angiotensin converting enzyme inhibitors and the allergist. *Ann. Allergy.*, **64**, 503–506.

Okuonghae, H. O., Ighogboja, I. S., Lawson, T. O. and Nnawa, E. J. (1992). Diethyleneglycol poisoning in Nigerian children. *Ann. Trop. Paeditr.*, **12**, 235–238.

Oliver, L. K. and Chuang-Stein, C. (1993). Laboratory data in multicenter trials: monitoring, adjustment and summarization. In: G. S. Gilbert (ed.) *Drug Safety Assessment in Clinical Trials.* 111–124 (Marcel Dekker, New York).

O'Mahony, B. (1993). Interactions between a general practitioner and representatives of drug companies. *Br. Med. J.*, **306**, 1649.

O'Mahony, M. S. and Woodhouse, K. W. (1994). Age, environmental factors and drug metabolism. *Pharmacol. Ther.*, **61**, 279–287.

O'Neill, R. T. (1988). Assessment of safety. In: *K. E. Peace* (ed.) *Biopharmaceutical Statistics for Drug Development.* 543–604 Marcel Dekker; New York.

Orme, M. H. J. (1991). Drug interactions of clinical importance. In: D. M. Davis (ed.) *Textbook of Drug Reactions*, 4th edn. (Oxford Medical Publication, Oxford).

Orme, M. H. J., Routledge, P. A. and Harry, J. D. (1991). The safety of phase 1 studies: A study of healthy volunteer studies in Great Britain over a 12–month period. *Drug Inf. J.*, **25**(2), 171–181.

Orme, M., Harry, J., Routledge, P. A. and Hobson, S. (1989). Healthy volunteer studies in Great Britain: the results of a survey into 12 months activity in this field. *Br. J. Clin. Pharmacol.*, **27**, 125–133.

Osterhaus, J. T. *et al.* (1994). Measuring the functional status and well-being of patients with migraine headache. *Headache*, **34**(6), 337–343.

Oswald, I. (1989) Triazolam syndrome 10 years on. *Lancet*, **ii**, 451–452.

Oswald, I. (1989). Rules for drug trials. *Br. Med. J.*, **299**, 1103.

Ottervanger, J. P., Van Witsen, T. B., Valkenburg, A., Grobbee, D. E. and Stricker, B. H. Ch. (1995). Differences in reporting of ADR to a specific drug between general practitioners and consumers. Abstract 057. *Pharmacoepidemiol. Drug Safety*, **4**, S25.

Owen, S. (1997). The role and responsibilities of the investigator in ensuring quality laboratory data. *Drug Inf. J.*, **31**, 723–727.

Owens, N. J., Fretwell, M. D., Willey, C. and Murphy, S. S. (1994). Distinguishing between the fit and frail elderly, and optimising pharmacotherapy. *Drugs Aging*, **4**, 47–55.

Pallen, M. (1997). Information in practice. *Br. Med. J.*, **310**, 954.

Pallot, P. (1996) The caring prescription is a hard pill to swallow. *Daily Telegraph*, 24th January, 29.

Palmer, C. R. (1993). Ethics and statistical methodology in clinical trials. *J. Med. Ethics.*, **19**, 219–222.

Pardo (1995). Interferon in hepatitis. *Drug Safety*, **13**(5), 310–312.

Park, B. K., Kitteringham, N. R., Pirmohamed, M. and Tucker, G. T. (1996). Relevance of induction of human drug-metabolizing enzymes: pharmacological and toxicological implications. *Br. J. Clin. Pharmacol*, **41**, 477–491.

Park, B. K., Pirmohamed, M. K. and Kitteringham, N. R. (1992). Idiosyncratic drug reactions. *Br. J. Clin. Pharmacol.*, **34**, 377–395.

Parker, B. M., Cusak, B. J. and Vestal, R. E. (1995). Pharmacokinetic optimisation of drug therapy in elderly patients. *Drugs Aging*, **7**, 10–18.

Parker, S. G. (1991). Transient hyerphosphataseaemia in association with acute infection in adults. *Postgrad. Med. J.*, **67**, 638–642.

Parkin, D. M., Henney, C. R., Quirk, J. and Crooks, J. (1976). Deviation from prescribed drug treatment after discharge from hospital. *Br. Med. J.*, **2**, 686–688.

Parrott, A. C. and Hindmarsh, I. (1978). Factor analysis of a sleep evaluation questionnaire. *Psychol. Med.*, **8**, 325–329.

Paterson, M. (1983). Measuring the socio-economic benefits of auranofin. In: G. Telling-Smith (ed.) *Measuring the Social Benefits of Medicine*. 97–110 (Office of Health Economics).

Patient Information Leaflet, ABPI. July 1993.

Paton, A. (1976). Diseases of the alimentary systems. Drug Jaundice. *Br. Med. J.*, **2**, 1126–1127.

Patterson, R. and Anderson, J. (1982). Allergic reactions to drugs and biologic agents. *JAMA*, **248**, (20), 2637–2645.

Payne, J. T. and Loken, M. K. (1975). A survey of the benefits and risks in the practice of radiology. *CRC Crit. Rev. Clin. Radio. Nuc. Med.*, **6**, 425–439.

Péré, J.-C., Bégaud, B., Albin, W. and Dangoumau, J. (1981). Effets indésirables non-descrits de l'observation aux données de la literature. *Thérapie*, **31**, 237–240.

Péré, J.-C., Bégaud, B., Haramburu, F. and Albin, H. (1984). Notions de fréquence et de gravité des effets indésirables. *Thérapie*, **39**, 447–452.

Peace, K. E. (1987). Design, monitoring, and analysis issues relative to adverse events. *Drug Inf. J.*, **21**, 21–28.

Peacock, S., Murray, V. and Turton, C. (1995). Respiratory distress and royal jelly. *Br. Med. J.*, **311**, 1473.

Peat, M., Ellis, S. and Yates, R. A. (1981). The effect of level of depression on the use of visual analogue scales by normal volunteers. *Br. J. Clin. Pharmacol.*, **12**, 171–178.

Pedersen-Bjergaard, U., Andersen, M. and Hansen, P. B. (1997). Drug-induced thrombocytopenia: clinical data on 309 cases and the effect of corticosteroid therapy. *Eur. J. Clin. Pharmacol.*, **52**, 183–189.

Perez, V., Schaffner, F. and Popper, H. (1972). Hepatic drug reactions. In: H. Popper and F. Schaffner (eds.) *Progress in Liver Disease*. 597–625 (Grune and Stratton, New York, London).

Perrillo, R. P. (1989). Treatment of chronic hepatitis B with interferon: experience in western countries. *Semin. Liver Dis.*, **9**(4), 240–247.

Perry, H. J., Sakamoto, A. and Tan, E. M. (1967). Relationship of acetylating enzymes to hydralazine toxicity. *J. Lab. Clin. Med.*, **70**, 1020–1021.

Perry, P. J. and Alexander, B. (1986). Sedative/hypnotic dependance: patient stabilisation, tolerance testing and withdrawal. *Drug Intell. Clin. Pharm.*, **20**, 532–537.

Perucca, E. and Richens, A. (1979). Reduction of oral bioavailability of lignocaine by induction of first pass metabolism in epileptic patients. *Br. J. Clin. Pharmacol.*, **8**, 21–31.

Pessayre, D. and Benhamou, J.-P. (1981). Est-il possible et souhaitable de détecter l'hepatotoxicité d'un médicament avant sa commercialisation? *Gastroenterol. Clin. Biol.*, **5**, 560–563.

Peterson, P. H., Klitgaard, N. A. and Blaabjerg, O. (1994). Do external quality assessments improve quality in clinical laboratories? *Drug Inf. J.*, **28**, 1207–1211.

Peto, V., Jenkinson, C., Fitzpatrick, R. and Greenhall, R. (1995). The development and validation of a short measure of functioning and well being for individuals with Parkinson's disease. *Qual. Life Res.*, **4**, 241–248.

Petri, H., Leufkens, H., Naus, J., Silkens, R., Van Hessen, P. and Urquhart, J. (1990). Rapid method for estimating risk of acutely controversial side-effects of prescription drugs. *J. Clin. Epidemiol.*, **43**(5), 433–439.

Petrie, W. M. and Levine, J. (1978). The assessment of adverse reactions in clinical trials. *Int. Pharmacopsychiat.*, **13**, 209–216.

Pfeiffer, M. (1998). Handling and analysing post marketing case reports, the German view. *DIA conference, February 23–27, 1998. Monitoring safety through the life-cycle of a pharmaceutical product.*

Pharmacology Journal Leader. (1994). Self-rating scale to detect neuroleptic side effects. *Pharmac. J.*, **253**, 695.

Pieters, M. S. M., Schoemaker, H. C., Breimer, D. D. and Cohen, A. F. (1992). Is the healthy volunteer 'normal'? A personality study of volunteers participating in pharmacological research compared with other students. *Br. J. Clin. Pharmacol.*, **31**(5), 611–612.

Pincus, T., Summey. J. A., Soraci, S. A., Wallston, K. A. and Hummon, N. P. (1983). Assessment of patient satisfaction in activities of daily living using a modified Stanford Health assessment questionnaire. *Arthr. Rheum.*, **26**(11), 1346–1353.

Piper, J. M., Ray, W. A., Daugherty, J. R. and Griffin, M. R. (1991). Corticosteroid use and peptic ulcer disease: role of nonsteroidal ant-inflammatory drugs. *Ann. Intern. Med.*, **114.**, 735–740.

Pisciotta, V. (1978). Drug-induced agranulocytosis. *Drugs*, **15**, 132–143.

Pitts, N. E. (1993). Laboratory parameters and drug safety. In: G. S. Gilbert (ed.) *Drug Safety Assessments in Clinical Trials*. Statistics, Textbooks and Monographs, Volume, 138. (Marcel Dekker, New York).

Platt, R. (1991). More automation does it make a difference? *D. I. A. Conference*. June 19th.

Plaut, D. (1978) Biochemical evaluation of liver function, *Am. J. Med. Tech.*, **44**, 3.

Pochin, F. E. (1975). The acceptance of risk. *Br. Med. Bull.*, **31**(3), 184.

Pocock, S. J. (1992). When to stop a clinical trial. *Br. Med. J.*, **305**, 235–40.

Podrebarac, T., Tugwell, P. and Hébert, P. C. (1996). A reader's guide to the evaluation of causation. *Postgrad. Med. J.*, **72**, 131–136.

Pogge, R. C. (1963). The toxic placebo. *Med. Times*, **91**(8), 773–776.

Poggiolini, D. *Pharmaceutical Regulating Activities in Italy.* (EIS, Gladbach, Germany).

Pohl, L. R., Satoh, H., Christ, D. D. and Kenna, J. G. (1988). The immunological and metabolic basis of drug hypersensitivities. *Ann. Rev. Pharmacol.*, **28**, 367–387.

Pollock, B. (1996). Clinical relevance of pharmacogenetic variations for geriatric psychopharmacology. *Drug Inf. J.*, **30**, 669–674.

Pollock, I., Young, E., Stoneham, M., Slater, N., Wilkinson, J. D. and Warner, J. O. (1989). Survey of colourings and preservatives in drugs. *Br. Med. J.*, **299**, 644–651.

Porta, A and Hartzema, A. G. (1987). The contribution of epidemiology to the study of drugs. *Drug Intell. Clin. Pharm.*, **21**, 741–747.

Porter, J. and Jick, H., (1977). Drug-related deaths among medical in-patients. *JAMA*, **237**, 879.

Posner, J. and Burke, C. A. (1985). The effects of naloxone on opiate and placebo analgesia in healthy volunteers. *Psychopharmacology*, **87**, 468–472.

Powell, J. R. (1986). Healthy volunteers, risk and research. *Drug Intel. Clin. Pharm.*, **20**, 776–777.

Pratley, N. (1996). Biotech setback despite new drug. *Daily Telegraph.*, 5th November, 25.

Prescott, L. F. (1982). Assessment of nephrotoxicity. *Br. J. Clin. Pharmacol.*, **13**, 303–311.

Price, J. (1997). Prescription information and labelling of medicines used in the workplace. *Int. J. Pharm. Med.*, **11**, 23–28.

Pryor, J. P. and Castle, W. M. (1982). Peyronie's disease associated with chronic degenerative arterial disease and not with beta-adrenoceptor blocking agents. *Lancet*, **1**, 917.

Pullar, R., Wright, V. and Feely, M. (1990). What do patients and rheumatologists regard as an 'acceptable' risk in the management of rheumatoid disease. *Br. Med. J.*, **29**, 215–218.

Pusey C. D., Saltissi, D., Bloodworth, L., Rainford, D. J. and Christie, J. L. (1983). Drug associated acute interstitial nephritis: clinical and pathological features and the response to high dose steroid therapy. *Quart. J. Med.*, NSL11, **206**, 194–211.

Putnam, R. K. (1990). *Analysis of Drug Prescribing Changes by Physicians. Report to the Pharmaceutical Manufacturers Association of Canada, Ottawa.*

Rabkin, J.G. and Markowitz, J.S. (1986). Side effect assessment with SAFTEE: Pilot study of the instrument. *Psychopharm. Bull.*, **22**(2), 389–398.

Ragg, M. (1993). MaLAM and Augmentin. *Lancet.*, **342**, 487.

Raghuprasad, P. K. (1979). Venepuncture and cardiac arrest. *JAMA*, **241**(2), 134–135.

Rainer, C., Scheincat, N. and Lafeber, E. J. (1991). Neuroleptic malignant syndrome when laevodopa withdrawal is the cause. *Postgrad. Med.*, **89**, 175–180.

Ramsay, I. (1985). Drug and non-thyroid induced changes in thyroid function tests. *Postgrad. Med. J*, **61**, 375–377.

Ramsay, L. (1990). *Br. J. Clin. Pharmacol.*

Ramsay, L. E. (1997). Commentary: placebo run ins have some value. *Br. Med. J.*, **314**, 1193.

Ramsay, L. E. and Yeo, W. W. (1995). ACE inhibitors, angiotensin II antagonists and cough. *J. Hum. Hypertens.*, **9**, Suppl. 5, 551–554.

Ramsey, L. (1990). *The Guardian*, 3rd June.

Ranek, L. (1978). Halothane hepatitis. *Arch. Toxicol.*, Suppl. 1, 137–139.

Raschetti, R., Menniti-Ippolito, F., Morgutti, M., Belisari, A. and Rossignoli, A. (1997). Adverse drug events in hospitalized patients. *JAMA*, **277**, 1351–1352.

Rawlins, M. D. (1984a). Doctors and the drug makers. *Lancet*, **2**, 276–278.

Rawlins, M. D. (1986). Regulatory decisions and consumers. *Med. Toxicol.*, 1 Suppl. 1, 128–129.

Rawlins, M. D. (1987). Risk–benefit decisions in licensing changes. In: S. W. Walker and A. W. Asscher (eds.) *Medicines and Risk/Benefit Decisions.* 137–141, (MTP Press Ltd).

Rawlins, M. D. (1988). Spontaneous reporting of adverse drug reactions 1: The data *Br. J. Clin. Pharmacol.*, **26**, 1–5.

Rawlins, M. D. (1988). Spontaneous reporting of adverse reactions 11: Uses. *Br. J. Clin. Pharmacol.*, **26**, 7–11.

Rawlins, M. D. (1989). Trading risk for benefit. In: R. D. Mann (ed.) *Risk and Consent to Risk in Medicine.* 193–202. (The Parthenon Publishing Group, Carnforth, Lancs).

Rawlins, M. D. (1995). The challenge to pharmacoepidemiology. *Pharmacoepidemiol. Drug Safety*, **4**, 5–10.

Rawlins, M. D. (1997). Predicting the future from the lessons of the past. *Int. J. Pharm. Med.*, **11**, 37–40.

Rawlins, M. D. and Dollery, C. T. (1977). Postmarketing surveillance of adverse reactions to new medicines. *Medico-Pharmaceutical Forum Publication.*, no. 7, 40.

Rawlins, M. D. and Jefferys, D. B. (1993). United Kingdom product licence applications involving new active substances, 1987–1989: their fate after appeals. *Br. J. Clin. Pharmacol.*, **35**, 599–602.

Rawlins, M. D. and Payne, S. (1997). Pharmacovigilance under the Commission. *Scrip*, February, 54–56.

Rawlins, M. D. and Thompson, J. W. (1977). Pathogenesis of adverse drug reactions. In: D. M. Davies (ed.) *Textbook of Adverse Drug Reactions* 10–31 (Oxford University Press, Oxford).

Rawlins, M. D., Fracchia, G. N. and Rodriguez-Farré, E. (1992). EURO-ADR: Pharmacovigilance and research. A European perspective. *Pharmacoepidemiol. Drug Safety*, **1**, 261–268.

Rawson, N. S. B., Pearce, G. L. and Inman, W. H. W. (1990). Prescription-event monitoring: methodology and recent progress. *J. Clin. Epidemiol.*, **43**(5), 509–522.

Ray, W. (1991). Medicaid databases and pharmacoepidemiology: What lies ahead? *D. I. A. Conference.* 19th June.

Ray, W. A. and Giffin, M. R. (1989). Use of Medicaid data for pharmacoepidemiology. *Am. J. Epidemiol.*, **129**, 837–849.

RCP. (1986). A report of the Royal College of Physicians. Research on healthy volunteers. *J. R. Coll. Physicians. Lond.*, **20**(4), 243–257.

Reactions (1994). Rules violated in Fialuridine trial. 21st May.

Read, P. R. and Stonier, P. D. (1995). Ethics and the promotion of medicines. *Pharm. Med.*, **9**, 49–53.

Redmond, G. P. (1985). Physiological changes during pregnancy and their implications for pharmacological treatment. *Clin. Invest. Med.*, **8**(4), 317–322.

Rees, J. K. H. (1980). Availability of amidopyrine preparations. *Lancet*, **13**(2), 581–582.

Rees, M. M. C. (1989) An approach to summarizing laboratory data from multi-center studies. Presented at the *10th Annual Meeting for Clinical Trials*.

Reidenberg, M. M. and Lowenthal, D. T. (1968). Adverse non-drug reactions. *N. Engl. J. Med.*, **279**(13), 678–679.

Rennie D. (1997). Thyroid storm. *JAMA*. **277**(15), 1238–1244.

Rheingold, P. D. (1968). The MER 29 story – an instance of successful mass disaster litigation. *Californian Law Reform.*, **56**, 116, 19–68.

Rich, M. L., Rittehof, R. J. and Hoffmann, R. J. (1950). A fatal case of aplastic anaemia following chloramphenicol (chloromycetin) therapy. *Ann. Intern. Med.*, **33**, 1459–1467.

Richman, V. (1996). Early warnings about drugs. *Lancet*, **347**, 1699.

Rickels, K. R. and Downing, R. W. (1970). Side reactions in neurotics. II: Can patients judge which symptoms are caused by their medications. *J. Clin. Pharmacol.*, **10**, 298–305.

Rieder, M. J. (1994). Mechanisms of unpredictable adverse drug reactions. *Drug Safety*, **11**, 196–212.

Riegelman, R. (1984). Clinical Trials. *Ann. Int. Med.*, **3**, 455.

Ritravato, C. A. and Dinella, C. (1995). The representation of women in clinical drug trials. *Drug Inf. J.*, **29**, 147–154.

Roberts, D. E. and Gupta, G. (1987). *N. Engl. J. Med.*, *316, 550.*

Roberts, R. (1996). Studies in pediatrics: special issues. *DIA Conference, 15–16 April 1996, Assessing Safety of Investigational Drugs.*

Roberts, R. J., Sandifer, Q. D., Evans, M. R., Nolan-Farrell, M. Z. and Dais, P. M. (1995). Reasons for non-uptake of measles, mumps, and rubella catch up immunisation in a measles epidemic and side effects of the vaccine. *Br. Med. J.*, **310**, 1629–1932.

Robson, J. (1997). Information needed to decide about cardiovascular treatment in primary care. *BMJ*, **314**, 277–280.

Rocklin, R. E. (1978). Drug allergy. *Spec. Immunol. Dis.*, 454–458.

Roddy, S. N., Ashwal, S. and Schneider, S. (1979). Venepuncture fits, a form of reflex anoxic seizure. *Pediatrics*, **72**(5), 715–716.

Rogers, A. and Tilson, H. (1984). Postmarketing surveillance. The sponsor's viewpoint. *Proceedings of the DIA Meeting, June, San Diego*, 101–105.

Rogers, A. S., Porta, M. and Tilson, H. H. (1990). Guidelines for decision making in post-marketing surveillance of drugs. *J. Clin. Res. Pharmacoepidemiol.*, **4**, 241–251.

Ronco, P. M. and Flahault, A. (1994). Drug-induced end-stage renal disease. *N. Engl. J. Med.*, **331**, 1711–1712.

Rose, G. (1982). Bias. *Br. J. Clin. Pharmacol.*, **13**, 157–162.

Rosenberg, F. (1985). A new international adverse reaction reporting system. *Drug Information Association Workshop. Arlington, December.*

Rosenberg, L. (1985). Postmarketing surveillance. The approach of the drug epidemiology unit. *Drug Inf. J.*, **19**, 263–268.

Rosenzweig, P., Brohier, S. and Zipfel, A. (1993). The placebo effect in healthy volunteers: influence of experimental conditions on the adverse events profile during phase 1 studies. *Int. J. Clin. Pharmacol. Ther.*, **54**(5), 578–583.

Rosenzweig, P., Brohier, S. and Zipfel, A. (1995). The placebo effect in healthy volunteers: influence of experimental conditions on physiological parameters during phase 1 studies. *Br. J. Clin. Pharmacol.*, **39**(6), 657–664.

Ross, C. (1994). New drug approval process under scrutiny. *Lancet*, **344**, 1075.

Rothman, K. J. (1996). Placebo mania. *Br. Med. J.*, **313**, 3–4.

Rothman, K. S. (1986). *Modern Epidemiology* (Little Brown).

Roujeau, J. C. and Stern, R. S. (1994). Severe adverse cutaneous reactions to drugs. *N. Engl. J. Med.*, 1272–1285.

Roujeau, J. C., Beani, J. C., Dubertret, L., Guillaume, J. C., Jeanmougin, M., Danan, G., Lagier, and Bénichou, C. (1989). Photosensibilité cutanée médicamenteuse. *Thérapie*, **44**, 223–227.

Routledge, P. A. (1986). The plasma protein binding of basic drugs. *Br. J. Clin. Pharmacol.*, **22**, 499–506.

Routledge, P. A. (1988). The Smith Kline and French lecture 1987. Clinical pharmacology and the art of bespoke prescribing. *Br. J. Clin. Pharmacol.*, **26**, 339–345.

Routledge, P. A. (1994). Pharmacokinetics in children. *J. Antimicrob. Chemother.*, **94**, Suppl A, 19–24.

Routledge, P. A. (1994b). Therapeutic drug monitoring. In: D. Wild (ed.), *The Immunassay Handbook* (Stockton Press, New York).

Routledge, P. A. and Shand, D. G. (1981). Drug interactions. In: A. M. Dawson, N. Compston and G. M. Besser (eds.) *Recent Advances in Medicine*, **18**, 39–54 (Churchill Livinstone, Edinburgh).

Royal College of General Practitioners (1974). *Oral Contraceptives and Health*, Pitman.

Royal College of General Practitioners and the British Medical Association Joint Computing Group. (1987). Guidelines for extraction of data from general practice computer systems by organisations external to the practice. (RCGP/BMA, London).

Royal College of Physicians (1986). Research on healthy volunteers. *J. R. Coll. Physicians Lond.*, **20**(4), 243–257.

Royal College of Physicians of London Committee on Ethical Issues in Medicine. (1996). J. Tripp, (ed.) *Guidelines on the Practice of Ethics Committees in Medical Research involving Human Subjects.* (Royal College of Physicians of London, London).

Royal, B. W. (1973) Moitoring adverse reactions to drugs, WHO Chronicle, **27**, 469–475.

Royer, R. J. (1990). Pharmacovigilance. The French system. *Drug Safety*, **5** Suppl. 1, 137–140.

Royer, R. J. (1997). Mechanism of action of adverse drug reactions: An overview. *Pharmacoepidemiol. Drug Safety.* **6**, S43–50.

Royer, R. J. and Bénichou, C. (1991). International reporting of adverse drug reactions. Final report of CIOMS ADR Working Group. *Thérapie*, **46**(3), 173–178.

Royer, R. J., Vidrequin, A., Trechot, Ph., Boissel, P. and Netter, P. (1990). Evaluation du coût d'un effet secondaire d'un médicament. *La Presse Médicale.*, **19**(26), 1240.

Royle, J. M. and Snell, E. S. (1986). Medical research on normal volunteers. *Br. J. Clin. Pharmacol.*, **21**, 548–549.

Rubin, J. D. (1995). *Prescribing in Pregnancy*, 2nd edition. 1–2 (Br. Med. J., Publishing Group, London).

Rubin, J. D., Ferencz, C. and Loffredo, C. (1993). Use of prescription and non-prescription drugs in pregnancy. *J. Clin. Epidemiol.*, **46**(6), 581–589.

Ruggeri, A., Carmignoto, F. and Matano, A. M. R. (1996). Development and evaluation of a knowledge-based system to assess a drug's safety profile from laboratory data. *Drug Inf. J.*, **30**, 413–419.

Ruskin, A. (1985). In: *The Detection of New Adverse Drug Reactions*. Ed. M. D. B. Stephens, pp 235, Macmillan Press, London.

Ryback, R. S., Eckardt, M. J., Rawlings, R. R., and Rosenthal, L. S. (1982) Quadratic discrimant analysis as an aid to interpretive reporting of clinical laboratory tests. *JAMA*, **248**, 2342–2345.

Rylance, G. and Armstrong, D. (1997). Adverse drug events in children. *Adv. Drug React. Bull.*, **184**, 699–702.

Sachs, L. (1984). (translated by Z. Reynarowych) *Applied Statistics, A Handbook of Techniques*, 2nd edition. 281–284. (Springer-Verlag, New York).

Sachs, R. M. and Bortnichak, E. A. (1986). An evaluation of spontaneous ADR monitoring systems. *Am. J. Med.*, **81**, Suppl. 5B, 49–55.

Sackett, D. L. (1979). Bias in analytical research. *J. Chron. Dis.*, **32**, 51–63.

Sackett, D. L. (1996). Evaluation of clinical method. In: D. J. Weatherall, G. G. Ledingham and D. A. Warrell, (eds.) *Oxford Textbook of Medicine*, 3rd edition. 15–21. (Oxford Medical Publications, Oxford).

Sackett, D. L. and Gent, M. (1979). Controversy in counting and attributing events in clinical trials. *N. Engl. J. Med.*, **301**(26), 1410–1412.

Sackett, D. L., Haynes, R. B. and Tugwell P. (1985). Deciding whether your treatment has done harm. In: *Clinical Epidemiology: A Basic science for Clinical Medicine* 230 (Little, Brown. Boston).

Sackett, D. L., Shannon, H. S. and Browman, G. W. (1990). Fenoterol and fatal asthma. *Lancet*, **1**, 46.

Safety Assessment of Marketed Medicines (SAMM) guidelines (1994). *Br. J. Clin. Pharmacol.*, **38**, 95–97, and *Pharmacoepidemiol. Drug Safety*, **3**, 1–6.

Sahli, H. R. (1989). Switzerland's drug surveillance. *Lancet*, **2**, 678.

Sakurai, Y., Kugai, N., Kawana, T., Fukita, T. and Fukumoto, S. (1995). A comprehensive adverse events management system for the pharmaceutical industry: The Takeda TRAC system. *Drug Inf. J.*, **29**, 645–659.

Salisbury, D. and Begg, N. (1996). In: *Immunisation against infectious diseases. Edward Jenner bi-centenary edition*. Ed. D. Salisbury and N. Begg. H. M. S. O. St Clement's House, 2–16 Colegate, Norwich.

Salsburg, D. S. (1993). The use of hazard functions in safety analysis. In: G. Sogliero-Gilbert (ed.) *Drug Assessment in Clinical Trials*. (Marcel Dekker, New York).

Salzman, C. (1990). Mandatory monitoring for side-effects. *N. Engl. J. Med.*, **323**, 827.

Sampson, H. A. (1996). Managing peanut allergy. *Br. Med. J.*, **312**, 1050–1051.

Sanchez, J., Costa, A., Fresquet, A., Abadia, S. and Bartlett, A. (1994). HIV screening 'healthy volunteers' and ethical committees. *Br. J. Clin. Pharmacol.*, **37**, 469.

Sanders, G. L., Davies, D. M., Gales, G. M., Rawlins, M. D. and Routledge, P. A. (1979). Comparison of methyl-dopa and labetalol in the treatment of hypertension. *Br. Clin. Pharmacol.*, **S**(S3), 148–153.

Sanford-Driscoll, M. and Knodel, L. C. (1986). Induction of haemolytic anemia by nonsteroidal antiinflammatory drugs. *Drug Intell. Clin. Pharm.*, **20**, 925–934.

Sannerstedt, R., Lundberg, P., Danielsson, B. R., Kihlström, I., Alván, G., Prame, B. and Ridley, E. (1996). Drugs during pregnancy, an issue of risk classification and information to prescribers. *Drug Safety*, **14**(2), 69–77.

Santé à Vendre: le Marché des Médicaments dans le Tiers-monde. (1984). (Peuples Solidaires, Rennes).

Savulescu, J., Chalmers, I. and Blunt, J. (1996). Are research ethics committees behaving unethically? Some suggestions for improving performance and accountability. *Br. Med. J.*, **313**, 1390–1393.

Schardein, J. L. (1993). In: *Chemically Induced Birth Dejects*, 2nd Ed. Marcel Dekker.

Scheifele, D. W. (1989). Postmarketing surveillance of adverse reactions to ProHIBit vaccine in British Columbia. *Can. Med. Assoc. J.*, **141**, 927–929.

Scherer, J. C., and Wiltse, C. G. (1996). Adverse events: After 58 years, do we have it right yet? *Biopharmaceut. Rep.*, **4**(3), 1–5.

Schimmel, E. M. (1968). Diagnostic procedures in liver disease. *Med. Clin. North Am.*, **52**(6), 1407–1416.

Schindel, L. (1972). Placebo-induced side effects. In: L. Meyer and H. M. Peck (eds.) *Drug Induced Diseases.* 323–330 (Excerpta Medica, Amsterdam).

Schmaurs, C., Apelt, S. and Emrich, H. M. (1987). Characteristics of benzodiazepine withdrawal in high and low dose dependant psychiatric in-patients. *Brain Res. Bull.*, **19**, 393–400.

Schneeweiss, S. G., Goettler, M. and Hasford, J. (1997). Adverse drug events in hospitalized patients. *JAMA*, **277**, 1352.

Schneider, P. J., Gift, M. G., Lee, Y.-P., Rothermich, E. A., Sill, B. E. *et al.* (1995). Cost of medication-related problems at a university hospital. *Am. J. Health-System Pharm.*, **52**, 2415–2418.

Schneiweiss, F. (1989). Capture and analysis of spontaneous adverse event data at AH Robins. *Drug Inf. J.*, **23**, 179–182.

Schoen, I. and Brooks, S. H., (1970). Judgement based on 95% confidence limits, *Am. J. Clin. Path.*, **53**, 190–195.

Schonhofer, P. (1981). *Scrip.*, no. 638, 2.

Schüppel, R., Boos, B., Bühler, G., Lataster, M. and Peters, T. (1996). *Eur. J. Clin. Pharmacol.*, **51**, 215–219.

Schulz, H. (1996). A new partner to join sponsor and CRO: The centralised laboratory and its role. *Pharm. Med.*, **10**, 87–94.

Schwartz. (1986). *Scrip.*, no. 1103, 19.

Scott, A. W. (1989). The importance of causality: an industry perspective. A paper presented at the Drug Information Association Conference entitled: *The Management of Adverse Experience Information Phase I through Epidemiology.* October 23–25.

Scott, E. and Cambell, G. (1998). Interpretation of subgroup analyses in medical device clinical trials. *Drug Inf. J.*, **32**, 213–220.

Scott, H. D., Thacher-Renshaw, A., Rosenbaum, S. E., Waters, W. J., Green, M., Andrews, L. G. and Faich, G. A. (1990). Physician reporting of adverse drug reactions. Results of the Rhode Island Adverse Drug Reaction Reporting Project. *JAMA*, **263**, 1785–1788.

Scott, J. and Huskisson, E. C. (1976). Graphic representation of pain, *Pain*, **2**, 175–184.

Scott, J. and Huskisson, E. C. (1979a). Vertical and horizontal visual analogue scales. *Ann Rheum Dis.*, **38**, 560.

Scott, J. and Huskisson, E. C. (1979b). Accuracy of subjective measurements made with and without previous scores: an important source of error in serial measurements of subjective rates. *Ann. Rheum. Dis.*, **38**, 558–559.

Scrip. (1987) no. 1194, 7.

Scrip. (1987) no. 119879, 6.

Scrip. (1989) no. 1450, 3.

Scrip. (1990). no. 1479, 18–19.

Scrip. (1991). no. 1637, 7.

Scrip. (1993). UK Medicines Information Bill blocked. *Scrip.*, **9**, 2–3.

Scrip. (1994) FDA faults Lilly, NIH on FIAU. 1925, 24–5.

Scrip. (1995). Pharma objects to new ADR rules. no. 1998, 15.

Seedat, Y. K. and Varoda, F. I. (1968). The Coombs test and methyl dopa. *Lancet*, **1**, 427–428.

Selby, P. (1985). Measurement of the quality of life after cancer treatment. *Br. J. Hosp. Med.*, **33**(5), 226–271.

Selby, P., Chapman, J. A. W., Etazadi Amoli, J., Dailey, D. and Boyd, N. F. (1984). The development of a method for assessing the quality of life of cancer patients. *Br. J. Cancer*, **50**, 13–22.

Seligmann, H., Podoshin, L., Ben-David, J., Fradis, M. and Goldshier, M. (1996). Drug-induced tinnitus and other hearing disorders. *Drug Safety*, **14**(3), 198–212.

Senard, J.-M., Montastruc, P. and Herxheimer, A. (1996). Early warnings about drugs from the stock market. *Lancet*, **347**, 987–988.

Sengupta, R. P., Chiu, J. S. P. and Brierley, H. (1975). Quality of survival following direct surgery for anterior communicating artery aneurysm. *J. Neurosurg.*, **43**, 58–64.

Senn, S. (1988). How much of the placebo 'effect' is really statistical regression? (letter to the editor) *Stat. Med.*, **7**, 1203.

Senn, S. (1997). Are placebo run-ins justified?. *Br. Med. J.*, **314**, 1191–1193.

Seventh European Symposium on Clinical Pharmacological Evaluation in Drug Control, Deidesheim, 1978. (WHO Euro Reports and Studies, WHO, Copenhagen, 13).

Shah, R. (1997). Annual meeting of the Society of Pharmaceutical Medicine. *Pharmaceutical Medicine.*, **11**, 351.

Shapiro, S. (1977a). General discussion. In: F. H. Gross and W. H. W. Inman (eds.): *Drug Monitoring*: Academic Press. 153.

Shapiro, S. (1977b). Postmarketing assessment of drugs. In: *Post-marketing Surveillance of Adverse Reactions to New Medicines.* (Medico-Pharmaceutical Forum, Publication no. 7).

Shapiro, S. (1984). The epidemiological evaluation of drugs. *Acta. Med. Scand.*, Suppl. 683, 23–27.

Shapiro, S., Slone, D., Lewis, G. P. and Jick, H. (1971) Fatal drug reactions amongst medical inpatients. *JAMA*, **216**, 467–472.

Shaughnessy, A. F. and Slawson, D. C. (1996). Pharmaceutical representatives. *Br. Med. J.*, **312**, 1494.

Shear, N. H. (1990). The skin as a target for adverse drug reactions. In: *C. A. Naranjo and J. K. Jones (eds.) Idiosyncratic Adverse Drug Reactions: Impact on Drug Development and Clinical Use after Marketing. 99–113 (Excerpta Medica, Amsterdam).*

Shedden, W. I. H. (1982). Side effects of benoxaprofen. *Br. Med. J.*, **284**, 1630.

Sherlock, S. (1972). Oral contraceptive cholestatic jaundice high in Scandinavian and Chilean women.

Sherlock, S. (1979). Progress report. Hepatic reactions to drugs. *Gut.*, **20**, 634–648.

Sherlock, S. (1986). The spectrum of hepatotoxicity due to drugs. *Lancet*, 440–444.

Sherman, L. A. (1996). Women in clinical trials: An FDA perspective. *Drug Information Association Conference, Assessing Safety of Investigational Drugs, April 15–16th.*

Sibille, M. (1990). Selection of healthy volunteers for phase I studies. *Fundam. Clin. Pharmacol.*, **4**, Suppl. 2, 167s-176s.

Sibille, M., Bresson, V., Janin, A., Boutouyrie, B., Rey, J. and Vital-Durand, D. (1997). Critical limits to define a lab adverse event during phase 1 studies: a study in 1134 subjects. *Br. J. Clin. Pharmacol.*, **52**, 81–86.

Sibille, M., Bresson, V., Janin, A., Rey, J., Boutouyrie, B. and Vital-Durand, D. (1994). Clinical limits to define laboratory adverse experiences in healthy volunteer studies. Abstract. *Clin. Trials Meta-analysis*, **29**, 283.

Sibille, M., Deigat, N., Janin, A., Kirkessezi, S. and Vital-Durand, D. (1998). Adverse events in phase I studies: a report on 1015 healthy volunteers. *Eur. J. Clin. Pharmacol.*, **54**, 13–20.

Sibille, M., Deigat, N., Olagnier, V., Vital-Durand, D. and Levrat, R. (1992). Adverse events in phase one studies: a study in 430 healthy volunteers. *Eur. J. Clin. Pharmacol.*, **42**, 389–393.

Sibille, M., Lassonary, L. G., Janin, A., Deigat, N., Boutouyrie, B. and Vital-Durand, D. (1995). Upper limit of plasma alanine amine transferase during Phase I studies. *Eur. J. Clin. Pharmacol*, **47**, 417–421.

Sikorski, R. and Peters, R. (1997). Internet anatomy 101, Accessing information on the World Wide Web. *JAMA*, **277**, 171–172.

Silverman, M. and Lydecker, M. (1980). Disclosures of hazards in international drug promotion. In: T. Soda (ed.) *Drug-induced Sufferings.* Medical, Pharmaceutical and Legal Aspects. 359–364 (Excepta Medica, Amsterdam).

Silverstein, M., Trinh, D. and Petterson, T. (1994). Adverse drug reactions resulting in hospitalisation in the elderly: a population-based study. Abstract 083. *Pharmacoepidemiol Drug Safety*, **3**, suppl. 1, S31.

Simmons, V. (1998). Clinical trial safety data management. *DIA conference, February 23–27, 1998. Monitoring safety through the life-cycle of a pharmaceutical product.*

Simpson, G. M. and Angus, J. W. (1970). A rating scale for extrapyramidal side effects. *Acta. Psychiatr. Scand. Suppl.*, **212**, 11–19.

Simpson, R. J., Tiplady, B. and Skegg, D. C. G. (1980). Event recording in a clinical trial of a new medicine. *Br. Med. J.*, **280**, 1133–1134.

Sjoquist, F. and Boethius, G. (1986). Attitude to development of drug therapy in Scandinavia. *Br. J. Clin. Pharmacol.*, **22**, 19S-26S.

Skegg, D. C. G. (1977). Medical record linkage. In: W. H. W Inman (ed.) *Monitoring for Drug Safety*, 1st edition. (MTP Press).

Skegg, D. C. G. (1979). Adverse reaction monitoring in the future. In: N. Macleod (ed.) *Pharmaceutical Medicine.* 144 (Churchill Livingstone).

Skegg, D. C. G. and Doll, R. (1977). The case for recording events in clinical trials. *Br. Med. J.*, **2**, 1523–1524.

Skegg, D. C. G. and Doll, R. (1981). Record linkage for drug monitoring. *J. Epidemiol. Commun. Health*, **35**, 25.

Skinner, J. B. (1991). On combining studies. *Drug Inf. J.*, **25**, 395–403.

Slater, E. E., Merrill, D. D., Guess, H. A., Roylance, P. I., Cooper, W. D., Inman, W. H. W. and Ewan, P. E. (1988). Clinical profile of angioedema associated with ACE inhibitors. *JAMA.*, **260**(7), 967–97.

Slovic, P. (1987). Perception of risk. *Science*, **236**, 280–285.

Smego, R. A. and Durack, D. T. (1982). The neuroleptic malignant syndrome. *Arch. Intern. Med.*, **142**, 1183–1185.

Smith, A. and Givens, S. V. (1993). Dealing with and defining abnormalities in laboratory data. *Drug Inf. J.*, **27**, 771–778.

Smith, J. M. (1985). Adverse reactions to pharmaceutical excipients. In: D. M. Davies, (ed.) *Textbook of ADR*, 3rd edition. Appendix **2**, 726–742.

Smith, M. W. (1981). The case control or retrospective study: in retrospect. *J. Clin. Pharmacol.*, **21**, 269–274.

Smith, P. M., Wilton, A. and Routledge, P. A. (1991). Jaundice associated with amoxycillin–clavulanate potassium therapy. *Eur. J. Gastroenterol. Hepatol.*, **3**, 95–96.

Smith, R. (1986). Doctors and the drug industry: too close for comfort. *Br. Med. J.*, **293**, 905–6.

Smith, R. B. (1979). Cardiac arrest or bradycardia following venepuncture. *JAMA*, **242**(2), 142.

Smyth, R. L., Ashby, D., O'Hea, U., Burrows, E., Lewis, P., Van Velsen, D. and Dodge, J. A. (1995). Fibrosing colonopathy in cystic fibrosis: results of a case–control study. *Lancet*, **346**, 1247–1251.

Sneader, W. (1986). In: *Drug Development from Laboratory to Clinic.* (Wiley).

Snell, N. J. C. (1990). Adverse reactions to inhaled drugs. *Resp. Med.*, **84**, 345–348.

Sniderman, A. D. (1996). The governance of clinical trials. *Lancet*, **347**, 1387–1388.

Sogliero-Gilbert, G., Mosher, K. and Zubkoff, L. (1986). A procedure for the simplification and assessment of lab parameters in clinical trials. *Drug Inf. J.*, **20**, 279–296.

Solal-Céligny, P., Bénichou, C., Boivin, P., Castot, A., Coulombel, L., Danan, G., Degos, L., Evreux, J. C., Lagier, G., Lavarenne, J. M., Soubrie, C., Tchernia, and Tobelem, G. (1987). Critère d'imputation d'une cytopenie granuleuse ou plaquettaire à un médicament. Résultats de réunions de consensus. *Thérapie.*, **29**, 265–270.

Spiers, C. J., Griffin, J. P., Weber, J. C. P. and Glenn-Bott, M. (1984). Demography of the UK adverse reactions register of spontaneous reports. *Health Trends.*, **16**, 49–52.

Spilker, B. (1984). *Guide to Clinical studies and Developing Protocols.* 45 (Raven Press).

Spilker, B. and Schoenfelder, J. (1990). In Chapter 7, Adverse Reactions. *Presentation of Clinical Data.* (Raven Press).

Spiro, T. E., Malya, P. A. G., Breuer, J., Delwai, P., Tryding, N., Tognoni, G., Galteau, M. M., Salway, J. and Siest, G. (1987) Drug interferences and drug effects in clinical chemistry, Part 5, Laboratory tests during clinical trials. *J. Clin. Chem. Clin.*

Spitzer, W. O. and Buist, A. S. (1990). Case–control study of prescribed fenoterol and death from asthma in New Zealand, 1977–81 *Thorax,* **45**, 645.

Sporer, K. A. (1995). The Serotonin syndrome. *Drug Safety.,* **13**(2), 94–104.

Spriet, A. and Simon, P. (1977). Questions à se poser pour verifier un protocole d'essai thérapeutique avant d'entreprendre l'execution. *Thérapie,* **32**, 633–642.

Spriet-Pourra, C. (1991). Postmarketing surveillance by the drug industry. Discussion on postmarketing surveillance of drug effects organised by the Drug Surveillance Research Unit on behalf of the European Community, Southampton, 10 April,.

Spriet-Pourra, C. and Auriche, M. (1988). Drug withdrawals from sale: an analysis of the phenomenon and its implications. *Scrip report.* PGB Publications.

Spriet-Pourra, C. and Auriche, M. (1994). Drug withdrawal from sale *Scrip Report,* 2nd edition, PGB Publications Ltd.

Spriet-Pourra, C., Spriet, A., Soubrie, C. and Simon, P. (1982). Les méthodes d'étude des effets indésirables des médicaments, II: *Thérapie,* **37**, 13–22.

Sriwatanakul, K., Kelvil, W., Lasagna, L., Calimlim, J. F., Weis, O. F. and Mehta G. (1982). Studies with different types of visual analogue scales for measurement of pain. *Clin. Pharmacol. Ther.,* **34**, 234–239.

St George, D. A. B. (1996). Data from several sources are needed to show numbers taking drugs. *Br. Med. J.,* **312**, 1419.

Standardization of definitions and criteria of causality assessment of adverse drug reactions. Drug-induced cytopenia. (1991). *Int. J. Clin. Pharmacol. Ther. Toxicol.,* **29**(2), 75–81.

Stanley, F. J. and Bower, C. (1986). Teratogenic drugs in pregnancy. *Med. J. Aust,* **145**, 596–599.

Start, R. D., Bury, J. P., Strachan, A. G., Cross, S. S. and Underwood, J. C. E. (1997). Evaluating the reliability of causes of death in published clinical research. *Br. Med. J.,* **314**, 271.

Statland, B. E. and Winkel, P. (1977). Effects of pre-analytical factors on the inter-individual variation of analytes in the blood of healthy subjects: Consideration of preparation of the subject and time of venepuncture. *Crit. Rev. Clin. Lab. Sci.,* **8**, 105–144.

Statland, B. E. and Winkel, P. (1979). Sources of variation in laboratory measurements. In: J. B. Henry *Clinical Diagnosis and Management by Laboratory Methods,* 16th edition. (W. B. Saunders). 3–28.

Stephen, P. J. and Williamson, J. (1984) Drug-induced parkinsonism in the elderly. *Lancet,* 1082–1083.

Stephens, M. D. B. (1983). Deliberate drug rechallenge. *Hum. Toxicol.,* **2**, 573–577.

Stephens, M. D. B. (1984). Assessment of causality in industrial setting. *Drug. Inf. J.,* **18**, 307–313.

Stephens, M. D. B. (1985). *The Detection of New Adverse Drug Reactions,* 1st edition. 116 (Macmillan, London).

Stephens, M. D. B. (1987). The diagnosis of adverse medical events associated with drug treatment. *Adv. Drug. React. Ac. Pois. Rev.*, **1**, 1–35.

Stephens, M. D. B. (1988). *Detection of New Adverse Drug Reactions*, 2nd edn, Macmillan, London.

Stephens, M. D. B. (1994). Asymptomatic abnormal liver function tests in clinical trials. *Pharmacoepidemiol Drug Safety*, **3**, 91–103.

Stephens, M. D. B. (1995). Dechallenge revisited. *Drug Inf. J.*, **29**, 335–338.

Stephens, M. D. B. (1997). From causality assessment to product labelling. *Drug Inf. J.*, **31**, 849–856.

Stern, R. S. (1994). Drug promotion for an unlabeled indication—the case of topical tretinoin. *N. Engl. J. Med.*, **331**, 1348–1349.

Stern, R. S. (1995). Drug promotion. *N. Engl. J. Med.*, **332**(15), 1033.

Stern, S. (1978). Extreme sinus bradycardia following routine venepuncture. *JAMA*, **239**(5), 403–404.

Stern, S. L. and Mendels, J. (1980). Withdrawal symptoms during the course of imipramine therapy. *J. Clin. Psych.*, **41**, 66–67.

Stewart, P and Beeley, L. (1988). Drug-induced skin disorders (1). *Pharma. J.*, 212–214.

Stewart, R. B. and Cooper, J. W. (1994). Polypharmacy in the aged: Practical solutions. *Drugs Aging*, **6**, 449–461.

Stewart, R. B., Hale, W. E. and Marks, R. G. (1984). Drug use and ADR in an ambulatory elderly population: a review of the Dunedin program. *Pharm. Int.*, 149–152.

Stewart, R. B., May, I. E., Moore, M. T., Hale, W. E. and Marks, R. (1990). Changing patterns of therapeutic agents in the elderly: a 10 year overview. *J. Clin. Res. Pharmacoepidemiol.*, **4**, 110.

Stinson, J. C., Pears, J. S., Williams, A. J. and Cambell, R. W. F. (1995). Use of 24 h ambulatory ECG recordings in the assessment of new chemical entities in healthy volunteers. *Br. J. Clin. Pharmacol.*, **39**, 651–656.

Stolley, P. D. (1981). Prevention of adverse effects related to drug therapy. In: D. W. Clarke, and M. McMahon, (eds.) *Preventative and Community Medicine*, 2nd edition 141–148. (Little Brown).

Stolley, P. D. (1989). A public health perspective from academia. In: B. L. Strom, (ed.) *Pharmacoepidemiology*. 53–54 (Churchill Livingstone).

Stolley, P. D. (1990). How to interpret studies of adverse drug reactions. *Clin. Pharmacol. Ther.*, **48**(4), 337–339.

Stone, D. H. (1993). How to design a questionnaire. *Br. Med. J.*, **307**, 1264–1266.

Stonier, P. D. (1992). Nomefensine and haemolytic anaemia—experience of a post-marketing alert. *Pharmacoepidemiol. Drug Safety*, **1**, 177–185.

Strand, L. M. (1985). Drug epidemiology resources and studies: The Saskatchewan data base, *Drug Inf. J.*, **19**, 253–256.

Strandberg, K. (1985). Experience from the WHO collaborating centre for international drug monitoring. *Drug Inf. J.*, **19**, 385–390.

Strathman, I. (1986). Experience with the WHO adverse reaction terminology at Searle, Seattle. *Drug Inf. J.*, **20**, 179–186.

Strom, B. L. (1988). Overview of different logistical approaches to post-marketing surveillance. *J. Rheumatol.*, **15**, Suppl. 17, 9–13.

Strom, B. L. (ed) (1989). *Pharmacoepidemiology.* 200 (Churchill Livingstone).

Strom, B. L. (1994). Study designs available for pharmacoepidemiologic studies. In: B. L. Strom (ed.) *pharmacoepidemiology.* John Wiley and Sons, Chichester.

Strom, B. L. and Carson, J. L. (1990). Medicaid billing data used to study the effects of marketed drugs. *Drug Inf. J.*, **24**, 477–483.

Strom, B. L., Carson, J. L., Morse, M. L. and Leroy, A. A. (1985). The computerised on-line Medicaid pharmaceutical analysis and surveillance system. A new resource for postmarketing drug surveillance. *Clin. Pharmacol. Ther.*, **38**(4), 350–364.

Stryer, D. B. and Bero, L. A. (1995). Drug promotion. *N. Engl. J. Med.*, **332**, 1032.

Stubbs, D. F. (1979). Visual analogue scales. *Br. J. Clin. Pharmacol.*, **7**, 124.

Sturk, A. (1994). Laboratory testing at a distance. *Drug Inf. J.*, **28**, 373–377.

Suissa, S., Spitzer, W. O., Heinemann, L. A. J., Lewis, M. A., Blais, L., Cusson, J. and Ernst, P. (1997). Risk profiles of venous thromboembolism and the use of newer oral contraceptives. Abstract 191. *Pharmacoepidemiol. Drug Safety.*, **6**, Suppl. 2, S91.

Swafford, S. (1997). Older people take too many drugs. *Br. Med. J.*, **314**, 1369.

Sylvestri, M. F., (1996). Water under the bridge: postmarketing concerns as related to pediatric populations. *Drug Inf. J.*, **30**, 1163–1171.

Szarewski, A. (1997). Third generation pill warnings were premature. *Lancet*, **350**, 497.

Taggart, H. M. and Aldedice, J. M. (1982). Fatal cholestatic jaundice in elderly patients. *Br. Med. J.*, **284**, 1372.

Talbot, J. C. C. (1989). Database management and reporting systems foreign based companies, The Glaxo approach. *Drug Inf. J.*, **23**, 189–196.

Talbot, J. C. C. and West, L. J. (1992). Information Sources. In: *Drug Safety. A Shared Responsibility*, 109–116. Churchill-Livingstone.

Tallercio, C. P. and Olney, B. A. (1985). Myocarditis related to hypersensitivity. *Mayo Clin. Proc.*, **60**, 453–468.

Tamarin, F. M., Conetta, R., Brandsetter, R. D. and Chadow, H. (1988). Increased muscle enzyme activity after yoga breathing during an exacerbation of asthma. *Thorax*, **43**, 731–732.

Tamblyn, R. M., McLeod, P. J., Abrahamowicz, M. and Laprise, R. (1996). Do too many cooks spoil the broth? Multiple physician involvement in medical management of elderly patients and potentially inappropriate drug combinations. *Can. Med. Assoc. J.*, **154**, 1174–1184.

Tangrea, J. A. and Morge, J. M. (1985). An improved method for adverse experience reporting in a multinational clinical trial. *Contr. Clin. Trials*, **6**(3) 235.

Tangrea, J. A., Adrianza, M. A. and Helsel, W. E. (1994). Risk factors for the development of placebo adverse reactions in a multicenter clinical trial. *Ann. Epidemiol.*, **4**, 327–331.

Tangrea, J. A., Adrianza, M. E. and McAdams, M. (1991). A method for the detection and management of adverse events in clinical trials. *Drug Inf. J.*, **25**, 63–80.

Tangrea, J., Edwards, B., Hartman, A., Taylor, P., Peck, G., Salasche, S., Menon, P., Winton, G., Mellette, R., Guill, M., Robinson, J., Guin, J., Stoll, H. and The ISO-BCC Study Group. (1990). Isoretinoin-Basal Cell Carcinoma Prevention Trial Design, recruitment results, and baseline characteristics of the trial participants. *Contr. Clin. Trials*, **11**, 433–450.

Taylor, A. (1998). Violations of the international code of marketing of breast milk substitutes: prevalence in four countries. *BMJ*, **316**, 1117–1122.

Teeling Smith, G. (1986). The economics of drug development and use. *Br. J. Clin. Pharmacol.*, **22**, Suppl. 1, 47s.

Temple, R. (1977). General discussion. In: F. H. Gross and W. H. W. Inman (eds.) *Drug Monitoring* 156 (Academic Press).

Temple, R. (1987). The clinical investigation of drugs for use by the elderly. Food and drug guidelines. *Clin. Pharmacol. Ther.*, **42**(6), 681–685.

Temple, R. J. (1991a). Access, science, and regulation. *Drug Inf. J.*, **25**(1), 1–11.

Temple, R. J. (1991b). The regulatory evolution of the integrated safety summary. *Drug Inf. J.*, **25**, 485–492.

Temple, R. J. (1996). The clinical pharmacologist in drug regulation: the US perspective, *Br. J. Clin. Pharmacol.*, **42**, 73–79.

Terol, M. J., Cervantes, F., Pereira, A. and Rozman, C. (1991). Autoimmune hemolytic anaemia after 9 years of treatment with alphamethyldopa. *Med. Clin. Barc.*, **10**, 598.

Tharakan, J., Bannerjee, D. A., Smith, D. A. and Carroll, S. (1993). Amiodarone-induced hepatic failure. *Hospital Update*, 180–182.

The International Agranulocytosis and Aplastic Anaemia Study. (1986). Risks of agranulocytosis and aplastic anaemia. A first report of their relation to drug use with special reference to analgesics, *JAMA*, **256**(13), 1749–1757.

The International Study of Agranulocytosis and Aplastic Anaemia (1983). The design of a study of the drug aetiology of agranulocytosis and aplastic anaemia. *Eur. J. Clin. Pharmacol.*, **12**, 653–658.

The Society of Pharmaceutical Medicine, Pharmacovigilance Group Working Party (October 1997). (1998). Monitoring drug safety in commercial licensing situations in Europe: a commentary. *Int. J. Pharm. Med.*, **12**, 55–70.

The WHOQOL Group. (1995). Position paper from WHO. *Soc. Sci. Med.*, **10**, 1403–1409.

Thomas, C. B. and Murphy, E. A. (1958). Further studies on cholesterol levels in the John Hopkins medical students, The effect of stress at examination. *J. Chronic. Dis.*, **8**, 661.

Thomas, M. (1998). Personal communication.

Thompson, M. S. (1986). Willingness to pay and accept risk to cure chronic disease. *Am. J. Publ. Health*, **76**, 392–396.

Thompson, M., Haynes, W. G., Webb, D. J. (1993). Screening for human immunodeficiency virus: a survey of British clinical pharmacology units. *Br. J. Clin. Pharmacol.*, **36**, 293–301.

Thompson, R. (1982). Side effects and placebo amplification. *Br. J. Psychiat.*, **140**, 64–68.

Thompson, W. L., Brunelle, R. L., Enas, G. G., Simpson, P. J., and Walker, R. L. (1988). Routine laboratory tests in clinical trials. In: A. E. Cato (ed.) *Clinical Drug Trials and Tribulations*, 119–172 (Marcel Dekker, New York).

Tierney, S. (1977). The testing of new drugs and the responsibility for their unforeseen effects. *J. Roy. Coll. Phys. Lond.*, **11**(3), 237.

Tilson, H. (1985). Methodologic issues in postmarketing surveillance. Pharmaceutical industry's view Burrough Wellcome. *Drug Inf. J.*, **19**, 275–283.

Tilson, H. H. and Bruppacher, R. (1990). A working group on epidemiology in the pharmaceutical industry (EPI). *J. Clin. Res. Pharmacoepidemiol.*, 4, 91–97.

Tizer, R. (1976). Cardiac arrest following routine venepuncture. *JAMA*, **236**(16), 1846–1847.

Tombes, M. B., Arzoomanian, R. Z., Alberti, D. B., Storer, B. and Spriggs, D. (1990). A comparative analysis of three commonly used toxicity grading tools. (World Health Organization Standards).

Toogood, J. H. (1980). What do we mean by 'usually'? *Lancet*, **i**, 1094.

Torrance, G. W. (1986). Measurement of health state utilities for economic appraisal. *J. Health Econom.*, **5**, 1–30.

Tramèr, M. R., Reynolds, D. J. M., Moore, R. A. and McQuay, H. J. (1997). Impact of covert duplicate publication on meta-analysis: a case study. *Br. Med. J.*, **315**, 635–639.

Trechot, P. F., Royer, R. J., Gaire, M., Gaspard, M. C. and Netter, P. (1990). A 30–month study of the calls to the Regional Drug Monitoring Center in Lorraine (Nancy). *Thérapie*, **45**(1), 43–46.

Tremmel, L. (1996). Describing risk in long-term clinical trials. *Biopharmaceut. Rep.*, **2**, 5–8.

Trost, D. C. (1996). The quantitative basis of laboratory medicine. *Adverse Events Workshop, Oct. 1996*. Washington D.C.

Trussel, J., Hatcher, R. A., Cares, W., Stewart, F. H. and Kost, K. (1990). Contraceptive failure in the United States: an update. *Stud. Fam. Plann.*, **21**(1), 51–54.

Tsubaki, T., Homma, Y. and Hoshi, M. (1971). Epidemiological study related to clioquinol as etiology of SMON. *Jpn. Med. J.* **2448**, 29–34.

Tubert, P., Bégaud, B., Haramburu, F. and Péré, J. C. (1991). Spontaneous reporting: how many cases are required to trigger a warning? *Br. J. Clin. Pharmacol.*, **32**(4), 407–408.

Tucker, J. and Menzies Smith, I. (1994). Electronic data transfer for clinical trials. *Drug Inf. J.*, **28**, 391–397.

Tucker, W. B. (1954). Effects of placebo administration and occurrence of toxic reactions, *JAMA*, **155**, 339.

Turk, J. L. (1994). Leonard Colebrook: the chemotherapy and control of streptococcal infections. *J. Roy. Soc. Med.*, **87**, 727–728.

Turk, J. L. (1994). Sir James Simpson: leprosy and syphilis. *J. Roy. Soc. Med.*, **87**, 549–551.

Turner, P. (1978). Future trends in pharmaceutical medicine. In: *N. Macleod (ed.) Pharmaceutical Medicine*. 156. (Churchill Livingstone).

Turner, W. M. (1984). The Food and Drug Administration algorithm, Special Workshop, Regulatory. *Drug Inf. J.*, **18**, 259–266.

Turner, W. M., Milstien, J. B., Faich, G. A. and Armstrong, G. D. (1986). The processing of adverse drug reaction. FDA. *Drug Inf. J.*, **20**, 147–158.

Twomey, C. E. J. and Griffin, J. P. (1983). The information lag—has it improved? *Pharmacy Intern.*, **4**, 57–61.

Tyrer, J. H., Eadie, M. J., Sutherland, J. M. and Hooper, W. D. (1970). Outbreak of anticonvulsant intoxication in an Australian city. *Br. Med. J.*, **iv**, 271–273.

Tyrer, P., Rutherford, D. and Huggett, T. (1981). Benzodiazepine withdrawal symptoms and propanolol. *Lancet*, **1**, 520–522.

Uchegbu, I. F. and Florence, A. T. (1996). Adverse drug events related to dosage forms and delivery systems. *Drug Safety*, **14**, 39–67.

Uetrecht, J. P. (1992). The role of leukocyte-generated reactive metabolites in the pathogenesis of idiosyncratic drug reactions. *Drug. Metab. Rev.*, **24**(3), 299–366.

US Cooperative Groups (1989/90). In: *Manual of Oncological Therapeutics*. Ed. Wittes, R. E., Philadelphia, Lippincott, Appendix A.

US Department of Health, Education and Welfare, Public Health Service Food and Drug Administration. General Considerations for the Clinical Evaluation of Drugs, Sept., 1977, p. 10. The establishment of the side effect profile of a new drug.

US Dept of Health, Education and Welfare, FDA. (1990). *National Adverse Drug Reaction Directory COSTART, Coding Symbols for Thesaurus of Adverse Reaction Terms*, 2nd edition. (1985 and update 1990).

Van Arsdel, P. P. (1982). Allergy and adverse drug reaction. *J. Am. Acad. Dermatol.*, **6**(5), 833–845.

Van Arsdel, P. P. (1986), Drug reactions: allergy and near-allergy. *Ann. Allergy*, **57**, 305–311.

Van Der Kroef, C. (1979). Reactions to trazolam. *Lancet.*, **2**, 526.

Vandenburg, M. J. (1987). Difficulties of a visual analogue scale in the assessment of angina. *Br. J. Clin. Pharmacol.*, **23**(i), 109–110.

Veatch, R. M. (1993). Benefit/risk assessment: What patients can know that scientists cannot. *Drug Inf. J.*, **27**, 1021–1029.

Venning, G. R. (1981). Priorities in the benefit–risk assessment of new drugs. *Adv. Drug. React. Ac. Pois. Rev.*, **3**, 113–121.

Venning, G. R. (1982). Validity of anecdotal reports of suspected adverse drug reactions: the problem of false alarms. *Br. Med. J.*, **284**, 249–252.

Venning, G. R. (1983). Identification of adverse reactions to new drugs: 4. Verification of suspected adverse reactions. *Br. Med. J.*, **286**, 544–547.

Venning, G. R. (1983). Identification of adverse reactions to new drugs: 1. What have been the important adverse reactions since thalidomide? *Br. Med. J.*, **286**, 199–202.

Venning, G. R. (1983). Identification of adverse reactions to new drugs: 3. Alerting processes and early warning systems. *Br. Med. J.*, **286**, 458–460.

Venning, G. R. (1991). How much drug in the tablet. *Lancet*, **337**, 670.

Venulet, J. (1977). Monitoring adverse reactions to drugs. In: E. Jucken (ed.) *Progress in Drug Research*. (Berghausen Verlag, Basle).

Venulet, J. (1983). Publishing adverse drug reaction data. *Arch. Intern. Med.*, **143**, 182–183.

Venulet, J. (1984). The Ciba-Geigy approach to causality—Special Workshop Industrial. *Drug Inf. J.*, **18**, 315–318.

Venulet, J. (1985). Informativity of ADR data in medical publications. *Drug Inf. J.*, **19**, 357–365.

Venulet, J. (1988). Early recognition of potential drug safety problems. *Drug Inf. J.*, **22**, 609–617.

Venulet, J. (1993). The WHO drug monitoring programme: the formative years (1968–1975). In: Z. Bankowski and J. F. Dunne (eds.) *Drug Surveillance: International Cooperation Past, Present and Future*. 13–22. (CIOMS, Geneva).

Venulet, J., Blattner, R., Von Bülow, J. and Bernecker, G. C. (1982). How good are articles on ADR? *Br. Med. J.*, **284**, 252–254.

Venulet, J., Ciucci, A. and Berneker, G. C. (1980). Standardized assessment of drug-adverse reaction associations-rationale and experience. *Int. J. Clin. Pharmacol. Ther. Toxicol.*, **18**, 381–388.

Venulet, J., Ciucci, A. G. and Berneker, G. C. (1986). Updating of a method for causality assessment of adverse drug reactions. *Int. J. Clin. Pharmacol. Therap. Toxicol.*, **24**(10), 559–568.

Vere, D. W. (1976). Drug adverse reactions as masqueraders. *Adv. Drug React. Bull.*, **60**, 208–211.

Vervaet, P. and Amery, W. K. (1992). An integrated causality assessment system. Abstracts. *Third International APWI Meeting. Paris.*

Vessey, M. P. (1984). Case–control studies in the assessment of drug safety. *Acta. Med. Scand.*, Suppl. 683, 29–33.

Vickers, J., Painter, M. J., Heptonstall, J. Yusof, J. M. H. and Craske, J. (1994). Community Disease Report. Hepatitis B outbreak in a drugs trial unit. Investigation, Recommendations. *Commun. Dis. Rep. CDR Rev.*, **4**, 1, R1–5.

Vinar, O. (1969). Dependence on a placebo: a case report. *Br. J. Psychiat*, **115**, 1189–1190.

Vinar, O. (1971). Scale for rating emergent symptoms in psychiatry DVP. *Activ. Nerv.*, Suppl., 238–240.

Vincent, P. C. (1986). Drug-induced aplastic anaemia and agranulocytosis, incidence and mechanisms. *Drugs*, **31**, 52–63.

Vomvouras, S. and Piergies, A. A. (1995). Gender differences in study events during phase 1 trials. *Clin. Pharmacol. Ther.*, **136**, PI-3.

Von Kries, R. (1998). Neonatal Vitamin K Prophylaxis: the Gordian knot still awaits untying. *BMJ.* **316** (1126), 161–162.

Von Kries, R., Göbel, U., Hachmeister, A., Kaletsch, U. and Michaelis, J. (1996). Vitamin K and childhood cancer: a population based case–control study in Lower Saxony, Germany. *Br. Med. J.*, **313**, 199–203.

Wade. G. L. (1972). In: D. J. Richards and R. K. Rondel. (eds.) *Adverse Drug Reactions* (Churchill Livingstone, Edinburgh).

Wadstein, J. and Skude, G. (1979) Serum ethanol, hepatic enzymes and length of debauch in chronic alcoholics, *Acta. Med. Scand.*, **205**, 317–318.

Wagner, A. K., Kosinski, M., Kellar, S. and Ware, J. C. (1994). Influence of a patient completed symptom checklist on the subsequent reporting of AE in a clinical trial interview. Abstract 53A. *Contr. Clin. Trials.*, **15**(35), Suppl.

Wakefield, A. J., Murch, S. H., Linnell, A. A. J., Casson, D. M., Malik, M., Berelowitz, M. *et al.* (1998). Ileal-lymphoid-nodular hyperplasia, non-specific colitis and pervasive developmental disorder in children. *Lancet*, **351**, 637–641.

Walden, R. J. and Prichard, B. N. C. (1978). Postmarketing drug surveillance, *Br. J. Clin. Pharmacol.*, **6**, 191–192.

Walker, A. M. (1989). Large linked data resources. *J. Clin. Res. Drug Dev.*, **3**, 171–175.

Walker, R. S. and Linton, A. L. (1959). Phenethyldiguanide: A dangerous side-effect. *Br. Met. J.*, **2**, 1005–1006.

Wallander, A. M.-A. and Palmer, L. S. (1986). A monitoring system for adverse drug experience in a pharmaceutical company—the integration of pre and postmarketing data. *Drug Inf. J.*, **20**, 225–235.

Wallander, M.-A., Dimenäs, E., Svärdsudd, K. and Wiklund, I. (1991). Evaluation of three methods of symptom reporting in a clinical trial of felodipine. *Eur. J. Clin. Pharmacol.*, **41**, 187–196.

Wallander, M.-A., Lundberg, P. and Svärdsudd, K. (1992). Adverse event monitoring in clinical trials of felodipine and omeprazole. *Eur. J. Clin. Pharmacol.*, **42**, 517–522.

Walle, J. K., Fagan, T. C., Topmiller, M. J., Conrad, E. C. and Walle, T. (1994). The influence of gender and sex steroid hormones on the plasma binding of propanolol enantiomers. *Br. J. Clin. Pharmacol.*, **37**, 21–25.

Waller, P. C. (1991a). P.M.S.: the viewpoint of a newcomer to pharmacoepidemiology. *Drug Inf. J.*, **25**(2), 181–186.

Waller, P. (1991b). P.M.S.: A regulator's tale, *Rostrum Conference, November 6th.*

Waller, P. C., Wood, S. M., Langman, M. J. S., Breckenridge, A. M. and Rawlins, M. D. (1992). Review of company postmarketing surveillance studies. *Br. Med. J.*, **304**, 1470–1472.

Waller, P. (1998). UK viewpoint. *DIA conference, February 23–27, 1998. Monitoring safety through the life-cycle of a pharmaceutical product.*

Wallerstein, R. O., Condit, P. K., Kasper, C. K., Brown, J. W. and Morrison, R. (1969). Statewide study of chloramphenicol therapy and fatal aplastic anaemia. *JAMA.*, **208**, 2045–2050.

Ward, J. (1995). Phase I clinical trials, conduct, objectives and data management. *Appl. Clin. Trials*, **4**(7), 44–47.

Warner, J. O. (1995). Review of prescribed treatment for children with asthma in 1990. *Br. Med. J.*, **311**, 663–666.

Watson, N. and Wyld, P. J. (1992). The importance of general practitioner information in selection of volunteers for clinical trials. *Br. J. Clin. Pharmacol.*, **33**, 197–199.

Watson, N., Wyld, P. J. and Nimmo, W. S. (1990). Abstract 24–22. *7th International Conference on Pharmaceutical Medicine* 125.

Wax, D. M. (1995). Elixirs, dilutents and the passage of the 1938 Federal Food, Drug and Cosmetics Administration. *Ann. Intern. Med.*, **15**, 456–461.

Weber, J. C. P. (1980). Storage and retreival of data on adverse reactions to drugs. *Interphex Symposium*, Brighton.

Weber, J. C. P. (1984). Epidemiology of adverse reactions to non-steroidal antiinflammatory drugs. In: K. D. Rainsford and G. P. Velo (eds.) *Advances in Inflammatory Research*, Vol. 6. 1–7 (Raven Press).

Weber, J. C. P. and Griffin, J. P. (1986). Prescriptions, adverse reactions and the elderly. *Lancet*, **1**, 1220.

Weber, W. W. (1997). *Pharmacogenetics*. (Oxford University Press, Oxford).

Weeks, R. A., Pitts, N. E., Siegel, A. M., Zubkoff, L. A. and Hopp, D. I. A., (1986) S.A.S. based system for reporting laboratory data from clinical trials. *Drug Inf. J.*, **20**, 311–313.

Weinberger, M. M. (1995). Placebo-controlled versus comparative studies of drug effects. *J. Paediat.*, **126**, 680–681.

Weintraub, M. (1978). Recording events in clinical trials. *Br. Med. J.*, **i**, 581.

Weissman, L. (1981) Multiple dose phase 1 trials. Normal volunteers or patients; one viewpoint. *J. Clin. Pharmacol.*, **21**, 385–387.

Weitzman, S. A. and Stossel, T. P. (1978). Drug-induced immunological neutropenia, *Lancet*, 1068–1071.

West, S. L., Savitz, D., Koch, G., Strom, B. L., Guess, H. and Hartezema, A. (1995). Demographic health behaviors and past drug use as determinants of recall accuracy for previous medication use, Abstract 075. *Pharamacoepidemiol. Drug Safety*, **4**, Suppl. 1, S33.

Westland, M. M. (1991). Coding: The mortar in the bricks of data analysis. *Drug Inf. J.*, **25**, 197–200.

Westlin, W. F., Cuddihy, R. V., Bursik, R. J., Seifert, B. G. and Koelle, J. G. (1977). One method for the systematic evaluation of adverse drug experience data within a pharmaceutical firm. *Methods Inf. Med.*, **16**(4), 240–247.

White, J. P. and Ward, M. J. (1985). Drug-induced adverse pulmonary reactions. *Adv. Drug React. Ac. Pois. Rev.*, **4**, 183–211.

WHO Collaborating Centre for International Drug Monitoring (1989). *International Monitoring of Adverse Reactions to Drugs Adverse Reaction Terminology*.

WHO Letter. (1991). M10/372/2(A), 1991.

WHO. (1972). *WHO Technical Report No. 498*.

WHO. (1979). *Handbook for Reporting Results of Cancer Treatment*. (WHO, Geneva, (1979). Offset Publication no. 48.

Widmann, F. K. (1987) *Clinical Interpretation of Laboratory Tests*. (F. A. Davis).

Wierenga, D. E. and Beary, J. F. (1995). The drug development and approval process. *Office of Research and Development, Pharmaceutical Research and Manufacturers of America*. January.

Wiholm, B.-E. (1984). The Swedish drug-event assessment method. *Drug Inf. J.*, **18**, 267–9.

Wiholm, B.-E. (1990). The impact of drug discontinuations: medical, social, pharmaceutical, legal, etc. In: C. A. Naranjo, and J. K. Jones (eds.) *Idiosyncratic Adverse Drug Reactions: Impact on Drug Development and Clinical Use after Marketing*. 71–2. (Excerpta Medica), Amsterdam.

Wiholm, B.-E. (1991). Weighing risk/benefit assessment: views of a Swedish 'regulator'. In: W. Van Eimerson (ed.) *Improving Drug Safety—A Joint Responsibility*. 131–135 (Springer-Verlag).

Wiklund, I., Dimenäs, E. and Wahl, H. (1990). Factors of importance when evaluating quality of life in clinical trials. *Cont. Clin. Trials.*, **11**, 169–179.

Wild, R. N. (1992). Micturin and torsades de pointe—experience of a post-marketing alert. *Pharmacoepidemiol Drug Safety*, 3, 147–150.

Wilkes, M. S., Doblin, B. H. and Shapiro, M. F. (1992). Pharmaceutical advertisements in leading medical journals: experts' assessments. *Ann. Intern. Med.*, **116**, 912–919.

Wilkinson, M. (1994). Carrier requirements for laboratory samples. *Drug Inf. J.*, **28**, 381–385.

Williamson, J. and Chopin, J. M. (1980). Adverse reactions to prescribed drugs in the elderly: a multicentre investigation. *Age Ageing.*, **9**, 73–80.

Wilson, A. B. (1977). Postmarketing surveillance of adverse reactions to new medicines. *Br. Med. J.*, **2**, 1001–1003.

Wilson, C. O. (1996) Abortions rise after pill scare. Daily Telegraph 22 November 1996.

Wilson, C. O. (1996). Midwives braced for baby boom. *Daily Telegraph*, 25th May.

Wilson, J. G. (1977). Teratogenic effects of environmental chemicals. *Fed. Proc.*, **36**, 1698–1703.

Wilson, J. T. (1996). Strategies for pediatric drug evaluation: A view from the trenches. *Drug Inf. J.*, **30**, 1149–1162.

Wilton, L. V., Pearce, G. L., and Mann, R. D. (1996). A comparison of ciprofloxacin, norfloxacin, ofloxacin, azithromycin and cefixime examined by observational cohort studies. *Br. J. Clin. Pharmacol.*, **41**, 277–284.

Wilton, L. V., Pearce, G. L., Edet, E., Freemantle, S., Stephens, M. D. B. and Mann, R. D. (1996). The safety of finasteride used in benign prostate hypertrophy: a non-interventional observational cohort study in 14,772 patients. *Br. J. Urol.*, **78**, 379–384.

Windhorst, D. B., Pun, E. F. C. and Zubkoff, L. A. (1987). Data on drugs and adverse experience: moving from the specific to the general. *Drug Inf. J.*, **21**, 39–46.

Wise, J. (1996). Baby milk companies accused of breaching marketing code. *Br. Med. J.*, **314**, 167.

Wise, J. (1997). Research suppressed for seven years by drug company. *Br. Med. J.*, **314**, 1149.

Witt, A., Williams, R. L. and Pierce, L. (1993). *Fialuridine: Hepatic and Pancreatic Toxicity. Report of an FDA Task Force.* 1–90.

Woggon, B., Linden, M., Backman, H., Krebs, E., Kufferle, B., Müller-Oerlinghausen, B., Pflug, B. and Schied, H. W. (1986). The AMDP system in international clinical trials: A double-blind comparison of fluperlapine and haloperidol. *Psychopharm. Bull.*, **22**(1), 47–51.

Wolf, S. (1950). Effects of suggestions and conditioning on the action of chemical agents in human subjects: the pharmacology of placebos. *J. Clin. Invest.*, **29**, 100.

Wolf, S. (1959a). Placebos. *Ass. Res. Nerv. Dis. Proc.*, **37**, 147–161.

Wolf, S. (1959b). The pharmacology of placebos. *Pharmacol. Rev.*, **II**, 689.

Wolf, S. and Pinsky, R. H. (1954). Effects of placebo administration and occurrence of toxic reactions. *JAMA*, **155**(4), 339–341.

Wood, K. L. (1994). The medical dictionary for drug regulatory affairs (MEDDRA) project. *Pharmacoepidemiol. Drug Safety*, **3**, 7–15.

Wood, S. (1989). Adverse drug reaction online information tracking (ADROIT). Development of a new computer system to support adverse drug reaction monitoring. *Pharm. Med.*, **4**, 139–148.

Wood, S. (1991). Post-marketing surveillance viewpoint from regulatory authorities. *Drug Inf. J.*, **25**, 191–195.

Wood, S. (1992). Handling of drug safety alerts in the European community. *Pharmacoepidemiol. Drug Safety*, **1**, 139–142.

Woodford Williams, E., Alvarez, A. S., Webster, D., Kandless, B. and Dickson, M. P. (1964). Serum protein pattern in normal and pathological ageing. *Gerontologia*, **10**, 86–99.

World Medical Association. (1992). Declaration of Helsinki IV: In: *Nurenberg Code: Human rights in Human Experimentation.* Oxford University Press, 339–342.

Wright, P. E. (1974). Skin reaction to practolol. *Br. Med. J.*, **2**, 560.

Wright, P. (1975). Untoward effects associated with practolol administration: oculo-mucocutaneous syndrome. *Br. Med. J.*, **1**, 595–598.

Wyngaarden, J. B. (1988). The use and interpretation of laboratory-derived data. In part XXV laboratory reference range values of clinical importance. Cecil's Text-book of Medicine, 17th edition. 2317–2320. W. B. Saunders Co.

Young, A. L. and Rave, N. L. (1993). Product liability considerations in prescription drug labeling. *Drug Inf. J.*, **27**, 915–920.

Young, E. J., Fainstein, V. and Masher, D. M. (1982). Drug-induced fever: Cases seen in the evaluation of unexplained fever in a general hospital population. *Rev. Infect. Dis.*, **4**(1), 69–77.

Young, G. A. R. and Vincent, P. C. (1980). Drug-induced agranulocytosis. *Clin. Haematol*, **9**, 483–504.

Yuen, W. C., Peck, A. W. and Burke, C. A. (1985). The subjective effects of dextromethorphan codeine and diazepam in healthy volunteers. *Proc. B. P. S.*, 290. April 10th–12th.

Yunginger, J. W. (1992). Anaphylaxis. *Ann. Allergy*, **69**, 87–96.

Zaccara, G., Muscas, G. C. and Messori, A. (1990). Clinical features, pathogenesis and management of drug-induced seizures. *Drug Safety*, **5**(2), 109–115.

Zarafonetis, C. J. D., Riley, P. A., Willis, P. W., Power, L. H., Werkbelow, J., Farhat, L., Beckwith, W. and Marks, B. H. (1978). Clinically significant events in a phase I testing program. *Clin. Pharmacol. Ther.*, **24**(2), 127–132.

Zbinden, G. (1990). Safety evaluation of biotechnology products. *Drug Safety*, **5**, Suppl. 1, 58–64.

Zeally, A. V. and Aitken, R. C. B. (1969). *Proc. Roy. Soc. Med.*, **62**, 993–996.

Zerbe, R. L. (1989). Concerns of causality in coding clinical trial events. In: *The Management of Adverse Experience Information Phase 1 through Epidemiology*. Abstract. Drug Information Association Conference.

Ziegler, M. G., Lew, P. and Singer, B. C. (1995). The accuracy of drug information from pharmaceutical sales representatives. *JAMA.*, **273**, 1296–1298.

Zilva, J. F., Panall, P. R., and Mayne, P. D. (1988). In: *Clinical Chemistry in Diagnosis and treatment*, 5th edition. 447 (Edward Arnold).

Zimmerman, H. J. (1990). Update of hepatotoxicity due to classes of drugs in common clinical use—non-steroidal drugs, anti-inflammatory drugs, antibiotics, antihypertensives and cardiac and psychotropic agents. *Semin. Liver Dis.*, **10**(4) 322–338.

Zipursky, A. (1996). Vitamin K at birth. *Br. Med. J.*, **313**, 179–180.

Zogg, W., Koch, U., Holsboer, E., Hemmeter, U., Seifritz, E., Meyer, J. W., Fromm, U., Knecht, T., Koller-Leiser, A. and Bandle, E. F. (1993). Clinician's assessment and patient's self-ratings by computer, a feasibility study with the antidepressant paroxetine. *Br. J. Clin. Res.*, **4**, 211–218.

Index